Sims' Symptoms in the Mind

Textbook of Descriptive Psychopathology

7th Edition

Sims' Symptoms in the Mind

Textbook of Descriptive Psychopathology

Femi Oyebode, MBBS, MD, PhD, FRCPsych, FRCPsych (Honorary)
Honorary Professor of Psychiatry
University of Birmingham
Birmingham, UK

For additional online content visit ExpertConsult.com

ELSEVIER

First edition 1988
Second edition 1995
Third edition 2005
Fourth edition 2008
Fifth edition 2015
Sixth edition 2018

Notices

Practitioners and researchers must always rely on their own experience and knowledge in evaluating and using any information, methods, compounds or experiments described herein. Because of rapid advances in the medical sciences, in particular, independent verification of diagnoses and drug dosages should be made. To the fullest extent of the law, no responsibility is assumed by Elsevier, authors, editors or contributors for any injury and/or damage to persons or property as a matter of products liability, negligence or otherwise, or from any use or operation of any methods, products, instructions, or ideas contained in the material herein.

ISBN: 978-0-7020-8525-3
Printed in India
Last digit is the print number: 9   8   7   6   5   4   3   2

Content Strategist: Trinity Hutton
Content Project Manager: Arindam Banerjee
Design: Bridget Hoette
Marketing Manager: Belinda Tudin

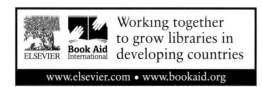

Contents

Preface to the Seventh Edition

In this new seventh edition, as in the previous editions, I have retained the original structure of the book but made some changes and many additions. I have added a new chapter on abnormalities of aesthetic perception and praxis. This new chapter deals with a little discussed but nonetheless important aspect of human existence, namely, our sense of the beautiful, which is fundamental to social life and that is very definitely affected by psychopathology. Other notable additions include an expanded description of Ganser State, Charles Bonnet syndrome, autoscopy, jealousy, erotomania and thought disorder. I have also included a section on musical hallucinations and on the nature of gestures and gestural abnormalities. These additions, like the additions in earlier editions, are prompted by my desire to ensure that readers fully appreciate that psychopathology is not a dead subject but one that is alive and is constantly in need of revision in response to conceptual changes or new empirical findings.

It is my belief that descriptive psychopathology, as a method, is the pre-eminent foundation for the practice of clinical psychiatry. This method allows us to observe and describe abnormal subjective phenomena and behaviours, and to categorize these in order to communicate more precisely about the world that patients inhabit. The clinician trained in the phenomenological approach is all the more aware of the need for empathic understanding, for assuming an atheoretical stance and finally of the provisional status of our understanding and explanations regarding psychopathology. Descriptive psychopathology is today even more relevant to the endeavours of clinicians and researchers. The standard psychiatric nomenclature is under strain. This means that the fundamental abnormal phenomena, the infrastructure of nosology, must of necessity assume greater importance in clinical practice. Otherwise the ability to communicate meaningfully across the profession will markedly deteriorate.

I am indebted to many more people than I can list. The Birmingham Philosophy Group has been meeting regularly since 1992. Its members (Theo Arvantis, Lenia Constantine, Simon O'Loughlin, Kate Robertson, Sandy Robertson and Persephone Sextou) continue to influence my thinking about psychiatric phenomena as do the members of the European Psychiatric Association Section of Psychopathology including Guenda Bernegger, Paolo Colavero, John Cutting, Maria Luisa Figueira, Mircea Lazarescu, Luis Madeira, Michael Musalek, Gilberto di Petta and Pedro Varandas. Finally, without the patients who experience and endure these abnormal phenomena, and the students and psychiatric trainees who ask awkward questions and out of curiosity enquire into the nature of these phenomena, this book would definitely be the poorer.

Femi Oyebode

Additional Materials Within Accompanying Electronic Version

The searchable full text for Sims' Symptoms in the Mind, seventh edition, is available at www.expertconsult.com, accessible via the enclosed pin code. Please follow the instructions on the inside front cover of this book. Additional materials integrated within this enhanced electronic version include the following:

- Four patient scenarios (videos with transcripts), exploring:
  1. auditory verbal hallucinations,
  2. persecutory delusion,
  3. low mood and
  4. obsessive compulsive phenomenon.

Look out for ▶ alongside the related sections within this book.

- Nine author podcasts on the following topics:
  1. What is psychopathology?
  2. Consciousness
  3. What are hallucinations?
  4. Critique of the nature of delusions
  5. Embodiment
  6. The self in psychopathology
  7. Affect, mood and emotions
  8. Shame and Guilt
  9. The nature of obsessions

Look out for 🌎 alongside the related sections within this book.

- Interactive question-and-answer sections for each chapter to test your understanding of key topics.

For my father, Jonathan Akinyemi Oyebode (1918–71)
FEMI OYEBODE

CONCEPTS AND METHOD

Chapter 1

Fundamental Concepts of Descriptive Psychopathology

KEYWORDS

Descriptive psychopathology
Phenomenology
Norms
Subjectivity

Summary

Descriptive psychopathology is the precise description, categorization and definition of abnormal experiences as recounted by the patient and observed in their behaviour. It relies on the method of phenomenology by focusing on experienced phenomena to establish their universal character. The aim is to listen attentively, to accurately observe and to understand the psychological event or phenomenon by empathy so that the clinician can, as far as possible, know what the patient's experience must feel like:

How the mind should be conceived for the purposes of psychopathology, what its faculties, functions or elements are (if there are any), how these can be distinguished, and how mental disorders can be comprehended by an application of these concepts are philosophic questions.

Manfred Spitzer (1990)

Psychiatry is that branch of medicine that deals with morbid psychological experiences. By definition, in the medical conditions that are central to psychiatric practice, psychological phenomena are important as causes, symptoms and observable clinical signs and also as therapeutic agents. The scope of psychiatry can be said to include minor emotional disturbances that are meaningful reactions to environmental or psychosocial stress; profound psychological change that is unheralded by significant or meaningful stress; disturbances of personality that have a pervasive influence on behaviour such that the person or others suffer;

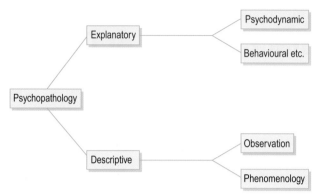

Fig. 1.1 The psychopathologies.

psychological changes that are directly the consequences of demonstrable organic brain change; and psychological and behavioural consequences of the use of substances such as alcohol, cannabis, cocaine or heroin. To describe, delineate and differentiate these conditions, the morbid psychological phenomena that constitute the subjective experience of patients need to be carefully assessed, elicited and recorded. This is the territory of descriptive psychopathology. In other words, descriptive psychopathology is concerned with the selection, delimitation, differentiation and description of particular phenomena of experience, which, through the use of accepted terminology, become both defined and capable of repeated identification.

It can be said that descriptive psychopathology is the fundamental professional skill of the psychiatrist; it is, possibly, the only diagnostic skill unique to the psychiatrist. It is considerably more than just carrying out a clinical interview of a patient or even listening to the patient, although it necessarily involves both of these. Its accurate application involves the deployment of *empathy* and *understanding* (we shall return to these later). Of course, for the rational practice of psychiatry there is a need for knowledge of the basic neurosciences; appropriate factual knowledge of psychology, sociology and social anthropology is also required. With these, there is a need for a comprehensive working knowledge of general medicine, especially neurology and endocrinology. This could be considered to be the minimum knowledge base that is essential for practising psychiatry. However, it is descriptive psychopathology that provides the foundation of clinical psychiatric practice. The subjective phenomena that are revealed during the clinical assessment, coupled with observable behaviours, ultimately determine the clinical judgements that influence treatment and management decisions.

What Is Psychopathology?

Psychopathology is the systematic study of abnormal experience, cognition and behaviour—the study of the products of a disordered mind. It includes the *explanatory psychopathologies* in which there are assumed explanations according to theoretical constructs (for example, on a cognitive, behavioural, psychodynamic or existential basis and so on) and *descriptive psychopathology*, which is the precise description, categorization and definition of abnormal experiences as recounted by the patient and observed in their behaviour (Fig. 1.1).

Descriptive psychopathology, as distinct from other forms of psychopathology, eschews explanation of the phenomena that it describes. It simply describes, thereby avoiding arguments about causation. Hence, descriptive psychopathology guards against and avoids theory, presupposition or prejudice. This constraint of descriptive psychopathology acts to secure the conceptual framework of phenomenology, restricting it to the actual experience of the patient. It is important to distinguish psychopathology from nosography, which is the description of single illnesses with provisional and characteristic features that lay the foundation for diagnosis (Stanghellini and Fuchs, 2013). Neither is it merely symptomatology nor pathology of the psyche (Stanghellini and Fuchs, 2013; Stanghellini and Aragona, 2016). It is, as elaborated later, a highly formalized and methodical system designed to inquire into and describe abnormal mental phenomena.

Explanatory psychopathologies, in contrast, often assume that mental phenomena are meaningful. In psychoanalysis, for example, at least one of several basic mechanisms are assumed to be taking place, and the mental state becomes understandable within this framework. Explanations of what occurs in thought or behaviour are based on these underlying theoretical processes, such as *transference* or *ego defence mechanisms*. For example, with a delusion, descriptive psychopathology tries to describe what it is that the person believes, how they describe their experience of believing, what evidence they give for its veracity and what the significance of this belief or notion is to their life situation. An attempt is made to assess whether this belief has the exact characteristics of a delusion and, if so, of what type of delusion. Having made this phenomenological evaluation, the information gained can be used diagnostically, prognostically and hence therapeutically. Some of the contrasts between descriptive and psychoanalytic psychopathology are summarized in Table 1.1.

Analytical or dynamic psychopathology, however, would be more likely to attempt to explain the delusion in terms of early conflicts repressed into the unconscious and now able to gain expression only in psychotic form, perhaps on a basis of projection. The content of the delusion would be considered an important key to the nature of the underlying conflict,

which has its roots in early development. Descriptive psychopathology makes no attempt to say why a delusion is present; it solely observes, describes and classifies. Dynamic psychopathology aims to describe how the delusion arose, its psychological origins and why it should be that particular delusion, on the evidence of that person's experience in early life.

There are other radically different models of psychology that regard mental experience, including thoughts, moods and drives, as *epiphenomena*, that is, as no more than froth on top of the beer. In these models (radical materialism or eliminative materialism), mental life is illusory; it is only the material, organic processes that are real. The significance the thinker attaches to subjective experience is regarded as purely illusory. Such a position poses difficulties for psychological enquiry and treatment and in any case is outside of the scope of this book.

Berrios (1996) has described two formulations of descriptive psychopathology in the 19th century. Psychologists and brain scientists predominantly tended to regard morbid phenomena as quantitative variations on normal mental functions—the *continuity* view. Psychiatrists working directly with the mentally ill (alienists) considered that some symptoms were too bizarre to have a counterpart in normal behaviour—the *discontinuity* view. Both formulations have contributed to the current state of descriptive psychopathology. Undoubtedly, the quality of empathy shown by the doctor contributes to the extent of understanding of the patient that is achieved. However, there is a theoretical

TABLE 1.1	Psychopathology: Descriptive Versus Psychoanalytic	
	Descriptive	**Psychoanalytic**
Summary	Empathic evaluation of patient's subjective experience	Study of the roots of current behaviour and conscious experience through unconscious conflicts
Terminology	Description of phenomena	Theoretical processes demonstrated
Methods	Understanding the patient's subjective state through empathic interview	Free association, dreams, transference
Differences in practical application	Makes distinction between understanding and explanation: understanding through observation and empathy	Understanding in terms of notional, theoretical processes
	Form and content clearly separated: form of importance for diagnosis	No distinction made; concerned with content
	Process and development distinguished: process interferes with development basis	No distinction made; symptoms seen as having unconscious psychological basis

limit to the psychological understanding that an interviewer can reach for some abnormal phenomena. It is often true that certain psychotic phenomena are such that the patient's notions and behaviour may no longer be psychologically comprehensible through the use of empathy. In these situations, the patient and doctor may have difficulty establishing a mutual understanding that, usually, readily underpins reciprocity and shared understanding. One of the consequences is that patients may find that their experiences are not fully comprehended by the clinician involved in their case. This fact underlines how alienating psychotic experiences can be. These two formulations, the continuity and discontinuity views, continue to influence how abnormal phenomena are conceptualized even today.

There are two distinct parts to descriptive psychopathology—the empathic assessment of the patient's subjective experience and the observation of the patient's behaviour. *Empathy* is an important psychiatric term that literally means 'feeling oneself into' and in psychiatric practice emphasizes the imaginative experiencing of another person's inner, subjective world. It can be distinguished from sympathy, which is 'feeling with'. A way to appreciate the distinction between 'empathy' and 'sympathy' is to recognize the role of an objective stance towards the patient coupled with an active attempt to fully understand how certain thoughts rise from particular moods, wishes or fears and the nexus of connections between different aspects of the patient's experiences that is integral to empathy.

In descriptive psychopathology, the concept of empathy is like a clinical instrument, conceptual in mode but no less incisive for that matter, that needs to be used with skill to explore, measure and represent to oneself another person's internal subjective state. The observer's own capacity for imaginatively representing another person's emotional and cognitive experience to themselves acts as the necessary instrument in this clinical task. Empathy is achieved by precise, insightful, persistent and knowledgeable questioning until the doctor is able to give an account of the patient's subjective experience that the patient recognizes as their own. If the doctor's account of the patient's internal experience is not recognized by the patient as their own, then the questioning must

continue until the internal experience is recognizably described. Throughout the process, success depends on the capacity of the doctor as a human being to experience something like the internal experience of the other person, the patient; it is not an assessment that could be carried out by a microphone and computer. It depends absolutely on the shared capacity of both doctor and patient for human experience and feeling. It is empathy that allows the doctor to come to *understand* the patient's experiences. In this sense, it is empathy that makes it possible for us to know what it is like for another person, another subject of experience, to be in a particular mental state. When empathy fails to render a patient's subjective experience understandable, we can then talk about that experience as being *un-understandable*. In other words, the farthest reaches of our intuitive comprehension of a phenomenon have been exceeded. This conclusion only ought to be reached after careful and exhaustive exploration and in-depth analysis.

Accurate observation of behaviour is the other component of descriptive psychopathology. Subjective human experience becomes available to us for examination and exploration not only through verbal communication but also through meaningful gestures, bodily stance, behaviour and actions. Observation of the objective expression of subjective experience, that is, of behaviour is extremely important and is a much more useful exercise than simply counting symptoms; the slavish use of a symptom checklist for their presence or absence is often an obstacle to genuine clinical observation, if not to the quality of doctor–patient communication. The objectivity that is facilitated by checklists is crucial, but there is a need also for the skilled observation of behaviour and for attentive and focused listening. Observation of behaviour includes observation of physical appearance, expressive gestures, facial emotional expressions, interpersonal stance and attitude, clothing, makeup and so on. It is a complex skill requiring an understanding of human conduct in context and the degree to which behaviour is influenced, accented and mediated by culture.

Phenomenology and Psychopathology

Psychopathology is concerned with abnormal experience, cognition and behaviour. *Descriptive psychopathology* avoids theoretical explanations for psychological events. It describes and categorizes the abnormal experience as recounted by the patient and observed in their behaviour. In its historical context, Berrios (1984) defines it as a cognitive system constituted by terms, assumptions and rules for its application, 'the identification of classes of abnormal mental acts'. *Phenomenology* is a term that is closely allied to descriptive psychopathology. It has a long tradition in philosophy and is associated with the name of Edmund Husserl (1859–1938). It is usually used to denote enquiry into one's conscious and intellectual processes, eschewing any preconceptions about external causes and preconceptions. The method of phenomenology aims to focus on experienced phenomena to establish their universal character. As used in psychiatry, phenomenology involves the elicitation and description of abnormal psychological events, the internal experiences of the patient and their consequent behaviour. An attempt is made to listen attentively, accurately observe and understand the psychological event or phenomenon so that the observer can, as far as is possible, know for oneself what the patient's experience must feel like.

How can one use the word *observer* about someone else's internal experience? This is where the process of *empathy* becomes relevant. Descriptive psychopathology therefore includes subjective aspects (phenomenology) and objective aspects (description of behaviour). It is concerned with the rich variety of human experience, but it is deliberately limited in its scope to what is clinically relevant; for example, it can say nothing about the religious validity of what James (1902) has called *saintliness*.

How does this work in practice? Mrs Jenkins complains that she is unhappy. It is the business of *descriptive psychopathology* both to elicit her thoughts and actions without trying to explain them and to observe and describe her behaviour—the listless sagging of her shoulders, the tense gripping and wringing of her hands or the strangely quiet and unrestrained sobbing. *Phenomenology* demands a very precise description of exactly how she feels inside herself: 'that horrible feeling of not really existing' and 'not being able to feel any emotion'.

Some psychiatrists have held the method of phenomenology in derision as archaic, hair-splitting or hare-chasing pedantry, but the diagnostic evaluation of symptoms is a task that psychiatrists omit at their own, and their patient's, peril. Studying phenomena whets diagnostic tools, sharpens clinical acumen and improves communication with the patient. Patients and their complaints deserve our scrupulous attention. If 'the proper study of mankind is man', the proper study of mental illness starts with the description of how the patient thinks and feels inside—'chaos of thought and passion, all confused' (Pope, 1688–1744).

A cavalier neglect of abnormal phenomena can have serious repercussions for care of the patient. Eight mentally well researchers were sent separately to 12 admission units in American mental hospitals on the pretence of complaining of hearing these words said aloud: *empty*, *hollow* and *thud* (Rosenhan, 1973). In all cases save one, they were diagnosed as suffering from schizophrenia. They produced no further psychiatric symptoms after admission to hospital but acted as normally as they could, answering questions truthfully except to conceal their name and occupation. The ethics and good sense of the experiment can certainly be questioned, but what comes out clearly is not that psychiatrists should refrain from making a diagnosis, but that their diagnosis should be made on a sound psychopathological basis. Rosenhan, his colleagues and the admitting psychiatrists gave no information as to what symptoms could reasonably be required for making a diagnosis of schizophrenia; this requires a method based on psychopathology. With adequate use of phenomenological psychopathology, this failure of diagnosis would not have occurred.

Jaspers (1997) wrote, 'Phenomenology, though one of the foundation stones of psychopathology, is still very crude'. One of the great problems in using this method is the muddled nature of terminology. Almost identical ideas may be assigned different names by people from different theoretical backgrounds, for example, the plethora of descriptions of how a person may conceptualize themself: self-image, cathexis, body awareness and so on.

There is considerable confusion over the meaning of the term *phenomenology*. Berrios has described four meanings in psychiatry:

P1 refers to its commonest clinical usage as a mere synonym for 'signs and symptoms' (as in 'phenomenological psychopathology'); this is a bastardized usage, and hence conceptually uninteresting. P2 refers to a pseudo-technical sense often used in dictionaries and which achieves spurious unity of meaning by simply cataloguing successive usages in chronological order; this approach is misleading in that it suggests false evolutionary lines and begs important questions relating to history of phenomenology. P3 refers to the idiosyncratic usage started by Karl Jaspers who dedicated his early clinical writings to the description of mental states in a manner which (according to him) was empathic and theoretically neutral. Finally, P4 refers to a complex philosophical system started by Edmund Husserl and continued by writers collectively named the 'Phenomenological Movement'.

Berrios (1992, p. 304)

Of these meanings, this chapter, and indeed this book, concentrates entirely on the Jaspersian meaning of phenomenology, P3 of Berrios. Jaspers defines *phenomenology* perhaps 30 to 40 times in his writings in subtly different ways but always implying the *study of subjective experience.* Walker (1988, 1993a, 1993b, 1994) has argued, very elegantly, that even though Jaspers himself thought that he had been influenced by Husserl and his system of phenomenology, this was not in fact so, and his psychopathology owed more to Kantian concepts such as form and content. Walker (1995a, 1995b) considers that Jaspers radically misconstrued Husserl's phenomenology. This view has been rebutted by others (Wiggins et al., 1992). The implication for what follows in this chapter, and in the rest of the book, is that the concept of phenomenology used here comes directly from Jaspers and was probably influenced by both Kant and Husserl.

Phenomenology, the *empathic* method for the eliciting of symptoms, cannot be learned from a book. Patients are the best teachers, but it is necessary to know what one is looking for—the practical, clinical aspects in which the patient describes themself, their feelings and their world. The doctor tries to unravel the nature of the sufferer's experience, to understand it well enough and to feel it so poignantly that the account of their findings evokes recognition from the patient. The method of phenomenology in psychiatry is entirely subjugated to its single purpose of rendering the patient's experience *understandable* (this is a technical word in phenomenology and is described in more detail in the Understanding and Un-Understandable section; however, it incorporates the capacity for putting oneself in the patient's place) so that classification and rational therapy may proceed.

It is not the assimilation of abstruse facts or the accumulation of foreign eponyms that is most difficult in phenomenology, although either of these may be hard: it is the comprehension of a method of investigation, a rigorous approach and the ability to use new concepts. In an attempt to avoid the obscure and obvious, some of these concepts are discussed in the rest of this chapter.

Concepts

DISEASE AND ILLNESS

Psychopathology concerns itself with *disease of the mind*, but what is disease? And, how does it differ from disorder and illness? This is a vast subject that has received discussion from philosophers, theologians, administrators and lawyers as well as from physicians. Doctors who spend most of their working time dealing with disease rarely ask this question and even less frequently attempt to answer it. Talk of disease by definition raises questions about the nature of health. But an even more pressing issue is whether it is possible for the mind to be diseased in the same way or manner that the liver or the kidneys can be diseased. These questions are outside of the scope of this book, but it is important to be aware of the varied approaches that different authorities take to this matter. I outline the basic arguments in the following text.

The most compelling model of a disease is that which grounds a medical condition such as pulmonary tuberculosis on the basis of a distinctive morbid anatomy demonstrable on examination of the lungs, is independent of any particular observer and is assumed to be value free. It is even better if there is an understanding of the detailed pathophysiology—how the causative agent, in tuberculosis for instance, results in the recognized, typical morbid anatomy of the lungs. It is obvious from the foregoing that, in most psychiatric diseases, no such typical morbid anatomy or pathophysiology has been described.

On the basis of the absence of demonstrable physical lesions, Szasz (1960) argued that psychiatric or mental diseases did not exist and that only behavioural deviance and moral or social judgements were at play in psychiatry. He also argued that *mental* is an abstract concept and not an objective, physical thing, and hence it could not be diseased. Brain diseases, in his view, are real, but mental diseases are a logical impossibility; thus Szasz uses the term *myth* to characterize mental diseases.

Other writers including Scadding (1967), Sedgwick (1973), Kendell (1975) and Boorse (1976) have put forward arguments that stand in opposition to Szasz. Scadding and Kendell use the combination of statistical deviance and biological disadvantage defined as reduced fertility to determine what a disease is. Boorse adds that a disease is any condition that interferes with any function of an organism (and in this view, mental functioning counts) that is necessary for its survival and reproduction. Additionally, a disease becomes an illness when it is deemed undesirable, a title for special treatment and a valid excuse for particular behaviours. Finally, Sedgwick makes the claim that all diseases start off as illnesses because the symptoms are negatively valued and hence become a focus of social and moral interest and that in this way the symptoms later attain disease status. In this account both the so-called *physical illnesses* and *mental illnesses* start off as negatively valued states afflicting human beings and there is no sharp distinction to be drawn between them. See Fulford et al. (2006) for further elaboration of these issues.

It is clear that there is no widely accepted view about the status of the conditions that fall under the interest of psychiatrists. A simple dictum is to regard disease as what doctors treat and illness as what persons suffer from. Although this distinction between normality and disease, health and illness is by no means trivial:

A large part of medical ethics and much of the whole underpinning of current medical policy, private and public, are squarely based on the notion of disease and normality. Left to himself the physician (whether he realizes it or not) can do very well without a formal definition of disease … Unfortunately, the physician is not left alone to work his common sense. He is attacked from two angles: the predatory consumers and the pretentious advisers.

Murphy (1979)

NORMS, NORMAL AND ABNORMAL

The subject of psychiatry is the person, not an organ such as the liver, kidney or even the brain. Psychiatric diseases are distinct from mere neurologic diseases in the sense that in neurology the disease process leaves the self, the personhood of an individual, intact. This means that we can speak of a person who suffers from multiple sclerosis or motor neuron disease. In psychiatry, the diseases afflict the self (i.e., affect the person in a deep and not superficial sense). Mood disorders and schizophrenia have a pervasive influence on aspects of the self in a way that strikes at what it means to be human.

The ability to experience and represent the world; the capacity to inhabit a social world including recognizing the rules and conventions that operate therein; the ability to form relationships and to imagine the world of the Other; the ability to communicate, to use language and to understand symbols, that is, to inhabit a world of meanings; the wherewithal to be an agent, the author of one's own projects and the drive and will to act; the capacity to operate in a world of moral and aesthetic values; and, the possibility of having an attitude to time, an orientation to the future—these manifold aspects of the person and many more yet to be fully described are influenced, if not impaired, by psychiatric diseases. Our understanding of these higher human functions is trivial. Abnormalities and pathology in these domains are manifest in social behaviour and are without independent or objective markers. So, talk of norms, normality and abnormality are integral to any discussion of psychiatric phenomena because to recognize impairments in these areas of function, we need an understanding of what normal function entails, but more fundamentally what it means to talk about norms, normality and abnormality.

The word *normal* is used correctly in at least four senses in the English language according to Mowbray et al. (1979). These are the *value* norm, the *statistical* norm, the *individual* norm and the *typological* norm. The *value* norm takes the ideal as its concept of normality. Thus the statement 'It is normal to have perfect teeth' is using normal in a value sense; in practice, most people have something wrong with their teeth. The *statistical* norm is, of course, the preferred use; the abnormal is considered to be that which falls outside the average range. If a normal Englishman is 5 feet 8 inches tall, to be either 6 feet 2 inches or 5 feet 2 inches tall is equally abnormal statistically.

The *individual* norm is the consistent level of functioning that an individual maintains over time. After brain damage, a person may experience a decline in intelligence that is certainly a deterioration from their previous individual level but may not represent any statistical abnormality from that of the general population (e.g., a decline in intelligence quotient from 125 to 105).

Typological abnormality is a necessary term to describe the situation in which a condition is regarded as normal in all the three meanings and yet represents *abnormality*, perhaps even disease. The example given by Mowbray et al. is the infective condition of *pinta*. The mottling of the skin of this condition is highly prized by the South American Indians who 'suffer' from it to the extent that 'nonsufferers' are excluded from the tribe. Thus having the condition is normal in a value, statistical and individual sense, and yet it is pathologic in the sense that it is the result of a spirochaetal skin infection. The pursuit of thinness by models and dancers in our society would be an everyday example.

In addition, one can talk about *social* norms by which we mean the rules, conventions and practices that determine in specific cultures what behaviours are acceptable and approved of. These include the etiquette, mores and ethics underpinning behaviour. In fact, for some people, psychiatric diseases are no more than behaviours classed as deviant by social rules, and psychiatrists are no more than social police officers.

There are other concepts implicit in discussions of norms, normality and abnormality. These are whether the discrete phenomena of interest to psychopathologists are categorically different from normal experience or whether the distinction between normal and abnormal phenomena is dimensional in nature. The distinction being drawn here is over and beyond whether psychopathological phenomena are statistically deviant. The question is whether the anxiety experienced by a psychiatric patient, for example, is only an exaggeration of that experienced by a 'normal' person or whether there is something categorically/qualitatively different about it.

UNDERSTANDING AND UN-UNDERSTANDABLE

It seems self-evident that understanding the patient's story, grasping the inner logic of the narrative and representing to oneself the patient's subjective experiences is fundamental to clinical practice. Understanding, in both an everyday and a phenomenological sense cannot be complete unless the doctor has a detailed knowledge of the patient's background culture and specific information about their family and immediate environment. Neither can phenomenology concentrate solely on the individual isolated in a moment of time. It must be concerned with the person in a social setting; after all, a person's experience is largely determined by their interactions with others. It must also be concerned with the mental state and environment of the individual before the event of immediate interest and with what occurs afterwards.

The method of phenomenology facilitates communication: its use makes it easier for the doctor to understand their patient. The patient is also helped to have confidence in the doctor, because they realize that their symptoms are understood and therefore accepted as 'real'. The precise description and evaluation of symptoms also helps communication between doctors.

Wilhelm Dilthey (1833–1911) argued that the natural sciences treat nature as objects and forces that can be explained through causal laws. In other words, the goal of such science is the formulation of general, universal laws, whereas the humanities, for example, history and psychology, have the human subject as their focus and causal laws do not apply in these circumstances. For Dilthey, science 'explains' natural phenomena by causal explanation. The humanities 'understand' human psychic phenomena through the interpretation of the meaning structures revealed in texts or through dialogue with another person. This distinction between 'explanation' and 'understanding' continues to be influential in our thinking even today (Phillips, 2004). In science, we come to know the object from outside, but in the humanities, we are able to 'know' the subject from inside. We are able to represent to ourselves, if not to 'know', the inner life of another person because we too have an inner life. We are able to understand the other person through the network of meanings associated with their behaviour. We start with the premise that behaviour means something; that is, it arises with internal consistency from psychological events. Wittgenstein (1953) stated, 'We explain human behaviour by giving reasons not causes'.

	Understanding	Explanation
Static	Phenomenological description	Observation through external sense perception
Genetic	Empathy established from what emerges	Cause and effect of scientific method

TABLE 1.2 Diagram of Understanding and Explanation

Jaspers drew on Dilthey's formulation and contrasted understanding (*verstehen*) with explaining (*erklären*). He has shown how these terms may be used in both a *static* and a *genetic* sense. *Static* implies understanding or explaining the present situation from information that is available now, whereas the *genetic* (an unfortunate term given contemporary use) sense considers how the situation reached its present state by examining antecedents, the evolving process and emerging situation. This is represented in Table 1.2.

Understanding and explanation are both necessary parts of the psychiatric investigation. *Explanation* is concerned with accounting for events from a point of observation outside them, understanding from inside them. One understands another person's anger and its consequences; one explains the occurrence of snow in winter. Explanations also can be described as static or genetic (Boxes 1.1 and 1.2).

Jaspers makes an important distinction between that which is *meaningful* and allows empathy and that which is ultimately *un-understandable*, the essence of the psychotic experience. There is thus a limit to understanding psychopathological phenomena. Although one can empathize with the *content* of a patient's delusion and thereby understand how that content of the belief originated, the occurrence of the delusion itself is, in this model, more recalcitrant to our empathy and understanding. It can be said that our understanding reaches its limit when it confronts the fact of the delusion itself. For that, we need to appeal to cognitive mechanisms or other natural science processes. We are in need of scientific explanation, not psychological understanding.

We can understand from a knowledge of the patient's background why, if their thinking is going to be disordered in form, the topic or content of that

BOX 1.1 STATIC AND GENETIC UNDERSTANDING

Understanding is the perception of personal meaning of the patient's subjective experience.
- If we want to find meaning at a particular moment in time, the method of phenomenology is appropriate. The patient's subjective experience is dissected out, and a *static* picture is formed of what that thought or event meant to them at that particular time. No comment is made on how the event arose, and no prediction is made as to what will happen next. The meaning is simply extracted as a description of what the patient is experiencing and what this signifies to them now. A person feels angry: static understanding uses empathy to describe in detail exactly what it is like for them to feel angry. Have I, the examiner, experienced phenomena like these? Are they known to me through the experiences I have had in my lifetime?
- *Genetic* understanding, as opposed to static understanding, is concerned with a *process*. It is understood that when this person is insulted, they react with violence; when that person hears voices commenting on their actions, they draw the curtains. For understanding the way that psychic events emerge one from another in the patient's experience, the therapist uses *empathy* as a method or a tool. He *feels himself into* the patient's situation. If that first event were to have occurred to him personally in the patient's total circumstances, the second event, which was the patient's reaction to it, might reasonably be expected to have followed. He understands the feelings he ascribed to the patient by the action that results from these feelings. So if I were the patient with the same history, do I feel that I would have the same experiences and behave in the same way? An example would help to demonstrate the humanity of this approach and the universality of human experience: I must put myself into the shoes of another young woman, aged 19, also raised in an isolated fishing community, the eldest of eight siblings who becomes stuporose during her second pregnancy. She is married to an alcoholic man aged 35, and her father is also alcoholic. I must understand how she dealt with her father's alcoholic behaviour as a child, what her pregnancy meant to her, how she regarded her mother's behaviour during her own pregnancies and so on.

thinking should be concerned with persecution by the Nazis—perhaps because their parents escaped from Germany in 1937. But we can have no understanding of why they should believe something that is demonstrably false (e.g., that their persecutors are putting a tasteless fluid into the drinking water that makes them feel ill). The delusion itself, as psychopathological

BOX 1.2 STATIC AND GENETIC EXPLANATION

- Static explanation is concerned with external sense perception, observing an event, for example, 'I witnessed the 1999 eclipse in Plymouth'.
- Genetic explanation consists of unravelling causal connections; it describes a chain of events and why they follow that sequence ('visual perception of the eclipse is the result of physiologic changes in my retina, which in turn produce changes in my occipital cortex that ultimately cause me to see the eclipse').

form, is *un-understandable*. Meaningful connections, then, show the linkage between different psychological events by understanding how these events emerge one from another by a process of empathy.

This is a controversial concept in that it implies that there are aspects of another person's mental life that are beyond our grasp and empathic understanding. It contradicts another axiom in psychiatric practice, namely that our purpose is to understand another person, and when understanding fails, it calls into question how conscientious and rigorous the psychiatrist has been in the pursuit of grasping the inner life of the patient.

EMPATHY

The classic method in medicine of gaining information about the patient is from the history and by physical examination. The use of phenomenology in psychiatry is an extension of the *history* in that it amplifies the description of the present complaint to give more detailed information. It is also *examination* in that it reveals the mental state. It is not possible for me, the doctor, to observe my patient's hallucination or in any direct way to measure it. However, what I can do to comprehend them is to use those human characteristics I hold in common with them: the fact that we inhabit the same world of meanings, that we communicate in language and that, like them, I have a rich inner life. It is also important to be intellectually curious and genuinely interested in the inner life of another person. The inquiries that arise from this stance should aim to re-create for oneself or represent to oneself the subjective experiences of another person with the aim of understanding and making sense of them. The aim is thus to explore and test, through dialogue, the patient's subjective experience. I endeavour

to create in my own mind what their experience must be like. I then test to see whether I am correct in my reconstruction of their experience by asking them to affirm or deny my description. I also use my observation of their behaviour—the sad expression of their face or their thumping the desk with their fist—to reconstruct their experiences.

Listening and observing are crucial for understanding. Great care must be taken with asking questions. Doctors, not infrequently, identify symptoms incorrectly and come to the wrong diagnosis because they have asked leading questions with which the patient, through their submissiveness to the doctor's status and anxiety to cooperate, are only too willing to concur.

The method of empathy implies using the ability to feel oneself into the situation of the other person by proceeding through an organized series of questions, rephrasing and reiterating when necessary until one is quite sure of what is being described by the patient. The sequence might proceed as follows.

Question: 'You describe your thoughts changing; what happens to them?'

Answer: The patient gives a description of how they have a recurring thought of killing people, and this results from a pain in the stomach.

Question (trying to isolate the elements of the patient's experience): 'What is your thought of killing people like?' (obsession, delusion, fantasy, is likely to be acted on, etc.). 'Do you believe that your stomach affects your thinking?' 'Is this different from people who know that they become irritable when hungry?' 'In what way is it different from that?' 'What causes your pain in the stomach?'

Answer: The patient describes the details, which include, among irrelevant material, the sort of information required for determining what symptoms are present.

Question (the invitation for empathy): 'Am I right in thinking that you are describing an experience in which rays are causing pain in your stomach and that your stomach, in some way quite independent of yourself, causes this thought, which frightens you so that you must kill somebody with a knife?' This is an account of the relevant symptoms that they have described in language they should be able to recognize as their own.

Answer: 'Yes' (we have then achieved our goal); 'No' (therefore I must try again to elicit the symptoms, experience them for myself and describe them back to the patient again).

To give examples of what this implies in practice, how do I, a clinician, decide whether an individual patient is depressed or not? This is not done by imitating a machine that might record units of vocal tone or of facial expression, adding up to a diagnosis of depression. For the clinical assessment, I go through the following process:

- I am capable of feeling unhappy, miserable and depressed and know what this feeling is like inside myself.
- If I were feeling as I observe the patient to be looking, speaking, acting and so on, I would be feeling miserable, depressed and unhappy.
- Therefore I assess the mood of the patient to be that of depression.

Of course, this mental process of diagnosis is not usually verbalized.

In another example, a patient says, 'The Martians are making me say swear words; it is not me doing it'. Empathic questioning reveals the false belief held by the patient that when swear words come from their mouth, they believe that the cause is actually outside themself, 'Martians', rather than from inside themself. Questioning would include 'Do you actually *hear* the Martians? How do you know that it is Martians and no one else?' and so on.

A further, nonpsychotic example would be a 20-year-old young woman who has fainting attacks when she is criticized at work. The clinician has to place oneself, even if he is a 55-year-old man from a different cultural background, into her position with knowledge not only of her social history but also of the way that she, in the present, perceives that history; only then may the development of her symptoms become understandable. For instance, when the clinician knows about her alcohol-abusing father; the rows her father had with her mother who suffered from epilepsy; the very restricted cultural background that they experienced in an isolated fishing village and how her mother would have a fit when rows became intolerable, then he may begin to understand something of the development of the patient's own symptom. This is not achieved solely by explanation as an outside observer

but by empathic understanding and the capacity for subjective experience by the doctor who puts himself into and therefore becomes the 20-year-old woman for the process of the psychiatric interview.

It is the purpose of the phenomenological method therefore to (1) describe inner experiences, (2) order and classify them and (3) create a reliable terminology. Empathy is also invaluable therapeutically in establishing a relationship with the patient. Knowing that the doctor understands and is even to some extent able to share her feelings gives the patient confidence and a sense of relief. This method of empathy is also useful as a way of extending knowledge more generally in the field of psychiatry because it allows a diagnostic terminology to be developed.

Empathy is nonetheless a problematic concept. It is unclear what Jaspers himself meant by it, and hence various potentially contradictory interpretations are possible including transferring oneself into another person's mind, sharing the patient's experience or actualizing the patient's experience for oneself (Fulford et al., 2006). The approach taken in this book is to emphasize the use of extended dialogue to discover and re-create a patient's subjective experience in oneself. Stanghellini and Aragona (2016) make the important point that empathic understanding is neither emotional fusion with the patient nor cold distance but always an attempt to modulate distance by continuous oscillation between the extreme of fusion and cold detachment.

FORM AND CONTENT

Form and content are distinct in phenomenology. For Jaspers:

Form must be kept distinct from content which may change from time to time, e.g., the fact of a hallucination is to be distinguished from its content, whether this is a man or a tree, threatening figures or peaceful landscapes. Perceptions, ideas, judgements, feelings, drives, self-awareness, are all forms of psychic phenomenon; they denote the particular mode of existence in which content is presented to us.

Jaspers (1997)

Thus, like warp and woof, form and content are essentially different but inextricably woven together.

One way to think of *form* is to regard it as the sense modality in which a perception is presented to us or the cognitive domain in which a particular aspect of psychic life is experienced or enacted. The *form* of a psychic experience is the description of its structure in phenomenological terms, for example, a delusion or, as Berrios (1996) says, 'Form refers to those impersonal aspects of the mental symptoms that guarantee its stability in time and space; that is, its "constancy" elements'. Viewed in this way, *content* is the subjective colouring of the experience. The patient is concerned because they believe that people are stealing their money. Their concern is that 'people are taking my money', not that 'I hold on unacceptable grounds a false belief that people are taking my money'. They are concerned about the content. Clearly, form and content are both important but in different contexts. The patient is concerned only with the content, 'that I am pursued by ten thousand hockey sticks'. The doctor is concerned with both form and content, but as a phenomenologist only with form, in this case a false belief of being pursued. As far as form is concerned, the hockey sticks are irrelevant. The patient finds the doctor's interest in form unintelligible and a distraction from what they regard as important, and often demonstrate their irritation.

In Chapter 7, a patient is described who said, 'When I turn the tap on, I hear a voice whispering in the water pipe, "She's on her way to the moon. Let's hope she has a soft landing."' The *form* of this experience is what demands the attention of the phenomenologist and is useful diagnostically. She is describing a *perception*; it is an auditory perception and a false or disordered auditory perception. It has the characteristics of a hallucination and specifically of a *functional* hallucination. This is the form. While the psychiatrist is busy clarifying the form, the patient might be getting irritated because 'he is not taking any notice of what I am saying'. She is worried that she is being sent to the moon. What will happen when she gets there? How will she get back? So, the *content* is all-important to her, and the doctor's absorption with form is incomprehensible and frustrating in the extreme.

The form is dependent on, and is therefore a diagnostic key to, the particular mental illness from which the patient suffers. For example, *delusional percepts* occur in schizophrenia, and when demonstrated as the form of the experience, they indicate this condition. The finding of a visual hallucination suggests the likelihood of an organic brain disease (Chapter 7). The nature of the content of these two examples is irrelevant in coming to a diagnosis. The content can be understood by the patient's life situation with regard to culture, peer group, status, sophistication, age, sex, life events and geographic location. For example, another patient described himself as having been sent to the moon and back during the night within a fortnight of the first landing by man on the moon. Describing one's thoughts as being controlled by television is necessarily confined to those people who have seen that invention.

Hypochondriacal content can occur in more than one form. It could take the form of an auditory hallucination in which the patient hears a voice saying, 'You have cancer'. It could be a delusion in that they hold, with conviction, the false belief that they have cancer. It could be an overvalued idea in that the patient has a conviction arising from prior experience of a mistaken diagnosis of cancer, and this results in them spending a major part of everyday checking on their health. It could be an abnormality of affect that manifests itself in extreme hypochondriacal anxiety or in depressive hypochondriacal despondency.

The significance of culture and individual variation in ascertaining the detailed complaint of the patient should be stressed. Because the psychiatrist needs to assess whether this notion of the patient demonstrates the specific psychopathological form of delusion, it does not diminish the parallel need to understand the patient's philosophic, religious, political and social beliefs and know how they fit, or fail to fit, into the patient's larger, national and more intimate, subcultural social contexts (Fabrega, 2000).

Alongside the need of the psychiatrist to acquire skills in psychopathology and the elucidating of mental symptoms is the parallel requirement for cultural education and sensitivity. Both aspects are necessary for every patient–doctor interaction. If anything, the painstaking and detailed study of phenomenology increases the awareness of the cultural context and how it influences cognition and behaviour.

PRIMARY AND SECONDARY PHENOMENA

Jaspers discusses the different meanings that can be given to the terms *primary* and *secondary* when applied to symptoms. The distinction may be in terms of understanding; what is primary is immediate and ultimate and therefore cannot be further reduced by understanding, for example, hallucinations. What is secondary is what *emerges* from the primary in a way that can be understood, for example, delusional elaboration arising from the healthy part of the psyche in response to hallucinations from the unhealthy part of the psyche. Again, the conceptual distinction of what is primary or secondary may be determined by the causal chain in that what is primary is the proximate cause, whereas what is secondary is the discernible distal effect. A cerebrovascular accident *causes* sensory aphasia and is therefore primary; the aphasia is the distal effect and is therefore secondary to the cerebrovascular accident.

These two distinct meanings of the term *primary* overlie the crucial distinction between meaningful connections and causal connections. For the avoidance of doubt in physics and chemistry, we make observations by experiment and then formulate causal connections and causal laws, whereas in psychopathology we experience another sort of connection in which psychic events emerge out of one another in a way that can be understood—so-called *meaningful connections*.

SUBJECTIVITY AND OBJECTIVITY IN PSYCHOPATHOLOGY

Objectivity in science has come to be revered as the ideal so that only what is external to the mind is considered to be real, measurable and valuable. This is a mistake, because objective assessments are necessarily subjectively value-laden in what the observer chooses to measure, and this subjective aspect can be made more precise and reliable. There are always value judgements associated with both subjective and objective assessments. The process of making a scientific evaluation consists of various stages: receiving a sensory stimulus, perceiving, observing (making the percepts meaningful), noting, coding and formulating hypotheses. This is a progressive process of discarding information, and it is the subjective judgement of what information is valuable that determines the small amount from each stage that is retained for transmission to the next part of the process. 'There is no such thing as an unprejudiced observation' (Popper, 1974).

Objective assessments in psychiatry have covered many aspects of life. A few examples are, in addition to many physiologic measures, the measurement of body movements, facial expression, patients' writings, learning capacity, responses to an operant conditioning programme, memory span, work efficiency and evaluation of logical content of the patients' statements. All these can be quantified and analysed objectively. Subjective analysis can be made, for example, from facial expression or from the patient's description of themselves, of their own writing or of their inner events. When a doctor says about a patient 'They look sad', they are not measuring the patient's facial expression in 'units of sadness' by some objective yardstick. They are going through this process: 'I associate their facial expression with the affect that I recognize in myself as feeling sad; seeing their expression makes me feel sad'. *Rapport* is the emotional quality of the relationship that the patient establishes with the doctor during the clinical encounter. For it to happen, the doctor has to be receptive to this communication. They have to be able to communicate in a genuine way, to be able to express an atmosphere of acceptance and to have a capacity for warmth and human understanding. This is necessarily a subjective experience for the doctor, but that is not to say that it is unreal or even that it cannot be measured. The method of phenomenology tries to increase our knowledge of subjective events so that they can be classified and ultimately quantified.

Aggernaes (1972) has defined subjectivity and objectivity for immediate everyday experiences.

When an experienced something has a quality of 'sensation', it is also said to have a quality of 'objectivity' if the experiencer feels that, under favourable circumstances, they would be able to experience the same something with another modality of sensation than the one giving the quality of sensation. When an experienced something has a quality of 'ideation', that is, it is not being directly sensed at the moment, it is also said to have a quality of 'objectivity' if the experiencer feels that under favourable circumstances, they would nevertheless be able to experience the same something with at least two modalities of sensation.

An experienced something has a quality of 'subjectivity' if the experiencer feels that under no circumstances they would be able to experience this something with two or more modalities of sensation.

Thus I can look at the table in front of me as a visual perception, or I can turn my head and still fantasize it as a visual image. As I 'see' it, in either way, the fact that I can imagine both hearing a sound if I were to hit it with a spoon and bruising my knuckles if I were to punch it confirms its quality of objectivity. If I use my imagination to create in my mind a visual image of a Chippendale chair that I have never actually seen but is a composite of objects and pictures I have seen, I know that I will never be able to feel or hear this actual chair; it is a subjective image without external, objective reality.

UNCONSCIOUS EXPERIENCE AND PHENOMENOLOGY

Phenomenology cannot be concerned with the unconscious because the patient cannot describe it, and so the doctor cannot empathize. Descriptive psychopathology has no theory of the unconscious, nor does it deny its existence. Strictly speaking, the unconscious is simply outside its terms of reference, and psychic events are described without recourse to explanations involving the unconscious. Dreams, the contents of hypnotic trance and slips of the tongue are described according to how the patient experienced them, that is, according to how they manifest in consciousness.

ORGANIC AND NEURAL SUBSTRATES AND PSYCHOPATHOLOGY

Psychopathology is the study of abnormal mental processes so that even when the organic causes of a condition are known, psychopathology remains involved in describing, defining and ordering the symptomatic phenomena and the experience of the patient rather than being preoccupied with its neural origin or pathophysiology. This is not to imply that underlying neural mechanisms are unimportant. To the contrary, they are undeniably important. However, the actual subjective experience of the patient is also important, and psychopathology concentrates on this.

There are established links between different abnormal phenomena and identifiable organic pathologies. However, it is not with these links that psychopathology is concerned, and its usefulness is not dependent on ultimately finding the localization in the brain of a delusion or any other psychic event. Early, organically oriented psychiatrists, such as Griesinger and Wernicke, were not concerned with

the psychopathological in psychiatry but much more with charting the diseased brain. This paid a rich dividend, for example, in elucidating the nature and treatment of cerebral syphilis. Similarly, some modern behaviourists have been uninterested in phenomenology. Phenomenology is not ultimately concerned with organic pathology or with behaviour per se but with the patient's subjective experience of their world.

For a long time, symptomatic psychiatry and descriptive psychopathology seemed to have lost contact with organic psychiatry in which evidence of mental illness is sought in disease of the brain. There has now developed what Mundt (2000) describes as a 'fresh wind from the experimental field of psychopathology, neuropsychology and biological neurosciences'. This linkage is still at an early stage, but it has potential for the future study of symptoms and brain pathology. But for these investigations to succeed and to come to fruition, a thorough appreciation of psychopathology is essential.

MIND–BRAIN DUALITY AND PSYCHOPATHOLOGY

Cartesian dualism is the view that mind and body are separate substances; the mind happens to be associated with a particular body but is ultimately self-sufficient and capable of independent existence. This view—expounded by René Descartes (1596–1650) in which he made a distinction between the material and physical world and the thinking human mind—continues to exert extraordinary influence. Husserl's philosophy, phenomenology, arose out of Husserl's rejection of many of Descartes' conclusions. There are a number of significant problems with Cartesian dualism, not least how an immaterial substance like the mind can influence a material substance like the body.

There are varied philosophic attempts to deal with the problem of dualism, and an account of these is beyond the scope of this book. What is important is that psychiatry is bedevilled by this problem: how to reconcile the phenomena that patients report with the materiality of the brain. Is it possible or plausible to reduce mental events to physical events in the brain? And how far can the changes observable during functional magnetic resonance imaging scanning be interpreted as products of certain mental phenomena? Phenomenology, as an approach, avoids this debate by leaving it to one side (bracketing it as Husserl would have said) while continuing to explore, investigate, describe, define and catalogue the mental events, the phenomena, reported by patients. Descriptive psychopathology is not concerned with causes but with descriptions of experience.

The philosophy of mind is a thriving area of research, in particular the elucidation of the nature of mind. The specific theories are outside the scope of this book (see *The Character of Mind: An Introduction to the Philosophy of Mind*; McGinn, 1997). That is not to say that those theories such as Spinoza's token identity theory, the type identity theory (also known as reductive materialism) or eliminative materialism or functionalism are not relevant to psychiatry or to experimental psychopathology, but merely to emphasise that psychopathology can develop in the absence of a full and final theory of the nature of mind.

REFERENCES

Aggernaes, A., 1972. The experienced reality of hallucinations and other psychological phenomena. Acta Psychiatr. Scand. 48, 220–238.

Berrios, G.E., 1984. Descriptive psychopathology: conceptual and historical aspects. Psychol. Med. 14, 303–313.

Berrios, G.E., 1992. Phenomenology, psychopathology and Jaspers: a conceptual history. Hist. Psychiat. 3, 303–327.

Berrios, G.E., 1996. The History of Mental Symptoms: Descriptive Psychopathology since the Nineteenth Century. Cambridge University Press, Cambridge.

Boorse, C., 1976. What a theory of mental health should be. J. Theory Soc. Behav. 6, 61–84.

Fabrega, H., 2000. Culture, spirituality and psychiatry. Curr. Opin. Psychiatry. 13, 525–530.

Fulford, K.W.M., Thornton, T., Graham, G., 2006. Oxford Textbook of Philosophy of Psychiatry. Oxford University Press, Oxford.

James, W., 1902. The Varieties of Religious Experience. Penguin, London.

Jaspers, K., 1997. General Psychopathology (J. Hoenig, M.W. Hamilton, Trans). The Johns Hopkins University Press, Baltimore.

Kendell, R.E., 1975. The concept of disease and its implications for psychiatry. Br. J. Psychiatry 127, 305–315.

McGinn, C., 1997. The Character of Mind: An Introduction to the Philosophy of Mind, second ed. Oxford University Press, Oxford.

Mowbray, R.M., Ferguson, R.T., Mellor, C.S., 1979. Psychology in Relation to Medicine, fifth ed. Churchill Livingstone, Edinburgh.

Mundt, C., 2000. Editorial. Psychopathology. 33, 2–4.

Murphy, E.A., 1979. The epistemology of normality. Psychol. Med. 9, 409–415.

Phillips, J., 2004. Understanding/explanation. In: Radden, J. (Ed.), The Philosophy of Psychiatry: A Companion. Oxford University Press, Oxford, pp. 180–190.

Popper, K., 1974. Unended Quest. Penguin, Harmondsworth.

Rosenhan, D.L., 1973. On being sane in insane places. Science 179, 250–258.

Scadding, J.G., 1967. Diagnosis: the clinician and the computer. Lancet 2, 877–882.

Sedgwick, P., 1973. Illness—mental and otherwise. Stud. Hastings Cent. 1, 19–40.

Spitzer, M., 1990. Why philosophy? In: Spitzer, M., Maher, B.A. (Eds.), Philosophy and Psychopathology. Springer-Verlag, New York.

Stanghellini, G., Aragona, M., 2016. Phenomenological psychopathology: toward a person-centred hermeutic approach in the clinical encounter. In: Stanghellini, G., Aragona, M. (Eds.), An Experiential Approach to Psychopathology – what Is it like to Suffer from Mental Disorders? Springer, Basel, pp. 1–43.

Stanghellini, G., Fuchs, T., 2013. Editors' introduction. In: Stanghellini, G., Fuchs, T. (Eds.), One Century of Karl Jaspers' General Psychopathology. Oxford University Press, Oxford. xiii–xxiii.

Szasz, T.S., 1960. The myth of mental illness. Am. Psychol. 15, 113–118.

Walker, C., 1988. Philosophical concepts and practice: the legacy of Karl Jaspers's psychopathology. Curr. Opin. Psychiatry 1, 624–629.

Walker, C., 1993a. Karl Jaspers as a Kantian psychopathologist. I. The philosophical origins of the concept of form and context. Hist. Psychiat. 4, 209–238.

Walker, C., 1993b. Karl Jaspers as a Kantian psychopathologist. II. The concept of form and context in Jaspers' psychopathology. Hist. Psychiat. 4, 321–348.

Walker, C., 1994. Karl Jaspers and Edmund Husserl: I: the perceived convergence. Philos. Psychiatr. Psychol. 1, 117–134.

Walker, C., 1995a. Karl Jaspers and Edmund Husserl: II: the divergence. Philos. Psychiatr. Psychol. 2, 245–265.

Walker, C., 1995b. Karl Jaspers and Edmund Husserl: III: Jaspers as a Kantian phenomenologist. Philos. Psychiatr. Psychol. 2, 65–82.

Wiggins, O.P., Schwartz, M.A., Spitzer, M., 1992. Phenomenology/descriptive psychiatry: the method of Edmund Husserl and Karl Jaspers. In: Spitzer, M., Uehlein, F., Schawartz, M.A., Mundt, C. (Eds.), Phenomenology, Language and Schizophrenia. Springer-Verlag, New York, pp. 46–69.

Wittgenstein, L., 1953. Philosophical Investigation (G.E.M. Anscombe, Trans). Blackwell, Oxford.

Chapter 2

Eliciting the Symptoms of Mental Illness

Chapter Outline

KEYWORDS

Diagnosis
History
Mental state examination

Summary

The clinical assessment of patients, which includes history taking, mental state examination, physical examination and the synthesis of the findings into a diagnosis that takes account of the patient's biological, psychological and social environment, is the basis of psychiatric practice. Without it, no adequate treatment and further clinical management is possible. At the heart of this task is the importance of focusing on the patient as the centre of clinical attention, recognizing the value of respect for the dignity of the patient and regarding the patient's narrative account as valuable, rich and privileged. The ascendancy of a tick-box approach to clinical assessment is to be deplored. It fails to grasp that, despite the fact that assessments have a structure to them and that they are systematic inquiries, assessments must be conducted in a conversational style and in a humane manner.

Human beings are like parts of a body,
Created from the same essence.
When one part is hurt and in pain,
The others cannot remain in peace and be quiet.
If the misery of others leaves you indifferent
And with no feelings of sorrow,
You cannot be called a human being.
                    Sa'adi, Persian (13th century)

Eliciting the symptoms and signs of emotional distress involves actively listening to a narrative account of the person's complaints and his internal state and observing the whole repertoire of behaviour and then reducing these to a few summarizing phrases. It is a difficult task, requiring an ability to listen and communicate, a sensitivity to the needs and feelings of a person who is bewildered and distressed and a knowledge of the possible conditions giving rise to the complaint. A genuine interest in the human condition and its manifold expressions, as well as a curiosity about intrapsychic experiences, is essential. This cannot be learned from a book alone, but a structure for case taking that suggests likely areas for exploration is invaluable. There are many comprehensive schemes, and they can often be traced to earlier textbooks with only slight modification. A summary of the scheme on which this chapter is based is shown in Box 2.1. A practical guide to history taking and evaluation of the mental state, diagnosis, formulation and management is found in the *Handbook for Trainee Psychiatrists* (Rix, 1987), *The Psychiatric Interview* (Carlat, 2005)

and *Kaplan and Saddock's Comprehensive Textbook of Psychiatry* (9th edition; Saddock et al., 2009). A useful approach to making the patient information available for diagnosis and planning treatment is *Making Sense of Psychiatric Cases* (Greenberg et al., 1986), and there are more in-depth texts on the psychiatric interview, such as *The Psychiatric Interview in Clinical Practice* (MacKinnon et al., 2006) and *The First Interview* (Morrison, 2008). A further account of the areas to be considered and the modifications of the history and examination required in particular circumstances is to be found in Sims and Curran (2001).

There is a significant conflict of interest between the patient and the interviewer. The patient describes untoward and distressing experiences. They want to be rid of these experiences. One patient may, for example, say that they are depressed and miserable, and another may complain that their thoughts

BOX 2.1 OUTLINE FOR PSYCHIATRIC EXAMINATION

Patient's name: _____
Age: _____
Occupation: _____
Marital status: _____
Address: _____
Source of referral: _____
- Reason for referral
- Present illness: symptoms and their chronology
- Previous medical history
  - i. Physical
  - ii. Psychiatric
- Family history: father, mother, siblings, other relations, atmosphere at home
- Personal history
  - i. Pregnancy
  - ii. Infancy
  - iii. Childhood and adolescence
  - iv. Education at school
  - v. Further education
  - vi. Occupation (and military service)
  - vii. Sexual history: puberty, menstruation
  - viii. Marital history
  - ix. Children
- Social data
  - i. Life situation: currently working, housing situation, financial problems, relationships

- ii. Crime, delinquency
- iii. Alcohol, drugs, tobacco
- iv. Social and religious affiliations and beliefs
- Premorbid personality
- Mental state
  - i. Appearance and behaviour
  - ii. Talk and thought
  - iii. Mood: subjective, objective, rapport
  - iv. Thoughts and beliefs: phobias, obsessions, compulsions, suicidal thoughts, delusions, misinterpretations
  - v. Experience and perception:
  - a. of the environment (hallucinations, illusions, derealization)
  - b. of the body (hypochondriasis, somatic hallucinations)
  - c. of the self (depersonalization, thought passivity)
  - d. cognitive state: orientation, attention, concentration and memory
  - e. insight
- Diagnosis and assessment
  - i. Diagnosis and differential diagnosis
  - ii. Evidence for diagnosis
  - iii. Aetiologic factors
  - iv. Management
  - v. Prognosis

are being sucked out of their head by the Martians. In both instances, the patient wants the symptom to be relieved and feels that describing it to the doctor in the way that it is affecting them is the first stage in achieving this. The doctor needs to learn a lot of things from the patient that the latter may consider irrelevant. They need to have a precise description of the symptoms and of the patient's state of mind. They need to know about the context of the patient's symptoms, including the patient's developmental history and about their adjustment to their social environment in general and to their symptoms in particular. To return to our examples, the doctor not only needs to know that the patient feels depressed, but also must enquire about the precise nature of the 'depression', what the word implies to the patient, how the affect disturbs the routine of their life and whether there are any other associated symptoms.

The person suffering at the hands of the Martians will be only too ready to talk about Martians. However, they are largely irrelevant to the interviewer, who is interested in exactly what the experience of 'thoughts being extracted' entails. What is the patient's evidence that this happens? What other abnormal mental phenomena are experienced? The reader can perhaps understand the patient's irritation if they can imagine that, after they had paid their gas bill, a final demand notice with an intimation that their gas supply was to be cut off came through the letterbox. On explaining to the authorities that the bill was already paid, they did not apologize or say that they would correct their computer, but they started interrogating the harassed consumer as to why they should be so upset about it, and what was their evidence that they had been especially picked on by the authorities. Understandably, there is a potential conflict of interest between the patient's wish for relief of symptoms and the doctor's need to start by making a diagnosis. This differing of perspectives, of priorities, is often at the root of the dissatisfaction that many patients experience about the clinical encounter. A solution to this dilemma, or indeed, a compromise is necessary.

The patient will quite quickly tire of the effort required to answer questions that are aimed at establishing the phenomenological status of subjective experiences. Several short interviews are preferable to a marathon session: 'never ask today what you can ask tomorrow'. This method should encourage the examiner to 'bracket out' all preconceptions and the patient to reflect on their experiences under guidance from the examiner, who should not be digging for phenomena like a dog at a rabbit hole. It is important for the examiner to distinguish clearly between observations and inferences.

Diagnosis and Labelling

Why make a diagnosis? The medical classification of diseases allows a cluster of symptoms to be brought under a single term that embodies the essence of a given condition. The diagnostic term carries information in an efficient manner. But there are disadvantages, including the unreliability of diagnostic terms as well as the risk of undue labelling and the associated stigma of a psychiatric diagnosis. It is central to the work of a professional that their first task is to carefully collect information so that they know exactly what clinical problem confronts them within their professional competence and therefore what action would be appropriate; this is what diagnosis implies. It is true that for many common medical diseases such as diabetes, the diagnostic term refers to underlying demonstrable pathophysiology for which independent markers exist, such as blood sugar levels. In psychiatry, practically all the major disorders are still recognized at a syndromal level, that is, by the cluster of signs and symptoms that are thought to be typical of the given disease. The assumption is that patterns of symptoms refer to discrete underlying anomalies yet to be systematically established. Sadly, diagnostic terms do not, as yet, refer to any well-described pathophysiology or indeed to any independent or reliable marker. This is a significant problem for the status of psychiatric diseases as bona fide medical diseases.

In psychiatry, a multifactorial approach to the understanding of a disorder is the rule rather than the exception. This is the basis of the biopsychosocial approach to psychiatric disorders. This means that a narrow diagnosis, in purely organic or purely behavioural terms, is inadequate. The diagnosis needs to be made in the context of an understanding of the biological, psychological and social antecedents, which, in turn, determine the biological, psychological and social management of the condition.

The Psychiatric History

This account is chiefly interested in the way that *taking the history* sheds light on the *mental state*. The nature and type of *referral* is noted and recorded, for example, from a general practitioner as an urgent problem, from a solicitor for a court report and so on. After recording the reason for referral, the history will usually begin with the patient's *verbatim* description of their *present symptoms,* including the duration of each symptom and an account of the development of the illness. Using the patient's own words is valuable in giving insight into their state of mind and how they themself view their symptoms. It is helpful after receiving a catalogue of complaints to ask, 'Which is the very worst of all these symptoms?' or 'What is your main concern?' This reveals how the patient conceptualizes the problem and also suggests a preliminary target for treatment.

Often the patient's history of their present complaint is literally their story; there is nothing wrong in recording this in narrative style provided this is accurate. A chronological account of the present illness reveals how the patient regards the development of their symptoms as well as giving information on the actual history. In the history, one wants to know about the sequence of symptoms and the effects these symptoms had on the patient's lifestyle, about changes in behaviour and about alterations in physical function. It is appropriate at this point to note psychiatric symptoms of which the patient has been aware in the past but for which they have never consulted a doctor or received treatment. They may have relevance in the total picture of how the illness developed, and it is known that the majority of people with psychiatric conditions of clinical severity do not seek medical consultation, let alone come to the attention of a psychiatrist (Andrews et al., 2001).

The patient feels it to be innately reasonable to describe chronologically and meticulously their previous *illnesses,* operations and accidents. They also will appreciate the logic of giving details of hospital and general practice treatment for mental illness and will usually give accurate information with regard to dates, duration, nature of the treatment, in what hospital and whether it was inpatient or outpatient. Treatment received from the family doctor is recalled less well; the dates are less reliable, and often the patient does not know the nature of the treatment or what it was for.

The *family history* is concerned with the patient's family of origin, the likelihood of genetic predisposition to mental illness, and the family relationships and their potential contribution to the patient's presentation. History of mental illness, suicide, nature of treatment and so on is relevant for the first-degree relatives (those sharing 50% of the genetic material with the patient: parents, siblings, children) and more distant relatives. It is important to know about the quality of relationships, emotional bonding and interpersonal conflicts, both for the family in which the patient was a child and for the family in which the patient may be a parent. Relationships between individual members of the family are described, as are the general emotional atmosphere and social and financial problems. The occupations of different family members give information about the social context; a record of health may be relevant, as may a description of their personalities. Of course, the family is seen through the patient's eyes; this means that it is not just a factual description but rather an account of the emotional impact the patient feels their family has had on them. If the history from the patient is supplemented by an account from another *informant,* this bias of the patient will itself give information that may be useful in subsequent treatment.

The *personal history* traces the stages of the patient's development, health and formation of relationships from conception, birth and infancy through childhood, school experiences, adolescence and further education to occupational, marital and sexual history. The factual details of these stages need to be recorded, as do the way they have influenced the personality development and attitudes of the patient, how he feels about them, how he has related to other people (e.g., teachers and workmates) and how all these details may be connected to the psychiatric condition. There are at least two processes at play in taking a history. There is the simple business of taking a factually accurate account of a patient's history of complaints as well as the family, personal and social history. In addition to this approach, there is the requirement to grasp the meaning of the patient's history, that is, their story, to understand how they see themself in relation to the world and how their development and circumstances have been influential in provoking, exacerbating or ameliorating their present illness.

The factual history is the foundation of the clinical diagnosis. Human beings live in a world of meanings, and the symbolic and social dimension of the history are the basis of an adequate and humane response to the patient's illness and distress. Accounts that emphasize, for example, the fact that the patient is an only child, a precious child, a victim of other people's malicious intentions, a fighter who has struggled against the odds or an unlucky individual for whom only failure and rejection characterize their life all say something about the dominant themes, the prism through which the individual analyses and perceives the world. So, although it is important to record the facts, the meanings and understanding that patients have of the trajectory of their life all communicate something that enriches the clinical encounter and potentially make possible a deeper doctor–patient relationship that should be satisfying for both doctor and patient.

Premorbid, Previous or Usual Personality

Assessment of personality is the most complex and problematic task that a psychiatrist faces. In clinical interviews, the doctor assesses the patient's personality using three areas of information. First, the examiner asks the patient to describe in detail their relationship with other people, their interests and activities. Second, the examiner studies the way in which the patient reacts to the examiner in the interview situation. Third, the examiner tries to help the patient describe and demonstrate what they, the patient, is like as a person; how they feel inside themself in different situations; and their interests, goals and standards.

Personality assessment is not the exclusive preserve of psychiatrists or psychologists but an important learned skill of many professionals who deal with people—for example, schoolteachers, lawyers and bank managers, although their terminology is different. Personality is that part of a person, excepting their physical characteristics, that makes them individual and unique, that is, different from other people. Personality is revealed by a person's characteristic behaviour, the enduring patterns of responding and reacting to given situations. If a clinician can attempt to predict how a patient will react in hypothetical situations, what their behaviour will be in particular circumstances, then the basis of that prediction is founded on a reasonable and relatively accurate evaluation of their personality. Subjectively, personality is shown in the totality of a person's aims and goals, formed of everything that they value and to which they aspire. Personality is not a *thing* but an abstraction, a model. It is simply a way of thinking about human character, temperament and conduct. Furthermore, it is multidimensional and is best defined in action. Verbal description is unlikely to exhaust the essence of any individual. Indeed, no description can exhaust the rich and complex essence of any individual person. It is a truism that human beings are full of potential and continue to surprise and astonish with the capacity for change, for transformation and for moral conduct including virtues and vices, which may not be readily identifiable on first contact.

Categorization into normal and abnormal personality requires a further level of abstraction. *Normal,* an ordinary word in everyday use, needs to be used more rigorously in this context (see Chapter 1). In medicine, the term *normal* is often used to denote a statistical norm, that is, what occurs in the majority of people. Equally, the term is also sometimes used to mean 'ideal' in the sense of a description that conforms to an 'ideal' type. In relation to personality, classification and definitions of personality disorders depend on deviance from the norm, but the definitions depend on 'ideal' descriptions of personality types or better still a typology. This can sometimes be difficult to grasp. We may have an ideal notion of what it is like to be 'extrovert' and then a particular individual is compared against this abstract notion. This comparison presupposes that the ideal notion, sometimes termed a *trait,* varies in a dimensional manner among people. An individual is more or less extroverted compared against this ideal notion. The implication is that abnormal personality has some characteristics that are either overdeveloped or underdeveloped compared with an ideal notion to such an extent as to significantly deviate from the mass of people. In other words, abnormalities of personality are differences of degree; the deviant traits are shared in common with others but exaggerated in expression.

In the clinical interview, there are various areas of dialogue with the patient that are likely to lead to useful information for depicting the detail and colouring of their personality—the *personality type*. Painting the picture and defining the type are both necessary clinical exercises. Social relations are investigated. How do they relate to their family? Are they detached or overly dependent? What sort of friendships do they form with what sort of people, and are they close-knit or superficial with an exclusive few or an unlimited crowd? How do their interests and leisure activities involve them with others? Are they sociable or solitary? Are their relationships structured or informal? How do they relate to bosses, workmates and employees at work? Are they a leader or a follower, an organizer or a loner? Are they pliant or truculent, cooperative, sympathetic or clubbable? Their sexual preferences and relationships should be noted.

The nature of their *interests* and activities is informative. What do they like doing in their spare time? If they are interested in sport, it is useful to know if they can feel partisan and involved and also whether they are a participant or an observer. Enquiry is made of their preference and interests in films and literature: how they observe, criticize and enjoy the material. To what social organizations do they belong? Religion requires more than a single word designating religious affiliation in the case notes. The phenomenological method is equally relevant for this area of life. What is the individual's self-experience of their religious beliefs, and how do these interact with psychiatric symptomatology (Sims, 1994)?

An account of the patient's predominant *mood* is explored and whether his mood is fluctuating or stable, responsive to precipitants or endogenously determined. Character traits imply a detailed adjectival list, for example, irritable, reserved, fussy and so on. It will, of course, be helpful to corroborate their description with an account from another person. Enquiry is made about their attitudes and values; their views about themself and their body; how they regard others close to them; their more general social values in religion, morality, politics and economics; how they feel events occur and can be made to occur. Drive and energy and the way these are expressed in ambition,

lethargy, effectiveness and persistence are all important aspects of personality.

Study of their *fantasy life* is made: the frequency and duration of daydreams and their content; whether these are goal-directed and realistic or dissociated from any expectation of fulfilment. Dreams and other supposed signs of unconscious psychic activity are useful, especially when the subject attempts to interpret them. We may comment on their habits of ingestion, inhalation and excretion—whether they are regular and to what extent they depend on this regularity. Is there an indication that there should be a more detailed history and exploration of current habits of eating, smoking, drinking alcohol and taking other drugs? As the patient unfolds the facets of their personality, so the overall emphases that they put on areas of description become illuminating in understanding them as a whole person.

Differentiation of Personality Disorder

Allocating the patient to a personality type without taking into account the infinite variability of individuals is inadequate. However, certain characteristics tend to occur together and are of clinical significance. Allocation to a particular category of personality disorder is made on the relative predominance of these different character traits. Having decided that a certain definite trait or traits are present in this individual to an abnormal extent, does the abnormality of personality cause the person themself or other people to suffer? That is, is personality disorder present?

More than one abnormal type of personality may be present in any individual; they are not mutually exclusive. In formulating the psychiatric history and evaluation of mental state, comment on premorbid personality should always be made, even if it is only to state that due to the ravages of the mental illness, it is impossible to accurately assess premorbid state. The predominant traits should be described, preferably with verbatim comments of the patient to illustrate them. The interviewer should decide whether these traits are there to a significantly abnormal extent and, if so, whether this amounts to personality disorder. The type of disorder should be differentiated.

THE MENTAL STATE EXAMINATION

The mental state examination is the special area of expertise of psychiatrists. It is the psychiatrist's equivalent of the neurologic examination. The mental state examination is guided by the same principles and communication skills as any other clinical interview (Box 2.2). It is dependent on facility with language because that is the tool with which psychiatric practice is conducted. The clinician uses 'open' questions at the beginning of clinical enquiries and utilizes 'closed' questions to clarify specific points. There are specific techniques for signalling active listening. These include the use of *summary statements* to summarize what the clinician has made of what the patient is saying and to provide the opportunity for the patient to correct any misapprehension on the part of the clinician. Furthermore, *normalizing statements* can be used to introduce difficult subjects; for example, the clinician could introduce the issue of suicidal thoughts by saying, 'It is not uncommon for people who are depressed to find that they feel hopeless and that life is not worth living; have you felt like that?' Statements that comment on the emotional aspects of the patient's communication or behaviour, such as 'I can see that it must be very difficult for you to talk about these experiences', may help to deepen the rapport between clinician and patient. Further practical advice on conducting the psychiatric examination is found in Leff and Isaacs (1990).

As the interviewer asks each question, they should be thinking what the possible answers to that question could be from a *reasonable* person in *this* context. In everyday conversations, one is conditioned to avoid asking embarrassing questions and so, when someone makes an odd remark, the tendency is to fill in the meaning of the response to make it ordinary, sensible and avoid asking further questions in this area. This is exactly the opposite of phenomenological investigation in which the interviewer is looking for ways into the patient's private way of thinking. When the patient says something unreasonable, odd or unexpected, the interviewer must note it and, without intending to embarrass or disturb the patient's equanimity, clarify the inner experience already partly revealed. This will entail the use of the empathic method described in Chapter 1. One of the difficulties for the aspiring phenomenologist is

BOX 2.2 COMMUNICATION SKILLS TECHNIQUES

- Introductory statements and setting the context: 'My name is Dr Smith. I have a letter from your GP informing me that you have been feeling low for the past 6 weeks.', etc.
- Open questions: 'Can I start off by asking how you have been feeling lately?'
- Closed questions: 'I understand that you have been hearing voices for several weeks now. Are these voices there all the time?'
- Summary statements: 'From what you have been saying, I understand that you have been feeling low for the past 6 weeks and that this has been steadily getting worse to the degree that you are now tearful all the time for no good reason and that your sleep has also been badly affected.'
- Normalizing statements: 'It is not uncommon for people in your kind of situation to feel so low that life no longer seems worth living. Have you felt like that?'
- Reflective and empathic statements: 'As I understand it, when your husband lost his job, you had a lot of money worries. That must have been quite difficult for you, especially with the new baby.'
- Concluding statements: 'I now have a good grasp of how things have been for you in the past year. Are there things that you wanted to tell me that you have not yet had the opportunity to bring up?'

to know when to pursue what the patient reveals in more detail—that is, when to make the incision for the psychopathological operation. Clinical wisdom involves knowing when to do what.

Words limit as well as liberate. The clinical interviewer needs to be careful not to restrain their patient's answers by imposing the shackles of psychiatric technical jargon. Careful attention must be paid to the patient's use of language, and, as far as possible, the clinician should use language that mirrors the patient's language. It is important to be certain that both clinician and patient are using words in the same sense. The question 'Do you hear voices?' is a good example of this. The patient may truthfully answer 'No' and yet be suffering from almost continuous auditory hallucinations. Although patients and their doctors quite often describe auditory verbal hallucinations as 'voices', the patient may regard phonemes in quite other terms. They may make no distinction at all between these auditory perceptions, 'voices' they hear for which an outside observer realizes there is an appropriate stimulus and auditory hallucinations. They may be largely oblivious of the form of the communication as *auditory* and *hallucinatory* because they are totally absorbed with its *content* (an order telling them to go to Strasbourg and preach). Obviously, another patient may answer the question 'Do you hear voices?' truthfully in the affirmative and yet have a quite different form of phenomenological experience from auditory hallucination (see Chapter 7).

Almost every *technical term* in general medicine has diagnostic implications. This is also true in psychiatry. A symptom may not be pathognomonic of a certain condition but nevertheless is predominantly found with that illness. If the doctor uses the term *perseveration* in describing their patient's mental state to a colleague, they are, by inference, suggesting a diagnosis of an organic psychiatric state. If this is not the diagnosis, they have some difficult explaining to do to justify the use of that word. Is it really perseveration or just the repetitive use of words and phrases in a person who has intellectual disability and shows poverty of expression? To avoid misunderstanding, it is best to use longer descriptions until the interviewer is sure that the symptom is truly present.

Observation of the *appearance* and *behaviour* of the patient is an invaluable supplement to their self-description. The observations of others and at times other than the interview need to be taken into account. As the interview proceeds, the interviewer more definitely pursues their real intention of finding out the meaning behind the words the patient uses. What is the patient feeling and experiencing? Their own account may be a blind to prevent other people, or even themself, from seeing how bad they really feel. The *empathic method* is invaluable in working out what they are implying. So also is acute, insightful and trained observation. *Observation* may reveal white lines across the knuckles of an anxious person talking about what upsets them most and which render them impotently angry. Empathy allows the observer to employ their own capacity for emotion as a diagnostic and therapeutic tool. Training and experience are essential for knowing in which areas delving will be rewarded with useful information; how to ask questions that are comprehensible to patients of different verbal abilities and cultural backgrounds and that will result in appropriate answers; and how to avoid damaging the patient still further with well-directed but blunt questions that are likely to be perceived as brutal

and emotionally traumatizing. Observation and empathy must always be used together in eliciting the mental state. Note also the double meaning of the word *observant:* it means not only noticing what is going on around oneself but also conforming with the cultural mores of the immediate society. A good phenomenologist will be observant in both senses of the word.

Systematic Enquiry

The *appearance* and *behaviour* of the patient are observed for the clinical medical information they carry. Does the patient look ill? Are they alert, oriented, fully conscious, fluctuating in their mental state? Are there any behavioural or neurologic abnormalities? Observation is also useful for assessing nonverbal communication (Argyle, 1975). From their posture, gestures, facial expression and so on, they betray their state of emotion, providing information about their personality and their attitude to the observer and to others despite their silence or contradictory verbal communication. Obviously, observation of behaviour also indicates psychiatric symptomatology such as tics, catatonic movements, possible hallucinatory perception, and feeding and excreting disorders. Posture can be revealing to the acute observer, for instance, the *pharaonic posture* and the slow deliberate movements of head and neck of the patient with schizophrenia. If the patient is mute, the observed behaviour is the only source of clinical information, but the importance of observation needs to be stressed also for those patients who do speak. Observation may be valuable to corroborate the patient's complaints, to make clear the degree of emotional involvement they have in their symptoms or sometimes to contradict their statement, for example, the person who manifests physically extreme anxiety yet denies any worries on enquiry.

Talk reveals *thought.* Listening to and studying the patient's utterances is usually the most important part of assessing their mental state. Thought disorder and the interpretation of abnormalities in the use of words, syntax and association of ideas are discussed in more detail in Chapter 9. The flow of talk merits notice. Do they talk volubly and easily or in taciturn monosyllables? Do they just answer questions or speak spontaneously? Is their conversation appropriate to the social context, and is it coherent? Is the train of thought readily distracted? Throughout the interview, as much of the patient's speech as possible should be recorded verbatim. This provides a clearer picture of this individual person's inner milieu, and the data of self-experience will allow another person to evaluate the diagnosis.

As the interviewer enquires about and forms their own assessment of *mood,* they have three areas for exploration: *subjective* and *objective* description of mood and evaluation of *rapport.* There is much more to mood than just depression or elation; the finer nuances of this person's *subjective* emotional experience must be carefully dug out like truffles, using a sensitive nose and delicate extraction. A person anticipating an event may be acutely apprehensive, exquisitely excited but rather anxious, hopelessly resigned and so on; 'afraid of the future' is not an adequate description. Mood can be studied for its direction (depression or elation), its consistency (stable or labile), its appropriateness, its amplitude and the degree of discrepancy between subjective description and objective observation.

Of course, there is really no such thing as wholly objective assessment of mood. The doctor comments on the mood state of their patient from their observation of the patient's demeanour and the general tone of their conversation during the interview. They make the comment, 'The patient appears depressed; they are agitated and tense'. In fact, this comment on the patient's emotion abbreviates the empathic process through which they go to make this judgement. The doctor observes the patient and picks up available cues for mood, relating these to their experience with other patients and other people through their life and ultimately to their knowledge of their *own* affective state. Their assessment runs as follows: 'If I felt how my patient looks, speaks and acts, I would feel profoundly depressed and agitated; they are, on observation, depressed and agitated'.

Rapport is a useful measure of the patient's ability to communicate their feelings to another person. The interviewer needs to make themself into a yardstick, a *constant rapport maker,* against which the patient's ability to make rapport can be measured. To do this, the doctor requires clinical experience and an objectivity in which they know how they react to and communicate with many different sorts of people. They know themself and their own competence well enough to exclude this from the assessment of rapport so that, as far as possible, it is only the patient's capacity for emotional communication that is being tested.

The *ideas* and *beliefs* the patient holds and *abnormalities of perception* they experience are ascertained and explored during the interview. In ordinary conversation, there is a great deal of filling in or editing to eliminate the deficiencies of communication. A person talks and comes to a halt halfway through a sentence for the loss of a word. The other person provides the word and thus continues the conversation to both parties' satisfaction. This is the nature of discourse. There is a tendency for those coming new to dialogue with the mentally ill to bring into their conversation these social niceties that are used to save embarrassment. The doctor tends to note what they think the patient meant to say, as if the latter's thinking processes were similar to their own, rather than concentrating on what the patient actually said. A lot of significant psychopathology is thus missed. Delusions and hallucinations are rarely, if ever, volunteered by the patient as symptoms for the obvious reason that they are not experienced as different from the rest of the person's thinking or perceiving. To the patient, subjectively, a delusion is indistinguishable from any other idea they have, a hallucination is indistinguishable from any other normal perception. Skill in interviewing therefore comes very much in knowing when to look for a delusion and how to make a clear distinction between what the person describes as experience and what it reveals phenomenologically.

Passivity or delusions of control, *obsessions, compulsions* and *depersonalization* may be obvious or only made plain with some difficulty. It is important to try to categorize the type of experience as early in the course of exposure to professional enquiry as possible, because patients' explanations tend to become contaminated on repeated questioning. When passivity, for example, is suspected, it is generally best to follow up the clues right away and decide once and for all whether the symptom is present.

Assessment of the *cognitive state* includes, at least briefly, testing for orientation, attention, concentration and memory. The Mini-Mental State Examination (Folstein et al., 1975) is a widely used standardized bedside test of cognitive function that is useful to administer in the clinical setting.

The doctor, from specific questions and from the interview in general, needs to form an idea of the patient's attitude towards their illness, difficulties and prospects. To what extent does the patient have *insight* into their condition? Any illness of some severity will alter the patient's world and view of the world. Insight assesses the awareness of this change by the patient and the accurate labelling of this change as originating from a mental illness that requires treatment. Insight is therefore highly complex as a function. It is the ability of the individual to be self-aware and to be sensitive to inner subjective change. The capacity to correctly attribute the subjective psychological change to pathologic causes is evidence of intact self-awareness despite evidence of mental illness. It is potentially an extremely valuable part of the mental state examination, as it is associated with compliance with treatment and also with the likelihood of treatment under compulsion. In summary, insight has three components: recognition of subjective psychological change, the labelling of this change as pathologic in nature and recognition of need for treatment as well as compliance with treatment (David, 1990; see Chapter 11).

Many textbooks and numerous psychiatric institutions have their own scheme for psychiatric interviewing. This account is a general commentary rather than yet another scheme. See Box 2.1 earlier in the chapter for a memorandum of key areas to be covered in the history and examination of a psychiatric patient.

REFERENCES

Andrews, G., Issakidis, C., Carter, G., 2001. The shortfall in mental health service utilisation. Br. J. Psychiatry 179, 417–425.

Argyle, M., 1975. Bodily Communication. Methuen, London.

Carlat, D.J., 2005. The Psychiatric Interview, second ed. Lippincott Williams & Wilkins, Philadelphia.

David, A.S., 1990. Insight and psychosis. Br. J. Psychiatry 156, 789–808.

Folstein, M.F., Folstein, S.E., McHugh, P.R., 1975. 'Mini-mental state'. A practical method of grading the cognitive state of patients for the clinician. J. Psychiatr. Res. 12, 189–198.

Greenberg, M., Szmuckler, G., Tantam, D., 1986. Making Sense of Psychiatric Cases. Oxford University Press, Oxford.

Leff, J.P., Isaacs, A.D., 1990. Psychiatric Examination in Clinical Practice, third ed. Blackwell Scientific, Oxford.

MacKinnon, R.A., Michels, R., Buckley, P.J., 2006. The Psychiatric Interview in Clinical Practice. American Psychiatric Publishing, Arlington, VA.

Morrison, J., 2008. The First Interview, third ed. Guildford Press, London.

Rix, K.J.B., 1987. Handbook for Trainee Psychiatrists. Baillière Tindall, London.

Saddock, B.J., Saddock, V.L., Ruiz, P., 2009. Kaplan and Saddock's Comprehensive Textbook of Psychiatry, ninth ed. Lippincott Williams & Wilkins, Philadelphia.

Sims, A., 1994. Psyche' – spirit as well as mind? Br. J. Psychiatry 165, 441–446.

Sims, A., Curran, S., 2001. Examination of the psychiatric patient. In: Henn, F., Sartorius, N., Helmchen, H., Lauter, H. (Eds.), Contemporary Psychiatry. Springer, Berlin, pp. 479–496.

CONSCIOUSNESS AND COGNITION

Chapter 3

Consciousness and Disturbed Consciousness

Chapter Outline

KEYWORDS

Consciousness
Delirium
Stupor
Twilight state
Automatism

Summary

Consciousness is a defining characteristic of animals, although conscious self-awareness may be particular to human beings. Abnormalities of consciousness are problematic from a phenomenology point of view because, by definition, self-reports of pathologic states of consciousness, unlike self-reports of conscious experience, are not immune from error. The unconscious state is not privileged because the subject is unable to report on the nature and quality of the experience, even in situations when there is only minimal impairment of consciousness; self-reports are still open to qualification and query. Hence, the terminology is determined by the observation of either the quantitative degree of abnormality or the apparent qualitative changes in conscious state. The terminology is imprecise, and often several terms are used for identical or frankly indistinguishable states. In this chapter, terms such as *vigilance, lucidity, clouding of consciousness, delirium, stupor, coma* and some others are introduced and defined:

Psychiatry and neuropathology are not merely two closely related fields, they are but one field in which only one language is spoken and the same laws rule.

Wilhelm Griesinger (1868)

I have always been intrigued by the specific moment when, as we sit awaiting in the auditorium, the door to the stage opens and a performer steps into the light, or, to take the other perspective, the moment when a performer who waits in semidarkness sees the same door open, revealing the lights, the stage, and the audience ... as I reflect on what I have written, I sense that stepping into the light is also a powerful metaphor for consciousness, for the birth of the knowing mind, for the simple and momentous coming of the self into the world of the mental.

Antonio Damasio (1999)

Consciousness is one of the most challenging philosophic problems of our times. In this chapter, the focus is on the subjective state of awareness of the sensible world, which terminates when we go to sleep, are comatose or are dead. It is important to emphasize that the term *consciousness* does not refer merely to the distinction between being asleep or awake. To be awake presupposes being conscious. The focus is on the process of being *conscious of* something, rather than merely being awake. In other words, it is the process of being conscious of something in the sense that one is aware that they can see a particular object or hear a particular conversation.

At the outset, it is important to distinguish consciousness from attention. Attention refers to the capacity to focus our interest or consciousness on specific aspects of the objective world. This might entail selecting, shifting and thereby focusing attention, for example, on a passing vehicle rather than on a lamppost. No doubt both processes are related, but there is empirical work to show that both processes can operate independently of one another. The global workplace theory, an influential psychological model of consciousness, uses a theatre metaphor in which attention resembles choosing a television channel and consciousness is the picture on the screen (Baars and Franklin, 2007). The distinction that is being drawn here is that between selecting an experience and being conscious of the selected event. It is a truism that we are only conscious of a fraction of the information processing going on in our brain at any one time. The function of attention seems to be to select some aspects of stimulus input defined by location in space, a given feature such as shape or by an object. In contrast, the function of consciousness pertains to summarizing all the information from the environment that we need to ensure that it is available for planning,

decision-making, language, rational thought and setting long-term goals (Tononi and Koch, 2008). This is what Jaspers (1997) refers to as 'the immediate experience of the total psychic state'.

Any theory of consciousness must attempt to explain certain basic facts about mental life, namely, (1) that consciousness has a subjective nature that is united by a unique individual's inner perspective; (2) that conscious awareness appears to have a quality that is recalcitrant to physical or materialist description, that is, that it cannot simply be reduced to physic–chemical processes; and (3) that conscious experience is directed towards objects, that is, it is intentional in nature. It is the particularly striking inner subjective aspect of conscious awareness that is of prime concern to psychiatrists.

Consciousness has a pivotal role in Husserl's (1859–1938) phenomenology. As previously described, phenomenology is the study or description of phenomenon and involves the description of things as one experiences them. In other words, phenomenology is concerned with subjective conscious experience. It is therefore the case that one must first be conscious to be able to experience the world. So the logical starting place for the study of symptoms, from a subjective standpoint, is that feature of mental life—namely, consciousness—that allows subjective experiences to exist. Until quite recently, studies of consciousness were looked on with suspicion by neuroscientists, thereby leaving clinicians, both neurologists and psychiatrists, in intellectual darkness. This has been rectified in the past two decades by combining and sharing the perspectives of different disciplines: philosophy, psychology, medicine and neurosciences (Bock and Marsh, 1993).

Although it is essential for our clinical work concerning disturbances in consciousness that we use the principles of descriptive psychopathology and applied phenomenology, we need to be aware of the limitations (Dennett, 1991). Dennett has pointed out that from Descartes via Locke, Berkeley and Hume, phenomenology has tended to describe consciousness from the first-person plural: 'according to longstanding philosophic tradition we all agree on what we find when we "look inside" at our own phenomenology'. We may not all be the same inside, and even if we are, we may get it wrong when we try to describe our inner experiences. He also questions the purely third-person perspective of behavioural psychology and advocates the 'Method of Heterophenomenology'. This depends, for its authenticity, on the meticulous precision of the questions asked, the objectivity of recording the transcript (three stenographers preparing separate documents from an audiotaped interview), adopting the 'intentional stance' (assuming that the subject of investigation was intending to make a statement about something) and scope for clarification. When this process has been followed, the text 'is taken to be *the* sincere, reliable expression and to be a *single, unified subject* of that very subject's beliefs and opinions'. It becomes clear that this process is similar, although more highly structured for research purposes, to the separate steps in the *method of empathy* as described in Chapter 1.

There is a further problem for phenomenological analysis as it concerns psychopathology, precisely in that it requires a description of subjective experience. However, abnormalities of consciousness, as usually construed in psychopathology, concern experiences that are characterized by demonstrable impairments of the capacity to accurately report subjective experiences.

Karl Jaspers (1883–1969) recognized this problem but was also additionally aware of another issue, namely, that in Husserl's phenomenology there is an inseparability of acts of consciousness such as attention, perception and so on and the actual objects of consciousness. Jaspers gave an account that treated consciousness as distinct from acts of consciousness. He identified three aspects of consciousness, namely (1) actual inner awareness, (2) a subject–object dichotomy and (3) knowledge of a conscious self. In this account, Jaspers used the metaphor of a stage, very reminiscent of the metaphor of a theatre that has currency today and that of a medium. These metaphors allowed Jaspers to refer to the idea that 'the stage can shrink (narrowing of consciousness) or the medium can grow dense (clouding of consciousness)' (Jaspers, 1997). For Jaspers, loss of actual inner awareness is synonymous with loss of consciousness. In Jaspers' conception, attention is conceived as either an active or passive turning towards an object, and the degree of clarity and distinctness of the content of consciousness is referred

to as the field of attention. Finally, Jaspers (1997) also commented on the role of attention for 'rousing further associations ... guiding notions, set tasks, target ideas' and so on.

In summary, consciousness is pivotal in Husserl's phenomenology, hence it is equally important in clinical psychopathology. Abnormalities of consciousness are problematic insofar as the terminology is appallingly confused. In this and subsequent chapters, I attempt to clarify the words used, sometimes at the expense of sacrificing altogether terms with a long history and sometimes lumping as a single concept words between which there are only minute differences of meaning. One major problem is that different disciplines and medical specialties use different terms to cover partly overlapping concepts and meanings. I propose to deal with abnormalities of consciousness under the following major headings: (1) dimensional changes in levels of consciousness and (2) qualitative changes of consciousness.

Disorders of Consciousness

It has proved complicated to describe exactly what is disordered in pathologic states of consciousness, hence this rather convoluted definition of a disturbed state of consciousness (DSC) by Aggernaes (1975):

A state in a person in which he has no experiences at all, or in which all of his experiences are deviant, concerning other or more qualities than tempo and mood colouring, from those he would have under similar stimulus conditions in his habitual waking state. The state is a DSC only if the individual cannot return to, and remain in, his habitual state by deciding to do so himself, and if others bring about a lasting return to his habitual state by the application of a simple social procedure.

DIMENSIONAL CHANGES IN LEVELS OF CONSCIOUSNESS

Impairment of consciousness can be seen as a continuum from alertness through to drowsiness and ultimately coma and death. In that sense, consciousness may be regarded as lying on a quantitative dimension (Fig. 3.1). Lishman (1998) makes the point that 'considerable difficulties can surround the conceptual levels of consciousness of patients with acute organic reactions, partly because of problems inherent in the use of certain terms and partly because of the expectation that impaired consciousness must necessarily be accompanied by decreased responsiveness to stimuli … In most conditions impairment of consciousness is accompanied by diminished arousal and alertness'.

Unconsciousness

Unconscious, according to Jaspers (1997), 'means something that is not an inner existence and does not occur as an experience; secondly, something that is

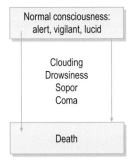

Fig. 3.1 Levels or stages of diminished consciousness.

not thought of as an object and has gone unregarded; thirdly, it is something which has not reached any knowledge of itself'.

In clinical practice, the term *unconscious* is used in three quite different ways that have in common only the phenomenological element in that there is *no* subjective experience (Fig. 3.2):

- A person suffering from serious brain disease may be unconscious; consciousness in this instance is seen as being on a continuum, with a normal state of consciousness at one end and death at the other.
- Someone who is asleep is unconscious; again, there is a continuum from full wakefulness to deep sleep.
- An alert and healthy person is aware of only certain parts of their environment both externally and internally; of the rest, they are unconscious. There is also a continuum here from full vigilance directed towards the immediate object of awareness to total unawareness.

The organic state of the brain as, for instance, demonstrated by the electroencephalogram is utterly different in these three situations.

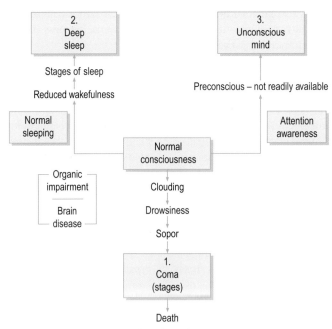

Fig. 3.2 Three dimensions of unconsciousness.

The third meaning of unconsciousness implies that certain mental processes cannot be observed by introspection alone, even when the brain is normal and healthy. Among such processes for which there is good evidence of their existence, frequency and complexity, there are some that have been, or may yet become, conscious. This is what Freud called the *preconscious* (Frith, 1979). Whereas there is a strict limit to the number of items available in the conscious state and that are therefore capable of being memorized (approximately seven, for example, a number with seven digits), there is much more information stored at the preconscious level. If a stimulus is ambiguous, only one interpretation is possible in consciousness at any one time; however, multiple meanings are available preconsciously. It is difficult to carry out more than one task at a time consciously, but undertaking parallel tasks is usual at a preconscious level. Preconscious processes are automatic, whereas conscious ones are flexible and strategic. This function of the preconscious was well known long before Freud, for example, Brodie (1854):

But it seems to me that on some occasions a still more remarkable process takes place in the mind, which is even more independent of volition than that of which we are speaking; as if there were in the mind a principle of order which operates without our being at the time conscious of it. It has often happened to me to have been occupied by a particular subject of inquiry; to have accumulated a store of facts connected with it; but to have been able to proceed no further. Then, after an interval of time, without any addition to my stock of knowledge, I have found the obscurity and confusion, in which the subject was originally enveloped, to have cleared away; the facts have all seemed to have settled themselves in their right places, and their mutual relations to have become apparent, although I have not been sensible of having made any distinct effort for that purpose.

Unconscious in the preceding sense is a theory that psychiatrists and psychopathologists have to explain some aspects of observable behaviour, whereas in the other two senses of the term *unconscious*, it is the fact that the individual is unconscious to the world—that

is, they are unrousable and unable to participate with this awareness of the sensory world intact—that is at stake.

The three dimensions of consciousness (contrasted with unconsciousness, as in Fig. 3.1) are vigilance, lucidity and self-consciousness.

Abnormalities of Vigilance

Vigilance is taken to mean the faculty of deliberately remaining alert when otherwise one might be drowsy or asleep. This is not a uniform or unvarying state but fluctuates. Factors inside the individual that promote or adversely influence vigilance are interest, anxiety, extreme fear or enjoyment, whereas boredom encourages drowsiness. The situation in the environment and the way the individual perceives that situation also affect one's position on the vigilance–drowsiness axis. Some abnormal states of health increase vigilance, whereas many diminish it.

In addition to the contrast between vigilance and drowsiness, there are qualitative differences in the nature of wakefulness. The vigilant state of mind of a person scanning a radar screen for a possible enemy interceptor is very different from the rapt attention of a music lover listening to a symphony. These aspects of attention and their abnormalities are discussed in Chapter 4.

Drowsiness is a persistent state and is the next level of progressive impairment of consciousness. The patient is 'awake' but will drift into 'sleep' if left without sensory stimulation. They are slow in actions, slurred in speech, sluggish in intention and sleepy on subjective description. There is an attempt at avoidance of painful stimuli. Reflexes, including coughing and swallowing, are present but reduced; muscle tone is also diminished.

In psychiatric practice, this is commonly seen after overdosage with drugs that have a central nervous system depressant effect (for example, tricyclic antidepressants). From the psychiatrist's point of view, it means, of course, that interviewing the patient is impossible. These levels of diminished consciousness are quite nonspecific and occur whatever the nature of the cause: head injury, tumour, epilepsy, infection, cerebrovascular disorder, metabolic disorder or toxic state.

In coma, the patient is unconscious, whereas the drowsy patient is conscious but lapsing at times into unconsciousness. In lighter states with strong stimuli, they may be momentarily rousable. There are no verbal responses or responses to painful stimuli. The righting response of posture has been lost; reflexes and muscle tone are present but greatly reduced; breathing is slow, deep and rhythmic; the face and skin may be flushed.

In later stages, the patient is no longer rousable; they are deeply unconscious. Distinct stages of coma have identifiable physical signs ultimately culminating in brain death, but these are not discussed further in this book—they are beyond psychiatry (Conference of Medical Royal Colleges and Their Faculties, 1976). Practical assessment of the depth and duration of impaired consciousness and coma has been quantified on the scale devised by Teasdale and Jennett (1974).

Abnormalities of Lucidity

Consciousness is inseparable from the object of conscious attention: lucidity can be demonstrated only in clarity of thought on a particular topic. The *sensorium*, the total awareness of all internal and external sensations presenting themselves to the organism at any particular moment, may be clear or clouded. Obviously, lucidity is not unrelated to vigilance: unless the person is fully awake, they cannot be clear in consciousness.

Clouding of consciousness denotes the lesser stages of impairment of consciousness on a continuum from full alertness and awareness to coma (Lishman, 1998). The patient may be drowsy or agitated and is likely to show memory disturbance and disorientation. In clouding, most intellectual functions are impaired, including attention and concentration, comprehension and recognition, understanding, forming associations, logical judgement, communication by speech and purposeful action. This represents the lesser stages of impairment of consciousness with deterioration in thinking, attention, perception and memory and, usually, drowsiness and reduced awareness of the environment. There are important differences between the reduced wakefulness before falling asleep and clouding in an organic state (Lipowski, 1967). Although the patient's awareness is *clouded,* they may be agitated and excitable rather than drowsy.

Clouding may be seen in a wide variety of acute organic conditions, including drug and alcohol intoxication, head injury, meningeal irritation caused by infection and so on. *Drowsiness* as a descriptive term simply means diminished alertness and attention that is not under the patient's control.

The term *clouding* should be used for the psychopathological state: impairment of consciousness, slight drowsiness with or without agitation and difficulty with attention and concentration. This will usually occur with organic impairment of function, for instance, with cerebral tumour, after head injury or with raised intracranial pressure. If it occurs in schizophrenia, it is as a part of the cognitive deficit that has been shown sometimes to occur in this disease (Frith, 1979). It is suggested that in this condition there is an awareness of automatic processes that normally occur below the level of consciousness. These processes are concerned with the selection of appropriate interpretation of stimuli and of response.

Heightened lucidity is the opposite of clouding of consciousness described earlier. Even though most abnormal states of consciousness show a lowering or diminution of consciousness but *heightened* lucidity of consciousness occurs in which there is a subjective sense of richer perception: colours seem brighter and so on; there are changes in mood, usually exhilaration, perhaps amounting to ecstasy; there is *subjective* experience of increased alertness and a greater capacity for intellectual activity, memory and understanding. Such states of heightening of consciousness may occur in normal, healthy people, especially in adolescence or at times of emotional, social or religious crisis: when falling in love, on winning a large sum of money, at sudden religious conversion and so on. Heightened lucidity is not uncommon with certain drugs, notably with the hallucinogens (e.g., lysergic acid diethylamide) and central nervous system stimulants (e.g., amphetamine). A similar state of awareness may occur occasionally in early psychotic illness, especially mania or, less often, in schizophrenia.

Abnormalities of Consciousness of Self

Alongside full wakefulness and clear awareness is an ability to experience self, and an awareness of self, that is both immediate and complex. This is considered in more detail in Chapter 12.

QUALITATIVE CHANGES OF CONSCIOUSNESS

Various other organic disturbances in brain function are recognized. These are virtually always associated with some degree of quantitative impairment. The use of terminology in this whole area of discourse is, unfortunately, muddled, with the same term sometimes having different meanings and similar phenomena being described by different words.

Delirium

Lipowski (1990) defines delirium as 'a transient organic mental syndrome of acute onset, characterized by global impairment of cognitive functions, a reduced level of consciousness, attentional abnormalities, increased or decreased psychomotor activity and a disordered sleep–wake cycle'. The *Diagnostic and Statistical Manual of Mental Disorders*, 5th edition (*DSM-5*), defines delirium as a condition in which there is a disturbance in attention that develops over a short period of time and that may include other disturbances in cognition, including in memory, orientation, language and spatial ability or perception. In addition, these disturbances are not the result of a pre-existing neurocognitive disorder, and investigation reveals that the disturbance is a direct result of physiologic consequences of another medical condition (American Psychiatric Association, 2013). It is important to conceptually distinguish between the term *delirium* in the sense of a subjective experience of a qualitatively altered state of consciousness as against the term when it refers to a nosologic entity as described in the *DSM-5*. This chapter's focus is on the subjective experience of the altered state of consciousness denoted by the term *delirium*. A detailed account of delirium as a condition is outside the scope of this book but can be found in Maldonado (2015).

Subjective accounts of delirium are rare, and the few published descriptions are open to criticism given the established fact that consciousness is impaired in delirium and the descriptions have had to be constructed with hindsight. Nonetheless, Crammer's (2002) account confirmed partial states of arousal during which some memory functions and belief

formation can be present, despite apparent unconsciousness. He wrote:

During the period 26–30 November I was, for the most part, completely unconscious, unaware of the passage of time, the presence of visitors, the attention of nurses and doctors or my transfer by trolley or ambulance from ward to ward and hospital to hospital. However, within that period there were several brief fluctuations (perhaps 5 min or so) in degree of awareness, and subsequently I could recall having some human contact and some idea (partly mistaken) about my whereabouts and state of health in these episodes. In the first two episodes I accepted that I was ill in some quite unspecified way and thought that I was to be transferred for operation (unspecified) first to India and then to Australia; in the fourth episode, although much the same in feeling, I thought that I was changing planes on the flight home from Australia.

Crammer describes his subjective experiences and also attempts to explain them in retrospect:

I come half-awake lying on a vague bed in a very vague room with two young women (in white coats?) standing by my side. I identify them as physiotherapists. One is dark-haired (Indian?) and says nothing; the other is fair, does the talking and laughingly tells me that I need an operation and it will be best for me to transfer to India for it, perhaps to a Christian Mission hospital, possibly called Vellore, with which they have a staff exchange programme (clearly the dark-haired girl). I receive this information passively without curiosity: I do not know or care where I am, or what is wrong with me, although I am prepared to believe I have something requiring treatment and am reassured that it will be well done. I fail to be myself, not very aware of surroundings and with no recollection of any injury or hospitalization.

He continued, 'the idea of India may have been prompted by the (Indian?) nurse and perhaps by an unconscious memory of a fall in India 3 years earlier' and the idea of Australia by the fact that 'on admission to hospital I had been struck by the Australian accents of some of the nurses (and I had read previously in the local paper that Oxford hospitals had imported numbers of Australians to help), although all this was out of the conscious mind. Perhaps an Australian nurse helped me into the ambulance'.

Crammer attempts to make sense of his experience in retrospect. He is fully aware of the vagaries of memory and the likelihood of bias, but nonetheless his explanations demand our attention:

The impairment of understanding – disorientation, misidentification of others, development of false beliefs – which is the central disturbance in the confusional state, developed slowly as consciousness declined and was based in memory failure and inattention. I believed that I was living in Australia, presumably because of an overheard voice, and thereafter held to this belief and denied that I could be or ever had been in the John Radcliffe Hospital (in reality, previously I had been both an out-patient and an in-patient). I thought that I had been at a doctor's social and checking-in for a flight home. A woman in a white coat was a physiotherapist, not a doctor; the doctor who later inspected my monitors was a flight engineer and the nurse was a check-in girl … These are not absurd answers to the self-posed questions (who, where, what is this?) but near-misses based on brief, limited sensory impression with limited associative memory, a sort of guess without any uncertainty or any correction in relation to previous experience or immediately subsequent events, processes that go on all the time in normal life.

In his comments on Crammer's account, Fleminger (2002) drew attention to the fact that the experience of delirium is akin to dreaming but that delirium is remembered with greater vividness than dreams. Also, that whereas it is traditional to conceive of delirium as being a disturbance of consciousness, it might be more profitable to think of it as a disturbance of the sleep–wake cycle. This is why the experience of delirium is akin to dreaming and why there is evidence that delirium is more likely in individuals with sleep deprivation.

David Aaronovitch (2011) wrote another account of delirium in an intensive care ward setting. Although his account is similar to that of Crammer, there was a more obvious narrative structure to the account. This may, of course, be because Aaronovitch is a journalist and his account necessarily had this structure. Or it could be that even though delirium is experienced as isolated events occurring in the ward at the time of the experience, the tendency to structure experiences into a whole is retained and that this is what gives accounts of delirium their narrative quality. He wrote:

Every time I closed my eyes, the inside of my eyelids would display a kaleidoscope of red, black and yellow violent cartoon images. So for four days and nights I didn't sleep and much of that time didn't know if it was day or night. After a while I noticed the clock on the wall of the room opposite, so now I could see the time, but I didn't know which 12-hour cycle I was in – whether it was 7 am or 7 pm, lunchtime or four hours before dawn. All I did know was that the nurses came and went in shifts, handing over to each other every 12 hours in a rather cacophonous atmosphere of greetings, innuendo and consultations over the patients' notes, and that this handover was going on up and down the passageway.

In this passage, it is clear that Aaronovitch's time sense was compromised and that sleep disturbance was a characteristic aspect of his experience. In other parts of his account, he described heightened acuity of hearing, persecutory beliefs including that a cup of coffee was injected through a large syringe into his drip line and he had grandiose beliefs: 'I told her of my plan to sue the hospital and everyone associated with it. I'd get £1 million, I told her. Hadn't they nearly killed a leading journalist on one of Britain's top newspapers? We'd also reach a settlement in which the millionaire consultants were forced to give me their 2012 Olympic tickets'.

Both Aaronovitch's and Crammer's accounts point to the extreme vividness of the experience and the difficulty in distinguishing reality from an experience within an altered state of consciousness, namely delirium.

Fluctuation of Consciousness

Fluctuations in consciousness levels are seen in various conditions. It occurs in health, in sleep and in fatigue. In patients with epilepsy, there is fluctuation in relation to fits, and it may occur before, during or after the seizures. Alterations of consciousness level are described with third-ventricle tumours associated with variations in intracranial pressure (Sim, 1974). In delirious states, there may be considerable diurnal fluctuation of consciousness. Characteristically, the patient becomes more disorientated, disturbed in mood and distracted perceptually with illusions and hallucinations in the late evening and shows greatest lucidity mid-morning. Such variation of consciousness level is also described and observed with drugs, such as mescaline, in which there may also be fluctuations of time sense.

Confusion

The concept of *confusion* was originally developed in France (*confusion mentale*) and later in Germany (*Verwirrtheit*) in the 19th century (Berrios, 1981). It is a term, imprecisely defined, referring to subjective symptoms and objective signs indicating loss of capacity for clear and coherent thought. It is purely a descriptive word and does not only apply to clouding of consciousness. When physicians, psychiatrists and nurses were asked what *confusion* meant, marked discordance was found. The term should be used only if clearly defined (Simpson, 1984). It occurs with impairment of consciousness in acute organic states and with disruption of thought processes due to brain damage in chronic organic states, but it is also seen in nonorganic disturbance. Thus confusion of thinking may occur as part of the picture in functional psychoses and in association with powerful emotion in neurotic disorders. It should therefore be used simply to describe these disturbances of thought and not as a term pathognomonic of organic psychosyndromes.

To simplify, therefore *confusion* of thinking can be described as occurring either when the individual describes their own thinking as being confused or when the external observer considers that the thought processes are disturbed and confused. Phenomenologically, therefore, it is simply a description of the patient's self-experience or the doctor's observation.

OTHER TERMS

Twilight State

A twilight state is a well-defined interruption of the continuity of consciousness (Sims et al., 2000). It is usually an organic condition and occurs in the context of epilepsy, alcoholism (*mania à potu*), brain trauma and general paresis; it may also occur with dissociative states. It is characterized by (1) abrupt onset and end; (2) variable duration, from a few hours to several weeks; and (3) the occurrence of unexpected violent acts or emotional outbursts during otherwise normal, quiet behaviour (Lishman, 1998). If the term is reserved for these three features in combination, as a psychopathological entity, then it should be used whenever they concur, irrespective of cause.

The forensic implications of this condition are therefore important, and it has been used as a legal defence for violent behaviour for which the person had subsequent amnesia.

Consciousness may be markedly impaired or relatively normal between episodes. There may be associated dream-like states, delusions or hallucinations. It is sometimes associated with the temporal lobe seizures of epilepsy; it may occur with other organic states without epilepsy; similar behaviour may occur in apparent hysterical dissociation; and it is also described as an acute reaction to massive catastrophe. In the forensic context, it is important to demonstrate (1) the occurrence of similar episodes with inexplicable behaviour before the key happening and (2) other objective evidence of physical or mental illness. The *Ganser state* (described with memory disorders in Chapter 5) is, in practice, a sort of twilight state in which the organic element is often dubious.

Mania à Potu (Pathologic Intoxication)

This is one type of twilight state specifically associated with alcoholism. It is important to distinguish this syndrome of acute pathologic intoxication with alcohol from delirium tremens, which is a symptom of *withdrawal*. Keller (1977) has defined *mania à potu* as:

an extraordinarily severe response to alcohol, especially to small amounts, marked by apparently senseless violent behaviour, usually followed by exhaustion, sleep and amnesia for the episode. Intoxication is apparently not always involved and for this reason pathological reaction to alcohol is the preferred term. The reaction is thought to be associated with exhaustion, great strain or hypoglycaemia, and to occur especially in people poorly defended against their own violent impulses.

Coid (1979) describes four components:
1. the condition follows the consumption of a variable quantity of alcohol;
2. senseless, violent behaviour then ensues;
3. there is then prolonged sleep; and
4. total or partial amnesia for the disturbed behaviour occurs.

Because there is often doubt as to whether intoxication really followed the consumption of an inappropriately small amount of alcohol and because several of the other causal factors are diagnostic categories in their own right (hypoglycaemia, epilepsy), Coid would do away with the diagnostic category of *pathologic* intoxication in the preceding definition, leaving only acute drunkenness or another condition associated with alcohol intake.

Automatism

Automatism implies action taking place in the absence of consciousness. It has been defined by Fenwick (1990) as follows:

An automatism is an involuntary piece of behaviour over which an individual has no control. The behaviour itself is usually inappropriate to the circumstances, and may be out of character for the individual. It can be complex, co-ordinated, and apparently purposeful and directed, though lacking in judgement. Afterwards, the individual may have no recollection, or only partial and confused memory, of his actions.

Epileptic automatism may be defined as a state of clouding of consciousness that occurs during or immediately after a seizure and during which the individual retains control of posture and muscle tone and performs simple or complex movements and actions without being aware of what is happening (Fenton, 1975). It occurs as part of the clinical presentation of psychomotor epilepsy, most often arising from discharge in the temporal lobes. It was particularly common in those patients with chronic epilepsy who were resident in an epilepsy colony or a mental hospital.

An *aura* may be the first sign of an epileptic attack with temporal lobe automatism and may be manifested as abdominal sensations; feelings of confusion with thinking; sensations elsewhere in the body, especially the head; hallucinations or illusions (especially olfactory or gustatory); and motor abnormalities such as tonic contracture, masticatory movement, salivation or swallowing.

Behaviour during automatism is usually purposeful and often appropriate, for instance, continuing to dry the dishes. Awareness of the environment is impaired; the patient appears to be only partly aware of being spoken to and does not reply appropriately. Initially, activity is diminished, with staring eyes and slumped posture; it then becomes stereotyped, with repetitive movements, lip smacking, fumbling and other actions. Finally, more complex purposeful behaviour occurs, such as walking about, making irrelevant utterances, removing clothing and so on. Sometimes, the patient may continue during automatism with whatever they were doing before—for example, driving their car—although there is subsequent amnesia, and the behaviour or speech at the time never appears entirely normal.

Violence is rare during automatism, and when it occurs, it usually amounts to resisting restraint. However, automatism is, rarely, cited as an explanation for a person's violent and criminal action of which they are unaware afterwards. The legal definition then becomes 'The state of a person who though capable of action, is not conscious of what he is doing … it means unconscious, involuntary action and it is a defence because the mind does not go with what is being done' (Viscount Kilmuir, 1963). Clearly, when such violent behaviour occurs, automatism fulfils the criteria for the definition of *twilight state* as defined earlier.

Speech automatism occurs when there is utterance of identifiable words or phrases at some stage during the epileptic attack of which the patient has no memory later. Phenomenologically, then, automatism is action without any knowledge of acting, and it is the latter claim that requires careful investigation.

Dream-like (Oneiroid) State

This is an unsatisfactory term not clearly differentiated from twilight state or delirium. The patient is disorientated and confused and experiences elaborate hallucinations, usually visual. There is impairment of consciousness and marked emotional change, which may be terror or enjoyment of the hallucinatory experiences; there may also be auditory or tactile hallucinations. The patient may appear to be living in a dream world, and *occupational delirium* could be mentioned in this context, for instance, the ship's petty officer admitted to hospital after a head injury at sea (associated with excess alcohol intake), who kept shouting, 'Man the boats.'

It is important to look for other symptoms or organic states to make the important distinction between physical illness and a dissociative nonorganic condition.

Stupor

'Stupor names a symptom complex whose central feature is a reduction in, or absence of, *relational* functions: that is, action and speech' (Berrios, 1996). It is distinct from coma and does not lie on a continuum from wakefulness to coma. This term should be reserved for the syndrome in which mutism and akinesis occur; that is, the inability to initiate speech or action in a patient who appears awake and even alert. It usually occurs with some degree of clouding of consciousness but does not refer solely to a diminished level. The patient may look ahead or their eyes may wander, but they appear to take nothing in.

This syndrome is characteristic of lesions in the area of the diencephalon and upper brainstem and also the frontal lobe and basal ganglia, and the term *akinetic mutism* has sometimes been reserved by neurologists to describe a much more narrowly defined organic syndrome. A rare but specific condition involving the motor pathways in the ventral pons is called the *locked-in syndrome* in which there is quadriplegia and anarthria with preserved consciousness and vertical eye movement (Plum and Posner, 1972; Smith and Delargy, 2005). It is important to realize, however, that the symptoms of akinesis and mutism in a conscious patient also occur with schizophrenia, with affective psychoses (both depressive and manic) and in dissociative states.

The difference between psychogenic (so-called functional) and neurologic (organic) causes of stupor can be clinically extremely perplexing. Psychiatric definitions have demanded that the condition occurs when there is 'a complete absence, in clear consciousness, of any voluntary movements' (Wing et al., 1974). Of course, it is not possible at the time of observation to know whether consciousness is quite clear or not, and even for functional stupors, subsequent amnesia is common. A phenomenological definition of stupor must therefore exclude the state of consciousness of a mute patient, and diagnosis of stupor must then be followed by investigation of the differential diagnosis, which includes both organic and nonorganic conditions.

Sleep Disorders

These are discussed in Chapter 4.

REFERENCES

Aaronovitch, D., 2011. ICU psychosis—my nightmare in hospital. The Times. 12 November 2011.

Aggernaes, A., 1975. The concepts: disturbed state of consciousness and psychosis. Acta Psychiatr. Scand. 51, 119–133.

American Psychiatric Association, 2013. Diagnostic and Statistical Manual of Mental Disorders, fifth ed. American Psychiatric Publishing, Washington, DC.

Baars, B.J., Franklin, S., 2007. An architectural model of conscious and unconscious brain functions: global workspace theory and IDA. Neural Netw 20, 955–961.

Berrios, G.E., 1981. Delirium and confusion in the 19th century: a conceptual history. Br. J. Psychiatry. 139, 439–449.

Berrios, G.E., 1996. The History of Mental Symptoms: Descriptive Psychopathology since the Nineteenth Century. Cambridge University Press, Cambridge.

Bock, G.R., Marsh, J., 1993. Experimental and Theoretical Studies of Consciousness. John Wiley, Chichester.

Brodie, B.C., 1854. Psychological inquiries. In: A Series of Essays. Longman, Brown, Green & Longman, London.

Coid, J., 1979. Mania à potu: a critical review of pathological intoxication. Psychol. Med. 9, 709–719.

Conference of Medical Royal Colleges and Their Faculties, 1976. Diagnosis of brain death. Br. Med. J. 2, 1187–1188.

Crammer, J.L., 2002. Subjective experience of a confusional state. Br. J. Psychiatry. 180, 71–75.

Damasio, A., 1999. The Feeling of what Happens: Body and Emotion in the Making of Consciousness. William Heinemann, London.

Dennett, D., 1991. Consciousness Explained. Allen Lane, London.

Fenton, G.W., 1975. Epilepsy and automatism. In: Silverstone, T., Barraclough, B. (Eds.), Contemporary Psychiatry. Headley Brothers, Ashford, pp. 429–439.

Fenwick, P., 1990. Automatism. In: Bluglass, R., Bowden, P. (Eds.), Principles and Practice of Forensic Psychiatry. Churchill Livingstone, Edinburgh.

Fleminger, S., 2002. Remembering delirium. Br. J. Psychiatry. 180, 4–5.

Frith, C.D., 1979. Consciousness, information processing and schizophrenia. Br. J. Psychiatry. 134, 225–235.

Griesinger, W., 1868, 1941. Quoted in Zilboorg, G. In: Henry, G.W. (Ed.), A History of Medical Psychology. W.W. Norton, New York.

Jaspers, K., 1997. In: Hoenig, J., Hamilton, M.W., Trans (Eds.), General Psychopathology. The Johns Hopkins University Press, Baltimore.

Keller, M., 1977. A lexicon of disablements related to alcohol consumption. Edwards, G., Gross, M.M., Keller, M., Moser, J., Room, R., (Eds). In: Alcohol Related Disabilities. World Health Organization, Geneva.

Kilmuir, V., 1963. Bratty v Attorney General for Northern Ireland AC 386, 1961. 3WLR965; (1961) 3 All ER 523.

Lipowski, Z.J., 1967. Delirium, clouding of consciousness and confusion. J. Nerv. Ment. Dis. 145, 227–255.

Lipowski, Z.J., 1990. Delirium: Acute Confusional States. Oxford University Press, Oxford.

Lishman, W.A., 1998. Organic Psychiatry: The Psychological Consequences of Cerebral Disorder, third ed. Blackwell Scientific, Oxford.

Maldonado, J.R., 2015. Delirium – neurobiology, characteristics, and management. In: Fogel, B.S., Greenberg, D.B. (Eds.), Psychiatric Care of the Medical Patient, third ed. Oxford University Press, Oxford.

Plum, F., Posner, J.B., 1972. Diagnosis of Stupor and Coma, second ed. F.A. Davis, Philadelphia.

Sim, M., 1974. Guide to Psychiatry. Churchill Livingstone, Edinburgh.

Simpson, C.J., 1984. Doctors and nurses use of the word confused. Br. J. Psychiatry. 145, 441–443.

Sims, A., Mundt, C., Berner, P., Barocka, A., 2000. Descriptive phenomenology. In: Gelder, M.G., López-Ibor, J.J., Andreasen, N.

(Eds.), New Oxford Textbook of Psychiatry. Oxford University Press, Oxford.

Smith, E., Delargy, M., 2005. Locked-in syndrome. Br. Med. J. 330, 406–409.

Teasdale, G., Jennett, B., 1974. Assessment of coma and impaired consciousness: a practical scale. Lancet 2, 81–84.

Tononi, G., Koch, C., 2008. The neural correlates of consciousness: an update. Ann. N. Y. Acad. Sci. 1124, 239–261.

Wing, J.K., Cooper, J.E., Sartorius, N., 1974. The Measurement and Classification of Psychiatric Symptoms. Cambridge University Press, Cambridge.

Chapter 4

Attention, Concentration, Orientation and Sleep

KEYWORDS

Attention
Concentration
Sleep
Hypersomnia
Parasomnia
Hypnosis

Summary

Consciousness, attention, concentration and sleep are all interrelated phenomena. In the previous chapter, consciousness and its abnormalities were described. Attention is often likened to a beam of light that focuses on a limited area of interest within a general field, but it is best to conceive of it as a limited-capacity channel that is dynamic in the selection and inhibition of information for further processing (Broadbent, 1958; Smith and Kosslyn, 2007). It is important for an organism's ability to engage with aspects of its environment. It is required for orientating the organism within its environment. Abnormalities of impairment therefore underlie such disparate phenomena as disorientation and impairment of new learning. The sleep–wake cycle is a physiologic mechanism that determines the alteration from wakefulness, that is, consciousness and the special temporary state of unconsciousness that is manifest as sleep. Abnormalities of this cycle including disturbances of amount, quality and so forth are described in this chapter.

Come, Sleep! O Sleep, the certain knot of peace
The baiting–place of wit, the balm of woe,
The poor man's wealth, the prisoner's release,
Th' indifferent judge between the high and low.
     Sir Philip Sidney (1554–86), Astrophel and Stella,
               sonnet 39

The terms *attention*, *concentration* and *orientation* have often been used very loosely. It is suggested that their use is restricted to the following. *Attention* is the active or passive focusing of consciousness on an experience such as sensory inputs, motor programmes, memories or internal representations. It can be defined as the process that enhances some information and inhibits others, thereby allowing us to select some information for further processing (Smith and Kosslyn, 2007). The concept overlaps with the terms *alertness*, *awareness* and *responsiveness*. *Voluntary* attention occurs when the subject deliberately focuses his attention on an internal or external event; *involuntary* attention occurs when the event attracts the subject's attention without his conscious effort. *Concentration* is only one aspect of attention. It involves focused or selective attention. Other aspects of attention include sustained attention, or *vigilance,* divided attention and alternating attention. *Orientation* is an awareness of one's setting in time and place and of the realities of one's person and situation. It is not a discrete function but is closely bound up with memory and the clarity or coherence of thought.

This chapter is concerned with cognitive function, but it is not limited to the functions that are disturbed by organic lesions and covers a wider field than just consciousness and its disorders.

Attention, Awareness and Concentration

Attention is a different function from consciousness, but it is dependent on it. Thus variable degrees of attention are possible with full consciousness, but complete attention and concentration are impossible with diminished consciousness. William James' (1842–1910) (1890) account is still a good starting point:

Attention is … the taking into possession of the mind, in clear and vivid form, of one out of what seem several simultaneously possible objects or trains of thought. Focalization, concentration, of consciousness are of its essence.

There are passive and active modes of attention. In passive attention, the subject responds to, for example, a loud noise, whereas in active attention, an individual's prior expectations and goals determine in a top-down fashion what is attended to (for a fuller description, see Eysenck and Keane, 2010). A central feature of attention is its limited *capacity*. This refers to the fact that only so much cognitive processing activity can be carried out at any one time. Attentional capacity is usually tested by the digit span, and, although it is a relatively stable feature of attention, it is prone to influence by, for example, fatigue, depression and brain injury. Components of attention include orientating to sensory events, detecting signals for focused processing and maintaining a vigilant and alert state. It is important to recognize that knowledge, prior beliefs, goals and expectations can alter the speed and accuracy of the processes that select meaningful or desirable information from the environment.

There are four other aspects of attention. *Focused*, or *selective*, *attention* refers to the capacity to highlight the one or two important stimuli or ideas being dealt with while suppressing awareness of competing distractions. This aspect of attention is usually referred to as *concentration*. 'Serial sevens' are usually employed to assess this aspect of attention, and it requires focused attention as well as other cognitive processes. *Sustained attention*, or *vigilance*, involves the ability to maintain attentional activity over a period of time. It is usually measured by vigilance tests. *Divided attention* involves the ability to respond to more than one task at a time or to multiple elements within a task. *Alternating attention* allows for shifts in focus of attention and tasks (Lezak et al., 2004; Table 4.1).

Automatic cognitive processes, that is, those that occur without intention, that are involuntary and that do not interfere with other ongoing activities, exist in parallel with those that require attentive processes (Kolb and Whishaw, 1996). These automatic processes allow for the effortless extraction of features of a perception in a bottom-up fashion, whereas attentive processes allow for the top-down processing of information (Fig. 4.1).

ALTERATION OF THE DEGREE OF ATTENTION

Attention is decreased in normal people in sleep, dreams, hypnotic states, fatigue and boredom. It may be pathologically decreased in organic states, usually with lowering of consciousness, for instance, with head injury, acute toxic confusional states such as

TABLE 4.1	Aspects of Attention
Aspect of Attention	**Definition**
Focused attention	The capacity to highlight important stimuli while suppressing awareness of competing distractions
Sustained attention or vigilance	The capacity to maintain attentional activity over a prolonged period
Divided attention	The ability to respond to more than one task at a time, including taking account of the multiple elements within a complex task
Alternating attention	The ability to shift attentional focus from task to task
Attentional capacity	The extent of the processing ability inherent in the attentional system; it is often considered to be a form of working memory

drug- and alcohol-induced conditions, epilepsy, raised intracranial pressure and brainstem lesions. In psychogenic states, attention may be altered, for example, it may be diminished in dissociative disorders. Narrowing of attention is also prominent in depressive illness in which the morbid mood state results in attention being limited to a restricted number of themes—mostly unhappy or morbid ones.

A severe deficit of attention is a prominent feature in the hyperkinetic disorders in childhood (World Health Organization, 1992) but also occurs in adult life (see Chapter 3). Observation of the child's behaviour by adults such as parents or teachers concentrates on three aspects: inattention, impulsiveness and hyperactivity. Inattention is shown in that the child, most often a boy and usually aged between 3 and 10 years, fails to finish activities he starts, appears not to listen, is easily distracted, has difficulty concentrating on any task requiring sustained attention and has difficulty sticking to a play activity.

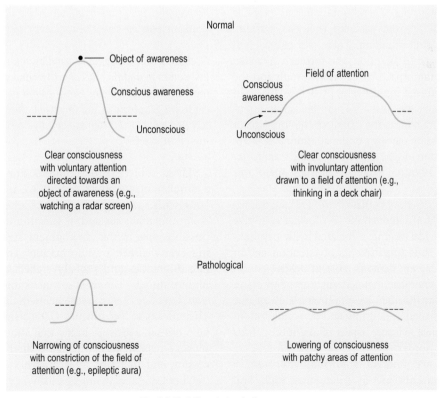

Fig. 4.1 Variations in level of awareness.

Impairment of focused attention and concentration denotes an inability to exercise attention on an object in a purposeful way, implying weakening of the *determining tendency*. This is a feature of mania and hypomania and also occurs in organic states. These features combine to show the symptoms of *distractibility*, which is prominent in mania and some organic states.

Narrowing of attention entails the ability of the subject to focus on a small part of the field of awareness and occurs in conditions in which involuntary attention is directed elsewhere—by hallucinations, by delusions or by strong emotion. After an unprofitable conversation with a patient with schizophrenia in which she repeatedly ignored questions, she said, 'I wish you would not interrupt when I am being given my instructions'.

DISORDER OF ATTENTION IN PSYCHOSIS

To recapitulate, attention is designed to present to the mind, with clarity and vividness, an appropriate selection, of only some of the objects in our environment where there are several simultaneous possible objects. It includes the capacity to focus, sustain, disengage and shift attention. There is a passive and an active element to attention, the former controlled in a bottom-up approach by external stimuli and the latter controlled in a top-down approach by the individual's goals or expectations. There is also an attentional capacity, which is the extent of the inherent or intrinsic processing capacity of the attentional system. A full description of the current cognitive neuroscience model of attention is outside of the scope of this chapter.

There is little doubt that there are attentional problems that are demonstrable on formal cognitive neuropsychological testing associated with psychiatric disorders. Thus impairments of attention and/or working memory are demonstrable in diverse conditions such as generalized anxiety disorder, depressive disorder, bipolar disorder, schizophrenia and organic brain disorders such as delirium and dementia. Attentional disturbance is a core aspect of attention deficit/hyperactivity disorder.

Subjective accounts of abnormal attention in early schizophrenia are at their most rich and detailed in the seminal studies of McGhie and Chapman (1961). In Chapman's (1966) later work, he gave several examples of problems with attention:

I can't shut things out of my mind and everything closes in on me. It stops me thinking and then the mind goes blank and everything gets switched off. I can't pick things up to memorize because I am so absorbing everything around me and take in too much so that I can't retain for any length of time – only a few seconds, and I can't do simple habits like walking or cleaning my teeth. I have to use all my mind to do these things. (Case 10).

At times there is nothing to hold the mind and this is when I go into a trance. (Case 15).

It happens when I'm watching the television as well and my concentration drifts away and focuses on any point in the room and I can't pick anything up that is going on. I go into a daze because I can't concentrate long enough to keep up the conversation and something lifts up inside my head and puts me into a trance. (Case 12).

Nothing settles in my mind – not even for a second. It just comes in and then it's out. My mind goes away – too many things come into my head at once and I lose control. I get afraid of walking when this happens. My feet just walk away from me and I've no control over myself. (Case 29).

These subjective descriptions draw attention to a number of cognitive difficulties, including problems with focusing attention, of disengaging from environmental cues and of selecting from a range of possible cues in the environment and thereby feeling overwhelmed by information. These are disparate difficulties and probably reflect distinct neural underpinnings. The most distinct subjective description refers to being overwhelmed by information. This speaks to Broadbent's (1958) theory in which he proposed a sensory buffer that allows only certain sensory data to pass through a filter for later processing and that this filter prevents overloading of the limited capacity mechanism beyond the filter.

McGhie and Chapman's (1961) own view is expressed as follows:

Now let us suppose that there is a breakdown in this selective–inhibitory function of attention. Consciousness would be flooded with an undifferentiated mass of incoming sensory data, transmitted from the environment via the sense organs. To this involuntary tide of impressions there would be added the diverse internal images, and their associations, which would no longer be coordinated with incoming information. Perception would revert to the passive and involuntary assimilative process of early childhood and, if the incoming flood were to carry on unchecked, it would gradually sweep away the stable constructs of a former reality.

John Cutting interprets these accounts differently. He makes the point that the patients had heightened attention rather than that the proposed sensory buffer was unable to streamline what information was available for processing (Cutting, 2011). Furthermore, Cutting used the term *lures* to describe features of the environment that seemed to capture the attention of patients with schizophrenia in such a manner that they were unable to disengage their attention. In his view, the potential lures are inanimate objects in the physical environment. In cognitive neuroscience terms, this implies an impairment of passive attention so that the patient is excessively liable to passive attentional capture. In addition, there are problems with disengaging and shifting attention.

There is well-established evidence that in mood disorders, including bipolar mood disorders, during the acute phase as well as in the euthymic state, there are demonstrable impairments in sustained attention and working memory (Clark et al., 2002; Marvel and Paradiso, 2004; Thompson et al., 2005). In addition, however, depressed mood is often associated with a preoccupation with gloomy thoughts to such an extent that concentration and attention are impaired. This suggests that attention, whether active or passive, can be in thrall to negatively valued features of the individual's inner or external world. In such a situation, misinterpretations of perception influenced by the mood state frequently arise. Every hearse is believed to be there to carry the patient to the graveyard, and a passing black car is noticed just sufficiently to be considered as strengthening this belief. Similarly, acute anxiety often results in diminished attention.

Cutting (2011) argues that, in mood disorder, what lures the individual's attention are people and not objects, in contrast to schizophrenia in which the reverse is true. The subjective description to support this view is drawn from Minkowski (1970):

I feel that, when you insist, I ought to submit to your will and do what you demand of me. It irritates me to be someone's fool, but I am incapable of resisting; I feel that you have control of me. I don't dare do anything unless you ask me to. I do everything unconsciously. If you insist that I go out, I will go out. I can't resist anymore. It is atrocious! After dinner, when the others get up from the table, I get up automatically, carried along by their movements. I am the reflection of others. In sum, I vibrate with people, I reflect their movements; it is their vibrations that make me vibrate myself.

Minkowski classifies this as an example of the influence of events, words and people on patients in depressive states. I am uncertain that this is an example of passive attention, namely, of what Cutting terms *lures*. Nonetheless, it is incontrovertible that depressed mood is associated with gloomy thoughts, memories of past morbid incidents to such a degree that there is marked impairment of concentration and attention. This suggests that both active and passive attention may be 'lured' by negative aspects of the patient's inner world.

As described earlier, schizophrenia is recognized as involving deficits of attention (Posner et al., 1988). However, there is considerable difficulty in establishing what aspects of attention are impaired in schizophrenia because the tasks that are used to assess attention may involve other cognitive functions, particularly given that attention is closely tied to concepts of working memory and to executive function. Current evidence suggests that schizophrenia is associated with significant impairment in the control of selection, the ability to identify and attend to task-relevant inputs, whereas there may not be impairment of the implementation of selection—the processes that determine the processing of relevant informational inputs (Luck and Gold, 2008).

It seems likely that in schizophrenia, on the basis of these reports, there is a greater susceptibility to lures within the environment that capture the passive attention of the patient. A good way to understand this is to imagine how a sudden, unexpected noise captures our passive attention. It does seem as if patients with schizophrenia are in thrall to irrelevant features of their environment.

HEMI-INATTENTION

A number of neuropsychiatric conditions illustrate the relationship between disorders of attention and impaired conscious awareness of objects. These conditions are complex and not completely understood. They include unilateral neglect, anosodiaphoria (lack of concern about hemiparesis), defective appreciation of hemiparesis with rationalization, denial of hemiparesis and unawareness of hemiparesis (anosognosia).

In their seminal paper, Paterson and Zangwill (1944) described unilateral neglect in a previously healthy male who suffered a penetrating injury of the right parietal occipital region after an explosion in 1943. He lost consciousness for 2 or 3 minutes and showed minimal post-traumatic and retrograde amnesia. On recovery his most significant deficit was a strong neglect of the left side of space. He collided with objects on his left and ignored food on the left side of his dish. It was concluded that the lesion was on the upper borders of the supramarginal and angular gyrus on the right side (Mattingley, 1996).

The aim in this section is not to examine in detail the varying hypothesis and findings regarding these disorders of conscious awareness but to draw out the fact that syndromes of unawareness exist, that these syndromes involve attentional systems and that these systems require intact brain function in particular hemispheres and regions. These conditions in which individuals demonstrate a degree of unawareness or denial of hemiplegia have been recognized for well over a century by, among others, Babinski (1857–1932), Lhermitte (1877–1959) and Critchley (1900–97).

Stuss and Benson (1986) described a classic case of denial of hemiplegia:

A 62-year old man suffered a subarachnoid haemorrhage. A right middle cerebral artery was demonstrated and successfully ligated, but the patient awoke with left hemiplegia. At first he vehemently denied the hemiplegia. At this time he was disoriented and had a retrograde amnesia covering at least 2 years prior to the surgery. When evaluated early one morning about 2 weeks postoperatively, he spontaneously described his paralysis, was oriented to both time and place, but had no memory of his cranial surgery.

In another case they described the extent to which individuals with anosognosia will go to deny their disability:

A 57-year old hypertensive man sustained an acute intracerebral haemorrhage involving the right putamen. On admission to hospital he was stuporous with profound left hemiplegia, left hemisensory loss, and left hemianopsia … He was disoriented for time and place, could not remember his doctors' names, and actively denied any physical disability. When asked if he could walk or dance, he would immediately say yes; when asked to raise his arms or legs, he would raise the right limbs and insist that both arms or legs had been raised. When his hemiplegia was demonstrated to him he would accept the obvious fact and repeat the examiner's statement concerning the cause of his disability but within minutes, if asked whether he had any disability, he would adamantly deny disability.

These accounts of unilateral neglect and anosognosia emphasize that the neural systems underpinning attention to both right and left visual fields are probably controlled by the right hemisphere, whereas the dominant hemisphere (the left hemisphere in right-handed individuals) only oversees the contralateral visual fields. Hence damage to the dominant hemisphere is not followed by unilateral neglect or anosognosia because the right hemisphere continues to monitor sensory information from all fields. Damage to the right hemisphere, on the other hand, is accompanied by hemineglect and anosognosia for the left visual field. However, these matters also pertain not merely to visual fields but also to how our bodies are experienced. This is made most manifest in a case that presented after embolism of the right cerebral artery reported by Critchley (1950):

It felt as if I was missing one side of my body (the left), but it also felt as if the dummy side was lined with a piece of iron so heavy that I could not move … I even fancied my head to be narrow, but the left side from the centre felt heavy, as if filled with bricks.

In summary, abnormalities of attention have a complex set of consequences, not merely inattentiveness or impaired concentration as measured by crude bedside tests but also significant abnormalities that would not normally be attributed to abnormalities of attention and that are demonstrable in schizophrenia, mood disorders and neuropsychiatric disorders.

Orientation

Orientation is the capacity of an individual to accurately gauge time, space and person in his current setting. This enables him to make sense of, and be at home in, his environment. This is virtually the same faculty as intellectual grasp in that various perceptual cues are used, and with correct sense of time and place, the person is able to come to appropriate conclusions from his context. A man suffering from an advanced dementia was being interviewed by a doctor in the presence of a dozen student nurses who were taking notes with pen and notebook. When asked where he was, he looked around the rather dingy hospital classroom and said, 'Well, we're waiting to see the doctor'. He had picked up certain clues that reminded him of a general practitioner's waiting room; he had totally missed the fact that all the nurses were in uniform, that they were taking notes and that he was being asked formal questions. He was disorientated in place and in person.

Orientation in *time* is labile and quite readily disturbed by rapt concentration, strong emotion or organic brain factors (for example, alcoholic intoxication). Milder degrees of disorientation are shown by inaccuracy of more than half an hour for the time of day or duration of interview. More advanced states are demonstrated with incorrect day of the week, year or period of day. Yet further disturbance is shown when the season of the year is not known correctly.

Orientation in *space* is disturbed later in the disease process than time. A patient may be unable to find his way, especially in an area that is relatively new to him. It may take him an inordinate length of time to learn his way to the dining table in the ward after admission. Disorientation in time and place are, when clearly established, evidence of an organic mental state; they may be the earliest signs in a dementing process.

In disorientation for *person*, the patient fails to remember his own name. Loss of knowledge of the patient's own name and identity occurs at a very late stage of organic deterioration. Loss of intellectual grasp (apprehension) occurs in organic states as a form of disorientation, usually combined with other evidence of deterioration. Such a person cannot understand the context of his present situation and connects outside objects and events with himself. Disorientation may occur with a disturbance of consciousness, attention, perception or intelligence. In severe intellectual defect and severe disturbances of memory, orientation is impaired even when consciousness is clear (Scharfetter, 1980).

DISORIENTATION

Orientation may fluctuate in some organic conditions; for example, a patient with delirium associated with congestive cardiac failure was disorientated in time every evening but quite clear mentally in the morning.

Disorientation in time and loss of intellectual grasp (situational disorientation) usually occur first in a progressive illness; disorientation in place usually occurs later and, in person, last of all. Disorientation for one's own identity occurs at a later stage than for that of other people. An elderly woman who knew who she was and her previous status as a professor's wife kept on referring to her daughter as 'that minx who comes in every time the doctor visits'.

Delusions that Mimic Disorientation

It is, of course, important to understand the phenomenological distinction between disorientation and a delusion that results in misinterpretation of place, of situation or of person. Disorientation is usually associated with other organic features, such as lowering of consciousness or disturbance of memory. Delusions of *misorientation* have the features of a delusion (see Chapter 8): a person on the ward may believe himself to be in prison, and a visiting relative may be considered to be an interrogator from the Gestapo.

Dissociation and Disorientation

Definite, undisputed disorientation is indicative of either an acute organic brain syndrome if coupled with lowering of consciousness or chronic organic deterioration. Dissociative disorders may mimic this, however, with apparent disorientation. Careful examination of the mental state is likely to reveal suggestive discrepancies; for example, disorientation for person may be much more marked than for time or may be bizarre to an excessive extent. A patient is described in the next chapter who lived in Birmingham, United Kingdom, but found himself after a dissociative fugue in Montreal. Although apparently disorientated, he actually showed an abnormality of memory as part of a dissociative state.

Sleep Disorders

Sleep—deep, satisfying and undisturbed—is conventionally associated with well-being and good health, as exemplified by the quotation with which this chapter begins; its absence or poor quality is equally held to account for disorder of mood and misery. There is a relationship between disturbed sleep and psychiatric disorder; mental illness may cause and manifest as sleep disturbance, disturbed sleep may precipitate psychiatric symptoms, or the two may occur together but independently. The *International Classification of Sleep Disorders* subsumes 85 sleep disorders into seven categories including:

1. insomnias,
2. sleep-related breathing disorders,
3. hypersomnias not due to a breathing disorder,
4. parasomnias,
5. sleep-related movements disorders,
6. other sleep disorders, and
7. isolated symptoms, apparently normal variants and unresolved issues.

For a fuller account, see American Academy of Sleep Medicine (2005).

The objective assessment of sleep is usually carried out electrophysiologically. Five stages of sleep can be identified (Rechtschaffen and Kales, 1968). Sleep is entered through non–rapid eye movement (NREM) sleep. NREM and rapid eye movement (REM) sleep alternate with a period near 90 minutes. NREM sleep accounts for approximately 75% to 80% of sleep, and REM sleep accounts for 20% to 25% of sleep, occurring in four to six discrete episodes (Pelayo and Dement, 2017). Using an electroencephalogram and electromyogram of the external ocular muscles, the duration of the various stages is recorded. It has been shown that REM sleep is associated with dreaming. With current neuroimaging techniques, it is possible, by showing changes in regional cerebral blood flow, to localize and represent visually altered activity, especially in the medial thalamus, which is associated with different stages of sleep from relaxed wakefulness to the slow-wave sleep of stage 4. There are also changes in the visual and auditory cortex, possibly associated with dreaming (Hofle et al., 1997). When considering the quality and duration of sleep and its stages and whether this amounts to a symptom, it is important to take into account the age of the patient, any medication he may be taking and whether he has slept during the day. The subjective experience, as described by the patient, may be very different from the objective findings of observation and measurement. The psychiatrist should investigate the meaning of this discrepancy phenomenologically and consider the consequences for diagnosis and treatment.

INSOMNIA

Insomnia implies subjective dissatisfaction with the duration or quality of sleep (Oswald, 1981); however, in many psychiatric conditions there is also objective disturbance of sleep. There are several approaches to the definition of insomnia from the subjective that merely specifies whether an individual has had trouble sleeping to the strictly formal that stipulates that there must be greater than 30 minutes of sleep-onset latency or wake time after sleep onset (Lichstein et al., 2017).

Formally, insomnia is defined as a complaint of dissatisfaction with sleep quality associated with difficulty initiating sleep, difficulty maintaining sleep that is characterized by frequent awakenings or problems returning to sleep after awakenings or early-morning awakening with inability to return to sleep (Ahmed and Thorpy, 2010; American Psychiatric Association, 2013). The individual may complain that the duration of sleep is too short; that sleep feels broken, less refreshing or insufficiently deep; or that the pattern of sleep has changed for the worse. Insomnia is more common in women and in older people and is more often associated with a feeling of excessive mental arousal than bodily disorder. Causes of dissatisfaction include unrealistic expectations from the elderly that they will sleep for as long as they did when they were younger and from the sedentary that they will sleep as deeply as after exhausting physical activity.

A discussion of primary insomnia is outside the scope of this book. It is well recognized that complaints of sleeping poorly are common and occur in many psychiatric disorders, including depression, generalized anxiety, panic and phobia, hypochondriasis and personality disorders. They are among the most frequent symptoms in anxiety-related disorders and affective disorders. Comparing those people with neuroses with a normal population, Jovanovic (1978) found that neurotic patients complained of more wakefulness in the first third of the night; they spent more time lying awake in bed, they awoke during the night more frequently, they spent a relatively short period in deep sleep and their sleep was more likely to be impaired by unfamiliar surroundings. Those with major depressive disorder suffer from disturbed sleep in which they take longer to fall asleep and spend less time asleep because of periods of wakefulness during the night and early-morning wakening.

Early insomnia, or difficulty in getting to sleep occurs in normal people who are aroused through anxiety or excitement. Their thoughts tend to dwell on the affect-laden experiences of the immediate past and also to rehearse ways of dealing with problems. Fatigue is experienced, but there is also a high level of arousal that prevents the necessary relaxation and withdrawal from perception that is required for sleeping. *Late insomnia,* or *early-morning wakening*, is particularly characteristic of the depressive phase of affective disorders. The patient may wake frequently in the night after getting off to sleep satisfactorily and thenceforward sleep only fitfully and lightly. Alternatively, he may wake early in the morning and be unable to get to sleep again. The important characteristic of depression is that there is a marked change in sleep rhythm from the normal pattern for that person. In depression, the early-morning wakening is often associated with marked diurnality of mood, with the most severe feelings of despondency and retardation occurring in

the early morning. There is also often a marked reduction of sleep requirement in mania.

The mean sleep requirement diminishes with increasing age. It is usually about 7 to 8 hours through the middle adult years but is markedly reduced from about 50 years of age onwards. With insomnia, intermediate stages of light, restless sleep occur. These are often associated with abnormal experience in the sleepy state, such as *hypnagogic* and *hypnopompic* hallucinations (Chapter 7). Pseudohallucinations also occur, as does vivid imagery that is difficult to distinguish from hallucination. Normally, passage into sleep is rapid and occurs passively rather than with active intention to sleep. Waking is also normally rapid, and the slowing of this process of becoming awake may be described as a symptom: a complaint of feeling drowsy and being incompetent and uncoordinated for an excessive time on wakening—in other words, *sleep drunkenness* or more accurately *confusional arousals* from NREM sleep in which confusion and disorientation and slowed speech and mentation occur (Lishman, 1997; Ahmed and Thorpy, 2010). Such patients may sleep for 17 hours or more and always require vigorous stimulation to wake them. The condition may persist throughout life.

HYPERSOMNIA

In hypersomnia the defining characteristic is daytime sleepiness. These cases are more often seen by a neurologist than a psychiatrist and are described only briefly here.

In the *Kleine-Levin syndrome,* attacks of somnolence occur, usually in adolescents. The condition is rare. In earlier accounts, the patient sleeps excessively by day and night but is rousable as from normal sleep. When awake, the patient eats voraciously (megaphagia) and may show marked irritability (Critchley, 1962). More recently it has become clearer that the condition is characterized by relapsing–remitting episodes of severe hypersomnia, cognitive impairment, apathy, derealization and psychiatric and behavioural disturbances. Boys are more frequently affected than girls. Slightly more than half of patients have hyperphagia, are hypersexual (mainly boys) or have depressed mood (mainly girls), and about a third have other psychiatric symptoms, such as anxiety, delusions or hallucinations. The hallucinations are usually brief and visual in nature—for example, of snakes near the bed or of a dangerous man with a bear in the hospital elevator (Arnulf, 2017). The delusions are said to be grandiose or persecutory in nature. Although some symptoms are similar to those in patients with encephalopathy, imaging and laboratory findings are unremarkable. The first episode of hypersomnia is often triggered by an infection, with relapses occurring every 1 to 12 months for a median of 14 years. Between episodes, patients generally have normal sleep patterns, cognition, mood and eating habits. During episodes, electroencephalography might show diffuse or local slow activity. Functional imaging studies have revealed hypoactivity in thalamic and hypothalamic regions and in the frontal and temporal lobes (Arnulf et al., 2012).

Narcolepsy is a form of hypersomnia and can occur either with or without cataplexy. Narcoleptic attacks are short episodes of sleep (10–15 minutes) that occur irresistibly during the day; they usually begin during adolescence and persist throughout life. Narcolepsy is often associated with *cataplexy*, during which the subject falls down because of a sudden loss of muscle tone provoked by strong emotion. *Hypnagogic hallucinations* and *sleep paralysis* may also occur but less commonly. Narcolepsy is associated with short sleep latency and sleep-onset REM periods. There is usually no structural brain disease present. Hypnagogic hallucinations are usually auditory but may be visual or tactile. They occur between wakefulness and sleep, less commonly between sleep and wakening (hypnopompic hallucination). Sleep paralysis is the inability to move during the period between wakefulness and sleep (in either direction).

In the *Pickwickian syndrome,* named after the fat boy of *The Pickwick Papers* (Dickens, 1837), or more specifically *obstructive sleep apnoea*, profound daytime somnolence is associated with gross obesity and cyanosis due to hypoventilation. Breathing is periodic during sleep and somnolence, with apnoeic phases that may last for up to a minute.

Sustained drowsiness may occur with organic lesions of the midbrain or hypothalamus from various causes. Hunger, weight gain, excessive thirst and polyuria may also occur. The most important conditions giving rise to secondary hypersomnia are brain tumours, neurosarcoidosis and Niemann-Pick type C disease.

Hypersomnia may also occur as a psychogenic symptom. There may be a state amounting to dissociative stupor, and other conversion symptoms may be present. Other patients with neurotic disorders complain persistently of daytime somnolence and an inability to concentrate.

PARASOMNIAS

The parasomnias are disorders of arousal and sleep-stage transition that consist of abnormal sleep-related movements, behaviours, emotions, perceptions, dreaming and autonomic nervous system functioning that accompany sleep (Ahmed and Thorpy, 2010). Sleepwalking is an example and consists of a series of complex behaviours arising during slow-wave sleep and resulting in walking during a period of altered consciousness. It is more characteristic of children than adults and of males than females. Activity is usually confined to aimless wandering and purposeless repetitive behaviour for a few minutes. The sleepwalker may reply monosyllabically to questions, and there is little awareness of the environment, but injury is unusual. Frequently there is a family history, and enuresis is often associated. As sleepwalking occurs in deep sleep (stages 3 and 4), usually during the first third of the night, it is unlikely to be the acting out of dreams. It is not the same phenomenon as epileptic automatism, which may also result in a person, who is apparently asleep, getting up and walking around. It is important to establish the diagnosis in each case.

Night terrors also occur in deep sleep early in the night and often in the same individual who sleepwalks. Intense anxiety is manifested, the subject may shout and there is rapid pulse and respiration. Usually there is complete amnesia for the experience on waking. It is not the same experience as a nightmare because the latter is a type of dream, occurring in lighter states of sleep, and is remembered vividly if the person awakes immediately after the experience. Most children grow out of night terrors and sleepwalking.

Claims have been made that automatic, violent behaviour has taken place during a night terror. A person who commits a criminal act while asleep is not conscious of his actions and cannot be held legally responsible for them; the law calls this *sane automatism* (Fenwick, 1986; Ebrahim and Fenwick, 2010). If the act—for instance, homicide—is remembered by its perpetrator as following a chain of psychic events ('being chased by Japanese soldiers'), these images are most likely to have occurred in the context of a nightmare, and the act therefore took place on waking from the dream and would be regarded as motivated. During the nightmare itself, sleep paralysis will prevent violent emotions being acted on. For the act to be convincingly ascribed to night terror, neither the act nor its antecedent storyline should be remembered, and all the evidence should point to the individual being asleep at the time. Previous evidence of night terror and sleep activity is important for corroboration.

Less known are the reports of *sexsomnia* in which sexual behaviour occurs during sleep. These cases seem to occur in the setting of disorders of arousal, the so-called NREM parasomnias that include confusional arousal, sleep terror and sleepwalking; REM sleep behaviour disorder; nocturnal partial complex seizures; and obstructive sleep apnoea (Ebrahim and Fenwick, 2010).

Dreams

How does phenomenology view dreams, their significance and their interpretation? First, phenomenology is concerned only with what is conscious; it cannot comment on that which is unconscious, although it may infer the existence of the unconscious insofar as it explains some observed behaviours and phenomena. Second, the meaning belongs to the dreamer and not to an interpreter or theorist. This has implications for the way in which the phenomenological approach will be used in therapy.

Phenomenology can make contributions to our understanding of dreaming but only in a limited way. Phenomenology is a study of the objects that are available to conscious subjective awareness. However, the content of dreams can only be recollected and described after the event. This has implications for the accuracy and verisimilitude of the recollected accounts. Graham Greene (1904–91) kept a dream diary from a very early age and always had a pencil and paper at hand on his bedside so that when he woke up from a dream, he could note down a few key words that he later used to reconstruct his dreams. His descriptions are vivid and highly detailed. These descriptions demonstrate that memory of the content of dreams can be accurate and detailed, sometimes very detailed indeed. And, once the premise of the dream is understood, the logic and reasoning become comprehensible. Even the bizarre elements become comprehensible. An example from Graham Greene's posthumous *A World of My Own* (Greene, 1992) illustrates these points:

I remember having a discussion with Sartre. I had made notes of various questions to ask him, and I tried to be very precise. I apologized for the badness of my French, which prevented me from being as precise as I wanted to be, and Sartre said kindly, 'You speak French very well, but,' he added, 'I don't understand a word you say.'

Then he became amiable and referred to a book of mine which Robert Laffont had published in France, the English title being The Origin of Brighton Rock. *It was a reproduction of a childish manuscript in brown ink – a story with animal characters – and it was illustrated by Beatrix Potter. Sartre very much admired her drawings, but he said nothing of my writing.*

The account of this dream is compelling, and it is difficult to fully grasp that it is not a description of a real encounter with Sartre in what Greene termed the *Common World* but an account of a dream event, or an experience in what he termed *A World of My Own*.

Orthodox sleep (stages 1–4) and *paradoxical* sleep (REM sleep) have been distinguished from each other through the use of sleep electroencephalographic tracings in human subjects (Oswald, 1980). Normal reflex activity occurs in the stages of orthodox sleep, but localized activity is seen in paradoxical sleep while other muscle actions are paralysed. REMs in paradoxical sleep are to some extent associated with dreaming. Nightmares are unpleasant dreams; often the particular horror of a nightmare is that there is nothing the sufferer can do about the terrifying experience. Dreaming occurs in REM (paradoxical) sleep, and the transfixed sensation of the nightmare is an accurate representation of the sleep paralysis that occurs in that phase.

Dreams have been used to establish elaborate psychiatric theories concerning the origins of conflict; it is outside the scope of this book to enter into any discussion of this area. It is, of course, a topic that was extensively written about by Sigmund Freud (1976). More recently, the meaning of dreams has been explored empirically by Kramer et al. (1976). Dreams are remembered and described as a psychic event: nightmares (unpleasant dreams) are often complained of and may be a prominent symptom, for instance, in depression. Dreams are highly complex experiences and, so far, have defied adequate analysis and explanation. However, certain characteristics can be described.

There is a loss of some of the structures of waking consciousness, thus there is a loss of self-awareness and awareness of the confines of one's own body. The margin between self and not-self becomes indefinite. The dreamer may dream of himself merging or transforming into someone else without contradiction. Time sense is also lost: there is no sense of progression of events but only immediate awareness of the present. Events occurring in the dream include those in which the dreamer himself is instrumental. There is often a loss of the sense of his having circumstances within his control, and there is also a loss of the physical and mental associations between the different parts of a whole experience. There are, therefore, gaps unaccounted for in space as well as in time and causation.

As well as the loss of temporal and spatial connections, there is a loss of the psychological associations between events. There is no progressive sequence of serial ideas or pictures. The dream is often like a group of short excerpts from very different films.

In addition to the loss of structure that is typical in the dreaming state, there are also elements that do not occur in the normal waking state. These are best called dream images because they are not accurately delusions, hallucinations, false memories or other abnormalities of perception or ideation characteristic of being awake. These images are more vivid than fantasy and have a characteristic of immediacy and importance, so it is not surprising that, from the beginning of time, people have acted on their dreams as if they were instructions.

To regard dreaming as a symptom rather than merely a remembered experience, it has to become invested with unpleasant affect. A patient may describe pleasant dreams if requested, but he does not usually complain of these as symptoms or ask for their removal. However, if the dream is associated with anxiety, terror, gloom or foreboding and especially if the content or the theme is recurrent, it will be complained of and will indicate a prevailing affect; possibly the areas of conflict that have precipitated the distress will be revealed in the content of the dream. Unpleasant dreams in which a part of the traumatic event is re-experienced are a diagnostic feature of post-traumatic stress disorder after major disaster or catastrophe.

Hypnosis

It has been suggested by Marcuse (1959) that we 'define hypnosis by what it does rather than by what it is'. At one extreme, hypnosis is considered to be a very different state of awareness from normal waking consciousness. At the other extreme, Merskey (1979) considers that 'the phenomena of hypnosis are identical with those of hysteria: they involve self-deception and the production of alternative symptoms or behaviour to solve a problem, even if not a conflict'. Merskey further goes on to propose as definition:

Hypnosis is a manoeuvre in which the subject and hypnotist have an implicit agreement that certain events (e.g., paralysis, hallucinations, amnesias) will occur, either during a special procedure or later, in accordance with the hypnotist's instructions. Both try hard to put this agreement into effect and adopt appropriate behavioural rules, and the subject uses mechanisms of denial to report on the events in accordance with the implicit agreement. This situation is used to implement various motives, therapeutic or otherwise, on the part of both participants. There is no trance state, no detectable cerebral physiological change and only such peripheral physiological responses as may be produced equally by nonhypnotic suggestions or other emotional changes.

Hypnosis in contemporary practice is defined as a psychophysiologic state of attentive, receptive concentration with a relative suspension of peripheral awareness, what is sometimes termed the *trance state*. It is thought that the ability to enter the trance state is widely distributed in the general population (Maldonado, 2015).

Superficially, hypnosis appears to resemble sleep, but there are no electroencephalographic findings to distinguish hypnosis from other states of relaxed wakefulness. The trance in hypnosis is therefore produced in a waking state by one person on another using suggestion with compliance (Marcuse, 1959).

It is understood that hypnosis involves three interconnected factors: *absorption, dissociation* and *suggestibility* (Maldonado, 2015). Absorption involves the tendency to engage in self-altering and highly focused attention with complete immersion in a central experience at the expense of contextual orientation such that the hypnotized subject can be intensely absorbed in their trance experience that they often choose to ignore environmental cues. Dissociation is the capacity to separate mental processes so that they seem to occur independently from each other, and thus a past memory may be dissociated from current events. Finally, suggestibility refers to the ability in a subject to be easily influenced because of heightened responsiveness to social cues including instructions given during the hypnotic trance.

Hypnosis has been claimed to occur in nonhuman species, but this state cannot necessarily be considered identical with hypnosis. Hypnosis has been used for the control of pain, in the treatment of hyperemesis gravidarum and especially in the control of anxiety (Waxman, 1984).

The induction of hypnosis requires the implicit contract that Merskey implies. The subject must be willing and cooperative; he or she relaxes and exercises imagination. The field of consciousness is narrowed to include only the instructions of the hypnotist. The subject relinquishes some degree of control to the hypnotist and accepts reality distortion. After the successful induction of hypnosis, autohypnosis can become established. Marcuse considers the following to be the characteristics of a hypnotic state:

- The subject ceases to make his own plans.
- Attention is selectively directed, for example, towards the voice of the hypnotist.
- Reality testing is diminished, and distortions are accepted.
- Suggestibility is increased.
- The hypnotized subject readily enacts unusual roles.
- Posthypnotic amnesia is often present.

Suggestion for the hypnotic subject is straightforward and obvious; it does not imply gullibility or loss of willpower. It describes the emotion of trust occurring within the implicit relationship in which the subject accepts the hypnotist's statements, acts on his commands and denies evidence from his own senses that would contradict those statements.

A capacity for fantasy is necessary for hypnosis to take place. The relaxation that accompanies hypnosis may progress to normal sleeping, even during a hypnotic session. The alteration in conscious awareness occurring in hypnosis is similar to that in dissociative states but different from the fluctuations of consciousness level occurring in organic psychosyndromes.

Suggestion has been used to produce many physical sequelae (e.g., blisters, alterations in pulse and blood pressure, levitation of an arm, opisthotonos, absence of pain sensation and so on). The psychological effects are equally variable and include alterations to perception, cognition, ideation, memory and affect. The subject enters a dramatically altered state in which he temporarily surrenders responsibility for his actions to the hypnotist. In his turn, the hypnotist retains the confidence of the subject only as long as he keeps within the limits of behaviour that the subject finds acceptable; beyond this, the subject will relinquish his dependent relationship and come out of the hypnotic state.

Hypnosis remains an enigma. There is now emerging evidence of the underlying neural correlates of hypnotizability and of the hypnotic state itself. These point to greater functional connectivity between the left dorsolateral prefrontal cortex, an executive-control region of the brain, and the salience network composed of the dorsal anterior cingulate cortex, anterior insula, amygdala and ventral striatum, involved in detecting, integrating and filtering relevant somatic, autonomic and emotional information in highly hypnotizable subjects compared with less hypnotizable subjects (Hoeft et al., 2012). As for the hypnotic state itself, during mental imagery for rehabilitation of neurodisability, functional magnetic resonance imaging signal increases exclusively related to hypnosis have been observed in the left superior frontal cortex, the left anterior cingulate gyrus and the left thalamus. Whereas the superior frontal cortex and the anterior cingulate were activated related more to movement performance than to imagery, the thalamus was activated only during motor imagery. These areas represent central nodes of the salience network linking primary and higher motor areas. This suggests hypnosis enhances motor imagery (Müller et al., 2012). Much work still needs to be done to unravel the physiology of hypnosis.

REFERENCES

Ahmed, I.M., Thorpy, M.J., 2010. Classification of sleep disorders. In: Pandi-Perumal, S.R., Kramer, M. (Eds.), Sleep and Mental Illness. Cambridge University Press, Cambridge.

American Academy of Sleep Medicine, 2005. International Classification of Sleep Disorders. American Academy of Sleep Medicine, Chicago, p. 2.

American Psychiatric Association, 2013. Diagnostic and Statistical Manual of Mental Disorders, fifth ed. American Psychiatric Publishing, Washington, DC.

Arnulf, I., 2017. Kleine-Levine syndrome. In: Kryger, M., Roth, T., Dement, W.C. (Eds.), Principles and Practice of Sleep Medicine, sixth ed. Elsevier, Philadelphia.

Arnulf, I., Thomas, J.R., Emmanuel, M., 2012. Diagnosis, disease course, and management of patients with Kleine-Levin syndrome. Lancet Neurol. 11, 918–928.

Broadbent, D.E., 1958. Perception and Communication. Pergamon, London.

Chapman, J., 1966. The early symptoms of schizophrenia. Br. J. Psychiatry. 112, 225–251.

Clark, L., Iversen, S.D., Goodwin, G.M., 2002. Sustained attention deficit in bipolar disorder. Br. J. Psychiatry. 180, 313–319.

Critchley, M., 1950. The body-image in neurology. Lancet 255, 335–341.

Critchley, M., 1962. Periodic hypersomnia and megaphagia in adolescent males. Brain 85, 627–656.

Cutting, J., 2011. A Critique of Psychopathology. The Forest Publishing Company, Forest Row.

Dickens, C., 1837. The Posthumous Papers of the Pickwick Club. Penguin, London.

Ebrahim, I., Fenwick, P.B., 2010. Forensic issues of sleep in psychiatric patients. In: Pandi-Perumal, S.R., Kramer, M. (Eds.), Sleep and Mental Illness. Cambridge University Press, Cambridge.

Eysenck, M.W., Keane, M.T., 2010. Cognitive Psychology: A Student's Handbook, sixth ed. Psychology Press, Hove.

Fenwick, P., 1986. Murdering while asleep. Br. Med. J. 293, 574.

Freud, S., 1976. The Interpretation of Dreams (J. Strachey, Trans). Penguin, Harmondsworth.

Greene, G., 1992. A World of My Own. Penguin, Harmondsworth.

Hoeft, F., Gabrieli, J.D.E., Whitfield-Gabrieli, S., et al., 2012. Functional brain basis of hypnotizability. Arch. Gen. Psychiatry. 69, 1064–1072.

Hofle, N., Paus, T., Reutens, D., et al., 1997. Regional cerebral blood flow changes as a function of delta and spindle activity during slow wave sleep in humans. J. Neurosci. 17, 4800–4808.

James, W., 1890. Principles of Psychology. Holt, New York.

Jovanovic, U.J., 1978. Sleep profile and ultradian sleep periodicity in neurotic patients compared with the corresponding parameters in healthy human subjects. Waking Sleep. 2, 47–55.

Kolb, B., Whishaw, I.Q., 1996. Fundamentals of Human Neuropsychology, fourth ed. W.H. Freeman, Basingstoke.

Kramer, M., Hlasny, R., Jacobs, G., Roth, T., 1976. Do dreams have meaning? An empirical enquiry. Am. J. Psychiatry. 133, 778–781.

Lezak, M.D., Howieson, D.B., Loring, D.W., 2004. Neuropsychological Assessment, fourth ed. Oxford University Press, Oxford.

Lichstein, K.L., Taylor, D.J., McCrae, C.S., Petrov, M.E., 2017. Insomnia: epidemiology and risk factors. In: Kryger, M., Roth, T., Dement, W.C. (Eds.), Principles and Practice of Sleep Medicine, sixth ed. Elsevier, Philadelphia.

Lishman, W.A., 1997. Organic Psychiatry: The Psychological Consequences of Cerebral Disorder, third ed. Blackwell Scientific, Oxford.

Luck, S.J., Gold, J.M., 2008. The construct of attention in schizophrenia. Biol. Psychiatry. 64, 34–39.

Maldonado, J.R., 2015. Hypnosis in psychosomatic medicine. In: Fogel, B.S., Greenberg, D.B. (Eds.), Psychiatric Care of the Medical Patient, third ed. Oxford University Press, Oxford.

Marcuse, F.L., 1959. Hypnosis: Fact and Fiction. Penguin, Harmondsworth.

Marvel, C.L., Paradiso, S., 2004. Cognitive and neurological impairment in mood disorders. Psychiatr. Clin. North Am. 27, 1–17.

Mattingley, J.B., 1996. Paterson and Zangwill's (1944) case of unilateral neglect: insights from 50 years of experimental inquiry. In: Code, C., Wallesch, C., Jonette, Y., Lecours, A.R. (Eds.), Classic Cases in Neuropsychology. Psychology Press, Brighton, pp. 243–262.

McGhie, A., Chapman, J., 1961. Disorders of attention and perception in early schizophrenia. Br. J. Med. Psychol. 34, 103–115.

Merskey, H., 1979. The Analysis of Hysteria. Baillière Tindall, London.

Minkowski, E., 1970. Lived Time: Phenomenological and Psychopathological Studies. Northwestern University Press, Evanston, IL.

Müller, K., Bacht, K., Schramm, S., Seitz, R.J., 2012. The facilitating effect of clinical hypnosis on motor imagery: an fMRI study. Behav. Brain Res. 231, 164–169.

Oswald, I., 1980. Sleep, fourth ed. Penguin, Harmondsworth.

Oswald, I., 1981. Assessment of insomnia. Br. Med. J. 283, 874–875.

Paterson, A., Zangwill, O.L., 1944. Disorders of visual space perception associated with lesions of the right cerebral hemisphere. Brain 67, 331–358.

Pelayo, R., Dement, W.C., 2017. History of sleep physiology and medicine. In: Kryger, M., Roth, T., Dement, W.C. (Eds.), Principles and Practice of Sleep Medicine, sixth ed. Elsevier, Philadelphia.

Posner, M.I., Early, T.S., Reiman, E., Pardo, P.J., Dhawan, M., 1988. Asymmetries in hemispheric control of attention in schizophrenia. Arch. Gen. Psychiatry. 45, 814–821.

Rechtschaffen, A., Kales, A., 1968. A Manual of Standardized Terminology, Techniques and Scoring System for Sleep Stages of Human Subjects. US Department of Health, Education, and Welfare, Bethesda.

Scharfetter, C., 1980. General Psychopathology: An Introduction. Cambridge University Press, Cambridge.

Smith, E.E., Kosslyn, S.M., 2007. Cognitive Psychology: Mind and Brain. Pearson Prentice Hall, Hoboken, NJ.

Stuss, D.T., Benson, D.F., 1986. The Frontal Lobes. Raven Press, New York.

Thompson, J.M., Gallagher, P., Hughes, J.H., et al., 2005. Neurocognitive impairment in euthymic patients with bipolar affective disorder. Br. J. Psychiatry. 180, 32–40.

Waxman, D., 1984. Psychological Influences and Illness: Hypnosis and Medicine. Macmillan, London.

World Health Organization, 1992. The ICD-10 Classification of Mental and Behavioral Disorders: Clinical Description and Diagnostic Guidelines. World Health Organization, Geneva.

Disturbance of Memory

Chapter Outline

KEYWORDS

Memory
Confabulation
Ganser state

Summary

Memory has a well-described and delineated architecture, namely, sensory memory, short-term memory and long-term memory. Short-term memory is itself subdivided into a central executive and the slave systems, termed the *visuospatial scratch pad* and the *phonological loop*. This architecture allows for a systematic understanding of the underlying processes at play in memory. It is helpful to conceptualize the memory processes as including *registration*, *retention*, *retrieval*, *recall* and *recognition*. These terms allow for an understanding of the anomalies that are exhibited in organic impairments of memory.

Cans't thou not minister to a mind diseas'd;
Pluck from the memory a rooted sorrow;
Raze out the written troubles of the brain;
And with some sweet oblivious antidote
Cleanse the stuff'd bosom of that perilous stuff
Which weighs upon the heart?

                    William Shakespeare (1606)

Disturbance of memory is always of significance for the sufferer; sometimes, however, forgetting is equally important and is an active process, as in the preceding quotation from Shakespeare. That memory disturbance was a specific feature after head injury and other conditions was recognized in neuropsychiatric writings in the mid-19th century. Hughlings Jackson (1835–1911; 1887) considered it to be an integral part of deterioration in organic mental functioning. The earliest detailed study of disordered memory from a psychological standpoint was by Théodule-Armand

Ribot (1839–1916; 1882). Sergei Korsakov (1854–1900; 1890) subsequently described his eponymous condition, pointing out that gross disorder of memory may occur in patients in whom other intellectual functions and judgement are preserved.

Mechanisms of Memory

One of the major justifications for using psychopathology in the description of memory disturbance is that there exists no good analogue of memory in animals. Conventionally, disturbance of memory is described by the length of time for which information has been retained. If one concentrates on the phenomenological aspects, the analysis of experience, it is in fact quite arbitrary to make a distinction between memory and perception because they are both stages in information processing (Weinman, 1981). Memory *storage* is organized in three ways.

SENSORY MEMORY

Sensory memory is the initial and early phase of memory. It holds large amounts of incoming information briefly. It is a selecting and recording system via which perceptions enter the memory system (Lezak et al., 2004). Fleeting visual image, *iconic* memory lasts up to 200 ms, whereas auditory, *echoic* memory lasts up to 2000 ms. The information selected and recorded at this level needs to be further processed as short-term memory, or it quickly decays and is lost.

SHORT-TERM MEMORY

Short-term memory is conceptualized as a limited-capacity system that operates as a set of subsystems. Although it is theoretically distinguishable from attention, in practice it is profitably equated with a simple span of attention limited to six or seven items and lasting 15 to 30 seconds unless the items are rehearsed. Baddeley and Hitch (1974) hypothesized a model of working memory comprising a *central executive, a visuospatial scratch pad* and a *phonological loop*. In this system, the *central executive* is the attentional controller assisted by the *visuospatial scratch pad* that allows for the temporary storage and manipulation of visual and spatial information. The *phonological loop* holds memory traces of verbal information for a couple of seconds combined with subvocal rehearsal (Baddeley, 1986, 2002).

LONG-TERM MEMORY

Long-term memory can be conceptualized into two retrieval systems: a *declarative* system, or *explicit* memory, which deals with facts and events and is available to consciousness for declaration, and a nondeclarative or implicit system (Lezak et al., 2004). The declarative system can be further divided into *semantic* (fact memory) and *episodic* (memory for specific autobiographical incidents) memory. In other words, *semantic memory* is the storage of information in pure form without specification of time or place ('*General Psychopathology* was written by Karl Jaspers'), whereas *episodic memory* refers to personally experienced events ('I had a kipper for breakfast today') (Baddeley, 1990). Long-term memory can hold information for periods of time from a few minutes to many decades, and the capacity is very large. Forgetting may be by loss of information or failure of retrieval. Normal forgetting rates are determined by such variables as personal meaningfulness of the material, conceptual style and age. Storage in and retrieval from the long-term memory are impaired in the *dysmnesic syndromes*. Information is stored in reorganized and sometimes distorted form.

Description of the requirements for memory is chiefly referable to long-term memory and can be subdivided *phenomenologically* into the following five functions:

1. *Registration* or *encoding* is the capacity to add new information to the memory store.
2. *Retention* or *storage* is the ability to maintain knowledge that can subsequently be returned to consciousness.
3. *Retrieval* is the capacity to access stored information from memory by recognition, recall or implicitly by demonstrating that a relevant task is performed more efficiently as a result of prior experience.
4. *Recall* is the effortful retrieval of stored information into consciousness at a chosen moment. It requires an active, complex search process. It is influenced by *primacy* (first item) and *recency* (last item) effects. The question 'What is the capital of France?' requires the recall function.
5. *Recognition* is the retrieval of stored information that depends on the identification of items previously learned and is based on either *re-*

membering (effortful recollection) or *knowing* (familiarity-based recollection). In this process, a stimulus triggers awareness; remembering or knowing then takes place. The question 'Which of the following is the capital of France: Paris, Lille or Lyon?' tests the recognition function.

Abnormality of memory may occur in any of these areas. In other words, there can be impairment of encoding, impairment of storage or impairment of retrieval.

Organic Impairment of Memory

Memory disturbances can be separated into those that are psychogenic, sometimes occurring in healthy people, and those that are organic, associated with disease of the brain. The latter are referred to as *organic* or *true* amnesias and can be described by the different functions of memory.

IMPAIRMENT OF REGISTRATION/ENCODING

In *anterograde amnesia*, the impairment is usually demonstrated in the failure of retrieval of information encountered after the onset of a clinical disorder. This impairment of retrieval may, of course, be due to problems at the registration (encoding) stage, particularly in patients with Korsakov's syndrome. There is evidence that these patients may have difficulty in spontaneously encoding the semantic features of information to a sufficient level at input, and this failure results in poor memory (Mayes, 2002). It is therefore problems in the initial analysis and representation of information and the inability to select the salient semantic features of information that underlie impairment of registration. In a list-learning test situation, for example, the semantic features of the words, such as the fact that the words are derived from a list of the names of flowers, fails to assist the subject to encode the new information.

IMPAIRMENT OF RETENTION

Retrograde amnesia is the loss of memory for events preceding the onset of brain injury. As with anterograde amnesia, the deficit is demonstrated in the impairment of retrieval, but it is thought to be due to impairment of retention (storage), particularly in cases of cerebral trauma. Usually, it is of short duration of

less than 30 minutes. Typically, it follows a temporal gradient in which newer memories are more vulnerable to loss than older ones. There is a dissociation between anterograde and retrograde amnesia such that registration may be impaired without any impairment of retention. This suggests that the anatomic structures involved in new learning and retention of old memories are distinct.

IMPAIRMENT OF RETRIEVAL OR RECALL

Retrieval is the capacity to access information from memory stores. Impairment of retrieval can be due to a deficit in either *direct retrieval*, in which a cue elicits a memory automatically or *strategic (indirect) retrieval* in which a cue provokes a strategic search process that produces a result. In *direct retrieval*, the question 'Have you ever been to Lagos?' acts as a cue that elicits a memory automatically. In *strategic retrieval*, the question 'Who won the World Cup before the current champions?' instigates a strategic process that frames the memory problem, initiates the search and constrains it, guiding it towards local, proximal cues that then activate associative memory processes. The memory output is then monitored for accuracy and placed in a proper temporal-spatial context in relation to other memories (Gilboa and Moscovitch, 2002). *Direct retrieval* is thought to be dependent on medial temporal lobes and related structures, whereas *strategic retrieval* is dependent on the ventromedial prefrontal cortex. Confabulation is a good example of a condition that is a result of impairment of retrieval. It results from a faulty memory system creating faulty cue–memory associations, faulty search strategies and defective monitoring of faulty memories (Gilboa and Moscovitch, 2002; DeLuca, 2009).

IMPAIRMENT OF RECOGNITION

Recognition is the retrieval of stored information that depends on the identification of items previously learned. In episodic memory, that is, memory for events that includes the context, time, place and emotions associated with the event, recognition can take the form of either conscious recollection (*remembering*) or *knowing* based simply on a sense of familiarity. This is the so-called *remember–know paradigm,* and it proposes a dual process memory system, one relying on conscious recollection and the other based on familiarity. In other words, the phenomenal experience that accompanies the recognition of a previously presented stimulus seems to take at least two forms. Recognition can occur when the stimulus evokes some specific experience in which the stimulus was previously involved, or alternatively the stimulus gives rise only to a feeling of familiarity without any recollective experience. A 'remember' response indicates that recognizing the stimulus brings back to mind some conscious recollection of its prior occurrence, whereas a 'know' response indicates that recognizing the stimulus is not accompanied by any conscious recollection of its prior occurrence (Dalla Barba, 1997; Tulving, 2000). Impairment of recognition has been described in Alzheimer's disease (Dalla Barba, 1997) and in schizophrenia (Drakeford et al., 2006).

Disturbances of Memory

NORMAL VARIATIONS
Déjà Vu and Related Phenomena (Paramnesia)

Déjà vu is not primarily a memory disorder but a disturbance in which the associated feeling of familiarity that normally accompanies previously experienced events occurs with a novel event, that is, when the event is experienced for the first time. An example might be having a strong feeling that one has been previously in a restaurant situated in a city that one is visiting for the first time. In *jamais vu*, an experience that the patient knows they have experienced before is not associated with the appropriate feeling of familiarity. An example might be that of visiting a museum in one's own hometown that one has visited several times in the past but, on this particular occasion, failing to have any sense of familiarity. The person may also have the feeling that some important memory is about to be recalled, although it does not actually arrive.

Déjà vu and *jamais vu* are relatively common, normal experiences but may also be significant symptoms of temporal lobe epilepsy or cerebrovascular disorder (Lishman, 1998). An epileptic patient said, 'I feel that I've done something terribly wrong'. However, these experiences on their own or associated only with vague feelings of depersonalization should not be accepted as evidence of temporal lobe epilepsy, as these symptoms are also frequently experienced both in patients with anxiety-related disorders and in normal individuals.

Selective Forgetting

In normal forgetting, there is loss of or diminished access to recently acquired and stored information. Rates of forgetting are influenced by the personal meaningfulness of the information, the conceptual style of the individual, the degree of processing and elaboration of the information and age. It is likely that normal forgetting is determined by disuse or interference by more recently learned or more vivid material and underpinned by physiologic or metabolic processes (Lezak et al., 2004). Additionally, there are two forms of interference: *proactive* and *retroactive*. In proactive interference, newly learned material interferes with the recall of previously learned material. In retroactive interference, previously learned material interferes with the recall of newly learned material (for a fuller discussion, see Eysenck and Keane, 2010).

The process of *repression* or *selective forgetting*, however, suggests that forgetting is not simply down to errors in the filing and retrieval mechanism. Forgetting is subject to the influence of affect: which sensations are registered, what is retained and for how long and what information is available for recall. In Freud's (1856–1939) account, traumatic or threatening memories are kept out of conscious awareness by the mechanism of repression. Other forms of active forgetting exist, including motivated forgetting, which subsumes repression as an example. Directed forgetting is the term for the process by which we actively use executive control processes within the prefrontal cortex to forget items that we do not wish to recall. It is obvious from the foregoing that forgetting is an important and normative process. The processes underlying directed forgetting are still being investigated. It is unclear to what degree intentional forgetting is an active process based on the inhibition of unwanted memory traces or reduction of selective rehearsal (Han et al., 2020). Furthermore, there is some evidence that depression may impair the capacity to forget negative material (Xie et al., 2018). In short, selective forgetting including directed forgetting involves unconscious and conscious mechanisms.

Falsification of Memory

False memories concern report of events that never happened or distorted memories of events that happened with the result that an individual claims that something happened and they believe and remember that it happened despite the fact their belief is erroneous (French et al., 2009). The mechanisms underpinning false memories in normal populations are relatively well established. First, false memories are commonplace in nonclinical populations as demonstrated by the significant numbers of people reporting alien abduction experiences. Second, studies of the *flashbulb memories* have shown that even for culturally significant and unique events such as the World Trade Centre attacks in New York in 2001, there is considerable distorted recall by witnesses of the event (French et al., 2009).

The mechanisms underlying the creation of false memories include exposure to postevent information and the role of misinformation in facilitating addition of nonexistent detail in reports. Susceptibility to false memory is at least partly determined by the quality of memory for the relevant observed event.

It is remarkable that it is practically impossible to distinguish between true and false memories in terms of the associated emotions or the degree of confidence with which the belief is held and, as French et al. (2009) suggest, this probably means that both kinds of memories are constructed in the same way. Both involve source monitoring and plausibility. Source monitoring involves determining the source of the experience whether it be internal (imagination) or external (actually experienced). Plausibility refers to the degree to which the event is likely to occur in the real world. Mazzoni et al. (2001) propose that there are three steps necessary for people to develop a false memory: (1) they must believe that the specific event could plausibly have happened, (2) they must develop a belief that the event actually happened to them and (3) they must make a source monitoring error and erroneously conclude that the details they remember must have come from a real experience.

The nature and origins of false memories in the normal population help to inform our understanding of false memories in clinical populations by drawing attention to the underlying mechanisms and to the similarities and differences in the nature, extent and behavioural consequences of false memories as described earlier. However, studies of false memories have not fully established any consistent findings either with regard to personality factors or to motivational factors. Yet these factors probably play a significant role in clinical populations.

In *pseudologia fantastica*—fluent, plausible lying—the untruthful statements are often grandiose and extreme. Questions are answered with fluency, and the story appears to be believed implicitly by the pseudologics themselves. Hence, it is often unclear the degree to which the patient believes the account. This usually occurs with an associated personality disorder and often when the individual is experiencing a major life crisis such as facing criminal proceedings. The picture is of a very isolated person, without family or friends, drifting into the accident and emergency department of a large hospital in a strange city late at night, with stories of their own exploits and importance and the unfortunate vicissitudes they have experienced. There is overlap with factitious disorder.

With personality disorders and also with affective disorders, especially at times of heightened emotion, memory is falsified and distorted, and events and circumstances can be misrepresented. The advice of doctors may be grossly misconstrued. An ophthalmic surgeon examined a depressed patient's eyes and informed her that her visual acuity was satisfactory and no treatment was required. She reported the following to her psychiatrist: her 'eyesight would be bad forevermore, and the surgeon has told me that nothing can be done about it'.

Inaccuracy of recall is sometimes called *paramnesia*. As well as occurring in the normal state and in personality disorders, it is a prominent feature of affective disturbances. A woman with depressive illness falsified the events of her life: 'I am not married. My children are illegitimate. We do not own this house. We are bankrupt.' All these statements were untrue, and the falsification of her memory occurred in response to her severe depressive mood. Memory itself was accurate, but on remonstrating on any particular point of fact, further depressive explanations of events would be given. For instance, the marriage licence was described as a forgery, and complicated legal explanations were given as to why the house did not belong to her and her husband. In mania, unacceptable events or opinions may be brushed aside as not having occurred and unrealistic goals pursued as though there were nothing to prevent their attainment.

MEANINGFUL DISTURBANCES OF MEMORY

Psychogenic Disturbance of Memory

Cryptomnesia can be described as a phenomenon in which what is objectively a memory is subjectively not recognized as such and is thus wrongly experienced by a person as a novel or original creation of their own mind. It can be regarded as unintended plagiarism (Taylor, 1965). There are a number of celebrated cases in the public domain which illustrate the nature of cryptomnesia including the so-called *twin poems* incident. Clifford Dyment, an English poet and journalist wrote a poem, *Saint Augustine at Thirty-Two*, first published in a journal in 1943 and included in a book of poems in 1944. The book was reviewed by Vita Sackville-West in 1944 after which she wrote to Dyment telling him how much she liked the poem. In 1949 at the invitation of the Poetry Review, Sackville-West submitted a poem for publication entitled *The Novice to her Lover*. Sackville-West's poem replicated 87 of the 100 words of Dyment's poem. Ironically, when Dyment's poem was once again included in another book in 1949, she wrote to draw his attention to the similarities between his poem and hers and she had no recollection of having previously reviewed his nor of having written to him about her appreciation of the poem (Taylor, 1965). The underlying mechanism of this phenomenon is yet to be fully elucidated.

Misnaming objects and momentary loss of memory for words in healthy subjects may result from faulty retrieval from short- and long-term memory stores rather than from the psychoanalytic explanation of repression. Such errors may be categorized as *acoustic* or *semantic*; acoustic errors tending to occur in short-term stores of up to 30 seconds and semantic ones in long-term stores after more than 5 minutes (Shallice and McGill, 1977).

Dissociative Focal Retrograde Amnesia

This is a condition in which there is focal retrograde amnesia for autobiographical events. There is no demonstrable anterograde amnesia. A 20-year-old student was found on the floor of his flat. The retrograde amnesia was for a period of approximately 3 years. He was conscious when discovered, and there was no history of head injury or any physical illness. His magnetic resonance imaging scan and other investigations including his electroencephalogram were reported as normal. The social context included the fact that his parents were separating. However, he said that there was not a significant or stressful event. He slowly made a full recovery. This condition can also occur in the context of a neurologic amnesia, but the extent and severity of the amnesia are judged to exceed what is expected (see McKay and Kopelman, 2009). The assumption here is that the focal amnesia results from psychological stressors that the individual is inappropriately attempting to deal with by virtue of amnesia. Usually it is assumed that there are unconscious processes at play.

Dissociative Fugue

The symptoms pertaining to dissociative (conversion) disorders in the *International Classification of Diseases* (10th revision *[ICD-10];* World Health Organization, 1992) are of two types: conversion and dissociation. In dissociation, there is a narrowing of the field of consciousness, with subsequent amnesia for the episode. In many ways, dissociative symptoms represent a layman's impression of 'madness'. In dissociative fugue states, there is narrowing of consciousness, wandering away from normal surroundings and subsequent amnesia. It involves loss of all autobiographical memories including identity. The person appears to be in good contact with their environment and usually behaves appropriately, maintaining basic self-care, although they sometimes display disinhibition. There is quite often loss of identity or assumption of another false identity. The duration of the episode can be very variable, from a few hours to several weeks, and the subject may travel considerable distances. A citizen of Birmingham, United Kingdom, described a state in which he 'came to' in a city he did not recognize and where people were speaking French. As he walked about the streets, he found he was near an airport terminal and, to his surprise, he discovered that he was in Montreal. Germane to his adventure was the history of a catastrophic row and the breakdown of his marriage just before he took off. Thus the features of dissociative fugue are dissociative amnesia, purposeful travel beyond the usual everyday range and maintenance of basic self-care (World Health Organization, 1992).

The predisposing factors include (1) precipitating stress resulting from relationship, marital or financial problems; (2) depressed mood including suicidal thoughts; and (3) a past history of transient organic amnesia (McKay and Kopelman, 2009).

Recovered Memory and False Memory Syndrome

This is one of the most hotly debated issues in psychiatry and clinical psychology. Those working with survivors of traumatic experiences noted in their patients the recovery of additional memories during clinical sessions after apparent psychogenic amnesia for a long time—sometimes decades. Recovered memory has been particularly associated with the return of memory for childhood sexual abuse. Brewin (1996) reviews the evidence for such events being 'forgotten' and then recalled after many years and the mechanisms that may account for this amnesia. He concludes that memories may be recovered from total amnesia, and they may sometimes be essentially accurate. Equally, such 'memories' may sometimes be inaccurate in whole or in part. An example of recovered memory is a 45-year-old male patient who was being investigated for possible colon cancer after presentation with blood in his stool. His general practitioner conducted a rectal examination, and immediately after this examination, the patient recalled incidents from his childhood of sexual abuse that caused him great distress and required specialized counselling.

The term *false memory syndrome* came into use in 1992, when the False Memory Syndrome Foundation was set up to represent the interests of parents who had been accused of abusing their children sexually. In the opinion of Merskey (1998), sufferers from false memory syndrome are typically female and are usually participating in some type of psychotherapy. They report sexual abuse in childhood that is claimed to have been forgotten and subsequently recovered only in adult life, having been repressed from 8 to 40 years. It is considered that these 'memories' have been implanted during therapy by a process of suggestion similar to that thought to occur in multiple personality disorder. Another situation in which false memories have been thought to develop has been in nursery day care, when caregivers have been subjected to grave and bizarre accusations.

There is empirical evidence demonstrating that there are differences between individuals whose recovered memories have been recalled inside therapy, those whose memories were recalled outside therapy and a third group whose memories of abuse were continuous from childhood into adulthood. In the first group, there was 0% corroborative evidence, whereas for the other two groups, it was 45% and 37%. Furthermore, those who had recovered memories outside therapy were able to suppress anxiety-provoking thoughts relating to those events compared with the groups with recovered memory from within therapy and the group with continuous memories, suggesting that women with recovered memories from outside therapy are especially adept at suppressing emotional memories when under laboratory conditions, confirming their liability to remain unaware of traumatic memories for long periods before their recovery (Geraerts et al., 2007, 2008).

MEMORY DISTURBANCE SECONDARY TO PSYCHIATRIC DISORDER

Confabulation

This is a falsification of memory occurring in clear consciousness in association with an organically derived amnesia (Berlyne, 1972). It is probably best to conceive of confabulation as a loose term that covers a wide range of qualitatively different memory phenomena. The term is used to describe mild distortions of an actual memory, such as intrusions, embellishments, elaborations, paraphrasing or high false alarm rates on tests of anterograde amnesia. It can also refer to highly implausible bizarre descriptions of false realities such as claiming to be a space traveller temporarily resident on earth (Gilboa and Moscovitch, 2002; Box 5.1). However, it is also true that the term *confabulation* has been extended, unhelpfully in my view, to include the following:

1. memory confabulations;
2. confabulations about intentions and actions as can occur in split-brain subjects or in hemiplegia of the left arm in which the subject denies their disability;
3. perceptual confabulations that occur in Anton syndrome characterized by unawareness of blindness; and
4. confabulation about emotions (for a fuller review, see Hirstein, 2009).

BOX 5.1 CHARACTERISTICS OF CONFABULATION

- It is a falsely retrieved memory, often containing false details within its own context.
- The patient is unaware that he or she is confabulating and often unaware of the existence of memory deficit. In other words, confabulations are not intentionally produced.
- Patients may act on their confabulation, confirming their belief in the false memory.
- Confabulation is most apparent in autobiographical memory.

From Gilboa, A., Moscovitch, M., 2002. Cognitive neuroscience of confabulation. In: Baddeley, A.D., Kopelman, M.D., Wilson, B.A. (Eds.), The Handbook of Memory Disorders, second ed. John Wiley, Chichester. With permission of John Wiley.

Bonhoeffer (1901, cited in Berlyne, 1972) observed that confabulation in Korsakov's syndrome could take two forms:

- Confabulation of *embarrassment* was a direct result of the memory loss and depended for its presence on a certain attentiveness and activity. This form of confabulation is *momentary,* a term introduced by Berlyne (1972), in nature. The momentary form of confabulation is often provoked by questions probing the patient's memory for particular events. The patient tries to cover an exposed memory gap by an ad hoc confabulated excuse relating to their recent behaviour. It does, therefore, reveal social awareness and some realization of the requirements of the situation in terms of social behaviour.
- In other cases, confabulation exceeded the needs of the memory impairment; the patient describes spontaneously adventurous experiences of a *fantastic* nature. The spontaneity is a key characteristic of this form of confabulation. Such memory disturbance may occur with organic deterioration after alcohol abuse and also in the 'organic amnesic syndrome, not induced by alcohol and other psychoactive substances' (*ICD-10;* World Health Organization, 1992), in which there is severe memory impairment, especially for recent memory; evidence for disorder of the brain; and absence of a defect in immediate recall, a disturbance of attention and consciousness, and global intellectual impairment.

The terms *momentary* and *fantastic* confabulation overlap somewhat with the terms *provoked* and *spontaneous* confabulation introduced by Kopelman

(1987). Provoked confabulation is said to be common in amnestic patients and resembles errors produced by healthy subjects at prolonged retention intervals during memory tests and may represent a normal response to a faulty memory. On the other hand, spontaneous confabulation is a rare pathologic phenomenon that probably results from the combination of frontal lobe pathology on an organic amnesia.

There is little doubt that the classification into subtypes of confabulation is work in progress. Schnider (2008) proposed an even more complex classification into four subtypes: (1) intrusions in memory, (2) momentary confabulations, (3) fantastic confabulations and (4) behaviourally spontaneous confabulations. This classification was developed to accommodate the empirical findings about the distinctions between the varying proposed categories but is, in my view, cumbersome.

Suggestibility is a prominent feature of the confabulating patient and was considered by Pick (1921, cited by Berlyne, 1972) to be dependent on clouding of consciousness, weakened judgement and the interplay of fantasy; it may, in fact, closely resemble daydreams. The confabulating patient may produce mutually contradictory statements consecutively and not make any attempt to correct them. The material of confabulations has been likened to dreams (Scheid, 1934, cited by Berlyne, 1972). It has also been explained, in terms of memory disturbance, that confabulations are actual experiences taken out of their chronologic order (Van der Horst, 1932) and that the individual's wishes and interests guide confabulation in the same way as in dreams and fantasy.

It seems probable that confabulation is related to the normal mechanisms of recollection. For example, say that all the owners of a certain model of car were asked by the police, as part of a large-scale murder hunt, what they were doing on a particular Monday about 9 months previously. To answer this question, an individual would have no recollection for that particular Monday, so they would re-create a typical programme with regular movements and times of appointments for a Monday from about that period. It would seem that the mechanism of *social confabulation* is of that order. To the question 'What did you do yesterday?', the confabulating patient might say, 'I pushed my baby in the pram down to the office to see my old workmates there'.

This could indeed have happened 12 years previously after she had resigned her job in that office during her pregnancy. The *fantastic* type of confabulation is also directly associated with memory. Normally, one has a clear memory of which sensations and events were experienced and which were fantasized, yet with confabulation it is probable that distant fantasies are remembered, but it is not remembered that they were fantasy rather than reality. Such confabulations, like the *momentary* type, are autobiographical. The momentary or embarrassment confabulation is very much more common than the fantastic type and is a true memory displaced in its time context (Berlyne, 1972).

Fantastic confabulation with persecutory content has been described by Roth and Myers (1969). This is a falsification of memory occurring in clear consciousness. Typically, the patient believes others are stealing their money or trying to defraud them. Memory falsifications of various types occur in schizophrenia, depressive illness, antisocial personality disorder and obsessional states. The more definite, fantastic and gap-filling features of organic confabulations are always associated with memory defect.

Central to the idea of confabulation is therefore a notion of false reports in the context of memory disorder. At a minimum, it involves distortions of both content and temporal context. The issue of distortions of temporal context has perhaps been understated in the literature. It refers to the finding that, in confabulation, there are often recollections of true events but that are incorrectly orientated in time and place. In other words, it is an impairment of the chronological order of events, what might be termed an *impairment of temporal order,* or *source monitoring.* The confabulatory recollection also often includes additions, distortions or elaborations that either actually or plausibly occurred (DeLuca, 2009):

Doctor: What did you do today?
Patient VR: Today I got up this morning and visited the rehabilitation unit … then I went home and was expecting some material and we received it. Then I came to the rehabilitation institute, no I actually went to Jimsburg store and we had a small meeting there. Then I came to the hospital and we had lunch and, then met with you.

The example first illustrates content distortion because the patient had been in hospital for several months without going home and, second, impaired temporal context because the patient had owned Jimsburg store many years before and had sold it.

The current view is that memory confabulation usually derives from dual lesions taking in basal forebrain areas and frontal executive systems. These lesions appear to result in impaired strategic retrieval of memory and disturbed verification/monitoring of the abnormal memory output (DeLuca, 2009).

Perseveration

Perseveration usually occurs in association with disturbance of memory and is a sign of organic brain disease, perhaps the only pathognomonic sign in psychiatry. Perseveration is defined as a response that was appropriate to a first stimulus being given inappropriately to a second, different stimulus. This may be demonstrated verbally or in motor activity. The interviewer, while conducting the mental state examination, asks, 'What is the capital of Italy?' The patient responds, 'Rome'. Subsequently the interviewer asks, 'What is the object that you wear that tells you the time?' The patient again responds, 'Rome'. Alternatively, the examiner asks the patient to put their right hand on their left shoulder, which they do correctly, and then, on asking them to put their left hand on their left knee, they again put their right hand on their left shoulder.

Memory Impairment in Schizophrenia

Earlier writers tended to play down the significance of intellectual impairment in schizophrenia (Bleuler, 1911; Kraepelin, 1913). However, decline in intellectual performance (Rogers, 1986), impairment in neuropsychological test batteries (Taylor and Abrams, 1984), sometimes a dementia-like syndrome (Liddle and Crow, 1984) and substantial memory deficit (Cutting, 1985; McKenna et al., 1990) have been demonstrated. Memory deficit has been shown not to be restricted to patients with chronic schizophrenia.

There are deficits in long-term memory, including evidence of impaired retrieval in both recall and recognition. There is also evidence of impaired short-term memory, demonstrated by deficit of forward digit span. Furthermore, there is evidence of impairment of working memory and semantic memory, but procedural or implicit memory is intact. The memory deficit has been shown to be associated with severity and chronicity of illness, negative symptoms and formal thought disorder (Tamlyn et al., 1992; McKenna et al., 2002).

Furthermore, in schizophrenia, remembered circumstances often take on a new meaning: 'I remember last week three red cars following me at the traffic lights in Stafford … I realized that I have become involved in politics'. This was stated by a patient who had quite suddenly come to believe that all her actions were being observed and, subsequently, her behaviour controlled. Memory is accurate, but its significance is distorted. A distinction should be made between delusional memories in which the primary delusional experience is a true memory with delusional interpretation and delusional retrospective falsification. This is a backdating of delusion to a time before the patient was ill, based on an admixture of remembered true events and delusional elaboration of the meaning of those events. This has been described by some authorities as a form of confabulation (Nathaniel-James and Frith, 1996). In the original study, when subjects were presented with narratives and asked to recall them, *confabulation* was defined as recall of information not present in the original narrative. The degree of confabulation was related to problems in suppressing inappropriate responses and formal thought disorder. In summary, there is little doubt that confabulation occurs in schizophrenia and is related to formal thought disorder, but it has a different signature compared to confabulation in the setting of neurological disease (Lorente-Rovira et al., 2007).

Affective Disorder of Memory

Memory is not only disturbed by organic damage to the brain itself, it is also affected by emotion. This is certainly true of normal, healthy people in whom the affective state strongly influences the processes of remembering and forgetting. It is also true of those with affective and schizophrenic psychoses, and of neuroses and personality disorders. Depression is linked to self-reported memory problems. There is also substantial evidence of an association between depression and generic memory impairment. It is thought that mood disorder, such as depression, reduces the amount of cognitive processing resources available for a given task, and in the memory domain this is manifest as deficits in the elaboration, organization, encoding and retrieval of material into and out of memory (Dalgleish and Cox, 2002). There is also evidence of memory bias for affectively toned material such that information that has an emotional valence is more likely to be retrieved if it is congruent with the individual's mood during retrieval. This *mood-congruent memory* effect is similar but distinct from *state-dependent memory*, which refers to the memory bias for material that is learned in a particular mood and is more easily retrieved if the individual is in that same mood during retrieval.

GANSER STATE

The original paper by Ganser (1898) has been much misunderstood. In it, he described four criminals who showed the following symptoms.

- *Vorbeigehen* ('to pass by'), or *approximate answers*, described by Ganser thus 'In the choice of answers the patient appears to deliberately pass over the indicated correct answer and to select a false one, which any child could *recognize* as such'.
- Clouding of consciousness with disorientation.
- 'Hysterical' stigmata.
- Recent history of head injury, typhus or severe emotional stress.
- 'Hallucinations', auditory and visual (from his description, they are more like pseudohallucinations).
- Amnesia for the period during which the preceding symptoms were manifest.

The Ganser state is rarely seen in English prisons, but, when it does occur, it is more likely in those awaiting trial than in those already sentenced (Enoch, 1990). A report of Ganser state in a man held in solitary confinement in prison both demonstrated the rarity of the condition in prison as well as the influence of the nature of the criminal charge, namely paedophilia in this case (Andersen et al., 2001). This case was only one of 268 remand prisoners and one of 33 held in solitary confinement for at least 2 months in the study period, all the others without developing Ganser state.

There has been considerable argument as to whether this condition is primarily dissociative in nature or an organic psychosis, with different authors supporting each contention (Latcham et al., 1978). A case that illustrated both the hysterical (dissociative) and organic elements was that of a female university student, aged 20 years, who experienced head injury with concussion when in Italy. Her premorbid personality was markedly histrionic and theatrical and, at the age of 13 years, she had developed a dissociative motor disorder in that she was unable to walk for a few weeks. After transfer from the Italian hospital to Britain, she demonstrated approximate answers:

Question: 'What is the capital of Italy?'
Answer: 'Naples'.
Question: 'How many legs has a centipede?'
Answer: 'Seven'.

This was accompanied by interference in the treatment of other patients, flirtatious behaviour towards male staff, lability of mood and a facetious manner. On serial testing of intellectual function on the Wechsler Adult Intelligence Scale, initial testing 12 days after head injury had to be abandoned; after 1 month, there was marked impairment, worse for performance than for verbal items. Intellectual function had eventually returned to her premorbid, superior level by 9 months. It is important to emphasize the point that the original description by Ganser already indicated the role of organic factors in Ganser state. To further underline this, Anupama et al. (2006) report a case associated with left-sided temporoparietal haemorrhage. Whitlock (1967) considers the distinction between the Ganser state and pseudodementia to lie in disturbed consciousness, present in the former and not the latter. However, sometimes clouding of consciousness in an organic state cannot be distinguished from the altered mental state of dissociative disorder in the absence of other organic signs.

Enoch and Trethowan (1979) have regarded the four main features of Ganser syndrome as:
- approximate answers,
- clouding of consciousness,
- somatic conversion features, and
- pseudohallucinations (not always present).

It should be noted that approximate answers are not the random inaccuracies of the quick guess but responses that appear deliberately to miss the correct answer. These authors regard the syndrome as a hysterical dissociative reaction and have pointed out the similarity of features with those exhibited by normal people asked to simulate mental disorder, the difference being that the Ganser subjects were subsequently amnesic for their abnormal behaviour. Ungvari and Mullen (1997) have classified Ganser syndrome with the controversial group of reactive psychoses so that a stressful life event is the usual predisposing factor. Cutting (2011) has a novel and original approach to Ganser syndrome. On the basis of examination of a number of cases including two of his own, he concludes that the Ganser syndrome is either part of a depressive illness or a transient disturbance in the left hemisphere's lexical or semantic knowledge. Cutting argues that the knowledge deficit demonstrable in Ganser syndrome is not hysterical on any account but a manifestation of a particular kind of cognitive impairment.

REFERENCES

Andersen, H.S., Sestoft, D., Lillebaek, T., 2001. Ganser syndrome after solitary confinement in prison: a short review and a case report. Nord. J. Psychiatry. 55, 199–201.

Anupama, M., Rao, K.N., Dhananjaya, S., 2006. Ganser syndrome and lesion in the temporoparietal region. Indian J. Psychiatry. 48, 123–125.

Baddeley, A.D., 1986. Working Memory. Clarendon, Oxford.

Baddeley, A.D., 1990. Human Memory: Theory and Practice. Erlbaum, Hove.

Baddeley, A.D., 2002. The psychology of memory. In: Baddeley, A.D., Kopelman, M.D., Wilson, B.A. (Eds.), The Handbook of Memory Disorders. John Wiley, Chichester, pp. 3–15.

Baddeley, A.D., Hitch, G., 1974. Working memory. In: Bower, G.A. (Ed.), Recent Advances in Learning and Motivation, vol. 8. Academic Press, New York, pp. 47–89.

Berlyne, N., 1972. Confabulation. Br. J. Psychiatry. 120, 31–39.

Bleuler, E., 1911. Dementia Praecox or the Group of Schizophrenias (J. Zikin, Trans, 1950). International Universities Press, New York.

Bonhoeffer, K., 1901. Die akuten Geisteskrankheiten der Gewohnheitstrinker. Gustav Fischer, Jena.

Brewin, C.R., 1996. Scientific status of recovered memories. Br. J. Psychiatry. 169, 131–134.

Cutting, J.C., 1985. The Psychology of Schizophrenia. Churchill Livingstone, Edinburgh.

Cutting, J.C., 2011. A Critique of Psychopathology. The Forest Publishing Company, Forest Row.

Dalgleish, T., Cox, S.G., 2002. Memory and emotional disorder. In: Baddeley, A.D., Kopelman, M.D., Wilson, B.A. (Eds.), The Handbook of Memory Disorders, second ed. John Wiley, Chichester.

Dalla Barba, G., 1997. Recognition memory and recollective experience in Alzheimer's disease. Memory 5, 657–672.

DeLuca, J., 2009. Confabulation in anterior communicating artery syndrome. In: Hirstein, W. (Ed.), Confabulation: Views from Neuroscience, Psychiatry, Psychology, and Philosophy. Oxford University Press, Oxford.

Drakeford, J.L., Edelstyn, N.M., Oyebode, F., Srivastava, S., Calthorpe, W.R., Murkhejee, T., 2006. Auditory recognition memory, conscious recollection, and executive function in patients with schizophrenia. Psychopathology 39, 199–208.

Enoch, M.D., 1990. Hysteria, malingering, pseudologia fantastica, Ganser syndrome, prison psychosis and Münchausen's syndrome. In: Bluglass, R., Bowden, P. (Eds.), Principles and Practice of Forensic Psychiatry. Churchill Livingstone, Edinburgh.

Enoch, M.D., Trethowan, W.H., 1979. Uncommon Psychiatric Syndromes. John Wright, Bristol.

Eysenck, M.W., Keane, M.T., 2010. Cognitive Psychology: A Student's Handbook, sixth ed. Psychology Press, Hove.

French, L., Garry, M., Loftus, E., 2009. False memories: a kind of confabulation in non-clinical subjects. In: Hirstein, W. (Ed.), Confabulation: Views from Neuroscience, Psychiatry, Psychology, and Philosophy. Oxford University Press, Oxford.

Ganser, S.J.M., 1898. A peculiar hysterical state. Archiv fuer Psychiatrie und Nervenkrankheiten. 30, 633 (C.E. Schorer, Trans, 1965. Br. J. Criminol. 5, 120–126).

Geraerts, E., McNally, R.J., Jelicic, M., Merckelbach, H., Raymaekers, I., 2008. Linking thought suppression and recovered memories of childhood sexual abuse. Memory 16, 22–28.

Geraerts, E., Schooler, J.W., Merckelbach, H., Jelicic, M., Haner, B.J.A., Ambadar, Z., 2007. Corroborating continuous and discontinuous memories of childhood sexual abuse. Psychol. Sci. 18, 564–568.

Gilboa, A., Moscovitch, M., 2002. Cognitive neuroscience of confabulation. In: Baddeley, A.D., Kopelman, M.D., Wilson, B.A. (Eds.), The Handbook of Memory Disorders, second ed. John Wiley, Chichester.

Han, Z., Yang, Y., Zhang, Q., Mo, L., 2020. Can you voluntarily forget what you are planning to forget? Behavioural evidence for the underlying truth of the cot-benefit principle. Psychol. Res. 85 (4), 1567–1582. https://doi.org/10.1007/s00426-020-01339-8.

Hirstein, W., 2009. Introduction: what is confabulation? In: Hirstein, W. (Ed.), Confabulation: Views from Neuroscience, Psychiatry, Psychology, and Philosophy. Oxford University Press, Oxford.

Jackson, J.H., 1887. Remarks on evolution and dissolution of the nervous system. In: Taylor, J. (Ed.), Selected Writings of John Hughlings Jackson, vol. 2. Hodder & Stoughton, London, p. 1931.

Kopelman, M.D., 1987. Two types of confabulation. J. Neurol. Neurosurg. Psychiatry. 50, 1482–1487.

Korsakov, S.S., 1890. Eine psych. Storung combiniert mit multipler Neuritis. Allgemeine Zeitschrift fuer Psychiatrie. 46.

Kraepelin, E., 1913. Dementia Praecox and Paraphrenia (R.M. Barclay, Trans, 1919). Livingstone, Edinburgh.

Latcham, R.W., White, A.C., Sims, A.C.P., 1978. Ganser syndrome: the aetiological argument. J. Neurol. Neurosurg. Psychiatry. 41, 851–854.

Lezak, M.D., Howieson, D.B., Loring, D.W., 2004. Neuropsychological Assessment, fourth ed. Oxford University Press, Oxford.

Liddle, P.F., Crow, T.S., 1984. Age disorientation in schizophrenia is associated with global intellectual impairment. Br. J. Psychiatry. 144, 193–199.

Lishman, W.A., 1998. Organic Psychiatry: The Psychological Consequences of Cerebral Disorder, third ed. Blackwell Scientific, Oxford.

Lorente-Rovira, E., Pomarol-Clotet, E., McCarthy, R.A., Berrios, G.E., McKenna, P.J., 2007. Confabulation in schizophrenia and its relationship to clinical and neuropsychological features of the disorder. Psychol. Med. 37, 1403–1412.

Mayes, A.R., 2002. Anterograde amnesia. In: Baddeley, A.D., Kopelman, M.D., Wilson, B.A. (Eds.), The Handbook of Memory Disorders, second ed. John Wiley, Chichester.

Mazzoni, G., Loftus, E.F., Kirsch, I., 2001. Changing beliefs about implausible autobiographical events: a little plausibility goes a long way. J. Exp. Psychol. Appl. 7, 51–59.

McKay, G.C.M., Kopelman, M.D., 2009. Psychogenic amnesia: when memory complaints are medically unexplained. Adv. Psychiatr. Treat. 15, 152–158.

McKenna, P.J., Ornstein, T., Baddeley, A.D., 2002. Schizophrenia. In: Baddeley, A.D., Kopelman, M.D., Wilson, B.A. (Eds.), The Handbook of Memory Disorders, second ed. John Wiley, Chichester.

McKenna, P.J., Tamlyn, D., Lund, C.E., Mortimer, A.M., Hammond, S., Baddeley, A.D., 1990. Amnesic syndrome in schizophrenia. Psychol. Med. 20, 967–972.

Merskey, H., 1998. Prevention and management of false memory syndrome. Adv. Psychiatr. Treat. 4, 253–262.

Nathaniel-James, D.A., Frith, C.D., 1996. Confabulation in schizophrenia: evidence of a new form? Psychol. Med. 26, 391–399.

Pick, A., 1921. Neues Zur Psychologie der Konfabulation Msschr. Psychiatr. Neurol. 49, 314–321.

Ribot, E., 1882. Diseases of Memory: An Essay in the Positive Psychology. Kegan Paul, Trench & Co., London.

Rogers, D., 1986. Cognitive disturbances: real or apparent? Psychiatry Pract. 5, 6–8.

Roth, M., Myers, D.H., 1969. The diagnosis of dementia. Br. J. Hosp. Med. 2, 705–717.

Scheid, W., 1934. Zur Pathopsychologie des Korsakow Syndroms. Zeitschrift fuer Neurologie und Psychiatrie. 151, 346–369.

Schnider, A., 2008. The Confabulating Mind—How the Brain Creates Reality. Oxford University Press, Oxford.

Shakespeare, W., 1606. Macbeth V, Iii, pp. 41–46.

Shallice, T., McGill, J., 1977. Attention and purpose. In: Requin, J., Bertelson, P. (Eds.), The Origins of Mixed Errors. Academic Press, New York.

Tamlyn, D., McKenna, P.J., Mortimer, A.M., Lund, C.E., Hammond, S., Baddeley, A.D., 1992. Memory impairment in schizophrenia: its extent, affiliations and neuropsychological character. Psychol. Med. 22, 101–115.

Taylor, F.K., 1965. Cryptomnesia and plagiarism. Brit. J. Psychiat. 111, 1111–1118.

Taylor, M.A., Abrams, R., 1984. Cognitive impairment in schizophrenia. Am. J. Psychiatry. 141, 196–201.

Tulving, E., 2000. Concepts of memory. In: Tulving, E., Craik, F.I.M. (Eds.), Oxford Handbook of Memory. Oxford University Press, Oxford.

Ungvari, G.S., Mullen, P.E., 1997. Reactive psychoses. In: Bhugra, D., Munro, A. (Eds.), Troublesome Disguises. Underdiagnosed Psychiatric Syndromes. Blackwell Science, Oxford.

Van der Horst, L., 1932. Ueber die Psychologie des Korsakowsyndroms. Monatsschr. Psychiatr. Neurol. 83, 65–84.

Weinman, J., 1981. An Outline of Psychology as Applied to Medicine. John Wright, Bristol.

Whitlock, F.A., 1967. The Ganser syndrome. Br. J. Psychiatry. 113, 19–29.

World Health Organization, 1992. The ICD-10 Classification of Mental and Behavioural Disorders: Clinical Description and Diagnostic Guidelines. World Health Organization, Geneva.

Xie, H., Jiang, D., Zhang, D., 2018. Individuals with depressive tendencies experience difficulty in forgetting negative material: two mechanisms revealed ERP data in the directed forgetting paradigm. Sc. Rep. 8 (1), 113. https://doi.org/10.1038/s41598-018-19570-0.

AWARENESS OF REALITY: TIME, PERCEPTION AND JUDGEMENT

Disorder of Time

KEYWORDS

Time
Circadian rhythm
Disorientation

Summary

Time is integral to how human beings experience the world. Although it is difficult to define, there are some overt aspects such as duration, sequence, synchrony, rhythm, past, present, future orientation and an arrow of time that are easily recognizable and understood by most people without the need for further elaboration. There is also an important relationship with space and with notions of the self. Abnormalities of time experience can, broadly speaking, be divided into those that affect objective time and those that affect the subjective aspects of time experience. There are also influences of circadian rhythms, seasons, monthly cycles and life epochs that are worthy of noting.

Space and time are always present in sensory processes. They are not primary objects themselves but they invest all objectivity. Kant calls them 'forms of intuition'. They are universal. No sensation, no sensible object, no image is exempt from them. Everything in the world that is presented to us comes to us in space and time and we experience it only in these terms.

Jaspers (1997)

In the preceding quotation, Jaspers draws attention to the way in which human beings live in space and time and how all subjective experience is mediated by space and time. Jaspers continues:

If we want to bring these primary things home to ourselves in some neat phraseology we may say that they both represent the sundered existence of Being, separated from itself. Space is extended being (the side-

by-side) and time is sequential being (the one-after-the-other).

A sense of time is clearly central to the concept of self and its relationship with the outside world. But what exactly is time, and how is it experienced? Barbara Adam (1995) in her book *Time Watch* interviewed a number of people about how they experience time and some of their responses are both instructive and helpful:

How time enters my life? I was born and now I am fifteen years old. We use the word when we ask what time it is. We talk about closing time, lunch-time, getting up time, and that time is up. What time is, that is more difficult to say. It is not a person, not a thing, not a vegetable. It's a period and units, the day chopped up into hours, minutes and seconds. But it also divides the past from the future … The time is now, this very second. But I do not know what it is we are chopping up into units. I think it's an illusion since there isn't anything to be chopped.

For me time is a dimension within which everything moves and happens. In conjunction with space it is a universal framework. We can't move through space without time and vice versa which means that we can't pass, spend, or allocate time without occupying space. Nothing exists and happens without time and space.

Adam herself emphasizes various aspects of time as follows:

Thinking about time, therefore, involves rhythm with variation, a dynamic structure of framing, timing, synchronization, duration, sequence, tempo and intensity. This cluster of time characteristics is implicated at all levels of being, from the most physical of planetary movements via physiological rhythms to patterns of social organization, from the taken for granted via the invisible to the obvious, from the imposed via the lived to the culturally constructed.

Entailed within those processes is an irreversible unidirectionality, an arrow of time. There can be no rejuvenation, no unknowing, no reconstitution of pollution back into aeroplane.

These accounts indicate that time is difficult to define but that there are some overt aspects such as duration, sequence, synchrony, rhythm, past, present, future orientation and an arrow of time. There is also an important relationship with space and with notions of the self, particularly with enduring self-identity that has been remarked upon by many thinkers including Immanuel Kant (1781/1929; see *Critique of Pure Reason*).

There is a sense in which time leaves a signature on the most diverse aspects of human life, yet in such a way that the influence of time is often unrecognized. Aside from the obvious, such as overt ways of measuring time, there is a time dimension in memory, in language (given the reliance on word sequence and order for manifest meaning), through rhythm and note order on music and in all actions including symbolic movements, dance, sports and so on. Covertly, time is involved in such concepts as expectation, desire, hope, prayer and even death. These latter ideas have evolved from the writings of Eugene Minkowski (1885–1972; 1970), a phenomenological psychiatrist.

Disturbance of sense of time or time-related disorder is a sensitive indicator that something is going wrong either in the self or its mechanisms. Sense of time and time-related disorders of biological rhythm will be considered separately in this chapter. There is no widely agreed classification of disorders of time. However, it is possible to divide the disorders of time into two broad categories: disorder of objective time and disorder of subjective time (Box 6.1).

OBJECTIVE (CLOCK) TIME AND SUBJECTIVE (PERSONAL) TIME

An important distinction is that between *objective (clock) time* and *subjective (personal) time*. Objective time—chronologic, physical or historical time—is quantitative and independent of the self. It depends on accurate measurement and is objective to the degree that it is shared with others and verifiable. Subjective time is the inner, subjective experience of time. Aspects of both kinds of time may be affected by psychiatric illnesses. Objective time may be altered so that the knowledge of time, that is, the orientation to time including age disorientation and appreciation of time duration and of chronology may be adversely affected. Subjective time may be altered so that the

BOX 6.1   CLASSIFICATION OF DISORDERS OF TIME

DISORDER OF OBJECTIVE TIME
- Disorder of knowledge of time: disorientation in time; age disorientation
- Disorder of duration of time
- Disorder of chronology (temporal order)

DISORDER OF SUBJECTIVE TIME
- Disorder of flow of time
- Disorder of direction of time
- Disorder of uniqueness of time
- Disorder of quality of time

experience of time duration, flow of time, meaning of time, uniqueness of time and succession of time may be affected.

BIOLOGICAL RHYTHMS AND TIME

Although our units of time are to some extent arbitrary, natural and biological, time operates within definite periods. The four periods that have the most relevance to mental illness are circadian rhythms (about 24 hours—night and day), monthly cycles, seasonal variations and life epochs (from birth to death). All these rhythms are important for the mental state in times of health and form the basis for such conditions as early-morning wakening in depression, premenstrual tension, seasonal affective disorder and involutional melancholia. Many of these biological rhythms with variation of mood are biochemically mediated through the endocrine system.

Personal time (and also, to a lesser extent, clock time) is often described in relation to these biological rhythms. Our whole notion of the progression of time is closely related to processes of physical function: birth, growth and decay.

Disorder of Objective Time

Disorder of objective time involves (1) the ability to separate events into past, present and future, even if limited, (2) the capacity to estimate duration and (3) the ability to put events in the correct sequence. These skills are necessary for intellectual processes to be carried out satisfactorily. Disorder of knowledge of time is closely associated with disturbance of consciousness, attention and memory.

DISORIENTATION IN TIME

Disorientation for time is demonstrated by the inability to correctly tell the time without recourse to a clock and to indicate the date, day and season. This impairment is closely associated with impairment of attention, concentration, consciousness and memory. It is a feature of delirium and dementia. It is also a good clinical criterion for distinguishing between organic and functional disorders (Cutting, 1997). The second abnormality is impairment of the ability to assess the *duration of time,* and this is also disturbed in organic states.

AGE DISORIENTATION

The term *age disorientation* was first used by Zangwill (1953) in relation to Korsakov's syndrome to describe a 'fixed, stable disorientation for age, which was impervious to logical correction'. *Age disorientation,* now defined as a 5-year discrepancy between the patient's actual age and what the patient states to be his own age, has been considered to correlate clinically with intellectual impairment in chronic schizophrenia (Crow and Stevens, 1978). Such patients were much less able than chronic schizophrenic patients without age disorientation to answer questions about date and the duration of time. They systematically underestimated the present year and the duration of their stay in hospital and sometimes their own age.

This gives quantitative support to the observation that for some chronic patients 'time stands still'; they remain in the cultural set of the time when they developed their illness. Such patients tend to use the idiomatic language, sing the popular songs, wear the modish clothes and tell the characteristic jokes of the time before their illness became established. It is a mistake to believe that they are indulging in nostalgia; their cultural life is still firmly fixed within that particular period. Not only in the back ward of an old-fashioned mental hospital, but also in a hostel in the community, these patients live in their own time capsule with invisible, but impregnable, walls.

DISORDER OF TIME DURATION

Estimation of time duration has been studied using various methods, but the results have been inconsistent. Objective measures of estimation of the passage of time, for example, show that patients with depressive illness tend to underestimate the passage of 30 seconds, on average, by 6 seconds. This is compared with overestimation of the passage of time by normal control subjects by, on average, 10 seconds (Kuhs et al., 1991). That is to say that depressed patients on average estimated 30 seconds' duration as 24 seconds and the normal controls estimated 30 seconds' duration as 40 seconds. In other words, time appeared to flow more slowly for patients with depression than it did for normal controls. It is important to emphasize that this refers to estimation of the passage of momentary time. Other investigations have demonstrated an overestimation of time duration in depression (Kitamura and Kumar, 1984; Munzel et al., 1988). There is more consensus on the subjective experience of time in depression, as discussed subsequently.

DISORDER OF CHRONOLOGY (TEMPORAL ORDER)

Memory of the temporal order of events is an aspect of time sense that is often ignored. There is evidence that patients with diencephalic lesions compared with those with medial temporal lobe lesions have distinct deficits in temporal order memory tasks. These patients are unable to correctly indicate the temporal order of learned words on a list or the sequence of presentation of particular stimuli. This has led to the suggestion that diencephalic structures may have a function in the encoding of temporal information (O'Connor and Verfaellie, 2002). Frontal lobe lesions are also associated with impairment of function on temporal order tasks. In addition to this, an aspect of temporal order coding, namely frequency estimation, which involves estimating how often an event has happened, is known to be impaired by left frontal but not temporal lesions (Baldoa and Shimamura, 2002).

Clinically significant disorders of temporal order for past and current events have been reported. These take the form of intact memory for autobiographical events but impaired appreciation of the duration and timing of these events. These impairments are associated with organic lesions in the cingulate gyrus, the parietal lobes and the left anterior frontal areas (Cutting, 1997).

Disorder of Subjective (Personal) Time

Disorder of subjective time is characterized by abnormalities in how time is experienced. This can involve the experience of (1) flow of time, (2) direction of time, (3) uniqueness of time and (4) quality of time. These disorders go to the heart of how the world is experienced. Any alteration in the way that time is experienced will by definition influence the experience of the objective world and may come to imbue perceptions of the objective world with an alien hue.

DISORDER OF FLOW OF TIME

The flow (passage) of time may slow down or speed up. In some instances, it may become arrested and standstill. Tolstoy's (1895) short story 'Master and Man' is true to life—or death. Lost at night in a Russian snowdrift, his character, Vasilii Andreich:

Got up and lay down a couple of dozen times. The night seemed it would never end. It must be getting on for morning now, he thought once as he raised himself and looked around. Let's have a look at my watch … He could not believe his eyes … It was only ten past twelve. The whole night still lay ahead.

Time, as a modality of personal experience, is disturbed in mood disorders. It has been observed both clinically and experimentally that those with depressive illness feel that time passes slowly (Wyrick and Wyrick, 1977). Lewis (1967) quotes a patient who was depressed with *affective functional psychosis*:

Everything seems very much longer. I should have said it was afternoon, though they say it is midday. They always tell me it is earlier than I think … and it looks as if I'm wrong and I can't help feeling I'm right … I cannot see any end to anything, only end to the world.

The flow of time can also be arrested such that time appears to stand still. The patient feels that time is standing still, that in some way everything temporal has come to an end. This is described not uncommonly with psychotic depression. A patient says, 'I have stopped being, I have just stopped, everything else has just stopped as well'. The incessant sequential march of events no longer impresses the person with its inevitability.

This feeling of time standing still may also be experienced in ecstasy states, in which the person may feel that he is existing in the past, the present and the future all at the same time. Such states may occur with mania, with some neurotic conditions or in normal people undergoing an exceptional psychological experience.

When the disturbance in the sense of the passage of time occurs in the setting of depression, the depressed mood is also apparent. Another of Lewis' (1967) patients said:

I never know any moment what is going to happen. It's the most terrible outlook I've ever had to look to. It's all perpetual. I've got to suffer perpetually.

And one of Minkowski's (1970) patients said:

I continue to live now in eternity; there are no more hours or days or nights. Outside things still go on, the fruits on trees move this way and that. The others walk to and fro in the room, but time does not flow for me. My watch runs just as before … Sometimes when people run quickly to and fro in the garden or if the wind stirs up the leaves, I would like to live again as before and be able to run interiorly with them in order that time would pass again.

In these examples, the patients are trying hard to describe the indescribable, the experience of time standing still. In addition to this experience there is also the related but distinct phenomenon of living in the instant, and this feeling is allied to the notion of finality and lack of continuity:

I live in instantaneousness. I don't have the feeling of continuity anymore … When I finish something, I have the feeling of not being able to do anything else afterwards and of doing this thing, going to dinner for example, for the last time.

Minkowski, 1970

This last sentence is perhaps the key to the abnormal psychopathology. It is the abnormal mood associated with time sense that is significant, so depressive inpatients were significantly more likely to feel that time was passing more slowly than healthy 'control' subjects (Kitamura and Kumar, 1982).

In mania, time passes rapidly, but the picture is uncertain in schizophrenia (Orme, 1966). The flow of time is also known to be affected in organic brain conditions. Patients with Korsakov's syndrome underestimate the passage of time, and subjects who have had thalamotomy experience the flow of time as speeded up (Cutting, 1997).

It is more usual to describe in dementias the disorientation for time, place and person. This disorientation refers to the disturbance in the appreciation of objective time. However, people who suffer from dementia also describe abnormalities of subjective experience of time. The most common is a disturbance in the flow of time. Christine Bryden (2005) described her experience as follows:

We have no sense of time passing, so we live in the present reality, with no past and no future. We put all our energy into now, not then or later. Sometimes this causes a lot of anxiety because we worry about the past or the future because we cannot 'feel' that it exists.

A distinct but related disturbance of the flow of time is the *Zeitraffer* phenomenon. This is literally a time-lapse phenomenon. It was first described in the German literature in the 1930s, and Cutting (1997) has now brought it to the attention of the English-speaking world. The characteristic features are as follows:

1. the speeding up or slowing down of events;
2. its association with increased speed, pitch and volume of auditory perceptions; and
3. alterations in the fluency of observed movements.

There may also be visual hallucinations, anomalous experience of space such as distortions of horizontal and vertical lines. This phenomenon invariably occurs in the setting of acute organic brain disease such as cerebrovascular accident.

The original case was described by Hoff and Potzl (1934, quoted in Cutting, 1997):

Doctors and nurses were first of all moving with a measured step, conspicuously, as if on a film. Then the tempo of things became very erratic, sometimes coming at a furious pace, 'like moving pictures speeded up' as if the people involved were 'running a race' … Music, whose source was to his left, sounded very loud and very fast, as if 'several radios were all blaring away together … as if all the instruments wanted to show how much noise they could make'. Sometimes, other people's speech seemed excessively fast and incomprehensible 'as if the doctors and nurses were practising for a world record'. However, if he were addressed directly, the rate appeared quite normal and he could understand it quite well. It was when someone was speaking away to the left that it sounded most peculiar – shriller, louder and faster than when to away to the right.

DISORDER OF DIRECTION OF TIME

It seems such a fundamental aspect of our experience of time that the arrow of time travels from the past through the present to the future. It is incomprehensible that anyone could experience time as if events were being played in 'rewind mode' backwards. This phenomenon was reported by one of Lewis' patients (1967):

Whenever anyone said anything to me, it referred back to some part of my life … One mind was living back and my mind forward.

Another of Minkowski's (1970) patients said:

There is no present anymore, only a sense of the past. Is there a future? There used to be, but now it is shrinking. The past is so obtrusive … I'll give you an example of what it's like. I'm like a machine that runs but does not move from its place. It goes at full speed, but it remains in place. I am like a burning arrow that you hurl before you; then it stops, falls back, and is finally extinguished as if in a space empty of air. It is hurled backwards.

DISORDER OF UNIQUENESS OF TIME

Part of our experience of time is the sense of uniqueness of the time, momentary or otherwise that we live through. This uniqueness of time experience is instantiated in the unique events that populate time. This means that every moment is given its singular identity by the context, by the events played out in a given place, by particular personalities and by association with specific emotions. These coordinates of time stamp each moment with its specific unique feeling.

The *déjà vu* experience can be conceptualized as an alteration of the feeling of uniqueness with which time and events are invested. When this sense of uniqueness is disrupted, novel events and the time and place in which they occur seem familiar. In this conceptualization, *déjà vu* is the experience of this feeling of familiarity for events and times that have not been previously encountered becoming associated with a novel situation. *Jamais vu* is the absence of this feeling of familiarity for events that have been previously encountered. In other words, even previously encountered situations are experienced as novel, that is, as unique. Although it is possible to conceptualize these experiences as disorders of time, it is probably more appropriate to regard them as aspects of memory disturbance (Chapter 5).

Déjà vu occurs in the normal state and in pathologic conditions. The composer Ralph Vaughan Williams, in describing his first hearing of the tune used in *Dives and Lazarus,* explained, 'I had that sense of recognition—here's something which I have known all my life, only I didn't know it' (Kennedy, 1964). Most people can recall similar *déjà vu* experiences. It is also commonly associated with temporal lobe epilepsy. A patient described his aura before a fit experienced in hospital: 'I went into the kitchen. The window looked as if I'd seen it before. I felt very peculiar'. *Déjà vu* and *jamais vu* are quite often described in schizophrenia.

Déjà vu has been produced with brain stimulation. Penfield and Kristiensen (1951) were able to reproduce a sensation of familiarity with stimulation of a brain electrode in epileptic patients. This stimulation clearly produced an abnormality of the feeling of familiarity, not an abnormality of memory. It was a disturbance of the feeling of recognition that accompanies recall in the process of memory. Janet considered *déjà vu* to be a form of loss of reality or negation of the present (Taylor, 1947), whereas Freud (1901) regarded it as being associated with the recall of unconscious fantasies.

In a more extreme form, the disorder of the uniqueness of time presents as *reduplication of time*. The term was first used by Weinstein et al. (1952). Petho (1985) described a case in which the patient's central symptom was the belief that she had lived through this life once before. The patient experienced a reduplication of every event and, in relation to attending the 1976 Olympic Games, said, 'It could happen that I will go;

I have a memory of it. But I also have a memory that I won't go to those Games so that that memory won't come back to me.'

DISORDER OF QUALITY OF TIME

In these conditions, the normal experience of the quality of time is either lost or distorted in some way. What is central to these experiences is that the 'taken for granted' aspect of time is replaced by a degree of alienation from it such that time becomes salient, obtrusive and even unreal.

In depersonalization and derealization, there can be a loss of the feeling of reality for time experience; there may also be alteration in the sense of duration or in the perspective of time (Freeman and Melges, 1977). The person can assess a time span quite accurately, and there is no loss of memory. However, he has no feeling that things are happening or time is passing; the abnormality is always one of experience. Time itself takes on a feeling of unreality, and he feels unable to initiate action.

This phenomenon can also occur in schizophrenia. One of Cutting's (1997) patients said:

Time is somewhat changed. Time isn't supposed to be the way it is. I don't know in what way.

Fischer described a number of cases (quoted in Cutting, 1997), of which one said:

Time stood still. Then it became different. Then it disappeared entirely … Then a new time emerged. This new time was endless, more manifold than the previous one, hardly deserving the name 'time' as we know it. Suddenly it came to me that this time did not only lie in front of and behind me, but spread out in all directions.

Biological Rhythms and Their Relation to Psychiatry

Daily, there are profound changes in the body and brain associated with the external rhythm of the world. During the waking day, we are active, and at night we sleep, recuperate and repair our body parts. This biological rhythm is driven by an internal clock. The primary internal body clock is located in the suprachiasmatic nuclei, a cluster of approximately 100,000 neurons located on either side of the midline above the optic chiasma, about three centimetres above the eyes (Hastings, 1998). There is strong evidence that the clock is an autonomous property of the suprachiasmatic nuclei, and individual cells, in vitro, continue to fire rhythmically for several weeks with only the slightest deviation from 24 hours. It is known that this clock can be desynchronized by jet lag, shift work and depression (Arendt, 1995). However, there is still a great deal of ignorance about the connections with different mental illnesses. In this section, brief reference is made to daily, monthly and annual rhythms and also to the association with the stage of life. Among psychiatric disorders, most information is available on affective disorder and its associations with daily and annual rhythms (Thompson, 1988).

CIRCADIAN RHYTHMS

Comparing internal time with clock time, repeated estimates of fixed time spans show a gradual increase in time of the estimate, suggesting that there is a slowing of the internal clock. Subjects were asked repeatedly to guess a fixed duration of time; their estimate started by being slightly longer than actual time and became progressively longer still. The intrinsic period of the circadian rhythm in humans is approximately 25 hours, but this is usually modified by external cues such as daylight (Wher and Goodwin, 1983). This has been likened to the finding in vigilance experiments in which there is a gradual decrease of efficiency. There was also found to be a greater overestimation of fixed intervals in the morning, compared with that in the afternoon, and this has been shown to correlate with body temperature. The internal clock accelerates when the body temperature is raised.

A number of circadian rhythm sleep disorders have been described including shift-work type and jet-lag type (Sack et al., 2007). These conditions are conceived as recurrent or persistent patterns of sleep disturbance due primarily to alterations in the circadian timekeeping system or a misalignment between the endogenous circadian rhythm and exogenous factors that affect the timing or duration of sleep. In the shift-work type, sleep is disrupted by a broad spectrum of nonstandard work schedules such as occasional on-call overnight duty, to rotating schedules, to steady and permanent night work. In the jet-lag type, the sleep disruption is generated by circadian misalignment, the inevitable consequence of crossing time zones too quickly for the circadian system to keep pace. Depending on the number and direction of time zones crossed, it may take days for the circadian rhythm to resynchronize (Sack et al., 2007).

The clinical features of jet lag include daytime somnolence, fatigue, impaired alertness and difficulty initiating and maintaining sleep. The sleep disturbance may be associated with impairment of work performance (Spitzer et al., 1999).

There is considerable circumstantial, but little direct, evidence that circadian rhythms are causally associated with affective disorders (Thompson, 1984). Early-morning wakening and diurnal variation in mood, with the mood most depressed in the early morning, are considered biological symptoms of depression and have been postulated as *phase advance* of the sleep–wake cycle; that is, each point of the rhythm occurs earlier than usual relative to the light–dark cycle. There is a change in depression in that rapid eye movement sleep occurs earlier, rather than later, in the night, and this also may point to phase advance of the circadian rhythm. Sleep deprivation has been used with variable success in the treatment of depression; there has been research into the genetic and familial aspects of sleep disturbance, into sleep disorders in depression and other neuropsychiatric conditions and into the relationship of sleep disturbance in depression and other neuroendocrine changes (Vogel et al., 1980; Linkowski and Mendlewicz, 1993).

Although diurnality of mood usually manifests itself by the subject feeling worse in the early morning, sometimes this is reversed. Styron (1991) describes this for his own severe depressive illness:

There was now something that resembled bifurcation of mood: lucidity of sorts in the early hours of the day, gathering murk in the afternoon and evening.

In depression, changes of body temperature and cortisol levels over 24 hours have also been interpreted as phase advance of the circadian rhythm, but the results are equivocal. The action of antidepressant drugs on the rhythm has been investigated by lengthening the intrinsic cycles of rest, temperature and sleep, but again, the evidence is not clear. Corroboration

studies of air travellers crossing time zones have suggested that travel from east to west is more likely to be associated with depression, and from west to east with hypomania (Jauhar and Weller, 1982). However, physiologic studies of jet lag would not support such an association (Arendt and Marks, 1982).

Thinking in relation to circadian rhythms in mood disorders was given further impetus because of the discovery of clock genes and cellular clocks, even though there is no consistent finding that disruption of these clocks exist in mood disorders (McCarthy and Welsh, 2012). It may be that clock gene expression outside of the suprachiasmatic nucleus is involved in mood regulation (McClung, 2007). This is a matter for future research.

It has been suggested that there may be a shortened rhythm, of less than 24 hours, in patients with long-term schizophrenia. Abnormalities of circadian rhythm have also been described, but not fully substantiated, in people with anorexia nervosa and with abnormal personalities.

MONTHLY CYCLES

Clearly, the most obvious human biological rhythm to recur monthly is the menstrual cycle, and this has been linked with changes in mental state, but premenstrual syndrome remains controversial in its definition, management and politicosocial implications (Bancroft, 1993). Similar psychological mood swings with a monthly cycle have been sought in the male but not convincingly found. Estimates for the frequency of *premenstrual syndrome* have varied in the general population between 30% and 80% of women of reproductive age (Clare, 1982). Psychological symptoms include lethargy, anxiety, irritability and depression, but many symptoms are both psychological and physical (headache, feeling bloated, loss of energy). It is the timing rather than the nature of the symptoms that indicates the diagnosis, and there are clearly differing constellations of complaint within the syndrome (Sampson, 1989).

Much numeric data have been provided by Dalton (1984) to support the contention that there is increased psychopathology of various types during the 8 days of the premenstruum and the menstrual period itself relative to the rest of the cycle. She stated that 46% of emergency psychiatric admissions, 53% of attempted suicides, 47% of admissions for depression and 47% of admissions for schizophrenia of women of reproductive age occur during these stages, but these figures have not yet been substantiated. However, reports of unusual manifestations of premenstrual syndrome include descriptions of auditory hallucinations and delusions of reference present only in the premenstrual period and hypomanic or manic states present in the 2- to 3-day period before the onset of menstruation (Hsiao and Liu, 2007).

The descriptions by Dalton (1984) are distinct from the careful analysis of cases drawn from a review of cases of menstrual psychosis over the past 300 years conducted and published by Ian Brockington (2005). These are cases that present with acute onset against a background of normality, of short duration with psychotic symptoms including confusion, stupor, mutism, delusions and hallucinations and occurring in a circa-menstrual periodicity and in rhythm with the menstrual cycle. The relationship with the menstrual cycle included cases where there was premenstrual onset and abrupt cessation at the beginning of menstrual bleeding and the so-called catamenial psychosis in which the onset of psychosis was associated with the onset of menstrual flow. It is the relationship with the menstrual cycle rather than the phenomenology of the cases that makes them remarkable.

SEASONAL VARIATION

Season of the year has been invoked for the onset of episodes of many psychiatric illnesses. Understandably, this is more pronounced at increasingly higher latitudes in the northern hemisphere. Similar associations of illness with summer or winter have been observed in the Southern Hemisphere.

In both Northern and Southern Hemispheres, patients with a diagnosis of schizophrenia are more likely to have been born in the winter months (Hare, 1988); this is most strikingly found for those without a family history of the illness (O'Callaghan et al., 1991). There is a higher rate for admission to psychiatric hospital during the summer months.

For every decade since 1921, suicide rates in England and Wales have been highest in the quarter comprising April, May and June (Morgan, 1979). There appears to be no association between season of birth and affective illness; however, the onset of depressive

illness and the administration of electroconvulsive therapy both become more common in spring and autumn (Rawnsley, 1982). Symonds and Williams (1976) found a peak for the admission of female manic patients in August and September.

Seasonal affective disorder (recurrent depressive disorder, F33 in the *International Classification of Diseases*, 10th revision; World Health Organization, 1992) is characterized by repeated episodes of depression, which may vary in severity from mild to severe and recur with an onset at the same time of year, most often late winter or spring. It is more common in women than in men and tends to start later in life, often about the fifth decade. There are often a large number of episodes of depression in seasonal affective disorder (10–17 per patient), each episode lasting from 17 to 23 weeks; anxiety, irritability, hypersomnia and gain in appetite and weight were prominent symptoms (Thompson and Isaacs, 1988). The distinctive symptoms of this condition have been measured using the Seasonal Pattern Assessment Questionnaire (Thompson et al., 1988). It occurs more frequently in higher latitudes in the northern hemisphere. In a study conducted in Finland (Saarijärvi et al., 1999) in which the prominent symptoms included lack of energy, hypersomnia, excessive eating, weight gain and a craving for carbohydrates in addition to other depressive symptoms, there was lower prevalence among Lapps, who are ethnically and genetically different from Finns living at the same latitude.

LIFE EPOCHS

Virtually the whole of psychopathology is mediated through, and influenced by, changes in situation and life epoch. It is important to take into account the relative preponderance of different factors: biological change, pressure of social context and individual perception of life situation. It is outside the scope of this book to chart these associations in detail, but an impressionistic sketch is offered in Fig. 6.1. The psychological effects of important life changes have been studied in primary care situations: birth of the first child (Jewell, 1984), starting school (Pitt and Browne, 1984), puberty (Howe and Page, 1984) and leaving school (Brown, 1984).

Some of the abnormal mental states associated with life changes of female gender could equally well be discussed with life epoch.

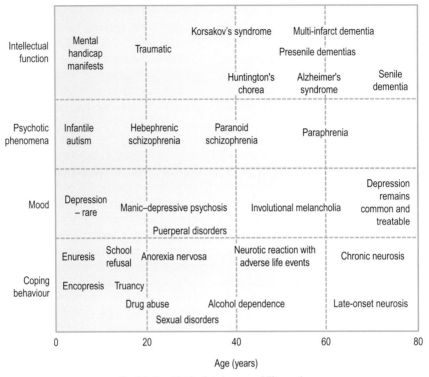

Fig. 6.1 Psychiatric disturbance and life epoch.

REFERENCES

Adam, B., 1995. Timewatch: The Social Analysis of Time. Polity Press, Cambridge.

Arendt, J., 1995. Melatonin and the Mammalian Pineal Gland. Chapman and Hall, London.

Arendt, J., Marks, V., 1982. Physiological changes underlying jet lag. Br. Med. J. 284, 144–146.

Baldoa, J.V., Shimamura, A.P., 2002. Frontal lobes and memory. In: Baddeley, A.D., Kopelman, M.D., Wilson, B.A. (Eds.), The Handbook of Memory Disorders, second ed. John Wiley, Chichester.

Bancroft, J., 1993. The premenstrual syndrome – a reappraisal of the concept and the evidence. Psychol. Med. Monogr. Suppl. 24, 1–47.

Brockington, I., 2005. Menstrual psychosis. World Psychiatr. 4, 9–17.

Brown, A., 1984. Leaving school. Br. Med. J. 288, 1884–1886.

Bryden, C., 2005. Dancing with Dementia: My Story of Living Positively with Dementia. Jessica Kingsley Publishers, London.

Clare, A.W., 1982. Psychiatric aspects of premenstrual complaint. J. Psychosom. Obstet. Gynaecol. 1, 22–31.

Crow, T.J., Stevens, M., 1978. Age disorientation in chronic schizophrenics: the nature of the cognitive deficit. Br. J. Psychiatry. 133, 137–142.

Cutting, J., 1997. Principles of Psychopathology: Two Worlds – Two Minds – Two Hemispheres. Oxford University Press, Oxford.

Dalton, K., 1984. The Premenstrual Syndrome and Progesterone Therapy, second ed. Heinemann, London.

Freeman, A.M., Melges, F.T., 1977. Depersonalization and temporal disintegration in acute mental illness. Am. J. Psychiatry. 134, 679–681.

Freud, S., 1901. The psychopathology of everyday life. In: Standard Edition of the Complete Works of Sigmund Freud, vol. 6. (J. Strachey, Trans, 1960). Hogarth Press, London, p. 151.

Hare, E., 1988. Temporal factors and trends, including birth seasonality and the viral hypothesis. In: Nasrallah, H.A. (Ed.), Handbook of Schizophrenia, vol. 3. Elsevier, Amsterdam.

Hastings, M., 1998. The brain, circadian rhythms and clock genes. Br. Med. J. 317, 1704–1707.

Howe, C., Page, C., 1984. Puberty. Br. Med. J. 288, 1809–1811.

Hsiao, M.C., Liu, C., 2007. Unusual manifestations of premenstrual syndrome. Psychiatry Clin. Neurosci. 61, 120–123.

Jaspers, K., 1997. In: Hoenig, J., Hamilton, M.W., Trans (Eds.), General Psychopathology. The Johns Hopkins University Press, Baltimore.

Jauhar, P., Weller, M.P.I., 1982. Psychiatric morbidity and time zone changes: a study of patients from Heathrow Airport. Br. J. Psychiatry. 140, 231–253.

Jewell, M.D., 1984. Birth of the first child. Br. Med. J. 288, 1584–1586.

Kant, I., 1781/1929. Critique of Pure Reason (N. Kemp Smith, Trans). MacMillan Press, London.

Kennedy, M., 1964. The Works of Ralph Vaughan Williams. Oxford University Press, London.

Kitamura, T., Kumar, R., 1982. Time passes slowly for patients with depressive state. Acta Psychiatr. Scand. 65, 415–420.

Kitamura, T., Kumar, R., 1984. Controlled study on time reproduction of depressive patients. Psychopathology 17, 24–27.

Kuhs, H., Hermann, W., Kammer, W., Tolle, R., 1991. Time estimation and the experience of time in endogenous depression (melancholia): an experimental investigation. Psychopathology 24, 7–11.

Lewis, A., 1967. The experience of time in mental disorder. In: Inquiries in Psychiatry. Routledge and Kegan Paul, London, pp. 3–15.

Linkowski, P., Mendlewicz, J., 1993. Sleep encephalogram and rhythm disturbances in mood disorders. Curr. Opin. Psychiatry. 6, 35–37.

McCarthy, M.J., Welsh, D.K., 2012. Cellular circadian clocks in mood disorders. J. Biol. Rhythms. 27, 339–352.

McClung, C.A., 2007. Role for the Clock gene in bipolar disorder. Cold Spring Harb. Symp. Quant. Biol. 637–644.

Minkowski, E., 1970. Lived Time: Phenomenological and Psychopathological Studies (N. Metzel, Trans, with Introduction). Northwestern University Press, Evanston.

Morgan, H.G., 1979. Death Wishes? the Understanding and Management of Deliberate Self-Harm. John Wiley, Chichester.

Munzel, K., Gendner, G., Steinberg, R., Raith, L., 1988. Time estimation of depressive patients: the influence of interval content. Eur. Arch. Psychiatry Neurol. Sci. 237, 171–178.

O'Callaghan, E., Gibson, T., Colohan, H.A., et al., 1991. Season of birth in schizophrenia. Evidence for confinement of an excess of winter births to patients without a family history of mental disorder. Br. J. Psychiatry. 158, 764–769.

O'Connor, M., Verfaellie, M., 2002. The amnesic syndrome. In: Baddeley, A.D., Kopelman, M.D., Wilson, B.A. (Eds.), The Handbook of Memory Disorders, second ed. John Wiley, Chichester.

Orme, J.E., 1966. Time estimation and the nosology of schizophrenia. Br. J. Psychiatry. 112, 37–39.

Penfield, W., Kristiensen, K., 1951. Epileptic Seizure Patients. Thomas, Springfield, IL.

Petho, B., 1985. Chronophrenia – a new syndrome in functional psychosis. Psychopathology 18, 174–180.

Pitt, G., Browne, M.J., 1984. Starting school. Br. Med. J. 288, 1655–1657.

Rawnsley, K., 1982. Epidemiology of affective psychoses. In: Wing, J.K., Wing, L. (Eds.), Handbook of Psychiatry 3: Psychoses of Uncertain Aetiology. Cambridge University Press, Cambridge, pp. 129–133.

Saarijärvi, S., Lauerma, H., Helenius, H., Saarilehto, S., 1999. Seasonal affective disorders among rural Finns and Lapps. Acta Psychiatr. Scand. 99, 95–101.

Sack, R.L., Auckley, D.A., Auger, R., et al., 2007. Circadian rhythm sleep disorders: part 1, basic principles, shift work and jetlag. Sleep 30, 1460–1483.

Sampson, G.A., 1989. Premenstrual syndrome. Baillières Clin. Obstet. Gynaecol. 3, 687–704.

Spitzer, R.L., Terman, M., Williams, J.B.W., et al., 1999. Jet lag: clinical features, validation of a new syndrome-specific scale, and lack of response to melatonin in a randomized, double-blind trial. Am. J. Psychiatry. 156, 1392–1396.

Styron, W., 1991. Darkness Visible. A Memoir of Madness. Jonathan Cape, London.

Symonds, R.L., Williams, P., 1976. Seasonal variations in the incidence of mania. Br. J. Psychiatry. 129, 45–48.

Taylor, W.S., 1947. Pierre Janet 1859–1947. Am. J. Psychol. 60, 637–645.

Thompson, C., 1984. Circadian rhythms and psychiatry. Br. J. Psychiatry. 145, 204–206.

Thompson, C., 1988. Biological rhythms and mental illness. Curr. Opin. Psychiatry. 1, 66–71.

Thompson, C., Isaacs, G., 1988. Seasonal affective disorder – a British sample: symptomatology in relation to mode of referral and diagnostic subtype. J. Affect. Disord. 14, 1–11.

Thompson, C., Stinson, D., Fernandez, M., Fine, J., Isaacs, G., 1988. A comparison of normal, bipolar and seasonal affective disorder subjects using the Seasonal Pattern Assessment Questionnaire. J. Affect. Disord. 14, 257–264.

Tolstoy, L., 1895. Master and Man (P. Foote, Trans, 1977). Penguin, London.

Vogel, D.W., Vogel, F., McAbee, R.S., Thurmond, A.J., 1980. Improvement of depression by REM sleep deprivation. Arch. Gen. Psychiatry. 37, 247–253.

Weinstein, E.A., Kahn, R.L., Sugarman, L.A., 1952. Phenomenon of reduplication. Arch. Neurol. Psychiatry. 67, 808–814.

Wher, T.A., Goodwin, F.K., 1983. Circadian Rhythm in Psychiatry. Boxwood Press, Pacific Grove.

World Health Organization, 1992. The ICD-10 Classification of Mental and Behavioral Disorders: Clinical Description and Diagnostic Guidelines. World Health Organization, Geneva.

Wyrick, R.A., Wyrick, L.C., 1977. Time experience during depression. Arch. Gen. Psychiatry. 14, 1441–1443.

Zangwill, O.L., 1953. Disorientation for age. J. Mental Sci. 99, 698–701.

Pathology of Perception

Chapter Outline

KEYWORDS

Imagery
Form constants
Synaesthesia
Illusions
Hallucination
Pseudohallucination
Autoscopy

Summary

Abnormalities of perception remain some of the most compelling experiences with which patients present. These experiences speak to the underlying structures of the perceptual world and the neural correlates that make perception itself possible. Sensory distortions and false perceptions between them point to the relative importance and the distinctions to be drawn between sensation and perception. Illusion, which is the misinterpretation of a normal perception, and hallucinations, the perception of an object in the absence of a stimulus, are the two most frequently encountered false perceptions in clinical practice.

For almost seven years – except during sleep – I have never had a single moment in which I did not hear voices. They accompany me to every place and at all times; they continue to sound even when I am in conversation with other people, they persist undeterred even when I concentrate on other things.

Daniel Schreber (1842–1911)

Disorders of perception, particularly auditory hallucinations or 'hearing voices', have a central place in psychopathology. Along with delusions (Chapter 8), they are thought of as synonymous with mental illness. This apparent association with mental illness has come to imply that 'hearing voices' is a sign of serious mental illness and that hallucinations portend madness. In this chapter, the nature of sensation, perception and imagery is discussed as a prelude to examining the nature of disorders of perception.

Sensation and Perception

Sensation is only the first stage in receiving information from outside the self. The sensory system includes the visual, auditory, tactile, olfactory, gustatory, kinaesthetic and proprioceptive pathways. These pathways deal with the receipt, transformation and transmission of raw and disparate sensory data from peripheral receptors to the central nervous system. The transformation of raw sensory stimuli into sensory information that is then decoded into meaningful perception at the cortical level involves active processes that are influenced by attention, affect, cultural expectations, context, prior experiences, memory and, most importantly, prior concepts. It is therefore the case that perception is not a passive process but an active one that involves the construction of an external world that depends on internal templates.

Much of what we know about sensation and perception derives from our understanding of the visual system. In the visual system, light sensation is received by the retina and transformed into a neural code that is transmitted from the retinal ganglion cells to the primary visual cortex via the lateral geniculate nucleus of the thalamus. Perception occurs when a stimulus has undergone processing according to its form, colour, motion and meaning.

The distinction between sensation and perception is well illustrated by the dissociation between intact sensation and impaired perception in the agnosias. In visual object agnosia, the subject is able to recognize that an object is in their field of vision (i.e., sensation is intact), but they are unable to recognize what the object or its function is (impaired perception). This visual model of perception is likely to have counterparts within the other sensory systems.

Oliver Sachs (1995) recounts the story of Virgil, a 51-year-old man who had been blind since infancy. He had a cataract extraction, but the return of visual sensation was unaccompanied by uncomplicated perception. Virgil was able to 'pick up details incessantly—but would not be able to synthesize them to form a complex perception at a glance. This was one reason the cat, visually, was so puzzling: he would see a paw, the nose, the tail, an ear, but could not see all of them together, see the cat as a whole'. This case is reminiscent of Gregory's (2004) patient, S.B., who, when he was first shown a lathe after recovering his sight, 'was quite unable to say anything about it, except he thought the nearest part was a handle … He complained that he could not see the cutting edge, or the metal being worked, or anything else about it, and appeared rather agitated … S.B. was allowed to touch the lathe. The result was startling … He ran his hands eagerly over the lathe, with his eyes shut. Then he stood back a little and opened his eyes and said: "Now that I've felt it I can see"'. These two cases underline the distinction between sensation and perception and confirm that 'we are not given the world: we make our world through incessant experience, categorization, memory, reconnection' (Sachs, 1995).

There are various competing models of the way that recognition is achieved by the visual system. A detailed description of these models is outside the scope of this chapter (see Smith and Kosslyn, 2007). Bottom-up processing consists of the primary processes that transform sensation into the perception of objects that have form, colour, motion and location in space. On the other hand, top-down processes involve the influence of our learned experience of perceiving objects to narrow the competition between the possible interpretations of the sensory information. The alternative models of the top-down processes that attempt to explain object recognition, that is, perception are (1) the template-matching model, (2) the feature-matching model, (3) the recognition-by-components model and (4) the configural models.

The template-matching model requires an internal template in memory to which an object can be matched. The weakness of this model is that the template must accommodate object size and orientation, for example, and must still be rapid and reliable. The feature-matching model requires only that a distinct and discriminating feature of an object on its own should specify what the object is. Trees need only be specified by the fact that they have a trunk and branches. The exact location of the branches and size of the trunk do not matter. The recognition-by-components model requires knowledge of the correct arrangement of parts in three-dimensional space. Thus irrespective of the perspective, a bicycle is still recognized as a bicycle. Finally, the configural model is a refinement of the recognition-by-components model. It deals with the mechanism whereby individual examples of a class are recognized. This is the distinction between different makes of cars, the variation that determines that one car is a Mercedes and another is a Volvo, for example.

IMAGERY

Imagery is the internal mental representation of the world and is actively drawn from memory. Imagery underlies our capacity for many crucial cognitive activities, such as mental arithmetic, map reading, visualising and imagining places previously visited and recollecting spoken speech. In day-to-day life, it is common to refer to 'seeing in the mind's eyes' or 'hearing in the mind's ears'. These terms refer to imagery. Jaspers (1997) described the formal characteristics of images as follows:

1. Images are figurative and have a character of subjectivity.
2. They appear in inner subjective space.
3. They are not clearly delineated and come before us incomplete.
4. Although sensory elements are individually the equal of those in perception, mostly they are insufficient.
5. Images dissipate and always have to be re-created.
6. Images are actively created and are dependent on our will (Table 7.1).

Functional imaging studies have demonstrated that the same cortical areas are implicated in visual imagery and visual perception (Kosslyn and Thompson, 2003), and transmagnetic resonance studies have also shown that transmagnetic stimulation applied repeatedly to visual areas reduces the capacity for visual imagery (Kosslyn et al., 1999). Furthermore, behavioural experiments have shown that participants are able to construct mental images that have perceptual qualities such as colour, size, shape and orientation. These images are uneven, with the level of detail depending on the degree of visual attention (Smith and Kosslyn, 2007).

The study of imagery remains a controversial area within cognitive neuroscience. Theories of visual imagery have borrowed from the language and model

TABLE 7.1 Formal Characteristics of Normal Perception and Imagery

Normal Perception	Imagery
Perceptions are of concrete reality.	Images are figurative and have a character of subjectivity.
Perceptions occur in external objective space.	Images appear in inner subjective space.
Perceptions are clearly delineated.	Images are incomplete and poorly delineated.
The sensory elements are full and fresh.	The sensory elements are relatively insufficient.
Perceptions are constant and remain unaltered.	Images dissipate and have to be re-created.
Perceptions are independent of our will.	Images are dependent on our will.

After Jaspers, K., 1997. General Psychopathology (J. Hoenig, M.W. Hamilton, Trans). The Johns Hopkins University Press, Baltimore.

of the camera; this is referred to as the *pictorial* or *depiction* theory of mental imagery. The foremost proponent of this approach is Kosslyn. A detailed account of the theory and its difficulties is outside the scope of this book (see Kosslyn, 2004; Pylyshyn, 2004). Kosslyn argues that a mental image is figuratively accurate, as each point of the image corresponds to each point on the represented object. This means that there is a point-to-point representation such that performing particular operations on the image takes as much time as it would take to perform the same operation on the object. In other words, the time to scan a mental image is the same as the time to scan the object. Pylyshyn, on the other hand, argues that there are decisive differences between retinal or cortical images and mental images.

Imagery is important for psychopathology because an understanding of the formal characteristics or nature of imagery is required for examining the nature of perceptions, hallucinations and pseudohallucinations. Functional imaging studies and case reports have shown that the mechanisms responsible for the visual perception of objects and those responsible for imagery may be similar. In other words, the neural substrates of perception and imagery at the very least overlap (Martin, 2006). Ultimately these investigations may shed light on the mechanisms uniting imagery and abnormal perceptions. In addition, there is an important relationship between mental images and imagination, a relationship that grounds mental operations such as perspective taking, 'as if' functions, mutual understanding in human culture and the discontinuities between fiction and reality in the capacity to have mental imagery (see Summa et al., 2018, for a fuller description).

FORM CONSTANTS, EXTENSION AND SYNAESTHESIA

Synaesthesia is a rare condition that is not regarded as an example of abnormal experience but nonetheless provides some understanding of elementary perceptual neural systems that may help to clarify and illuminate the problem of abnormal perception. Synaesthesia can be defined as the perception of an object presented in one sensory modality and at the same time experienced in a different sensory modality. This is best illustrated by giving an example of music to colour synaesthesia:

When I listen to music, I see the shapes on an externalized area about 12 inches in front of my face and about one foot high onto which the music is visually projected. Sounds are most easily likened to oscilloscope configurations – lines moving in colour, often metallic, with height, width and, most importantly, depth. My favourite music has lines that extend horizontally beyond the 'screen' area.

Cytowic and Eagleman, 2009

Various forms of synaesthesia have been reported including, most commonly, graphene to colour, time unit to colour, musical sounds to colour, general sounds to colour and phoneme to colour. Other forms are sounds to taste, sound to touch, vision to taste, etc. Another example of sound to colour synaesthesia:

One of the things I love about my husband are the colours of his voice and his laugh. It's a wonderful golden brown, like crisp, buttery toast, which sounds very odd, I know, but it is very real.

Cytowic and Eagleman, 2009

These experiences seem to be spatially extended but different from seeing or imagining. They are often experienced close to the body, within reach of limbs,

and within 'peri-personal space'. These experiences raise the question of whether the extended space in synaesthesia is akin to the space in which visual or auditory verbal hallucinations are experienced. Furthermore, the synaesthetic experiences are consistent over time and are elementary and specific in nature. The sensations do not evoke elaborate or complex perceptions, but rather elementary colours, shapes, bright-dark configurations and jagged-smooth sensations are provoked. Indeed, there is evidence that the sensations are examples or elaborations of *form constants*. Form constants in the visual domain are variations of tunnels and cones, central radiations, gratings and honeycombs and spirals. Variations in colour, brightness, symmetry, replication, rotation and pulsation provide further gradations of the subjective experience of these percepts. What is significant is that these form constants seem to be a property of the visual cortex itself and are more commonly experienced in the aura phase of migraine or in periods of sensory deprivation (for a more detailed discussion, see Cytowic and Eagleman, 2009).

In summary, synaesthesia introduces the possibility of understanding some abnormal perceptions as occurring within peri-personal space, which is neither like imagery nor a normal percept. In other words, a 'third space' might exist in which some experiences such as those in synaesthesia take place. A good way to understand this is to recognize that normal perceptions are projected into the objective shared space where they coincide with the material world that is their source. In cases where no material objective origin exists, the exact location of the perceived object becomes problematic. In some people, it appears in objective and external space, but in others the spatial configuration may be more ambiguous and indeterminate and that might be best considered as a 'third space'. Additionally, fundamental and elementary features of the neural underpinning of perception might be involved in determining the form of abnormal perception, that is, the nature and configuration of abnormal perceptions are not randomly determined.

PRIVATE SPEECH AND INNER SPEECH

In addition to understanding the nature of imagery, extended space and form constants, there is a need to comprehend why auditory hallucinations have the syntactical structure that they have, namely, command format and second- and third-person syntax. An approach is Vygotsky's (1896–1934) developmental model of thought and speech. He proposed that inner speech developed first from the internalisation of external dialogue into private speech and finally into inner speech (Vygotsky, 1934/1987; Fernyhough, 1996). For Vygotsky (1978) human forms of practical and abstract intelligence develop when speech and practical activity, two independent lines of development, converge. Egocentric or private speech is, in Vygotsky's view, a transitional form between external and inner speech. A child might, for example, be instructed by a parent to 'do this or that', and the child internalizes this instruction into private speech and later into inner speech. Or a child might use private speech to accompany action, to reflect in real time how a problem is being solved and ultimately the private speech becomes part of a planning process that precedes action. In other words, private speech is an overt, spoken language that is not aimed at communicating with others but is linked with thinking and action. This transformation of dialogic, external speech into inner speech may provide a basis for understanding the ubiquity of 'command' auditory hallucinations—the grammatical structure of private speech therefore serving as the template for the structure of command hallucinations. The message here is that the syntactical structure of auditory verbal hallucinations is not arbitrary but may be tractable to earlier development forms anticipated by language acquisition in childhood. A similar case may be made for second- and third-person auditory hallucinations. Second-person hallucinations take a similar form to the structure of language used by parents making evaluative statements about children's performance and behaviours, for example, 'you're a good boy' or 'you're a naughty girl', etc. Third-person auditory verbal hallucinations also have the structure of comments between parents about their children, for example, 'He's been good today'.

There are a number of things that stand out about Vygotsky's claim: (1) he draws attention to the role of language development as a separate entity that is linked to thought and action and (2) that inner speech and thinking derive from private speech and are built on fragmentary and condensed images. In my view this makes it possible to start to interrogate the formal structure of verbal hallucinations and to make sense of these.

In his classic text, *Phenomenology of Perception*, Merleau-Ponty (1962) proposes that to perceive is to see 'standing forth from a cluster of data, an immanent significance'. For Merleau-Ponty perception is irreducible to sensations, and the perceived object is given directly and is already full of meaning, which gives it a function in the world. In other words, the subject of perception is not a mere spectator, and the perception is not a spectacle. In Merleau-Ponty's schema, attention is important to perception because it creates a 'field' that can be surveyed. Objects of perception already have value and significance by being perceived. These ideas that are fundamental to Merleau-Ponty's conception of perception remind us that objects of perception are relevant to the individual who perceives them. When we come to look at hallucinations and illusions, it becomes even clearer that what is seen or heard is never neutral; it is already full of significance and relevance for the person who perceives. The perceived voice in verbal hallucination is not experienced as eavesdropping on matters that concern others but rather as hearing speech that has personal significance and importance.

Abnormal Perception

We will now divide abnormal perception into *sensory distortions* in which a real perceptual object is perceived in a distorted way and *false perceptions* in which a new perception occurs that may or may not be in response to an external stimulus. *Illusions, hallucinations* and *pseudohallucinations* will be included under false perceptions. The possibility of a neurologic deficit affecting perception also needs to be considered.

Subjectively, *hallucination* is similar to sense perception: it is experienced as a *normal* perception. In *vivid imagery*, the whole experience is imaginary. *Pseudohallucination* has a close affinity to imagery but also has some aspects that are characteristic of sense perception or hallucination: vividness, definition, constancy and apparent independence from volition.

SENSORY DISTORTIONS

Disturbance of the mental state, with or without organic brain pathology, may cause sensory distortion. This distortion may involve any of the components or elementary aspects of perception, such as uniqueness, size, shape, colour, location, motion or general quality. What is significant is that the perceived object is correctly recognized and identified yet there is a deviation from its customary appearance without prejudicing the knowledge of the kind of thing that it is (Cutting, 1997).

Elementary Aspects of Visual Perception

In visual perception, the recurrence or prolongation of a visual phenomenon beyond the customary limits of the appearance of the real event in the world is termed *palinopsia* (Cutting, 1997). Critchley (1951) gave a number of examples: a cat noticed in the street one day kept appearing at various times and various situations over the next few days, and the words 'Pullman Springs' noticed on the back of a van kept appearing on other vehicles over the next few months.

The size of the perception can be either larger (*macropsia*) or smaller (*micropsia*) than expected. In some cases, there can be apparent reduction in one hemifield of vision (*hemimicropsia*). These anomalies are common in temporal lobe epilepsy. Alteration in the customary shape of the perceived object is termed *metamorphopsia*. Usually, this may involve the appearance of things taking on a different aspect: 'One woman saw people upside down, on their heads' (Bleuler, 1950). This is an example of inversion. When metamorphopsia affects faces, it is referred to as *paraprosopia*. Typically, these perceptual distortions of faces are rapidly fluctuant and dynamic. Schreber (1955) describes his experience as follows: 'At the same time I repeatedly witnessed that [some patients] changed heads during their stay in the common room; that is to say without leaving the room and while I was observing them, they suddenly ran about with a different head'. Bleuler (1950) also describes, 'Wardmates change their faces the very moment that one looks at them'. One of Cutting's patients (1997) said, 'Man behind a lorry was pulling hideous faces'.

Different aspects of colour perception can be affected. The intensity of the colour (*visual hyperaesthesia*), the actual hue and the quality of the colour can all be affected. Cutting (1997) gives several examples:

- 'colours are brighter', 'colours more vivid—red, yellow, orange stood out';
- 'black looked brown sometimes', 'brown looked different; trouble with pink as it comes across as green'; and
- 'this colour looks like an old blue—something horrible'.

Bleuler (1950) describes 'one patient sees everything as coloured red; another sees everything as white', and Jaspers 'I only see black; even when the sun is shining, it is still all black'. These perceptual distortions of colour occur in schizophrenia. In organic conditions, *achromatopsia*, which is the complete absence of colour, has been described after unilateral or bilateral occipital lesions usually of the lingual and fusiform gyri. *Dyschromatopsia* refers to the perversion of colour perception and occurs after unilateral posterior lesions.

The spatial location of a perceived object may be distorted. *Teleopsia* involves the object appearing far away, and *pelopsia* involves the object appearing nearer than it should. *Alloaesthesia* is the term for when the perceived object is in a different position from what is expected, so that the patient, for example, experiences the transposition of objects from left to right.

Akinetopsia is the impairment of visual perception of motion in which the individual is unable to perceive the motion of objects. It is very rare and is said to follow bilateral posterior cortical damage. Zeki (1993) quotes Zihl's case:

She had difficulty, for example, in pouring tea or coffee into a cup because the fluid appeared to be frozen, like a glacier. In addition, she could not stop pouring at the right time since she was unable to perceive the movement in the cup (or a pot) when the fluid rose.

The general quality of perception can be affected. This usually involves an indefinable alteration in the visual appearance of the perceived world so that everything seems different from what it used to be: 'People [look] like toys—almost dead and lifeless, carrying out automatic movements with special meaning' (Cutting, 1997); 'people look dead, pale, cold' (Cutting, 1997);

'A factory-worker sees a grasshopper and becomes very disturbed and excited at the sight of this *very strange* [my emphasis] and unknown animal' (Bleuler, 1950). These experiences are examples of derealisation. Normally, perception is accompanied by affect, which may be a feeling of familiarity, of enjoyment, of dislike, of involvement, of proximity and so on. This is usually appropriate and so ignored. However, changes in these feelings may present as symptoms, for example, 'everything looks clear but it all looks miles away', 'I feel in seclusion. It is like looking through the wrong end of a telescope'. These and many other feelings are described under *derealisation* (Chapter 13). There is a feeling of unreality in the perceptual field, an alteration in the feelings associated with the objects of perception, but, significantly, the patient refers to these experiences with the preface 'as if', indicating both the difficulty in describing and the need to resort to analogous language.

A patient who exemplified both the loss of intensity of sensation and the change in feelings associated with perception in the context of a depressive illness was a 23-year-old Sri Lankan Buddhist priest. After a session of meditation, he became frightened on waking up to discover that he had assaulted another priest during the night. In the next few days, he felt that he had lost all sensation. Things he saw and heard he could not understand properly. He could see only the things that were nearby. He could not get any sensations from his skin. He said that he could not read nor understand nor feel sadness or happiness. He said that he could not feel anything: 'all is numbed, body and mind'. He admitted to feeling low, that life was not worth living and that he had thought of ending his life. There was no neurologic or other physical abnormality.

Elementary Aspects of Auditory Perception

The elementary elements of auditory perception that can be disturbed include the uniqueness of the experience, the intensity of the experience and the spatial position (Cutting, 1997). In *palinacousis*, the uniqueness of a perceptual experience is disturbed and there is persistence of sounds that are heard. A subject returned to answer the door several times during a 30-minute period after the doorbell had actually rung (Jacobs et al., 1973). The *intensity* of auditory perception may be altered so that it is either heightened or

diminished. For example, heightening in the auditory modality is called *hyperacusis*, a symptom in which the patient complains of everything sounding abnormally loud, saying, 'I can't bear the noise'. Ordinary conversation may sound intolerably noisy, and even whispering at a distance may be found uncomfortable. There is, of course, no true improvement of auditory perception but simply a lowering of the threshold at which noise becomes unpleasant. The symptom occurs in depression, migraine and some toxic states, for example, the hangover after acute alcohol excess. The spatial position of a sound may be disturbed so that the sound appears as if it was nearer, further away or displaced in position.

Elementary Aspects of Tactile Perception

Palinaptia is the experience of tactile sensation outlasting the stimulus so that an object held in the hand continues to be perceived well after it has been discarded. Stacy (1987) reports a case of a patient with biparietal lesions who could feel her toothbrush in her hand 15 minutes after putting it away. The palinaptic experience occurred in the setting of astereognosis and palpatory apraxia. The palinaptia can be conceived as a complex haptic hallucination. *Exosomesthesia* is the 'displacement of cutaneous sensation into extrapersonal space' (Shapiro and Fink, 1952; Shapiro et al., 1952). This is a curious condition in which the individual experiences direct cutaneous touch sensation when a distal object that is in the same room is touched.

If the palm of their hand was in contact with some object (bed, table, book) and the dorsum of that pricked with a pin, the patient insisted that the bed or table had been touched and not their hand. This phenomenon could be elicited only from the hand and only when the palm was in contact with some object.

This unusual phenomenon can be experimentally induced, and it has been suggested that the body image, despite its appearance of durability and permanence, is a transitory internal construct that can be altered by encountered stimulus contingencies and correlations (Ramachandran and Hirstein, 1998).

It is even possible to 'project' tactile sensations onto inanimate objects such as tables and shoes that do not resemble body parts. The subject is asked to place their right hand underneath a table surface (or behind a vertical screen) so that they cannot see it. The experimenter then uses their right hand to randomly stroke and tap the subject's right hand (under the table or behind the screen) and uses their left hand to simultaneously stroke and tap the table in perfect synchrony. After 10 to 30 seconds, the subject starts developing the uncanny illusion that the sensations are now coming from the table and that the table is now part of their body.

Alloaesthesia is a neurologic condition seen after right-sided vascular lesions of the putamen that is characterized by a sensory stimulus on one side of the body being perceived on the contralateral side. It can also occur after spinal cord lesions such as cervical tumours, cervical disc herniation and multiple sclerosis (Kawamura et al., 1987; Fukutake et al., 1993).

Splitting of Perception

This rare phenomenon is described sometimes with organic states and also with schizophrenia: the patient is unable to form the usual, assumed links between two or more perceptions. A patient watching television experienced a feeling of competition between the visual and auditory perceptions. She felt that the two were not coming from the same source but were competing for her attention and conveying opposite messages. *Splitting of perception* occurs when the links between different sensory modalities fail to be made, and so the sensations themselves, although in fact associated, appear to be quite separate and even in conflict. This anomaly reveals the underlying implicit nature and automaticity of the binding of disparate elements of any perception, namely the binding of colour, shape, texture, motion and position to form a coherent whole. Also it demonstrates the important principle that anomalies can act to reveal underlying mechanisms.

FALSE PERCEPTION

Now we turn from the altered perception of real objects to consider the perception of objects that are not there; these are *new perceptions* that include illusion, hallucination and pseudohallucination. Illusions were separated phenomenologically from hallucinations by Esquirol (1817) and later also by Hagen, who introduced the term *pseudohallucination* (Berrios,

1996). Esquirol described illusions as transformations of perceptions coming about by a mixing of the reproduced perceptions of the subject's fantasy with natural perceptions.

Illusion

In order to fully understand the nature of illusions, it is best to briefly consider the contributions of Gestalt psychology to our understanding of visual perception. Gestalt psychology emphasized that we perceive entire patterns or configurations not merely individual component parts. The aim of the project was to discover the principles underlying how sensory information is interpreted, that is, how we come to create, perceive and experience a coherent pattern that is more than its parts. The proponents of Gestalt psychology, Wolfgang Kohler (1887–1967) and Kurt Koffka (1886–1941), argued that there are regular and predictable ways that we structure incoming sensory information and these included processes such as proximity, similarity, continuity, closure, part–whole relationship and common fate. *Proximity* refers to how sensory elements that are close together in space or time come to be perceived together. *Similarity* refers to how similar figures tend to be grouped together. *Continuity* refers to the process by means of which smooth and continuous patterns are perceived rather than discontinuous ones. *Closure* is the tendency to perceive closed figures rather than open or incomplete ones and this accompanied by the tendency to supply missing information to close an incomplete figure. *Part–Whole Relationship* refers to the fact that, irrespective of the elements that make up the parts of a pattern, the pattern remains recognisable. This explains our capacity to recognize a melody despite the fact that it is played on differing instruments. And finally, *Common Fate* refers to the tendency for elements that are seen to be moving together are perceived as belonging together. For example, a group of people running in the same direction are seen as belonging together, unified in their purpose. A critique of Gestalt theory is outside the scope of this book. Nonetheless, there are a number of problems with the theory, in particular the degree to which it is capable of precise description and measurement. Wagemans et al. (2012) examined the conceptual and theoretical aspects of Gestalt theory after a century and attempted a reformulation in terms of information-processing

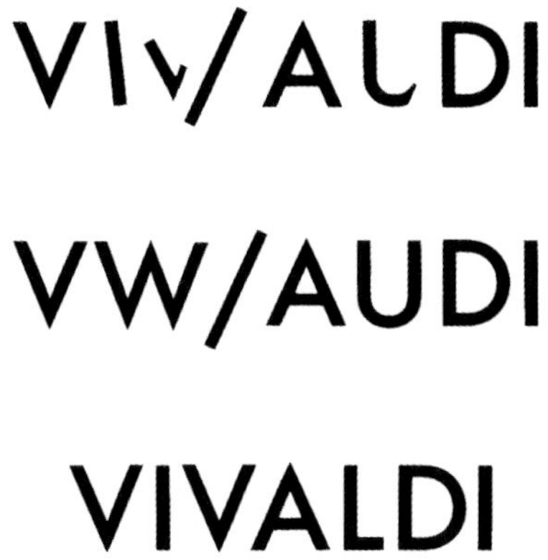

VI√ALDI

VW/AUDI

VIVALDI

Fig. 7.1 Illusion.

framework. This reformulation demonstrates that it is possible to reconceptualize Gestalt theory without losing the essential elements of its insights.

In psychopathology three types of illusions are normally described: *completion illusion, affect illusion* and *pareidolic illusion*. Completion illusions depend on inattention for their occurrence. The faded lettering of an advertisement outside a garage is represented in Fig. 7.1. Being more interested in music than cars, this can be misread this as 'Vivaldi'. We commonly miss the misprints in a newspaper because we read the words as if they were written correctly. As soon as our attention is drawn to the mistake, our perception alters. An incomplete perception that is meaningless in itself is filled in by a process of extrapolation from previous experience and prior expectation to produce significance.

Very clearly, completion illusion demonstrates the principle of *closure* in Gestalt psychology. It is necessary for us to make sense of our environment, so when the sensory cues are incomplete, we fill in the gaps and a whole perceptual experience becomes meaningful.

When *illusion* arises through *affect*, the perception of everyday objects is changed. The illusion can be understood only in the context of the prevailing mood state. A child who is frightened of the dark wakes up in the half-light and mistakes a towel hanging by the wall for a person moving. The influence of emotion on perceptual experience derives from the relationship between emotion and meaning in determining what a percept is. Even though this is not directly

discussed in Gestalt theory, it is well recognized that form perception, which refers to the separation of perceived objects (the figure) from the surroundings (the ground), allows for the emergence of a meaningful form from the ground. In situations of ambiguity, such as in figure-ground reversal, attentional shifts allow for reversal of the figure and ground. In affect illusions, emotion determines the identification of the perceived object, but focused attention clarifies the error.

Pareidolia occurs in a considerable proportion of normal people. Pareidolia can also be provoked by psychomimetic drugs. Typically, identifiable figures are seen in random or formless sensory stimuli such as cloud formations or ambiguous reflections on polished glass windows. Many of the Gestalt principles may be at play in determining what is perceived, including such principles as ambiguity between figure and ground, continuity, similarity, etc.

Pareidolic illusions are created out of structureless sensory stimuli. The percept takes on a full and detailed appearance: 'A Victorian lady with a crinoline and frilled bloomers'. The person experiencing it, like someone seeing a photograph, knows that it is not truly there as an object and that it is figurative. However, they cannot dismiss what they see. Completion and affect illusions occur during inattention; they are banished by attention, which will, on the other hand, increase the intensity of pareidolic illusions as they become more intricate and detailed.

Pareidolic illusion occurs in children more than in adults. It should be distinguished from the following conditions.

- *Perceptual misinterpretation,* that is, simply making a mistake as to the nature of perception without that perception being particularly influenced by emotion mixed with fantasy.
- *Functional hallucination,* which occurs when a certain percept is necessary for the production of a hallucination, but the hallucination is not a transformation of that perception. For example, the patient hears voices when the tap is turned on; they hear voices in the running water, but the voices and the noise of water are quite distinct and can be heard separately and synchronously like any other voice that is heard against a background noise. The perception of hearing running water is necessary to produce the hallucination,

but the hallucination is not a transformation of that perception.
  • *Fantastic interpretations* or elaborate *daydreaming* can be very similar to pareidolic illusions and, as we have already discussed, there is a large admixture of fantasy in such illusions.

⊗ Hallucination

Hallucinations are the most significant type of false perceptions. Here are five definitions of hallucination.
  • A perception without an object (Esquirol, 1817).
  • Hallucinations proper are false perceptions that are not in any way distortions of real perceptions but spring up on their own as something quite new and occur simultaneously with and alongside real perception (Jaspers, 1997).
  • A hallucination is an exteroceptive or interoceptive percept that does not correspond to an actual object (Smythies, 1956).
  • According to Slade (1976a), three criteria are essential for an operational definition: (1) percept-like experience in the absence of an external stimulus; (2) percept-like experience that has the full force and impact of a real perception; and (3) percept-like experience that is unwilled, occurs spontaneously and cannot be readily controlled by the percipient. This definition is derived from Jasper's formal characteristics of a normal perception (see Table 7.1).
  • A hallucination is a *perception without an object* (within a realistic philosophic framework) or the *appearance of an individual thing in the world without any corresponding material event* (within a Kantian framework), according to Cutting (1997).

One of the simplest facts about hallucinations is often one of the most difficult to comprehend: what the doctor calls a hallucination is a *normal perceptual experience* to the patient. Although the standard definitions of hallucination imply that, subjectively, a hallucination is indistinguishable from a normal percept, some authors argue that hallucinatory percepts may be distinct from normal percepts (as discussed later). One of the clues that the sufferer uses to grasp the fact that they might be hallucinating is that there is no corroborative evidence for the percept in other modalities. A person hears voices giving a commentary on their

activity: 'They are going to the sink. They are putting the coffee on'. They see no one else in the room but recognize the voices of their neighbours. They cannot understand how they can be hearing them, but they are so convinced by the reality of the voices that they draw the curtains and take the mirrors off the walls. There is some conflict in their mind: they hear voices but can see no person to account for them. However, they resolve this conflict in what is a rational way, assuming that they believe implicitly in the genuineness of the perception: 'someone must have fixed a device or altered my sense of hearing'. What is notable is that they do not doubt the reality of the percept.

Horowitz (1975) has investigated hallucinations using a cognitive approach, looking at each of the following four constructs in terms of coding, appraising and transforming information.

Hallucinations are mental images that (1) occur in the form of images, (2) are derived from internal sources of information, (3) are appraised incorrectly as if from external sources of information and (4) usually occur intrusively. Each of these four constructs refers to a separate set of psychological processes, although together they comprise a holistic experience.

This provides a conceptual framework for investigating the phenomena of hallucination.

This idea has been further developed by Bentall (1990), who considers that hallucinations represent faulty judgements about the origin of their perceptions, tending to attribute them to an external source. The content of hallucination was thought to be explained, at least in part, by the need to defend the individual's own self-esteem. Hallucinations may result from a failure of the metacognitive skills involved in discriminating between self-generated and external sources of information. This explanation was given further support by the finding that hallucinators more often misattributed auditorily presented answers to difficult clues from an experimenter than either a deluded but not hallucinated group of patients or normal control subjects (Bentall et al., 1991).

The current, most influential, explanatory model of verbal auditory hallucinations is the misattribution of inner speech model. In this model, inner speech is assumed to be involved in cognitive planning, self-monitoring and in reflecting on action. Furthermore, there are possible roles for inner speech in regulating emotions and behaviour. Although, in many respects, inner speech is akin to spoken language, it can also be an abbreviated version of spoken language, taking on a more condensed and telegraphic form. A full description of the dialogic model of inner speech and its proposed relationship to auditory verbal hallucination is outside the remit of this book but can be found in Fernyhough's book, *The Voices Within* (2016). The importance of this model is that it points to the ubiquity of inner speech and lays the foundation for understanding the links between inner speech and the obvious abnormalities demonstrated in verbal hallucinations. Furthermore, it draws attention, implicitly, to the distinctions that may exist between verbal hallucinations and hallucinations in other modalities. Misattribution, in this model, implies that there is impairment of self-monitoring with the result that patients are unaware that the perceived auditory verbal hallucinations are indeed their own self-generated thoughts/inner speech (Upthegrove et al., 2015).

Other theoretical explanations include alterations in the mechanisms for language production, speech production and perception. These mechanisms are implicated because of findings that demonstrate activation of left superior temporal cortex during auditory verbal hallucinations in patients with schizophrenia. Aberrant memory functions may also be at play, especially in those patients whose auditory hallucinations occur as a failure of inhibition of recall and unintended memory activation. This mechanism is thought to be more likely in those patients in whom auditory verbal hallucinations are best conceptualized as intrusive memories that arise out of context and are linked to past trauma. Finally, it is also possible that auditory verbal hallucinations occur as a result of faulty auditory processing in which auditory stimuli are misinterpreted as 'voices'.

Attempts to explain hallucinations by underlying neurochemistry and neuropathology have so far not made much progress. An attempt has been made to incorporate concepts of biological vulnerability and psychological influences in the aetiology and clinical presentation of hallucinations, but research has produced no single mechanism to account for them (Asaad and Shapiro, 1986).

Hallucinations take place at the same time as normal sensory stimuli are perceived. In this way, they are unlike dreams, which in fact have more of the characteristics of illusions. Hallucinations are like normal percepts of which several can be perceived simultaneously or in rapid succession. Thus the patient can hear hallucinatory voices at the same time as they are seeing their interviewer and listening to them speak.

The sense of reality experienced by patients when they hallucinate was studied by Aggernaes (1972), developing the concepts of Rasmussen. He pointed out six qualities of which normal people can be aware when they experience a sensation, which also occurred in more than 90% of a series of hallucinations.

- With normal sensation, we are able to distinguish *perceiving* with our sense organs from *imagining* the same objects; hallucinations similarly are experienced as *sensation* and not as *thought* or *fantasy*.
- When a subject experiences something, they realize its possible *relevance* for their own emotions, needs or actions; hallucinations also have this quality of behavioural relevance.
- Normal sensation has a quality of *objectivity* in that the experiencer feels that, under favourable circumstances, they would be able to experience the same something with another modality of sensation; this is also the experience of the hallucinator.
- An object is considered to *exist* if the observer feels certain that it still exists even though nobody else is experiencing it at that time; perceived objects and hallucinations share this quality.
- Experience of object perception and hallucination is *involuntary* in that the experiencer feels that it is impossible or extremely difficult to alter or dismiss the experience simply by wishing to do so.
- Normally, the experiencer is aware, or through simple questioning becomes aware, that their experience is not simply the result of being in an unusual mental state; this quality of *independence* is present with normal perception and with hallucination.

One further quality of normal object perception was found to be absent more often than not with hallucination. This is the quality of *publicness* in which the experiencer would be aware that anybody else with normal sensory faculties would be able to perceive this something. Often, the hallucinator does not believe that others could share their experience (delusional explanation may be given for this).

Clearly, cultural factors influence the manner in which subjects describe their abnormal perceptions. It has been claimed by Andrade (1988) that because patients in India were more prepared to accept paranormal explanations for phenomena, false perceptions or 'true hallucinations' are more likely to be ascribed with objectivity and veridicality. Even if this is so and it is not proven, the qualities described by Aggernaes would still be useful in distinguishing hallucination from other abnormalities of perception.

Cutting (1997) has argued that hallucinatory experiences are hardly plausible everyday occurrences and that therefore it is not that hallucinatory percepts are indistinguishable from normal percepts, but rather that they are taken for reality despite the fact that they are distinct from everyday reality. He makes the point that, for example, Lilliputian hallucinations in delirium and complex hallucinations involving comic characters are obviously not plausible perceptions in the real world yet they are taken as real. However, Cutting ignores the fact that it is precisely because hallucinatory phenomena have the quality of a normal experience that they are taken for reality despite being, as he points out, implausible. Other authors, such as Spitzer (1994), argue that hallucinations are not like normal perceptions, in that patients can distinguish between real perceptual experiences and their hallucinatory experiences. This is one reason why patients are able to understand the reference to 'hearing voices' in interactions with clinicians; both parties know what this way of speaking stands for. Indeed, Wernicke (1906) had already drawn attention to when he pointed out that the notion of 'hearing voices' was not invented by psychiatrists but rather was used by patients to indicate that somehow their experience was akin to hearing other people talk but also different from this as well. Junginger and Frame (1985) showed that a substantial proportion of patients (40%) rated the voices they heard as more akin to inner speech than to external spoken or heard speech, thus emphasizing that hallucinations may not always have the hallmark of normal perception.

AUDITORY HALLUCINATION

An additional video for this topic is available online ▶

Hallucinations can occur in any of the areas of the five special senses and also with somatic sensation. We will start by discussing *auditory hallucinations* because they are most often of supreme diagnostic significance. In acute organic states, the auditory hallucinations are usually unstructured sounds—*elementary hallucinations*; for example, the patient hears whirring noises or rattles, whistling, machinery or music. Often the noise is experienced as unpleasant and frightening. Of interest are musical hallucinations, which tend to occur in older women with deafness or brain disease and no history of psychiatric illness (Berrios, 1990). There are, therefore, similarities with Charles Bonnet's syndrome, which is described later in the section on visual hallucinations.

Hearing voices is characteristic of schizophrenia, but it also occurs occasionally in other conditions, such as *chronic alcoholic hallucinosis* or *affective psychoses*. These voices are sometimes called *phonemes* (confusion exists, unfortunately, because the word is used with a totally different meaning in linguistics, in which phonemes are the units of speech-sound from which words are made). Usually in *organic states*, the phonemes are simple words or short sentences often spoken to the patient in the second person as either peremptory orders or abusive remarks. These abusive or imperative phonemes also occur in schizophrenia, but other more complicated speech is also heard; the voices may be single or multiple, male or female or both and from people known and recognized by the patient or not known. They are experienced as coming from outside their head or their self. The voice is clear, objective and definite and is assumed by the patient to be a normal percept that, at the same time, may be baffling and incomprehensible in its import. Particularly characteristic of schizophrenia are voices that say the patient's *own thoughts out loud*, which give a *running commentary* on the patient's actions or voices, which *argue* or *discuss* vigorously *with each other*. They refer to the patient in the third person (Schneider, 1959).

In a series of 100 current patients experiencing auditory verbal hallucinations, all of whom were described as 'hearing voices', 61 suffered from schizophrenia and 78 from schizophrenia-related conditions (Nayani and

David, 1996). Fifty-two percent of the patients had an experience of sadness, and 45% experienced churning or butterfly sensations in the stomach at or before onset. Most voices spoke in conversational tones, but a few whispered and a few shouted; half of the sample heard their voices through their ears as external stimuli. Most voices were male, often a middle-aged man, usually speaking in a different accent from the patient, for example, 'an upper-class voice'. Subjects heard a mean of 3.2 different voices and usually knew the identity of at least one; in half of the subjects, the voices signified forces of Good or Evil. Half of the subjects were able to exert some control over their voices, and two-thirds had developed coping mechanisms to deal with them; high levels of distress were found among those with little control and few means of coping. The majority of subjects ascribed reality characteristics to their voices. A long history of auditory hallucinations tended to be associated with more hallucinated words, more voices, a greater range of emotional expression and grammatical style and greater likelihood of delusional interpretations of the voices.

In a qualitative study of 25 subjects, Upthegrove et al. (2016) reported that the research participants experienced the verbal hallucinations as an entity that was able to socially interact with them and had a well-developed character of its own. The experience was often real in the sense that the participants found it difficult to distinguish between their experiences and reality and were surprised that other people could not hear the same 'voices'. The voices were described as 'demanding' rather than 'commanding'. The voices could also influence the participant's emotions by being threatening, blaming or mocking and tricking or manipulating the participants. Participants found the voices disruptive to the degree that their concentration was affected and simple tasks became arduous.

Auditory verbal hallucinations in schizophrenia are generally private events, but several early writers observed vocalizations that corresponded with the content of the voices taking place at the same time as the hallucinations. Normal people occasionally vocalize their own thoughts *sotto voce*; in the psychotic equivalent of this, it seems that sometimes those with schizophrenia are vocalizing their hallucinations at the same time as they experience them. Green and Preston (1981) increased the audibility of the whispers of

such a patient to an intelligible level using auditory feedback.

Sometimes patients with schizophrenia describe abnormal perceptions in both the visual and the auditory modalities. The examiner should be careful not to assume that there are both auditory and visual hallucinations present; there may be a different *form*, particularly for the visual experience. A man aged 45 years described his experience as follows: 'I hear my nephews talking [about me]. "He is a poofter [homosexual] and a pervert" … I see them as well. The curtains move and I know that it is them moving them'. This is a description of a persecutory auditory hallucination, but the visual experience is a delusional interpretation of a normal perception, not a visual hallucination.

Patients' descriptions of their phonemes vary greatly. Sometimes, patients talk openly and quite blandly about their 'voices'. Not uncommonly, a patient may deny voices but assert that they hear 'spoken messages' or 'transmissions' or some other spoken sound, and it may be difficult to decide whether this is a real perception or an auditory hallucination. The phonemes may be so insistent, compelling and interesting that ordinary conversation with the doctor is found boring and even unreal in comparison. The voices may form an insistent background to life that is so ensuring that a large part of the patient's speech and behaviour is occupied in answering and obeying the voices. Psychiatric nurses often observe that the auditory hallucinations described by patients are as real to them as any other remembered conversations, and both hallucinatory and real auditory perceptions form the memories on which patients base their life and behaviour in the present.

Auditory hallucinations occur when there is a combination of vivid mental imagery and poor reality testing in the auditory modality (Slade, 1976b). This has been investigated using a battery of tests including the *verbal transformation effect*. The word *tress* was repeated on a tape recorder to the subjects for 10 minutes. After a time, subjects began to hear other words and syllables. Normal subjects and patients with schizophrenia who were not auditorily hallucinated usually heard words that were phonetically linked to the original monosyllable, but patients who experienced auditory hallucinations heard words that were quite different phonetically as often as those that were linked.

It appears that auditory hallucinations are dependent on the meaningfulness of sensory input. When various types of auditory input were presented to patients with schizophrenia who experienced hallucinations, it was found that it was not the degree of external stimulation that was required to diminish hallucinations but the nature of the stimulus and the degree of attention it received. When the subject was required to actively monitor the experimental material by reading aloud a prose passage and deciding the content afterwards, this produced a greater decrease of hallucinatory experience than any of the conditions in which sounds were played to the subject through earphones (Margo et al., 1981). Morley (1987) reported the psychological treatment of a 30-year-old man with auditory hallucinations. Distraction by means of music presented by a portable cassette produced a transient reduction in the frequency and clarity of hallucinations. Subsequently, these hallucinations were totally abolished by the unilateral placement of a wax earplug: attention was considered more effective than distraction. The patient located the hallucination 'about a foot away from my right ear', and the plug was only effective in the right ear.

Patients with schizophrenia experiencing auditory hallucinations were found to be impaired in cognitive processing in the aspects of tolerance of ambiguity and availability of alternative meanings. *Tolerance of ambiguity* was tested by asking the patient to recognize a spoken word, which was obscured by a masking noise of people reading. The masking noise was gradually reduced in volume until recognition occurred. *Alternative meanings* tests the subject's knowledge of less familiar meanings of words. These two processes reduced the quality of perception (resulting in hallucination) by introducing errors of premature judgement without the safeguard of subsequently considered alternatives (Heilbrun and Blum, 1984).

Some auditory hallucinations are considered to be 'first rank symptoms of schizophrenia' (Schneider, 1959); these are *audible thoughts*, *voices* heard *arguing* with each other and *voices commenting* on the patient's behaviour. These three perceptual disturbances, as other first rank symptoms, each represent a massive interference with the boundaries of self-image, the discrimination of what is 'I' from what is 'not I' (Sims, 1991).

The mechanisms used by patients with chronic schizophrenia to cope with persistent auditory hallucinations were discussed by Falloon and Talbot (1981). The strategies used to cope with intrusive voices could be classified as changes in behaviour, in sensory or affective state and in cognition. Changes in behaviour included alteration of posture, such as lying down, or seeking out the company of others. Physiologic arousal was altered to cope with hallucinations through relaxation or physical exercise such as jogging. Cognitive methods included control of attention or active suppression of hallucinations. These authors believe that the common sense application of strategies used by patients can be beneficial in the control of these distressing symptoms.

Finally, there is a vigorous debate about the presence of auditory/verbal hallucinations in disorders other than the psychoses such as borderline personality disorders and also in normal populations (McCarthy-Jones, 2012). In a recent report from the Adult Psychiatric Morbidity survey, it was reported that, overall, 12.6% of individuals with a mental disorder reported hallucinations compared with 3.7% of individuals who did not have a mental disorder. Surprisingly, hallucinations were prevalent in agoraphobia, specific phobia, social phobia, obsessive compulsive disorder, panic disorder, depression, borderline personality disorder and generalized anxiety disorder (Kelleher and DeVylder, 2017). The question that remains to be answered is whether the form of these verbal hallucinations is identical to the form of the verbal hallucinations in schizophrenia, for example. Further, there is some evidence derived from functional neuroimaging suggesting that the neural underpinning of auditory verbal hallucinations in schizophrenia may involve altered dopamine synthesis and reduced functional lateralisation (Upthegrove et al., 2015).

It is important to emphasise that not all auditory hallucinations are verbal in nature. Musical hallucinations, for example, are reported in individuals with deafness and are often thought of as the auditory equivalent of Charles Bonnet syndrome, a condition that is associated with visual hallucinations in the context of visual impairment. Musical hallucinations often involve familiar melodies such as ballads and hymns. The melodies can be repetitive including a single line or verse and can be present in both ears. Stewart et al. (2006) make the point that the phenomenology of musical hallucinations, especially the fact that the perceptions are of complex patterned sequences that are in line with the previous musical listening experience of the subject, suggests that there is amplification of normal imagery that is usually suppressed by inputs from the external sensory world that decrease in the context of deafness (Stewart et al., 2006). The proposition is that the decreased signal-to-noise ratio in auditory transmission in the deaf leads to inappropriate activation of cortical networks usually involved in perception and imagery, and the networks involved are also those involved during musical perception and imagery in the absence of deafness. Furthermore, there is the claim that the auditory perception in the context of deafness is not verbal in nature because the fundamental aspects of music are more predictable and repetitive compared to speech such that hearing a few notes of music is sufficient to predict the coming notes. Hence, the tendency to hear music rather than language in deafness is more likely.

VISUAL HALLUCINATION

Visual hallucinations characteristically occur in *organic states* rather than in the functional psychoses. A 69-year-old married man was referred to the duty psychiatrist in a casualty department for assessment. He said that his life was at an end and he deserved to die, as he had been caught masturbating by his daughter-in-law and grandchildren that afternoon. His wife said that this was not true; he had become very agitated and distressed over 12 hours, and no one had visited the house that day. During the interview, he was intensely agitated and put his hands in front of his face. He claimed that he could see clearly a sheet of glass half a metre in front of him, which he attempted to move. Later, he described seeing dust falling down everywhere and was trying to catch it. He manifested clouding of consciousness. A diagnosis of viral encephalitis was made on the basis of the history of persistent headache, the neurological signs and the finding of lymphocytosis in the cerebrospinal fluid.

It is often difficult to decide whether the full criteria for the presence of a hallucination have been fulfilled in the visual modality. Distortion of visual percepts based on either sensation of external stimuli or internal interference with the visual pathway may produce disturbances that are similar to those occurring with entirely new perceptions. Sometimes the account of an experience given by the patient may sound like a sensory transformation rather than a hallucination, but the bizarre and complex nature of the experience can render the description of the phenomena difficult.

Visual hallucinations occur with *occipital lobe tumours* involving the visual cortex, for example, tuberculous granuloma in the left occipital lobe can cause a 'starburst' effect in the right visual field (Werring and Marsden, 1999). Hallucinations and other visual disturbances may occur with other physical lesions, such as *loss of colour vision, homonymous hemianopia* (loss of half of the field of vision, the same half in both eyes; Komel, 1985), *dyslexia* (inability to read at a level appropriate to the individual's age and intelligence), *alexia* (word blindness) in a dominant hemisphere lesion and *cortical blindness* (blindness due to a lesion of the cortical visual centre). They may, as in delirium tremens, be associated with an affect of terror or with an affect of hilarious absurdity. Similar visual hallucinations, illusions and changes in mood occur in other forms of delirium. Visual hallucinations also occur in the *post-concussional state,* in *epileptic twilight states* and in metabolic disturbances, for example, *hepatic failure.* Visual hallucinations have also been described in association with various dementing processes, including Alzheimer's disease (Burns et al., 1990), senile dementia (Haddad and Benbow, 1992), multi-infarct dementia (Cummings et al., 1987), Pick's disease (Ey, 1973), Lewy body dementia (Donaghy and McKeith, 2014) and Huntington's chorea (Lishman, 1989). Among referrals to a psychogeriatric service, visual perceptual disturbance occurred in 30% of patients; there was a strong correlation between the presence of visual hallucination and eye pathology (Berrios and Brook, 1984). In fact, visual hallucinations are common in elderly patients with a wide variety of medical conditions and often no psychiatric history (Barodawala and Mulley, 1997).

Hallucinations have also been described by individuals after sniffing glue and petrol. The drugs mescaline and lysergic acid diethylamide are potent causes of visual perceptual change. Visual hallucinations are infinitely variable in their content. They range from quite crudely formed flashes of light or colour (elementary hallucinations), through more organized patterns and shapes, to complex, full, visual perceptions of people and scenes. Visual and auditory hallucinations may occur synchronously in organic states. For example, in *temporal lobe epilepsy* a visual hallucination of a human figure was also heard to speak.

With psychomimetic drugs, there are alterations in spatial perception, in the perception of movement and in the appreciation of colour, and visual illusions and hallucinations may occur. Visual hallucinations are very uncommon in schizophrenia (although some of the earlier writers used the term *hallucination* for other visual abnormalities that occurred). Persaud and Cutting (1991) cautiously refer to 'anomalous perceptual experiences in the visual modality' in schizophrenic patients, for example, as in the patient who although still recognising a face considers it to be distorted. These authors report four such cases of perceptual disturbance in one visual field, always the left field. Visual hallucinations are not reckoned to occur in uncomplicated affective psychoses. It is common in schizophrenia for the patient to describe auditory hallucinations associated with visual *pseudohallucinations*. Although the phonemes are complete and appear to have all the characteristics, subjectively, of a normal percept, the visual experiences are often inferred on the basis of the auditory hallucinations and of contemporaneous delusions. It is possible to see, in most instances, how psychotically disordered fantasy accounts for the content of the visual experiences. Vivid elaborate scenic hallucinations have been described in *oneiroid* states of schizophrenia. In these states, there is also an altered state of consciousness, and the patient appears to lose contact with their environment and acts as if they were dreaming. The elements of the hallucinations are said to have a melodramatic quality including scenes of catastrophes, dangerous adventures, and glimpses of heaven and hell.

Sometimes, visual hallucinations do not appear to be associated with any other psychiatric abnormality. Charles Bonnet's syndrome (phantom visual images) is a condition in which individuals experience complex visual hallucinations in association with impaired vision without demonstrable psychopathology or disturbance of normal consciousness (Schultz and Melzack, 1991). Although more common in the elderly, it can occur at any age and is usually associated with central or peripheral reduction in vision. Episodes may last from days to years, with images of people, animals, buildings and scenery being most frequently reported, the images being static, moving in the visual field or animated. Clearly, this condition is of importance in the differential diagnosis.

In most cases of Charles Bonnet's syndrome and in musical hallucinosis in the deaf to which it has been likened, there is no demonstrable brain pathology (Fuchs and Lauter, 1992), although it has been reported in the context of central neurophysiological disturbance such as bilateral occipital infractions or in association with optic neuritis in multiple sclerosis. The features of this syndrome have been considered by Podoll et al. (1990) to be as follows:

- Elderly persons with normal consciousness experience visual hallucinations.
- None of the following are present: delirium, dementia, organic affective or delusional syndromes, psychosis, intoxication or neurological disorder with lesions of the central visual cortex.
- There is reduced vision resulting from eye disease in most cases.

Hallucinations in this condition are always located in external space, are usually coloured and are much more vivid and distinct than the patient's impaired vision would otherwise permit. The content is *elementary* in about one-third of cases, such as photisms or geometric patterns. Complex objects are most often human figures, less often animals, plants and inanimate objects; these objects may be fragmented and may change over time—figures gliding through the room. The percepts may be modifiable by voluntary control, for example, closing the eyelids, and there is usually insight concerning their 'unreality'.

It is becoming clearer that Charles Bonnet syndrome results from reduced visual sensory stimuli that leads to excessive excitability and spontaneous neural activity that manifest as a visual hallucinatory experience (ffytche, 2007). Furthermore, analysis of the visual percepts shows that there are three main types including (1) extended landscape scenes, (2) grotesque, disembodied and distorted faces with large eyeballs and (3) visual perseverations such as palinopsia (ffytche and Howard, 1999). These distinct types of perceptions typically arose from predictable neural lesion sites: extended landscape scenes derived from lesions in anterior temporal projections to the ventral

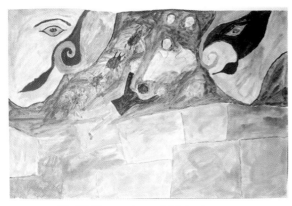

Fig. 7.2 The experience of delirium tremens.

visual pathways; distorted faces occurred from lesions in the superior temporal sulcus; and visual perseverations occurred following lesions in the visual parietal lobe. ffytche (2007) has argued that this demonstrates the utility of neurophenomenology.

The alcoholic withdrawal syndrome of *delirium tremens* is a specific form of acute organic syndrome and is characterized by gross changes in perception, mood and consciousness state (see Chapter 3). Pareidolic, or affective, illusions are often prodromal in delirium tremens, and these are followed by visual and haptic *Lilliputian* hallucinations, which are often of little animals or diminutive men. There is a bizarre intermingling of affect so that the patient experiences stark terror and, at the same time, a humorous response to absurd experiences especially common with these disorders.

The hallucinations in delirium tremens may change so rapidly that the patient has difficulty describing them. A patient experiencing such visual phenomena tried to portray this in Fig. 7.2. Illusions are frequently associated with hallucinations, especially affective illusions in which, through the predominant mood state of terror, cracks in the wall of the ward or curtains moving in the breeze may be misinterpreted in a frightening way. At the same time, such patients are highly suggestible and can form abnormal visual experiences as a result of suggestion.

HALLUCINATION OF BODILY SENSATION

It has been convincingly argued by Berrios (1982) that diverse 'perceptions without object' were brought together by Esquirol (1817) within the term *hallucination*, which was relevant for 'distance senses' such as vision, hearing and, to a lesser extent, smell and taste but not really applicable to touch. So-called *tactile hallucinations* appear to be different phenomenologically and to only superficially resemble hallucinations of the distance senses. It would seem for tactile hallucinations that the most important corroborating diagnostic factor is the concurrence of a delusional component. Berrios concludes that the concepts of hallucination and delusion may be closer to each other than has often been considered, especially in British psychiatry.

Hallucinations of bodily sensation may be *superficial, kinaesthetic* or *visceral.* Superficial hallucinations affecting skin sensation may be *thermic,* an abnormal perception of heat and cold ('my feet on fire'); *haptic,* of touch ('a dead hand touched me'); or *hygric,* a perception of fluid ('all my blood has dropped into my legs and I can feel a water level in my chest'). *Paraesthesiae* is the term describing the sensation of tingling or 'pins and needles'. These may be delusionally ascribed, although of course they are often neurologically mediated, for example, ulnar nerve compression causing pins and needles in the forearm.

Kinaesthetic hallucinations are those of muscle or joint sense. The patient feels that their limbs are being bent or twisted or their muscles squeezed. Such hallucinations in schizophrenia are often linked with bizarre somatic delusions. A man suffering from schizophrenia described the experience: 'I thought my life was outside my feet and made them vibrate'—he experienced kinaesthetic hallucinations of vibration. Kinaesthetic hallucinations may occur in organic states: 'a feeling of being rocked about'. Abnormal kinaesthetic perceptions have also been described in the withdrawal state from benzodiazepine drugs (Schopf, 1983) or from alcohol intoxication. A man, after recovery, described his episode of delirium tremens, saying, 'I felt as if I was floating in the air about 50 feet above the ground'. He illustrated this feeling with the picture in Fig. 7.2.

Visceral hallucinations are false perceptions of the inner organs. There is only a limited range of possible visceral sensation, for example, pain, heaviness, stretching or distension, palpitation and various combinations of these, such as throbbing. However, the possible range of bizarre schizophrenic false perceptions and interpretations is limitless. One man believed that he could feel semen travelling up his vertebral column into his brain, where it became laid out in sheets.

Hallucinations of bodily sensation are quite common in schizophrenia and are almost always delusionally elaborated, often by *delusions of control* (Chapters 8 and 12). Haptic hallucinations may be experienced as touch ('like a hand stroking me') or painful ('knives stabbing my neck'). A patient believed that the smoke sensor in the ward was an infrared camera, 'because I feel it warm on my neck'. Another patient described a haptic hallucination in which she experienced genital stimulation that she ascribed to having sexual intercourse simultaneously with 'both Kennedy brothers all the time'. It is important to realize that there is both a hallucinatory and a delusional component in such experiences. One particularly unpleasant form of haptic hallucination is called *formication* (Latin: *formica*, 'ant'), the sensation of little animals or insects crawling over the body or just under the skin. This is especially associated with some drug states and withdrawal symptoms, for example, cocaine addiction and alcohol withdrawal. It is often associated with *delusions of infestation*, but the latter may occur without hallucination.

OLFACTORY AND GUSTATORY HALLUCINATION

Hallucinations of smell and of taste frequently occur together, and it may be difficult or impossible to distinguish them from each other. This is not surprising, as a lot of what a layperson ascribes to taste is actually determined by smell: 'the eucalyptus fragrance of this wine from the Barossa Valley'.

Olfactory Hallucinations

Olfactory sensation or memory is often associated with powerful emotional resonances; it is not surprising, therefore, that hallucinations are also invested with a strong affective component. Olfactory hallucinations occur in schizophrenia, in epilepsy and in some other *organic* states. The patient has a hallucination of smell. The smell may or may not be unpleasant, but it usually has a special and personal significance (Aggernaes' quality of *relevance*); for example, it may be associated with the belief that people are pumping a poisonous or an anaesthetic gas into the house, which the patient alone can smell. Sometimes, patients have an olfactory hallucination relating to themselves: 'I smell repulsive, unbearable—like a corpse, like faeces'. This particular patient killed himself. He felt that he created such a stench that he was intolerable in any reasonable society. Sometimes patients misinterpret and *overvalue* normal body odours. A delusion in which a patient believes themself to smell malodorously without an accompanying olfactory hallucination is quite common in schizophrenia and related paranoid states.

A distinct condition in which olfactory hallucinations also occur is *olfactory reference syndrome*. It was originally codified by Pryse-Phillips in his seminal paper published in 1971 (Pryse-Phillips, 1971). He described 36 patients presenting with the belief that smells emanated from their bodies without the intervention of any external agency, what Pryse-Phillips termed *intrinsic hallucinations*. This belief was accompanied by a 'contrite' reaction manifest as a deep sense of shame, embarrassment, self-abasement and a sensitivity to the reaction of people around them. There were also behavioural responses to this belief including excessive washing, excessive changing of clothing and social withdrawal. This condition was distinguished from olfactory hallucinations in the context of schizophrenia, mood disorder and epilepsy.

Pryse-Phillips makes the point that olfactory reference syndrome has been previously described in the literature and given different names including *délire à bâse olfactive,* parosmia and bromidrosiphobia. What is significant is that in describing olfactory reference syndrome, Pryse-Phillips was focusing on olfactory hallucinations as the presenting complaint in the absence of other primary psychiatric or neurological condition. Current definitions of olfactory reference syndrome concentrate on the following criteria: (1) a persistent false belief that one emits a malodorous smell; this belief may encompass a range of insight; (2) the belief causes clinically significant distress and is time consuming or results in significant impairment in social, occupational or other important areas of functioning; and (3) the belief is not accounted for by another mental disorder or a general medical condition (Begum & McKenna, 2011). In other words, the role of hallucinatory experience has been de-emphasized in the definition of olfactory reference syndrome even though a significant number of the reported patients make the claim that they can smell the odour.

Olfactory hallucinations also occur in epilepsy, especially in association with a temporal lobe focus, and commonly form the aura (or earliest phase) of such fits. A patient described a smell of burning rubber regularly just before he became unconscious. Visual, auditory, gustatory and visceral hallucinations also occur in temporal lobe epilepsy.

Gustatory Hallucinations

Gustatory hallucinations occur in various conditions. In schizophrenia, they sometimes occur with delusions of being poisoned. There may be a persistent taste, for example, 'onions', 'a metallic taste' or some more bizarre type of taste. In depression and in schizophrenia, the flavour of food may disappear altogether or become unpleasant. Changes in gustatory perception may occur with some organic states, such as temporal lobe epilepsy, and also with some psychotropic drugs, for example, lithium carbonate or disulfiram. A relatively common condition is *burning mouth syndrome*. This is a condition that is seen in dentistry and maxillofacial surgery. This condition presents with a burning sensation on the tongue, palate, inner aspects of the cheeks and gums. It is often associated with altered taste sensation. The patients report metallic taste, viscid or gritty saliva or dryness of the mouth. It is often difficult to describe how this disturbance of taste is mediated and, therefore, whether it is hallucinatory.

DIFFERENTIATION OF HALLUCINATIONS

Before deciding that a patient is hallucinated, the possibility of other perceptual experiences must be considered. These are not necessarily of pathologic significance. The differential diagnosis of hallucination includes illusion, pseudohallucination, hypnagogic and hypnopompic images and, of course, vivid imagery and normal perception.

Pseudohallucinations

Pseudohallucination is one of the least understood phenomena in psychopathology. As Berrios (1996) remarks, 'it has been used to refer to real perceptions perceived as "unreal", isolated hallucinations which do not fit into favoured diagnoses, side effects of drugs, withdrawal hallucinations, diabetic hallucinations, etc.' Berrios goes on to say:

Unrestrained, usage has strayed even wider, pseudohallucinations being sometimes applied to (i) phenomena which meet criteria for hallucinations or illusions, (ii) hallucinations in people without mental illnesses (e.g., the bereaved), (iii) the false perceptions of people recovering from psychotic illnesses, (iv) factitious hallucinations in malingerers, and (v) occasionally, normal but unusual perceptions which initially seem to be hallucinations (e.g., radio reception in dental amalgam or intracranial shrapnel fragments).

Furthermore, part of the confusion over the meaning of the term *pseudohallucination* has arisen because it is often used in two different and mutually contradictory ways, according to Kräupl Taylor (1981). On one hand it refers to hallucinations with insight (Hare, 1973), and on the other hand it refers to vivid internal images. Hallucinations with insight would be those hallucinatory experiences in which the subject is aware that the hallucinatory percepts do not correspond to external reality despite the perceptions being veridical and in external objective space. Vivid internal images are those phenomena that have all the clarity and vividness of a normal percept except that they occur in inner subjective space.

Jaspers (1997) identified pseudohallucination as similar to normal perception except that it occurs in inner subjective space. Pseudohallucination shares this characteristic with imagery. In other words, for Jaspers, pseudohallucination is a perceptual experience that is figurative and occurs in inner subjective space, not in external objective space, but it has all the vividness and clarity of a normal perception and can be retained unaltered. It occurs independently of the subject's will and therefore cannot be deliberately evoked. Jaspers derived this description of pseudohallucination from Kandinsky.

Kandinsky (1849–89) based his description of pseudohallucination on his own personal experiences. He died by suicide at age 40 years while a patient at St Nicholas Hospital, St Petersburg, where he had once been medical superintendent (Lerner et al., 2001). In 1885 he described *pseudohallucination* as a separate form of perception from true hallucination and wrote, 'subjective perceptions which in vividness and character are real hallucinations except that they do not have objective reality' (quoted in Berrios, 1996). Pseudohallucinations can be identified in the visual, auditory or tactile modalities.

Hare (1973) has given as an example of pseudohallucination the voice heard by an obsessional or depressed person. It is described by the patient as a voice but is actually recognized as their own thoughts. Pseudohallucinations are not pathognomonic of any particular mental illness. A patient with histrionic personality disorder saw a robed figure at the foot of her bed lifting his index finger to his mouth to caution her to silence. The image was sharp and vivid but was recognized as being seen with the inner eye. The patient knew that the figure was not at the foot of the bed and that other people in the room could not see him. When she tried to relate the figure in space to the background of her field of vision, in this case the walls and curtains of the room, she realized that she could not do so; it had no definite location in external space, that is, outside herself.

To summarize, the significance of hallucination is that it almost always denotes a morbid mental state. The significance of pseudohallucination is in its differential diagnosis from hallucination, as pseudohallucination is not necessarily psychopathologic.

Other Abnormalities of Perception

AUTOSCOPY

Autoscopy is the experience of seeing an image of oneself in external space and knowing that it is oneself (see also visual hallucination). It is sometimes called the phantom mirror image. It is one of the abnormalities of unity of self described in Chapter 12. Like so many topics of considerable phenomenological interest, the term *autoscopy* has been used with different meanings and definitions since its first use by Féré in 1891. The experience concerns how the individual regards the boundaries of self and is discussed further with other disorders of self-image. It has been suggested that it is best to reserve the term *autoscopy* for abnormalities of visual perception involving seeing oneself—'visual experiences where subjects see an image of themselves in external space viewed from within their own physical body' (Dening and Berrios, 1994).

However, it is also true that Brugger and colleagues (1997) describe the phenomenology of five main types of autoscopy, namely (1) autoscopic hallucination, (2) heautoscopy proper, (3) feeling of presence, (4) out-of-body experience and (5) negative autoscopy. Autoscopic hallucination involves the pure visual experience of seeing one's own body or its upper parts as if reflected in a mirror. In other words, in autoscopic hallucination, the percept is often but not always a mirror image of the patient. The hallucinatory experience is in natural colours and is usually of a motionless perception or the percept may imitate the gestures, movements or face expressions of the patient. Heautoscopy proper also involves visualization of the double but in addition there may be other anomalous experiences including a feeling of detachment, strangeness of one's body as well as lightness and occasionally the experience of vertigo. The double may appear transparent, grey or ghost-like. The double may imitate the patient's actions but may also act autonomously, not necessarily mirroring the patient's actions or movements. The term *feeling of presence* describes a feeling of the physical presence of another person close to the patient who is not seen but appears to be just out of sight. The patient may, in addition, experience altered or anomalous phenomena regarding their body. Out-of-body experience involves seeing one's body from an outside perspective. The core of this experience is the separation of the body from the experiencing self. Typically, the body is observed from a detached and an elevated spatial position. The body is usually motionless during the observation. The surrounding environment is also seen from an elevated perspective. There is an associated strong emotional accompaniment and significance to the experience and the emotions are more often positive except in cases where the experience is a precursor to a seizure. Negative heautoscopy refers to the failure to perceive one's own body in a mirror or when looked at directly. It is often accompanied by depersonalisation and the loss of awareness of one's own body, sometime termed *aschematia*.

Although this topic has been of considerable literary interest over the years, clinical cases with definite perceptual abnormality are not common. Dening and Berrios reviewed 56 cases, 53 from the literature and 3 of their own. Males predominated, with a ratio of two to one, and the mean age of subjects was 40 years.

Both neurological and psychiatric disorder occurred in about 60% of cases (different subjects), with epilepsy in approximately one-third. Decreased consciousness occurred in 45%, delirium in 18% and 9% of subjects were dead within 1 year. Visual imagery or narcissism was present in one-third of subjects and depersonalisation in 18%. The commonest psychiatric diagnosis was depression. Usually, autoscopic episodes lasted for less than 30 minutes. Almost always, the subject saw their own face; quite often, they were lying in bed at the time. The experience often provoked distress, fear, anxiety and depression. This subjective experience was complex, with different components and causes rather than unitary.

EXTRACAMPINE HALLUCINATION (CONCRETE AWARENESS)

'I know that there is someone behind me on the right all the time; he moves when I move', 'I keep on hearing them talking about my disease down in the post office' (half a mile away)—these hallucinations are experienced outside the limits of the sensory field, outside the visual field or beyond the range of audibility. They are not of diagnostic importance, as they occur in schizophrenia, epilepsy and other organic states and as *hypnagogic hallucinations* in healthy people. The phenomenon is quite definitely experienced as a perception by the patient and not just as a belief or an idea.

HYPNAGOGIC AND HYPNOPOMPIC HALLUCINATION

These are perceptions that occur while going to sleep (*hypnagogic*) and on waking (*hypnopompic*). According to Zilboorg and Henry (1941), hypnagogic hallucinations were first mentioned by Aristotle. It is known that the consciousness level fluctuates considerably in different stages of sleep, and both types of abnormal perception probably occur in a phase of increasing drowsiness: the structure of thought, feelings, perceptions, fantasies and, ultimately, self-awareness becomes blurred and merges into oblivion. These experiences occur in many people in good health. They are also described with *narcolepsy, cataplexy* and *sleep paralysis* to form a characteristic tetrad of symptoms (see Narcolepsy for descriptions). *Toxic states* such as glue sniffing, acute fevers (especially in children), postinfective *depressive states* and phobic anxiety neuroses

are other conditions that may be associated with these perceptions.

The perception may be visual, auditory or tactile. It is sudden in occurrence, and the subject believes that it woke them up, for example, a loud voice in the street below saying 'world war!', a feeling of someone pushing them over the bed or seeing a man coming across the bedroom. The importance of these phenomena in psychopathology is to recognize their nature and realize that they are not necessarily abnormal, even though they may be truly hallucinatory.

FUNCTIONAL HALLUCINATION

This is the strange phenomenon in which an external stimulus is necessary to provoke hallucination, but the normal perception of the stimulus and the hallucination in the same modality are experienced simultaneously. A schizophrenic patient heard hallucinatory voices only when water was running through the pipes of his ward. He heard no phonemes for most of the time, but when he heard water rushing through the pipes along the wall, he became very distressed by voices that told him to damage himself. He was terrified of the content of these voices because he was afraid he might act on them. He could readily separate the noise of water from the voices, and the latter never occurred apart from the former, but both perceptions were recognized as distinct and *real*. Another patient heard voices when the radio or television was switched on, alongside the broadcast voices; he had persecutory delusions that these activities were carried out deliberately to upset him and he became very distressed, and at times violent, as a result.

REFLEX HALLUCINATION

As a doctor was writing in his case notes during his interview of a female patient, she said, 'I can feel you writing in my stomach'. The patient saw and heard the act of writing and was quite sure that it accounted for the tactile sensation in her abdomen. A stimulus in one sensory modality producing a hallucination in another is called a *reflex hallucination*. This is, in fact, a hallucinatory form of *synaesthesia*, mentioned earlier as the experience of a stimulus image in one sense modality simultaneously producing an image in another, for example, the feeling of discomfort caused by seeing and hearing somebody scratch a blackboard with their fingernails. Another reflex hallucination occurred in a woman who experienced pain whenever certain words were mentioned. Functional and reflex hallucinations are not themselves of diagnostic or theoretical significance, but they require mentioning for completeness and recognition to identify other more important symptoms with confidence.

ABNORMAL IMAGERY

Mental imagery tasks are designed to assess a subject's capacity for mental representation of the perceived world. In cases of hemineglect, there has been interest in whether the observed deficits in imagery are due to inattention or to impairment of mental imagery. Bisiach and Luzzatti (1978) described abnormalities in individuals with hemineglect. Their patients were asked to describe the Piazza del Duomo in Milan from two standpoints: facing the cathedral and with their backs to the cathedral. From both standpoints, the subjects were unable to describe the right side of the scene despite having correctly described it from the previous standpoint. In other words, even in imagination the mental representation of the piazza was unilaterally deficient for the right side. In these cases, inattention influenced the capacity for imagery. Guariglia et al. (1993) reported a patient without hemineglect in whom impairment of imagery for objects in the left visual field was demonstrated. For the first time, this showed that without hemineglect, that is, visual inattention for space, failure of imagery was still possible.

SENSORY DEPRIVATION

Continuing perception is necessary for consciousness. The field of sensation varies all the time as individual sensations in different modalities from the outside world and from inside oneself compete for attention. *Consciousness* consists of the integration of this changing field to form a composite awareness of oneself in one's environment. The essential nature of sensation has been explored by studying its absence, as revealed by research on the effects of sensory deprivation (Zubek, 1969). This topic is only given brief mention, as it is somewhat peripheral to psychiatry.

Sensory deprivation was studied using Canadian college students as volunteers (Bexton et al., 1954). The subjects, wearing translucent goggles and gloves with cardboard cuffs, lay on a bed in a light but partially soundproof room; there was a continual background noise. This experience was found to be extremely unpleasant and, despite being paid, subjects were not prepared to remain in this state for more than 3 days.

This technique has been refined subsequently to blot out external sensations more completely. Various perceptual abnormalities are experienced. Visual hallucinations of varying complexity were described, but further study of these perceptual changes resulted in their being considered, more cautiously, to be 'reported visual sensations' and 'reported auditory sensations' (Zuckermann, 1969). These were classified into 'meaningless sensations' and 'meaningful integrated sensations'. Some of the latter are more like hallucinatory experiences. Depending on the completeness of deprivation of other sensations, abnormal perception occurs in modalities other than vision. Subjects show an altered affective state: they become panicky, restless, irritable or, alternatively, bored and apathetic.

Despite considerable neuropsychological research with valuable findings for investigating the sensory environment in growth and development, developing brain interconnections, neurochemistry and neurophysiology, the study of sensory deprivation has not so far made as big an impact on descriptive psychopathology as was initially expected. There are various difficulties to be accounted for. What part of the effects of deprivation is due to failure of development and what to loss of behaviours already established? How can one use animal work to explore subjective symptoms? How can one extrapolate from the experience of normal individuals in a highly abnormal environment to those who are psychiatrically ill? Many studies in sensory deprivation are described by Riesen (1975), who links the experimental data to neurological function and development.

The distinction has been made between *sensory deprivation* and *perceptual deprivation*. The latter is achieved by rendering the sensations patternless and meaningless, rather than by preventing sensations, by using such devices as translucent goggles and continuous 'white' noise. The deleterious effects of sensory deprivation have been considered by Slade (1984) as:

- inability to tolerate the situation,
- perceptual changes,
- intellectual and cognitive impairments,
- psychomotor effects, and
- physiologic changes in electroencephalograph and galvanic skin response measures.

Fantasy is often used as a means of reducing the unpleasant affective component of sensory deprivation. The subject may become disoriented and show increasing difficulty with problem solving and concentration. For perception and maintenance of the normal state of consciousness, it is necessary to have a variety of sensory stimuli available and for these stimuli to be changeable. If the objects of perception do not themselves change, the observer will move their point of observation to create change.

REFERENCES

Aggernaes, A., 1972. The experienced reality of hallucinations and other psychological phenomena. Acta Psychiatr. Scand. 48, 220–238.

Andrade, C., 1988. Free hallucinations as culturally sanctioned experience. Br. J. Psychiatry. 152, 838–839.

Asaad, G., Shapiro, B., 1986. Hallucinations: theoretical and clinical overview. Am. J. Psychiatry. 143, 1088–1097.

Barodawala, S., Mulley, G.P., 1997. Visual hallucinations. J. R. Coll. Physicians Lond. 31, 42–48.

Begum, M., McKenna, P.J., 2011. Olfactory reference syndrome: a systematic review of the world literature. Psychol. Medicine. 41, 453–461.

Bentall, R.P., 1990. The illusion of reality: a review and integration of psychological research on hallucinations. Psychol. Bull. 107, 82–95.

Bentall, R.P., Baker, G.A., Havers, S., 1991. Reality monitoring and psychotic hallucinations. Br. J. Clin. Psychol. 30, 213–222.

Berrios, G.E., 1982. Tactile hallucinations: conceptual and historical aspects. J. Neurol. Neurosurg. Psychiatry 45, 285–293.

Berrios, G.E., 1990. Musical hallucinations: a historical and clinical study. Br. J. Psychiatry. 156, 188–194.

Berrios, G.E., 1996. The History of Mental Symptoms: Descriptive Psychopathology since the Nineteenth Century. Cambridge University Press, Cambridge.

Berrios, G.E., Brook, P., 1984. Visual hallucinations and sensory delusions in the elderly. Br. J. Psychiatry. 144, 662–664.

Bexton, W.H., Heron, W., Scott, T.H., 1954. Effects of decreased variation in the sensory environment. Can. J. Psychol. 8, 70–76.

Bisiach, E., Luzzatti, C., 1978. Unilateral neglect of representational space. Cortex 14, 129–133.

Bleuler, E., 1950. In: Zinkin, J., Trans (Eds.), Dementia Praecox or the Group of Schizophrenias. International University Press, New York.

Brugger, P., Regard, M., Landis, T., 1997. Illusory reduplication of one's own body: phenomenology and classification of autoscopic phenomena. Cognit. Neuropsychiatry 2, 19–38.

Burns, A., Jacoby, R., Levy, R., 1990. Psychiatric phenomena in Alzheimer's disease 2. Disorders of perception. Br. J. Psychiatry. 157, 76–81.

Critchley, M., 1951. Types of visual perseveration: 'palinopsia' and 'illusory visual spread. Brain 74, 267–299.

Cummings, J.L., Miller, B., Hill, M.A., Neshkes, R., 1987. Neuropsychiatric aspects of multi-infarct dementia of the Alzheimer type. Arch. Neurol. 44, 389–393.

Cutting, J., 1997. Principles of Psychopathology: Two Worlds – Two Minds – Two Hemispheres. Oxford University Press, Oxford.

Cytowic, R.E., Eagleman, D.M., 2009. Wednesday Is Indigo Blue: Discovering the Brain of Synesthesia. The MIT Press, London.

Dening, T.R., Berrios, G.E., 1994. Autoscopic hallucinations: a clinical analysis of 56 cases. Br. J. Psychiatry. 165, 808–817.

Donaghy, P.C., McKeith, I.G., 2014. The clinical characteristics of dementia with Lewy bodies and a consideration of prodromal diagnosis. Alzheimer Res. Ther. 6 (4), 46. https://doi.org/10.1186/1lzrt274.

Esquirol, J.E.D., 1817. Hallucinations (Reprinted in Des Maladies Mentales, 1938). Baillière, Paris.

Ey, H., 1973. Traité Des Hallucinations. Masson, Paris.

Falloon, I.R.H., Talbot, R.E., 1981. Persistent auditory hallucinations: coping mechanisms and implications for management. Psychol. Med. 11, 329–340.

Féré, C., 1891. Note sur les hallucinations autoscopiques ou spéculaires et sur les hallucinations altruistes. C. R. Seances Soc. Biol. Fil. 3, 451–453.

Fernyhough, C., 1996. The dialogic: a dialogic approach to the higher mental functions. New Ideas Psychol. 14, 47–62.

Fernyhough, C., 2016. The Voices within: The History and Science of How We Talk to Ourselves. Profile Books Limited, London.

ffytche, D.H., 2007. Visual hallucinatory syndromes: past, present and future. Dialogues Clin. Neurosci. 9 (2), 173–189.

ffytche, D.H., Howard, R.J., 1999. The personal consequences of visual loss: positive pathologies of vision. Brain 122 (7), 1247–1260.

Fuchs, T., Lauter, H., 1992. Charles Bonnet syndrome and musical hallucinations in the elderly. In: Katona, C., Levy, R. (Eds.), Delusions and Hallucinations in Old Age. Gaskell, London.

Fukutake, T., Kawamura, M., Sakakibara, R., Hirayama, K., 1993. Alloaesthesia without impairment of consciousness after right putaminal small haemorrhage. Rinsho Shinkeigaku 33, 130–133.

Green, P., Preston, M., 1981. Reinforcement of vocal correlates of auditory hallucinations by auditory feedback: a case study. Br. J. Psychiatry. 139, 204–208.

Gregory, R.L., 2004. Recovery from blindness. In: Gregory, R.L. (Ed.), The Oxford Companion to the Mind, second ed. Oxford University Press, Oxford.

Guariglia, C., Padovani, A., Pantano, P., Pizzamiglio, L., 1993. Unilateral neglect restricted to visual imagery. Nature 364, 235–237.

Haddad, P.M., Benbow, S.M., 1992. Visual hallucinations as the presenting symptom of senile dementia. Br. J. Psychiatry. 161, 263–265.

Hare, E.H., 1973. A short note on pseudohallucinations. Br. J. Psychiatry. 122, 469–476.

Heilbrun, A.B., Blum, N.A., 1984. Cognitive vulnerability to auditory hallucinations: impaired perception of memory. Br. J. Psychiatry. 144, 508–512.

Horowitz, M.J., 1975. A cognitive model of hallucinations. Am. J. Psychiatry. 132, 789–795.

Jacobs, L., Feldman, M., Diamond, S.P., Bender, M.B., 1973. Palinacousis: persistent or recurring auditory sensations. Cortex 9, 211–216.

Jaspers, K., 1997. In: Hoenig, J., Hamilton, M.W., Trans (Eds.), General Psychopathology. The Johns Hopkins University Press, Baltimore.

Junginger, J., Frame, C.L., 1985. Self-report of the frequency and phenomenology of verbal hallucinations. J. Nerv. Ment. Dis. 173, 149–155.

Kandinsky, V., 1885. Kritische und klinische. Betrachtungen im Gebiete der Sinnestanschangen. St. Petersburg.

Kawamura, M., Hitayama, K., Shinohara, Y., Watanabe, Y., Sugishita, M., 1987. Alloaesthesia. Brain. 110, 225–236.

Kelleher, I., DeVylder, J.E., 2017. Hallucinations in borderline personality disorder and common mental disorders. Br. J. Psychiatry. 210, 1–2.

Komel, H.W., 1985. Complex visual hallucinations in the hemianopic field. J. Neurol. Neurosurg. Psychiatry. 48, 29–38.

Kosslyn, S.M., 2004. Mental imagery: depictive accounts. In: Gregory, R.L. (Ed.), The Oxford Companion to the Mind, second ed. Oxford University Press, Oxford.

Kosslyn, S.M., Thompson, W.L., 2003. When is early visual cortex activated during visual mental imagery? Psychol. Bull. 129, 723–846.

Kosslyn, S.M., Pascual-Leone, A., Felician, O., et al., 1999. The role of area 17 in visual imagery: convergent evidence from PET and rTMS. Science 284, 167–170.

Kräupl Taylor, F., 1981. On pseudohallucinations. Psychol. Med. 11, 265–272.

Lerner, V., Kapstan, A., Witztum, E., 2001. The misidentification of Clerambault's and Kandinsky–Clerambault's syndromes. Can. J. Psychiatry. 46, 441–443.

Lishman, W.A., 1989. Organic Psychiatry: The Psychological Consequences of Cerebral Disorder, second ed. Blackwell Scientific, Oxford.

Margo, A., Hemsley, D.R., Slade, P.D., 1981. The effects of varying auditory input on schizophrenic hallucinations. Br. J. Psychiatry. 139, 122–127.

Martin, G.N., 2006. Human Neuropsychology. Pearson Education, Harlow.

McCarthy-Jones, S., 2012. Hearing Voices: The Histories, Causes and Meanings of Auditory Verbal Hallucinations. Cambridge University Press, Cambridge.

Merleau-Ponty, M., 1962. In: Smith, C., Trans (Eds.), Phenomenology of Perception. Routledge, London.

Morley, S., 1987. Psychological modification of auditory hallucinations: distraction versus attention. Behav. Psychother. 15, 240–251.

Nayani, T.H., David, A.S., 1996. The auditory hallucination: a phenomenological survey. Psychol. Med. 26, 177–189.

Persaud, R., Cutting, J., 1991. Lateralized anomalous perceptual experiences in schizophrenia. Psychopathology 24, 365–368.

Podoll, K., Schwartz, M., Noth, J., 1990. Charles Bonnet-Syndrom bei einem Parkinson-Patientem mit beidseitigen Visusverlust. Nervenarzt 61, 52–56.

Pryse-Phillips, W., 1971. An olfactory reference syndrome. Acta Psychiatr. Scand. 47, 484–509.

Pylyshyn, Z.W., 2004. Mental imagery. In: Gregory, R.L. (Ed.), The Oxford Companion to the Mind, second ed. Oxford University Press, Oxford.

Ramachandran, V.S., Hirstein, W., 1998. The perception of phantom limbs: the D.O. Hebb lecture. Brain 121, 1603–1630.

Riesen, A.H., 1975. The Developmental Neuropsychology of Sensory Deprivation. Academic Press, New York.

Sachs, O., 1995. An Anthropologist on Mars. Picador, London.

Schneider, K., 1959. In: Hamilton, M.W., Trans (Eds.), Clinical Psychopathology, fifth ed. Grune and Stratton, New York.

Schopf, F., 1983. Withdrawal phenomena after long-term administration of benzodiazepines: a review of recent investigations. Pharmacopsychiatry 16, 1–8.

Schreber, D., 1955. In: Macalpine, I., Hunter, R.A., Trans (Eds.), Memoirs of My Nervous Illness. Dawson, London.

Schultz, G., Melzack, R., 1991. The Charles Bonnet syndrome: 'phantom visual' images. Perception 20, 809–825.

Shapiro, M.F., Fink, M., 1952. Exosomesthesia: the displacement of cutaneous sensation to extrapersonal space. Trans. Am. Neurol. Assoc. 56, 260–262.

Shapiro, M.F., Fink, M., Bender, M.B., 1952. Exosomesthesia or displacement of cutaneous sensation into extrapersonal space. Arch. Neurol. Psychiatry. 68, 481–496.

Sims, A.C.P., 1991. An overview of the psychopathology of perception: first rank symptoms as a localizing sign in schizophrenia. Psychopathology 24, 369–374.

Slade, P.D., 1976a. Hallucinations. Psychol. Med. 6, 7–13.

Slade, P.D., 1976b. An investigation of psychological factors involved in the predisposition to auditory hallucinations. Psychol. Med. 6, 123–132.

Slade, P.D., 1984. Sensory deprivation and clinical psychiatry. Br. J. Hosp. Med. 32, 256–260.

Smith, E.E., Kosslyn, S.M., 2007. Cognitive Psychology: Mind and Brain. Prentice Hall, Upper Saddle River, NJ.

Smythies, J.R., 1956. A logical and cultural analysis of hallucinatory sense-experience. J. Ment. Sci. 102, 336.

Spitzer, M., 1994. The basis of psychiatric diagnosis. In: Sadler, J.Z., Wiggins, O.P., Schwartz, M.A. (Eds.), Philosophical Perspectives on Psychiatric Diagnostic Classification. Johns Hopkins University Press, Baltimore.

Stacy, C.B., 1987. Complex haptic hallucination and palinaptia. Cortex 23, 337–340.

Stewart, L., von Kriegstein, K., Warren, J.D., Griffiths, T.D., 2006. Music and the brain: disorders of musical listening. Brain 129, 2533–2553.

Summa, M., Fuchs, T., Vanzago, L., 2018. Imagination and Social Perspectives: Approaches from Phenomenology and Psychopathology. Routledge, New York.

Upthegrove, R., Broome, M., Caldwell, K., Ives, J., Oyebode, F., Wood, S., 2015. Understanding auditory verbal hallucinations: a systematic review of current evidence. Acta Psychiatr. Scand. 133, 352–367.

Upthegrove, R., Ives, J., Broome, M.R., Caldwell, K., Wood, S.J., Oyebode, F., 2016. Auditory verbal hallucinations in first-episode psychosis: a phenomenological investigation. Br. J. Psych. Open 2, 88–95.

Vygotsky, L.S., 1978. Mind in Society: The Development of Higher Psychological Processes. In: Cole, M., John-Steiner, V., Scribner, S., Souberman, E. (Eds.), Harvard University Press, Cambridge, Massachusetts.

Vygotsky, L.S., 1934/1987. Thinking and Speech. The Collected Works of LS Vygotsky, vol. 1. Plenum, New York.

Wagemans, J., Feldman, J., Gepshtein, S., Kimchi, R., Pomerantz, J.R., van der Helm, P.A., 2012. A century of Gestalt Psychology in visual perception II: conceptual and theoretical foundations. Psychol. Bull. 138, 1172–1217.

Wernicke, C., 1906. Grundri Der Psychiatrie in Klinischen. Vorlesun Gen. Thieme, Leipzig.

Werring, D.J., Marsden, C.D., 1999. Visual hallucinations and palinopsia due to an occipital lobe tuberculoma. J. Neurol. Neurosurg. Psychiatry. 66, 684.

Zeki, S., 1993. A Vision of the Brain. Blackwell, Oxford.

Zilboorg, G., Henry, G.W., 1941. A History of Medical Psychology. Norton, New York.

Zubek, J.P., 1969. Sensory Deprivation: Fifteen Years of Research. Appleton-Century-Crofts, New York.

Zuckermann, M., 1969. Variables affecting deprivation results. In: Zubek, J.P. (Ed.), Sensory Deprivation: Fifteen Years of Research. Appleton-Century-Crofts, New York, pp. 47–84.

Chapter 8

Delusions and Other Erroneous Ideas

Chapter Outline

KEYWORDS

Delusion
Delusional misidentification syndrome
Koro
Overvalued idea

Summary

Delusions are false judgements that are held with extraordinary conviction and incomparable subjective certainty and are impervious to other experiences and to compelling counterargument. Usually delusions are easily recognized when out of keeping with the individual's educational and sociocultural background. Primary delusions have diagnostic significance, whereas the content of secondary delusions may signal the nature of the primary abnormal phenomenon from which they derive. Overvalued ideas are comprehensible beliefs that arise from the history and experiences of an individual. They are held with conviction and motivate behaviour that may cause the patient harm and suffering.

I cannot pretend to agree with him, when I know that his mind is working altogether under a delusion.

                        Anthony Trollope (1869)

Anthony Trollope, in his novel *He Knew He Was Right*, describes not only the totally destructive effect of delusional jealousy on the individual but also the extraordinary dilemma this poses for other people who come into contact with him: whether to humour the individual and risk reinforcement or to confront him and risk violence. Fundamental to clinical practice in psychiatry, using the phenomenological or empathic method is obtaining a clear account of the ideas or notions that the subject, the patient, actually holds. Although delusions are often referred to as beliefs, there is a growing literature questioning whether they are beliefs at all. There is a sense in which the term *belief* is being used to distinguish the nature of delusions from that of, for example, abnormal perceptions and other kinds of abnormal phenomena. In other words, the varying terms such as *judgement, beliefs, ideas* or *notions* that are used in connection with delusions are attempts to categorize the phenomena of delusions and to distinguish it from other abnormal phenomena. *False beliefs* include primary and secondary delusions, overvalued ideas and *sensitive ideas* of reference.

Ideas, Beliefs and Delusions

Rarely does anyone claim to be deluded, and usually what a delusional patient thought was true does not prove to be so. A delusion is a false, unshakeable idea or belief that is out of keeping with the patient's educational, cultural and social background; it is held with extraordinary conviction and subjective certainty. Subjectively, or phenomenologically, it is indistinguishable from a true belief. A man who is a bachelor of medicine of the University of London holds a delusion that he is being used as 'an envoy from Mars'. He believes that he is both a doctor and an envoy, and neither thought seems to him to be delusional or imaginary. He likes to imagine himself a rich man with an estate in Gloucestershire. He has not the slightest difficulty in identifying this latter idea as fantasy. To the man himself, a delusion is much closer to a true belief than imagination, and the reasons enlisted to support its veracity are produced in the same way that a person would prove any other notion on which he was challenged. Normally, fantasy is easily distinguished from reality, although the subject may show great reluctance in accepting his aspirations as 'mere fantasy'. Similarly, there is usually little difficulty for the external observer in deciding whether a false belief is a misinterpretation of the facts based on false reasoning or a delusion.

⊙ MEANING OF DELUSION

The English word *delude* comes from Latin and implies playing or mocking, defrauding or cheating. The German equivalent *Wahn* is a whim, false opinion or fancy and makes no more comment than the English on the subjective experience. The French equivalent, *délire*, is more empathic; it implies the ploughshare jumping out of the furrow (*lira*), perhaps a similar metaphor to the ironical 'unhinged'. As Bayne and Fernandez (2009) say:

On the face of things, it seems obvious that delusions involve departures – typically, quite radical departures – from the procedural norms of human belief formation. Delusions stand out as exotic specimens in the garden of belief, as examples of what happens precisely when the mechanisms of belief formation break down.

In this chapter, the complexity of delusions as concepts, experienced symptoms, and abnormal phenomena is explored, discussed and analysed.

Definition of Delusion

An additional video for this topic is available online. ⊙

There continues to be much debate and controversy about the definition of delusions. The standard approach is to follow Jaspers' (1997) claim that delusions are manifest in judgements and arise in the process of thinking and judging. For Jaspers, the characteristics of delusions are that:

- they are false judgements,
- they are held with extraordinary conviction and incomparable subjective certainty,
- they are impervious to other experiences and to compelling counterargument, and
- their content is impossible.

Each of these criteria has been subjected to criticism. Delusions may not be objectively false insofar as the content is concerned. This is best exemplified in delusional jealousy, whereby the belief may correspond to objective truth and is therefore not false. Delusions may not be held with extraordinary conviction but, equally, normal beliefs may be held with extraordinary conviction such that intensity of conviction cannot distinguish between normal and abnormal beliefs. Delusional beliefs may also be amenable to counterargument, although it is rare that this by itself will alter the belief. Finally, delusional content need not be impossible.

There is a growing body of opinion that delusions are not beliefs at all. Spitzer (1994), for example, argues this case. He makes the distinction between 'to know that' and 'to believe that'. In Spitzer's view, delusions make knowledge claims rather than belief claims. In other words, patients are asserting that they 'know such and such' rather than they 'believe such and such', which is why delusional statements are expressed with conviction and certainty and not subject to discussion and inquiry. Berrios (1996) comes to the same conclusions. He states that 'delusions are empty speech acts which assert themselves as beliefs'. Furthermore, he makes the point that the content of delusions is incidental to the fact of the phenomenon being a delusion. In Berrios' view, the content of delusions is randomly chosen; the content merely reflects whatever is in the environment at the time the delusion is formed. The content is lacking in informational quality and is not a 'symbolic expression of anything'. These critiques of the current definitions and understanding of delusions underline the complexity of the conceptual status of delusions and show that there is still fruitful theoretical work to be done in psychopathology.

It is important to emphasize that the tradition that locates delusions within the domain of thinking and judging derives very simply from the need to distinguish hallucinations (abnormalities of perception) from delusions (abnormalities of thinking and judging). In any case, arguing that delusions are not abnormalities of belief is like arguing that chorea (an involuntary movement) is not an abnormality of movement because the observed movements are not purposeful or intentional. Bortolotti (2010) has critically examined the arguments against the idea that delusions are beliefs and concluded that these arguments that she classed as procedural, epistemic and agential apply equally to normal beliefs. She therefore concluded that there is little reason to treat delusions as anything other than beliefs. With this in mind, it is profitable to continue to classify delusions as abnormal beliefs.

The decision to call a belief or judgement *delusional* is not made by the person holding the belief but by an external observer. There can be no phenomenological definition of delusion because the patient is likely to hold this belief with the same conviction and intensity as they hold other nondelusional beliefs about themself or as anyone else holds intensely personal nondelusional beliefs. In this respect, delusions are to ideation what hallucinations are to perception. Subjectively, a delusion is simply a belief, a notion or an idea. Stoddart's (1908) definition of a delusion—'a judgement which cannot be accepted by people of the same class, education, race and period of life as the person who experiences it'—has some advantages. However, it could include as delusional falling in love with a person others regard as unsuitable, having a minority religious belief or holding any unusual idea without acknowledging reasonable argument to the contrary.

Hamilton (1978) defined delusion as 'a false unshakeable belief which arises from internal morbid processes. It is easily recognizable when it is out of keeping with the person's educational and cultural background'. This definition makes the point that a belief can be a delusion even when it is not out of keeping with the patient's educational and cultural background.

Rather than suggest a unitary definition for delusion, Kendler et al. (1983) have proposed several poorly correlated dimensions or vectors of delusional severity:

- Conviction: the degree to which the patient is convinced of the reality of the delusional beliefs.
- Extension: the degree to which the delusional belief involves areas of the patient's life.
- Bizarreness: the degree to which the delusional beliefs depart from culturally determined consensual reality.
- Disorganization: the degree to which the delusional beliefs are internally consistent, logical and systematized.
- Pressure: the degree to which the patient is preoccupied and concerned with the expressed delusional beliefs.

Two other dimensions that might also be considered are as follows:

- Affective response: the degree to which the patient's emotions are involved with such beliefs.
- Deviant behaviour resulting from delusions: patients sometimes, but not always, act on their delusions.

It is clear that no single definition of the term *delusion* is without problems. It may be that in clinical practice a pragmatic approach is employed that includes the probability that the statement is true and, plausibility of what the patient says. In addition, the manner of presenting the belief also matters. Parnas (2013) expresses this approach best when he writes: 'Something more global may be at stake, e.g. something that transpires through the patient's way of arguing. This gestalt-like whole comprises a fabric of branching, interconnected beliefs, attitudes, background assumptions, which ultimately inhere in the overall structure of consciousness and experiencing. It is these contextual aspects, surrounding the focal propositional content, which help the clinician to classify a given statement as an instance of delusion'. This approach will not satisfy anyone who seeks a simplistic definition, but nonetheless it captures the complexity of clinical judgements in the real world and concedes that the subjectivity of the clinician too is involved in decision-making.

Primary and Secondary Delusions

The confusing subject of primary and secondary delusions requires some explanation. It is probably most meaningful to use the term *primary* to imply that delusion is not occurring *in response* to another psychopathologic form such as mood disorder. *Secondary* delusion is used in the sense that the false belief is *understandable* in present circumstances because of the pervasive mood state or because of the cultural content. It is usual to consider delusions as secondary to another abnormal phenomenon.

Gruhle (1915) considered that a primary delusion was a disturbance of symbolic meaning, not an alteration in sensory perception, apperception or intelligence. Primary delusions occur in schizophrenia and not in other conditions; they include both delusional perception and delusional intuition (Cutting, 1985). However, delusional intuitions, notions or ideas are not pathognomonic of schizophrenia, because in any individual case there is too much scope for arguing whether this delusion is indeed *primary*, that is, ultimately un-understandable, or *secondary* in nature. Secondary delusions occur in many conditions other than schizophrenia and can sometimes be understood in relation to the person's background culture or emotional state.

Wernicke (1906) formulated the concept of an *autochthonous idea*, an idea that is 'native to the soil', aboriginal, arising without external cause. The trouble with finding supposed autochthonous or primary delusions is that it can be disputed whether they are truly autochthonous. For this reason, they are not considered of *first rank* in Schneider's (1957) classification of symptoms. It is too difficult to decide in many cases whether a delusion is autochthonous. Several writers

have claimed that all delusions are understandable if one knows enough about the patient.

THE ULTIMATELY UN-UNDERSTANDABLE

Jaspers' detailed exposition of delusion has been carefully reviewed by Walker (1991). Jaspers' concepts of the *un-understandable*, and of *meaningful connections*, are relevant here. If we ask an offender to describe the psychic world in which he lives—his attitudes, his feelings and how these developed through his childhood until now—we may be able to understand his sexual cruelty, which at first seemed quite incomprehensible: the behaviour becomes *meaningful* in the context of abuse by his stepfather and surviving as an adolescent in a harsh urban subculture with violence, humiliation and frustration. However, when we consider the middle-aged woman living on her own with a history of schizophrenia who believes that men unlock the door of her flat, anaesthetize her and interfere with her sexually, we find an experience that is ultimately not understandable. We can understand, on obtaining more details of the history, how her disturbance centres on sexual experience, why she should be distrustful of men, her doubts about her femininity and her feelings of social isolation. However, the *delusion,* her absolute conviction that these things really are happening to her, that they are true, is not understandable. The best we can do is to try to understand externally, without really being able to feel ourselves into her position (*genetic empathy,* see Chapter 1), what she is thinking and how she experiences it. We cannot understand how such a notion could have developed.

This is the core of the primary or autochthonous delusion: it is *ultimately un-understandable*. The patient described above also believed the police were using rays to observe her. One does not have to try to find which delusion came first, the anaesthesia or the observation by rays, to decide which is primary; *primary* is not dependent on temporal relationships. In that both delusions are not ultimately understandable, they are both primary delusions. A delusion can still be primary in Jaspers' sense, although it arises on the basis of a memory, an atmosphere or a perception. The protagonist in Gogol's (1809–52) *Diary of a Madman* (Gogol, 1972) says, 'There is a King of Spain. He has been found at last. That king is me. I only discovered this today.' This sudden and inexplicable belief arose autonomously and unpremeditated. Thereafter, it dictated the protagonist's every behaviour and influenced his view of the world.

HOW IDEAS AND DELUSIONS ARE INITIATED

A delusion is a belief, an idea, a thought, a notion or an intuition, and it arises in the same type of setting as any other idea—in the context of a perception, a memory or an atmosphere—or it may be autochthonous, appearing to occur spontaneously.

Ideas are initiated in the following ways:

- An example of an idea occurring on the basis of a *percept:* I smell food cooking and then form the idea that I will go and eat.
- Ideas may follow *memory:* I remember listening to a string quartet and form the idea of playing a compact disc.
- Ideas may arise out of an *atmosphere* or a mood state: I already feel irritable, and when I collect my car from the garage and it makes an unexplained noise, I become unreasonably angry and blame the mechanic for not repairing it satisfactorily.
- An idea may be *autochthonous.* I visit a ward of the hospital on an afternoon when I never normally go there. Although I accept that all behaviour has an explanation for its occurrence, I do not know why on this particular occasion I did this. Theoretical explanations may be given as to where such ideas come from, for example, the *unconscious,* but subjectively they seem to have occurred de novo. Delusions occur in similar settings on the basis of percept, memory, atmosphere or de novo—'out of the blue'.

In our discussion of primary delusions, we will see how the same four situations also account for the onset of delusions: percept, memory, mood or autochthonous. In this sense, delusion *is* an idea.

SECONDARY DELUSIONS

Primary delusions differ from secondary delusions in that the former are ultimately not understandable. Secondary delusions are understandable in the context of other abnormal phenomena such as abnormal mood, abnormal perception or indeed of a primary abnormal belief. A manic patient claimed to be Mary, Queen of Scots. She accepted that the queen in question lived and died centuries ago but claimed descent from her

and felt fully entitled to say that she *was* Mary, Queen of Scots. The belief could be understood in relation to her elated and expansive mood and disappeared as her affective state subsided. A depressed patient believed that they had committed the 'unforgivable sin'. Discussion and persuasion, even with a person whose religious views they respected, was of no avail in giving them relief. The belief could be seen as an integral part of their depressed mood. Depressive delusions may remain after treatment has resulted in improvement from retardation, and they account for suicide occasionally occurring in the recovery phase of depression. It has been suggested that there may be a decline in the prevalence of delusion occurring with depressive illness, but Eagles (1983), studying admissions to hospital in Edinburgh from 1892 to 1982, considered there to be no genuine reduction.

Secondary delusions can be distinguished from *overvalued ideas* (discussed later). Whereas secondary delusions are derived from another abnormal phenomenon, overvalued ideas are comprehensible in the light of the patient's personal history or some identifiable historical event whose value has become heightened for some reason. No prior abnormal phenomenon explains the presence of an overvalued idea.

Types of Primary Delusion

Kurt Schneider (1957) discusses the dilemma of primary symptoms in schizophrenia extremely lucidly by giving six different possible meanings for the term *primary,* but he still leaves us in doubt as to whether the belief is primary or not. He makes it clear, however, that primary symptoms are not the same as *first-rank symptoms* of schizophrenia. Primary symptoms are those that arise without understandable cause in the context of the psychotic illness. They are therefore the necessary manifestations of the underlying psychopathology in the same way that swelling and redness are a necessary consequence of physical trauma. First-rank symptoms, on the other hand, are, according to Schneider, simply a useful empirical list of symptoms that are found commonly in schizophrenia and not in other conditions. Describing their presence makes no claim as to how they arose.

True delusions, or *delusions proper*, are distinguished by Jaspers from *delusion-like ideas. True delusions* therefore become synonymous with primary delusions, and delusion-like ideas with secondary delusions. Delusion-like ideas can be seen to *emerge* understandably from the patient's internal and external environment, especially from their mood state. True delusions cannot be so explained; they are psychologically irreducible. They have, according to Jaspers, the following types:

- autochthonous delusion (delusional intuition),
- delusional percept,
- delusional atmosphere, and
- delusional memory.

AUTOCHTHONOUS DELUSION (DELUSIONAL INTUITION)

These are delusions that appear to arise suddenly 'out of the blue'; they are phenomenologically indistinguishable from the sudden arrival of a normal idea. The patient gropes for explanations for the occurrence of their delusion in answering the interviewer's question in the same way that a healthy person would find it difficult to account for the arrival of any idea if they were asked to explain it. The difference lies in the ability of the observer to empathize with—to understand—a nondelusional idea even though it may be bizarre and destructive, but they cannot understand how a person can have come to *believe* their delusion.

Schneider regarded the term *delusional idea* as based on outmoded psychology, and he felt it should therefore be abandoned. It is often confused with *delusion-like idea,* even in some textbooks, and this is another good reason for abandoning it. *Delusional intuition* is perhaps the most satisfactory translation of the German *Wahneinfall*. Delusional intuition occurs as a single stage, unlike *delusional perception,* which occurs in two stages: perception and then false interpretation. Like delusional perceptions, delusional intuitions are self-referent and usually of momentous import to the patient.

DELUSIONAL PERCEPT

This is present when the patient receives a normal perception that is then interpreted with delusional meaning and has immense personal significance. It is a *first-rank symptom of schizophrenia*. Jaspers delineated the concept of delusional percept, and Gruhle (1915)

used this description to cover almost all delusions—he minimized the importance of delusional intuition. Schneider (1949) considered the essence of delusional perception to be the abnormal significance attached to a real percept without any cause that is understandable in rational or emotional terms; it is self-referent, momentous, urgent, of overwhelming personal significance and, of course, false.

It is often difficult to decide whether a delusion is truly a delusional percept or is being used to explain the significance of certain objects of perception within a delusional system. A woman said, 'every night blood is being injected out of my arms [sic]'. When asked for her evidence, she explained that she had little brown spots on her arms and therefore knew that she was being injected. The interviewer looked at the spots on her arms, rolled up his sleeve and showed her spots identical in appearance on his own arm. He said that they had been on his arm as long as he could remember and were called *freckles*. She agreed that both sets of spots looked similar and accepted his explanation of his own spots, but she still insisted that her freckles proved that she was being injected in her sleep. This was a delusional percept.

Another example of what was probably a delusional percept caused considerable problems in surgical management, ultimately resulting in the death of the patient (Porter and Williams, 1997). A 65-year-old woman had flooded her house by leaving all the taps on.

On admission she was unkempt with unwashed hair, wearing a dirty dress and vest. She was bringing up bile-stained vomit and was reluctant to be interviewed. She expressed delusional beliefs that her stomach had been blown up with ether over several weeks and that it was liable to burst as a result of a Citizens' Band (CB) radio that was located in her stomach. She believed that the IRA had been after her for years and experienced auditory hallucinations of voices, which she identified as coming from the CB receiver. One 'voice' told her not to let anyone examine her. There was no evidence of an acute confusional state, and the diagnosis was consistent with a long-term paranoid psychosis.

On physical examination her abdomen was soft but distended with a hard, craggy, immobile, central mass. The liver and spleen were of normal size, and the kidneys were not palpable. Bowel sounds were loud. A diagnosis of possible intra-abdominal malignancy was made.

She refused any investigation or treatment. She developed acute renal failure and ultimately died; ascitic fluid revealed adenocarcinomatous cells probably of ovarian origin.

Another patient, who had other delusional symptoms, believed that many of the patients in the hospital were well-known citizens cunningly disguised with wigs, makeup and false beards. She recognized that they did not look like the people whom she presumed them to be but considered this to be part of a gigantic hoax in which she was herself involved to 'help people spiritually'. Although her percepts were normal and her interpretations delusional, this was not considered to be a delusional percept but a misinterpretation. All the circumstances in her life were explained by an immensely complicated delusional system, and these perceptions had no immediate personal significance beyond the significance that she found in all the objects and events around her.

In a delusional percept, there is a direct experience of meaning for this particular normal percept; it is not simply an interpretation of this percept to fit in with other established delusional beliefs. Delusional perception is therefore a direct experience of meaning that the patient did not have previously. Objects or persons take on new personal significance that is delusional in nature, even though the perception itself remains unchanged. This is different from a delusional misinterpretation in which the delusional system affects all aspects of the patient's life, and so every event or perception is interpreted as being involved with that delusion. A patient sees that a doorknob is missing; this is not the precipitant of immediate *new* personal significance of a delusional nature, but rather, it further confirms the belief they already held that people are trying to trap them and subject them to vivisection.

Perception, when considering delusional percept, can be understood in quite a wide sense. There is no difference in subjective experience between perceiving an object by means of a sense organ and perceiving or understanding the sense of written or spoken messages, although the perceptual routes are different. Thus delusional perception includes delusional significance attached to words and sentences as well as to purely sensory objects. For example, an inpatient at Rubery Hill Hospital walked to an entrance of the hospital and saw a dilapidated notice: 'RUBE … ILL'. She suddenly realized that this was a concealed message just for her—'Are you be(ing) ill?', that people were concerned to help her and that she would get better. The delusional interpretation was attached to the meaning of the letters of the notice.

There are two distinct stages in delusional perception:

1. The object becomes meaningful within a field of sensations and is perceived; this is usually visual perception (Mellor, 1991).
2. That object becomes invested with delusional significance.

These two stages need not be simultaneous for the experience to be a delusional percept. On occasions, they have been separated by an interval of years. A patient believed that his mind was being jammed by an electronic device. He claimed that this had started when, 5 years before, he had lifted the telephone receiver and heard an unusual clicking noise. The delusional belief he had held for only a few months.

DELUSIONAL ATMOSPHERE

For the patient experiencing delusional atmosphere, their world has been subtly altered: 'Something funny is going on', 'I have been offered a whole world of new meanings'. They experience everything around them as sinister, portentous, uncanny and peculiar in an indefinable way. They know that they personally are involved but cannot tell how. They have a feeling of anticipation, sometimes even of excitement, that soon all the separate parts of their experience will fit together to reveal something immensely significant. This is, in fact, what usually happens, as delusional atmosphere is part of the underlying process, and often, the first symptom of schizophrenia and the context in which a fully formed delusional percept or intuition arises. The mood of the atmosphere is important, and this experience is often referred to as *delusional mood*. The patient feels profoundly uncomfortable, often extremely perplexed and apprehensive. When the delusion becomes fully formed, resolving the inchoate nature of the delusional atmosphere, they often appear to accept it with a feeling of relief from the previous unbearable tension of the *atmosphere*.

In Gogol's *Diary of Madman*, the sudden and inexplicable delusional belief was expressed as follows: 'Today is a day of great triumph. There is a king of Spain. He has been found at last. That king is me. I only discovered this today. Frankly, it all came to me in a flash. I cannot understand how I could even think or imagine for one moment I was only a titular counsellor. I can't explain how such a ridiculous idea ever entered my head. Anyway, I'm rather pleased no one thought of having me put away yet. The path ahead is clear: everything is as bright as daylight'. It was preceded by a delusional atmosphere descried by the protagonist as follows: 'I don't really understand why, but before this revelation everything was enveloped in a kind of mist. And the whole reason for this, as I see it, is that people are under the misapprehension that the human brain is situated in the head: nothing could be further from the truth. It is carried by the wind from the Caspian Sea' (Gogol, 1972).

In a real-life example, a middle-aged man presented initially as a psychiatric outpatient with apparent obsessional symptoms. He kept checking that his neighbours could not hear what he was saying in his home. He had resigned from several jobs because he believed that his employers would not accept his religious beliefs. He felt that people around him were hostile and implacably opposed to him, although he could not define quite how—he just 'felt it'. He kept moving house, but the feeling stayed with him. This continued for several years, and he then arrived at a casualty department claiming that his neighbours were talking about his actions and controlling his thoughts. The atmosphere had developed insidiously over years, and eventually he manifested *auditory hallucinations* and *passivity of thought* (see Chapter 9).

German psychopathologists never used the term *delusional atmosphere* but always referred to *delusional mood,* according to Berner (1991), but he considers that atmosphere is to be preferred because it allows the distinction to be made between a cognitive, perceptual disturbance provoking an emotional response and a modification of mood causing a changed perception of the outside world. It is considered that delusional atmosphere is a common end state resulting from different pathways: vulnerability to cognitive disturbance, as in 'Bleulerian' schizophrenia; dynamic derailment, as in affective disorders such as puerperal depression or psychogenic vulnerability; or without either of the other two, with stressful life events. Berner considers that this state is not restricted to sufferers of schizophrenia.

The prodromal phases of schizophrenic illnesses are very variable in nature, and often another diagnosis has been given before the definitive symptomatology becomes established. In an instructive review of the literature on the simulation of psychosis and a study of six patients who were thought to be feigning a schizophrenic psychosis, Hay (1983) commented on the nature of *feigned psychosis*. In his opinion, simulation of schizophrenia is generally a prodromal phase of a schizophrenic psychosis occurring in people with extremely deviant premorbid personalities. All but one of his patients were found to be suffering from schizophrenia at the time of follow-up.

DELUSIONAL MEMORY

In much the same way that delusional percept is a delusional interpretation of a normal percept, delusional memory is the delusional interpretation of a normal memory. These are sometimes called *retrospective delusions*. An event that occurred in the past is explained in a delusional way. A man aged 50 whose mental illness had lasted for about 2 years claimed that his health had been permanently affected since age 16, when he had had 'an operation to remove his appendix'. He now believed that the operation had been an excuse to 'implant a golden convolvulus' in his bowels.

If delusional meaning is attached to a normal percept that is remembered, this then becomes a *delusional percept.* It has the two components that were described as being necessary for delusional percept: the image of the remembered percept and the attachment to this percept of delusional significance. A married woman remembered years previously seeing a man standing in a pub 'with a sad look on his face'. She 'realized', at the start of her schizophrenic illness 2 weeks before admission to the hospital, that he had been in love with her then, and she tried to locate his name in the telephone directory and make contact again, feeling that they were involved in a special relationship.

Of course, it is a mistake to expect phenomenological symptoms to reveal themselves tidily from the patient's conversation. There is no absolute demarcation between delusional memory and delusional percept or intuition. The patient describes a delusion. Did this occur 1 hour, 1 week or 10 years ago? At what point will this be delusional memory, not delusional intuition? Similarly, there is no absolute distinction between a normal event, perception or idea that occurred in the past and is remembered with a delusional interpretation and a delusional event, perception or idea that occurred in the past and is also remembered with a delusional interpretation. In other words, there are two senses to the term *delusional memory*. There is the sense in which a normal memory is misinterpreted in the present, and another sense in which the actual memory is itself a false memory that is imbued with delusional interpretation. Both of these are delusional memories, and it is not always possible to know how much of the event was factual and how much was delusional. A woman with schizophrenia, aged 34, described 12 years ago picking up a telephone to ring a man she liked very much: 'God moved my arm and made me put the telephone back'. It was not possible to decide exactly what part of this experience was factual and what was delusional and at what time the delusion occurred.

Fine distinctions are sometimes imposed on the classification of primary delusions but are more collector's items than features of useful clinical significance. *Delusional awareness* is an experience that is not sensory in nature in which ideas or events take on an extreme vividness as if they had additional reality. *Delusional significance* is the second stage of the occurrence of delusional perception. Objects and persons are perceived normally but take on a special significance that cannot be rationally explained by the patient.

The Origins of Delusion

What is the origin of delusions? This question drives at how far delusions are, by definition, different from normal beliefs, and, if they are different from normal beliefs, what mechanisms are involved in their development and manifestation. Jaspers' (1997) own view was that delusion was a primary phenomenon and that it implies a transformation in the total awareness of reality. This means that a delusional belief involves and implicates practical activity, behaviour, the meanings that are immanent in objects and radically transforms

BOX 8.1 FACTORS INVOLVED IN THE GERMINATION OF DELUSIONS

- Disorder of brain functioning
- Background influences of temperament and personality
- Maintenance of self-esteem
- The role of affect
- As a response to perceptual disturbance
- As a response to depersonalization
- Associated with cognitive overload

the basic experience of the world. A person who is deluded that they are loved by a celebrity approaches the world with this certainty and knowledge and acts accordingly by writing to, telephoning or attempting to visit the celebrity. This erroneous belief invests the patient's world with new meanings. In these terms, *reality* lies in the interpretation of or the significance attached to events that occur interpreted in the light of the primary erroneous belief.

An understanding of how delusions radically alter the patient's world as described does not help us to explain how delusions form in the first place. The factors involved in delusion formation have been summarized by Brockington (1991); see Box 8.1.

Fish (1967) developed a useful précis of the earlier German theories of the origins of delusion. Conrad proposed five stages in the development of delusional psychosis:

1. *Trema*: delusional mood representing a total change in perception of the world
2. *Apophany*: a search for, and the finding of, new meaning for psychological events
3. *Anastrophy*: heightening of the psychosis
4. *Consolidation*: forming of a new world or psychological set based on new meanings
5. *Residuum*: eventual autistic state

Gruhle (1915) considered *delusional perception* to be the most significant form of delusion, a normal percept taking on a new meaning. This results in a disturbed relationship of the understanding of events. Matussek (1953) considered that with delusional perception there is a change either in the significance of the words used or in the actual nature of the perception itself. These writers and Schneider regard *delusional perception* as the key to understanding the nature of delusional experience.

Hagen (1870) regarded *delusional atmosphere* as primary, arising for reasons unknown and resulting in a rearrangement of meanings in the world around the patient who gropes for an answer to this problem of understanding and finds it by creating a delusion. It is easier to bear the certainty of a delusion than the uncertain foreboding of the atmosphere. Jaspers considered that there is a subtle change of personality due to the illness itself, and this creates the condition for the development of the delusional atmosphere in which the delusional intuition arises.

All these theories assume that the delusion is *primary* and *ultimately not understandable* in the same sense that Jaspers considers the experience of reality to be primary. Experience holds a symbolic implication beyond the fact of the event itself; for example the doctor writing a prescription for their patient in the consulting room means much more to the latter than if the doctor were doodling on their prescription block. (A patient in North Africa in the 19th century ate the written prescription his doctor gave him, so great was his confidence in, and veneration for, the doctor; Sims, 1972.) It seems that the symbolic belief attached to events and perceptions is altered in delusion, and this is why the patient does not necessarily act on their delusions. The delusional atmosphere is not an essential prerequisite for a delusional intuition, as the latter may occur apparently de novo.

Some writers have not tried to explain delusions because they find them totally incomprehensible and consider that they are directly due to an abnormality of the brain (Schneider, 1949). Bleuler concentrated on the *alteration in affect* as primary rather than delusional atmosphere or perception. He considered that heightened affect loosens the capacity to form associations and thus facilitates the arrival of a delusion. At the beginning of a schizophrenic illness, there is extreme affect, perhaps in the form of anxiety or ambivalence, which the patient cannot express.

Kretschmer (1927) stressed the importance of the underlying personality. He described the *sensitive premorbid personality* occurring in a person who retains *affect-laden complexes* and has a limited capacity for emotional self-expression. Such a person is driven painfully by, for example, powerful sexual feelings, but they have great difficulty in communicating their passion and relating to other people. They are very much aware of social constraints and are rigidly controlled by their superego. Such a person, somewhat rigid, narrow-minded and suspicious in their views, readily forms *sensitive ideas of reference*. A key experience may occur in their life circumstances, and quite suddenly these ideas become structured as *delusions of reference*.

A girl was always shy, reticent and sensitive at school. Quite often, she was reluctant to go to school. She was meticulous in her attention to personal neatness and cleanliness. After leaving school, she remembered vividly several occasions as a child when she had felt humiliated. At age 18, when she was working in a factory, she was in the women's cloak-room brooding because her boyfriend had told her that he was leaving her for someone else. She heard one of the other women say, 'Ugh, doesn't she smell?' Immediately, she applied the statement to herself and to explain her boyfriend's behaviour. From then onwards, she was convinced that she smelt unpleasant all the time, although she could smell nothing herself. This delusion dominated her life, prevented her mixing and caused her great distress. This development of a delusion (*Sensitiver Beziehungswahn*) from sensitive ideas of reference, as the sequel to a *key experience,* is sometimes seen at the onset of schizophrenia but is not common. The key experience, as demonstrated in this case, has two important qualities. First, it has particular appropriateness to the patient's areas of conflict as sensitive ideas of reference. Second, it occurs at a time of marked emotional turmoil and distress so that the psychic ground is prepared for a catastrophic event.

Attempts have been made to find all delusions understandable in relation to the person's internal experience or social background. Westphal considered that if one knew all about the patient, the change in their view of themselves and the belief that they had become noticeable in some way would explain the delusion (Fish, 1967). Freud's (1907) theories on the development of delusions also attempted to make them ultimately understandable through the mechanisms of denial, projection and so on. Other authors have claimed that delusions are understandable in a social context. Laing (1961) considered the flight into madness as a necessary defence against a highly destructive family—not only understandable, but admirable, and even worth emulating.

When four psychological theories were appraised to explain paranoid phenomena, a basis of *shame-humiliation* was found to be the most consistent (Colby, 1977). Winters and Neale (1983) consider that existing theories of delusional thinking develop two main themes: *motivational* and *defect*. The motivational theme explains the arrival of a delusion to explain unusual perceptual experience or to reduce uncomfortable psychic states. Defect implies some fundamental cognitive-attentional deficit resulting in delusion.

The variety and range of explanations adduced as the origin of delusions attest the extent of our ignorance about the ultimate nature, structure and derivation of delusions. It is probably wise to regard *delusion* as a term describing a multitude of abnormalities of thinking that have merely a superficial familial relationship. To employ an analogy, *delusion* is like the term *ataxia*, a term that describes several abnormalities of movement with differing underlying lesions and mechanisms. The term *delusion* is not a description of a unitary, homogenous abnormality of thinking; it is most likely an umbrella term for a collection of disparate abnormalities of thinking.

COGNITION AND REASONING IN DELUSION

In trying to understand the role of cognition and reason in delusion formation, it is probably useful to think of the formation, elaboration and persistence of delusional beliefs as an expression of numerous causal influences converging; each exerts a different influence in the evolution of the belief (Roberts, 1992). The process of reasoning in order to come to conclusions about one's situation in the outside environment appears to be altered in those experiencing delusions. A 'jump-to-conclusions style' has been demonstrated in deluded subjects when asked to perform a probabilistic reasoning task (Huq et al., 1988). This was confirmed by Garety et al. (1991) in showing that 41% of deluded subjects but only 4% of controls reached a conclusion on the basis of only one item of information. A common cause in abnormality of information processing has been proposed for those subjects with abnormal reasoning and abnormal perception; failure to make use of previously acquired knowledge of regularities in the world, resulting in overreliance on information immediately present, may be a factor in delusion

formation (Garety, 1991). This model emphasizes the deviant nature of the thinking process that is associated with delusions in patients with schizophrenia. In Garety's model, judgemental processes involved in delusion formation include:

1. prior expectation that may be modified by emotion;
2. current information that we have at our disposal, such as the information reaching us by way of our perceptions; and
3. the nature of our information processing bias or style.

In this model, if perceptual abnormalities predominate the role of deviant information, then processing mechanisms will be underemphasized. In other words, when delusions are secondary to hallucinations, reasoning should remain intact. The advantage of this model is that it highlights the varying routes to delusion formation.

Attribution in Delusion

An alternative psychological explanation for delusion comes from *social attribution theory*. Kaney and Bentall (1989, 1992) found that deluded patients made excessively external, stable and global attributions for negative events ('The fact that I broke my leg proves yet again that the Wetherby freemasons are getting at me') and excessively internal, stable and global attributions for positive events ('Everyone smiles and nods when they see me because I have been sent by God to communicate with people about evil and I have a letter from the Pope as proof'). Deluded subjects were unwilling to attribute negative events of which they were the victim to their own cause; also, in judging the behaviour of other people they were reluctant to attribute negative events to the victims themselves. These and other studies suggest that persecutory delusions have a function in protecting the individual from low self-esteem (Bentall, 1993).

Deluded subjects were considered to evaluate their own causal statements in a distinctive manner, and this difference from depressed subjects was greater than the differences in the causal statements themselves; that is, the difference between deluded and other subjects in internality for positive and negative events does not reflect differences in the causal statements of these subjects but rather differences in their attributions (Kinderman et al., 1992). Once again, delusions are linked both to personal meaning and to boundaries of self. This investigation of attributional style was further extended using obvious and opaque tests of attributional style. Deluded subjects attributed negative outcomes to external causes in the obvious or transparent tests but a more covert testing to internal causes; this further supported the hypothesis that persecutory delusions function as a defence against underlying feelings of low self-esteem (Lyon et al., 1994). This psychological exploration is further supported by the clinical study that follows.

Delusion and Meaning in Life

Roberts (1991) has developed the thesis that delusions, in the context of schizophrenic illness, may not themselves be an affliction or illness but an adaptive response to whatever initiates the psychotic break. A group of chronically deluded subjects was compared with previously deluded patients now in remission and with two nonpatient groups. Persecutory delusions were common in both patient groups, but grandiose and erotic delusions and delusions of special knowledge were mostly found in the currently deluded group. The chronically deluded group scored much higher than the remitted patients for positive meaning in life and much lower for depression and suicidal intention. They had a very high level of perceived purpose and meaning in life. It is considered that, for some, the formation of delusions is adaptive in combating purposelessness, loneliness, sense of inferiority, hopelessness, isolation and painful awareness of broken relationships and provides a new sense of identity, a clearer sense of duty and responsibility, an experience of freedom, protection from past hurts and a change from fear, worry, depression and boredom towards feeling lively, enthusiastic, interested and peaceful. One patient described this: 'I've had a great time. I've got this one great thought in my mind that I am Jesus—that's enough … nothing hurts me now, I need nothing now.'

Content of Delusions

Delusions are, of course, infinitely variable in their content, but certain general characteristics commonly occur. Unlike the *form,* which is dictated by the type of illness, the *content* is determined by the emotional, social, cultural and biographical background of the patient: Napoleons are now rare in mental hospitals; schizophrenia sufferers from traditional societies may describe their thoughts as being interfered with by the spirits of their ancestors rather than by television. As computers and the Internet increasingly affect all aspects of our lives, we are beginning to have described by those with mental illness delusions of control concerning the Internet (Catalano et al., 1991).

DELUSIONS OF PERSECUTION

This is the most frequent content of delusion. It was distinguished from other types of delusion and from other forms of melancholia by Lasègue (1852). People who believe delusionally that their lives are being interfered with from outside more often feel this to be harmful than beneficial. A variant on the usual beliefs of persecution or malevolent intent are delusions of prejudice: the patient or victim believes that they are being slighted, overlooked or passed over in favour of someone else. The interfering agent in delusions of persecution may be animate or inanimate, other people or machines; it may be systems, organizations or institutions rather than individuals. Sometimes the patient experiences persecution as a vague influence without knowing who is responsible.

Persecutory delusions occur in many conditions: in schizophrenia, in affective psychoses of manic and depressive type and in organic states, both acute and chronic. The affect associated with the belief of persecution may vary from an inappropriate indifference and apathy in schizophrenia to stark terror, as commonly seen in delirium tremens.

Manic patients with persecutory delusions show gross overactivity and flight of ideas in attempting to express and deal with their beliefs. In depression, the persecutory delusions take on the characteristic colouring of the dominant mood state. Persecutory overvalued ideas are a prominent facet of the *litigious* type of paranoid personality disorder.

MORBID JEALOUSY AND DELUSION OF INFIDELITY

Morbid jealousy, a disorder of *content* described by Ey (1950), may be manifested in various forms, for example, as delusion, overvalued idea, or part of depressive affect or anxiety state. The feeling of jealousy, coupled with a sense that the loved object 'belongs to me' and therefore 'I belong to the other' is part of normal human experience; it is of social value in marital relationships for preserving the family. Various terms have been used to describe abnormal, morbid or malignant jealousy. Kraepelin (1905) used the term *sexual jealousy*. Enoch and Trethowan (1979) have considered it important to distinguish psychotic jealousy from other types, and this is dependent on the demonstration of a *delusion of infidelity*. It is sometimes difficult to distinguish understandable jealousy from that which is delusional.

Mullen (1997) classified morbid jealousy with *disorders of passion* in which there is an overwhelming sense of entitlement and a conviction that others are abrogating the subject's rights: 'The morbidly jealous believe that they are the victims of an infidelity that has deprived them of the fealty which is their due and they are driven to expose this disloyalty, reassert their control and punish the transgression'. The other two categories are the querulent, who are indignant at infringements of rights, and the erotomanic, who are driven to assert their rights of love.

Delusion of infidelity, that is, when the subject unreasonably believes themselves to be the victim of their partner's unfaithfulness, may occur without other psychotic symptoms. It has been described by Todd and Dewhurst (1955) and by Mullen (1990). This is identifiably delusional when the belief of the spouse is based on delusional evidence. Such delusions are resistant to treatment and do not change with time. A patient was very concerned that his wife was being unfaithful with numerous people, including his boss, her general practitioner and others. Four years later, despite various treatments, his belief was unchanged, but he said, 'I don't blame her now. She is much younger than I am and everyone does that sort of thing'. Delusions of jealousy are common with alcohol abuse; for instance, Shrestha et al. (1985) found sexual jealousy to be present in 35% of men and 31% of women who abused alcohol or had alcohol dependence syndrome. As jealousy appeared to be justified in some cases, *morbid jealousy* was considered to be present in 27% of men and 15% of women. Delusional jealousy, often associated with impotence, also occurs in some organic states, for example, the punch-drunk syndrome of boxers after multiple contrecoup contusions. Quite frequently, the spouse, wearied by continued accusations of infidelity, does form another sexual involvement, which may result in an acute exacerbation in the mental state of the patient and further marital conflict.

The sexual content of the delusion is obvious; however, Enoch (1991) regards the nature of the relationship between the two partners as the key aspect of the condition. Jealousy is directed towards the sexual partner. The deluded person is very attached to, and often emotionally utterly dependent on, the other; they may have a misplaced sense of owning them completely. The victim is often much more sexually attractive than the deluded partner, for instance, a young wife or a sociable and popular husband. The deluded person may have been promiscuous in the past and therefore resignedly expects their spouse to show similar behaviour. A male partner may have become impotent and projected the blame for his failure onto his wife. He may have homosexual fantasies directed towards the men with whom he claims his wife is consorting. Morbid jealousy arises with the belief that there is a threat to the exclusive possession of his wife, but this is just as likely to occur from conflicts inside himself, his own inability to love or his sexual interest directed towards someone else as from changing circumstances in his environment or his wife's behaviour. The jealous feeling is associated with intense feelings of anger, fear, sadness, envy and sometimes with sexual arousal. Checking behaviours that accompany jealousy can be engrossing and exhausting. The jealous partner checks for seminal stain, examining bedsheets or clothing for telltale signs of secret sexual liaisons. Husbands or wives may show sexual jealousy, as may cohabitees and homosexual couples.

Crimes of violence are notoriously associated with morbid jealousy; violence is more often vented on the partner than on the supposed rival, most often by men on women. Morbid jealousy makes a major contribution to the frequency of wife battering and is one of the commonest motivations for homicide (Mullen, 1990). Daly et al., (1982) show from their examination of homicide data from Detroit in 1972 that a substantial number of homicides resulting from social conflict were ultimately motivated by sexual jealousy. The risk factors predicting lethal violence in spousal homicide include a history of previous domestic violence, cohabiting, childhood victim of family violence, large age disparity, drug and alcohol misuse, sexual jealousy, threats of separation by the female spouse, and personality disorder (Aldridge and Browne, 2003).

DELUSIONS OF LOVE

The delusions associated with loving and being loved are quite different from the behavioural and affective abnormalities of *nymphomania,* the situation of a woman characterized by morbid or uncontrolled sexual desire, and *satyriasis,* the male equivalent of excessive sexual activity. Both these latter conditions exist initially in the opinion of an external commentator—the doctor.

Approximately twice as many schizophrenic patients had sexual preoccupations in the mid-20th century compared with in the mid-19th century (Klaf and Hamilton, 1961). The term *erotomania* has a long pedigree. It was first used by Jacques Ferrand (1640) in the title of his book *Erotomania or Treatise Discoursing of the Essence, Causes, Symptoms, Prognosticks and Cure of Love or Erotic Melancholy* (Hunter and MacAlpine, 1970). *Erotomania* was described by Sir Alexander Morrison (1848) as being:

characterized by delusions ... the patient's love is of the sentimental kind, he is wholly occupied by the object of his adoration, whom, if he approaches, it is with respect ... the fixed and permanent delusions attending erotomania sometimes prompt those labouring under it to destroy themselves or others, for although in general tranquil and peaceful, the patient sometimes becomes irritable, passionate and jealous.

Erotomania is commoner in women than in men, and a variety was called *old maids insanity* by Hart (1921) in which persecutory delusions often develop. These have sometimes been classified as paranoia rather than paranoid schizophrenia; these delusional symptoms sometimes occur in the context of manic-depressive psychosis (Guirguis, 1981). Trethowan (1967) demonstrated the social characteristics of erotomania, relating the patient's previous difficulties in parental relationships to the present erotomania.

A variation of erotomania was described by, and retains the name of, de Clérambault (1942). Typically, a woman believes a man who is older and of

higher social status than she is in love with her. The victim has usually done nothing to deserve her attention and may be quite unaware of her existence; sometimes he is a well-known public figure quite remote from the patient. In a case of the author's, the victim was a previous employer of the patient. She believed that he was the father of her child (although at another time she agreed that there had been no sexual relationship with her employer). She also believed that he was sending her money, and she would write letters thanking him for his generosity and affirming her gratitude for the evidence of his love (Sims and White, 1973). Ellis and Mellsop (1985) proposed operational criteria for erotomania derived from Clérambault and these are (1) delusional conviction of amorous communication, (2) a love object of higher rank, (3) the love object being the first to fall in, (4) the love object being the first to make advances, (5) sudden onset within a 7-day period, (6) the love object remains unchanged and if other love objects occur they are only of transitory significance, (7) the patient rationalizes the paradoxical behaviour of the love object, (8) there is a chronic course and (9) there is an absence of hallucinations.

In a series of 16 erotomanic cases, Mullen and Pathé (1994) tried to distinguish between those cases in which there is a morbid belief in being loved and those with morbid infatuation. They found that in most cases both notions were described: a mixture of being loved and loving in return. It is notable that erotomania is associated with stalking behaviour including cyberstalking and violence.

DELUSIONAL MISIDENTIFICATION

Delusional misidentification syndromes include a number of discrete but related syndromes that have in common the concept of the double. These syndromes include *Capgras'* syndrome (Capgras and Reboul-Lachaux, 1923), *Frégoli's* syndrome (Courbon and Fail, 1927), the syndrome of *intermetamorphosis* (Courbon and Tusques, 1932) and the syndrome of *subjective doubles* (Christodoulou, 1978).

Capgras' syndrome is regarded by Enoch and Trethowan (1979) as 'a rare, colourful syndrome in which the person believes that a person, usually closely related to them, has been replaced by an exact double'. It is a specific delusional misidentification of a person with whom the subject usually has close emotional ties and towards whom there is a feeling of ambivalence at the time of onset. The belief in Capgras' syndrome has the full characteristics of delusion (Enoch and Trethowan, 1979). The basic concept of this syndrome is prominent in all cultures, hence the delusion is universal (Christodoulou, 1991). Like other delusions, *delusion* describes the form; the explanatory content is culture-dependent. A recent patient believed his mother had been replaced by an impostor after falling through a time warp to a parallel universe, and this explained the horrible things that had happened in the past 3 weeks.

Frégoli's syndrome is the delusional misidentification of an unfamiliar person as a familiar one, even though there is no physical resemblance. The syndrome of intermetamorphosis is the delusional belief that others undergo radical changes in physical and psychological identity, culminating in a different person altogether. The syndrome of subjective doubles is the delusional belief in the existence of physical duplicates of the self, and these duplicates are usually thought to have different psychological identities (for review, see Moselhy and Oyebode, 1997).

In a series of cases reviewed by Berson (1983), 55% (70 patients) were unquestionably diagnosed as suffering from schizophrenia, and a further 8 patients (totalling 61%) were probably suffering from schizophrenia; 13% were suffering from bipolar mood disorder and 24% were considered to have an organic diagnosis. Of 133 patients, 57% were female; the age range was from 12 to 78 with a mean of 42.8 years. Majority opinion would not favour denoting this as a separate disease but rather as a symptom that colours the clinical state and dominates the symptomatology. The four varieties of delusional misidentification have in common psychopathologically the form of a delusion. Capgras' syndrome, when it occurs in schizophrenia, can be based on a delusional percept (Sims, 1986) but the fundamental problem is misidentification of a familiar person as a double. In Capgras' syndrome, there is no outward change in the appearance of the object, and there is no false perception, for the patient often admits that the double exactly resembles the original (Enoch and Trethowan, 1979), but careful questioning usually reveals that there are distinguishing stigmata. Sometimes patients will say, 'I know that

it is not my mother because she would never stand like that' or 'this person moves too slowly to be my father'.

The ambivalence towards the object of misidentification may be expressed in the history, with a clear account of both negative emotions, such as hostility, fear or contempt, and affection and dependence. On those few occasions when an object, rather than a person, is wrongly identified, that object has important emotional connotations for the patient, for example home or a letter from a relative. The subjects of misidentification in Berson's (1983) review of 133 patients comprised 60 spouses and 2 lovers; on 29 occasions, a child or children; 40 parents; 24 siblings; 13 therapists; four grandparents; three in-laws; two neighbours; two domestics; and one each of fiancé, cousin, stepson, employer and priest. On eight occasions, the self was misidentified either solely or with other evidence of the syndrome; on two occasions, animals, and eight times inanimate objects were misidentified. Thus in 31% of occasions, the delusional misidentification refers to a marital partner, and in 46% to a first-degree relative; in only 4% was the misidentification of the patient themself.

There is growing evidence that delusional misidentification syndromes are associated with organic disorders, including dementia, acquired brain injury, epilepsy and cerebrovascular accidents in 25% to 40% of cases, and neuroimaging studies reveal association with right hemisphere abnormalities, particularly in the frontal and temporal regions (Edelstyn et al., 1999). Furthermore, neuropsychological investigations have consistently shown impairments of face processing in delusional misidentification syndromes (Ellis et al., 1993; Edelstyn et al., 1996; Oyebode et al., 1996). These findings underpin the assumption of right hemisphere abnormalities in delusional misidentification syndromes, because the right hemisphere is implicated in face processing and recognition.

GRANDIOSE DELUSIONS

Primary grandiose delusions occur in schizophrenia. The patient may believe themself to be a famous celebrity or to have supernatural powers. They may believe themself to be involved in some special and secret mission about which they have not yet been fully briefed but in anticipation of which they are waiting with excitement for the dénouement. Beliefs of this sort are sometimes called *delusions of special purpose* and are of the form of delusional intuition.

Expansive or grandiose delusional beliefs may extend to objects. Sometimes a psychotic patient demonstrates delusions of invention in which, for example, they build a machine that they believe to have special capabilities, considering themself to be a creative prodigy. Secondary grandiose delusions, or delusion-like ideas, occur in manic states. A patient said that there was no life on Mars because 'if there had been I would have been able to get in touch by telepathy using my great genius'. He showed no evidence of true passivity experiences. A manic patient, mentioned earlier, believed that she was descended from the royal Stuart line and therefore was actually in some way Mary, Queen of Scots. She invited the queen and the prime minister to a party in her student flat because she thought they would be honoured to be invited: 'It is only fair that they should have an invitation.' The expansive affect of mania can be clearly seen to render this delusion understandable.

RELIGIOUS DELUSIONS

Religious delusions are common. However, they formed a higher proportion of all delusions in the 19th century than in the 20th century: three times as many patients with schizophrenia of both sexes had religious preoccupation in the 19th century (Klaf and Hamilton, 1961). Decision as to whether beliefs are delusional must rest on the principles described earlier—that is, on the way the belief is held and the evidence produced in its support. Because a religious belief is bizarre and at variance with those held by the interviewer does not necessarily make it a delusion. Religious delusions may be grandiose in nature, for example, a patient in the United Kingdom who believed that she was an emissary of God to the Birmingham Housing Department. They may also be secondary to depressive mood, as in the patient of Emil Kraepelin (1905) quoted at the beginning of Chapter 16: 'I cannot live and I cannot die, because I have failed so much, I shall bring my husband and children to hell'

The religious nature of the delusion is seen as a disorder of content dependent on the patient's social background, interests and peer group. The form of the delusion is dictated by the nature of the illness.

So religious delusions are not caused by excessive religious belief or by the wrongdoing that the patient attributes as cause, but they simply accentuate that, when a person becomes mentally ill, their delusions reflect, in their content, their predominant interests and concerns.

Sometimes, it can be difficult to make the distinction between religious delusion and the experience of an unusual religious belief or practice. Psychiatric morbidity would be suggested by the following (Sims, 1992):

- Both the subjective experience and the observed behaviour conform with psychiatric symptoms, that is, the self-description of this particular experience is recognizable as being the symptomatology of a known psychiatric illness—it has the form of delusion.
- There are other recognizable symptoms of mental illness in other areas of life: other delusions, hallucinations, disturbance of mood, thought disorder and so on.
- The lifestyle, behaviour and direction of personal goals of the individual subsequent to the event or religious experience are consistent with the natural history of mental disorder rather than with a personally enriching life experience, compatible with the conditions in which delusions occur.

DELUSIONS OF GUILT AND UNWORTHINESS

Such delusions are common in depressive illness. They often lead to suicide and, rarely, to homicide, when the killing of a close relative may be followed by the patient's suicide. Affective illness may be followed by the killing of children by depressed mothers or the killing of their wife or sometimes also children by husbands; suicide may follow immediately or later (Higgins, 1990).

The beliefs about guilt may totally dominate the patient's thinking. An elderly woman spent the day rushing round the house wringing her hands and telling her worried family that she was wretched, worthless and only deserved to die. She told her married daughters that they were illegitimate and that the house she lived in was not hers but stolen, and she told her husband of 30 years' standing that they were not legally married. When it was suggested to her that she come into hospital, she assumed that she would be killed on arrival, and she asked whether this could take place there and then so that she could receive her just desserts.

DELUSIONS OF POVERTY AND NIHILISTIC DELUSIONS

Delusions of poverty are common in depression; an elderly patient believed that 'the nurses' had been systematically raiding her purse and that she was destitute. *Cotard's syndrome* contains features typical of psychotic depression in the elderly: nihilistic and hypochondriacal delusions that are often bizarre, dramatic and tinged with grandiosity; depressed mood with either agitation or retardation and a completely negative attitude. According to Griesinger (1845), 'the patient confuses the subjective change in his own attitude to outside things … the real world seems to the patient to have disappeared completely, or to be dead'. This was graphically depicted by Cotard (1882):

I would tentatively suggest the name 'nihilistic delusions' (délire de negations) to describe the condition of the patients to whom Griesinger was referring, in whom the tendency towards negation is carried to its extreme. If they are asked their name or age, they have neither – where were they born? They were not born. Who were their father and mother? They have no father, mother, wife or children. Have they a headache or pain in the stomach, or any other part of the body? They have no head or stomach and some even have no body. If one shows them an object, a rose or some other flower they answer, 'that is not a rose, not a flower at all'. In some cases negation is total. Nothing exists any longer, not even themselves.

The central character in Patrick McGrath's novel, Spider, said, 'I was contaminated by it, it shrivelled me, it killed something inside me, made me a ghost, a dead thing, in short it turned me bad'. Elsewhere, the same character says, 'a single pipe takes water from my stomach … and this pipe alone drops through the void and connects to the thing between my legs that hardly resembles a formed male organ at all anymore' (McGrath, 1990).

Nihilistic delusions are the reverse of grandiose delusions in which oneself, objects or situations are expansive and enriched; there is also a perverse grandiosity about the nihilistic delusions themselves. Feelings of guilt and hypochondriacal ideas are developed to their most extreme, depressive form in nihilistic delusions.

HYPOCHONDRIACAL DELUSIONS

A very depressed man said that he was full of water, that there was nothing else inside him, and that he could not pass water but that if he did, that would be the end of him. He could not drink or the water would flood the room. Other less striking hypochondriacal beliefs and delusions occur in depression, and Schneider (1920) has considered that locating the experience of depression as a sensation in a bodily organ is equivalent to a 'first-rank symptom' of depressive psychosis (see Chapter 16). An elderly woman with depression who had had a mitral valve replacement for rheumatic heart disease said that she felt worthless and hopeless and described her physical functions as 'nothing is working'.

Hypochondriacal delusions may also occur in schizophrenia and have the characteristics of other schizophrenic ideas. They are more likely to be given a persecutory than a nihilistic explanation. Thus a patient believed that his bodily functions were being interfered with by rays emitted from a planet and that this was part of a plot to control his thoughts and behaviour. Hypochondriacal delusions are discussed further in association with hypochondriasis in Chapter 14; however, other features of hypochondriasis, such as bodily preoccupation, disease phobia and conviction of the presence of disease with nonresponse to reassurance, are in fact more common than delusion (Pilowsky, 1967). Facial pain is described in Chapter 15 and other delusion-like ideas and overvalued ideas of the body in Chapter 14. Delusions concerning the patient's origins are sometimes described and have some affinity to hypochondriacal delusion. The patient believes, on delusional evidence, that they are not their parent's child, or perhaps that they are of royal birth, part animal or supernatural. Alternatively, they may believe that they do not exist and were never born.

Hypochondriacal delusions are commonly associated with delusional disorder in the *International Classification of Diseases*, 10th revision (previously known as paranoia; World Health Organization, 1992). Munro (1988) has described *delusional disorder* as an encapsulated monodelusional disorder with several subtypes, such as erotomanic, grandiose, jealous, persecutory, somatic and unspecified; the concept has developed from the older term *paranoia* (Munro, 1997). He has described the somatic type as *monosymptomatic hypochondriacal psychosis* and, of 50 cases, the three main groups were:

1. delusions of body odour and halitosis;
2. infestation delusion (insects, burrowing worms or foreign bodies under the skin); and
3. delusions of ugliness or misshapenness (dysmorphic delusions).

In a factor analysis of the features of delusional disorder, four independent factors were identified, suggesting considerable heterogeneity of the condition (Serretti et al., 1999). The first factor incorporated core depressive symptoms, which may be either a depressive syndrome reactive to stresses deriving from delusional ideation, a comorbid mood disorder or both. Other factors were hallucinations, delusions and symptoms of irritability.

The complaint was always presented with great intensity, and patients were utterly convinced of the physical nature of the disorder. Hypochondriacal delusions may also occur with administration of drugs, both prescribed and those of abuse.

Koro (Lapierre, 1972) is an unusual condition that has been described as an example of hypochondriacal delusion. This view is probably incorrect. The features of koro include:

- the belief that the penis is shrinking into the abdomen;
- the belief that when the penis disappears into the abdomen, death will ensue; and
- extreme anxiety accompanying this belief.

Yap (1965) describes this as a culture-bound depersonalization syndrome and considers it to be a manifestation of acute anxiety associated with folk beliefs concerning sexual exhaustion. It has occurred in epidemic proportions among Malays in Singapore (Gwee, 1963) but has also been described in individual cases in a French Canadian (Lapierre, 1972), in a West Indian, in a Greek Cypriot (Ang and Weller, 1984) and in an Englishman (Berrios and Morley, 1984). Oyebode et al. (1986) have shown in a single case study that

this belief is accompanied by real penile shrinkage as measured by plethysmography. This suggests that the belief is based on physiologic changes that are likely to be due to anxiety. In essence, the penile change is similar to tachycardia, hyperhidrosis or other features of sympathetic arousal associated with anxiety.

A group of patients who, in some respects, are intermediate between those suffering from somatic delusions and delusions of infestation are those who were described by Videbech (1966) as suffering from chronic olfactory paranoid syndromes; these have also been referred to as having *olfactory reference syndrome* (Pryse-Phillips, 1971). Characteristically, these patients have a fixed and unalterable belief that they smell but do not have hallucinations or other olfactory experience. It is usually seen in the context of sensitive, paranoid personality development. There is a severe phobic reaction, with the behaviour of other people interpreted as finding their smell offensive and aversive.

Delusions of Infestation

Delusions of infestation have been described by Hopkinson (1970) and by Reilly (1988). In *Ekbom's syndrome* (Ekbom, 1938), the patient believes that they are infested with small but macroscopic organisms. Freudenmann and Lepping (2009) describe the nature of the imaginary pathogens reported by patients as including vermin, insects, parasites, 'small animals'. Often the nature of the infestation is surmised from an itch that is ascribed to mites, scabies, lice, worms, bugs, fleas, flies, ticks or spiders. Sometimes, microscopic pathogens such as bacteria or viruses are identified as the cause of the patient's problems. In the Mogellons phenomenon, inanimate materials such as filaments, threads, fibres and pigments may be identified as responsible for the sensory experiences. The most common sources of the imagined infestation are other human beings, plants, animals, pets and parts of the home. The identified affected sites on the body include the skin of the hands, arms, feet, lower legs, scalp, the upper back and the breast and genitals. Bodily orifices including the nose, ears, mouth, anus, urethra and the gastrointestinal tract have all been identified as locations of infestation. There are a number of behaviours associated with delusional infestation. These include attempts to remove the identified pathogen or object by digging into the skin, producing excoriations or lacerations. Sometimes patients will self-mutilate using tweezers, knives or other sharp instruments.

The patient's experience may take the form of a tactile hallucinatory state, a delusion or an overvalued idea. The aetiology is also variable. It is probably most common as a symptom of circumscribed hypochondriasis in affective psychosis, along with other depressive symptoms, but it also occurs in paranoid schizophrenia, in monosymptomatic hypochondriacal psychosis (delusional disorder), in organic brain syndromes or with neurotically determined conditions. This topic is reviewed by Berrios (1985) and by Morris (1991).

Patients have believed that they had a spider in their hair, worms and lice beneath the skin or infestation with various insects. The delusion may be accompanied by other depressive delusions or overvalued ideas of being dirty, guilty, unworthy or ill. These delusions may also occur in schizophrenia, in which condition they characteristically take on a bizarre character and are accompanied by other schizophrenic symptoms. A 49-year-old mother of four children, one of whose sons had developed a schizophrenic illness, complained of recurrent pain in her vagina that she explained as being caused by a parasite that had migrated from her stomach, where it had been responsible for epigastric pain diagnosed earlier as hiatus hernia (McLaughlin and Sims, 1984). She described the parasite as wandering through her bloodstream and as having been responsible for various aches and pains she had experienced in the past. She related having passed multiple small red worms and worm casts in her faeces and, on one occasion, a two-inch green frog.

Delusions of infestation may occur in organic states with tactile hallucinations, in delirium tremens during alcohol withdrawal and in cocaine addiction. They may be described in cerebrovascular disease, in senile dementia and in other brain disease, and they have been ascribed to disorder of the thalamus. Overvalued ideas and delusion-like ideas of infestation sometimes occur in people with personality disorder of anankastic or paranoid type with no psychotic illness.

Characteristically, these ideas occur in patients older than 50 years. Typically, those with delusions of infestation have always had a particular concern for personal cleanliness. Sometimes, the condition is precipitated by a skin disease and becomes a delusional elaboration of existing tactile symptoms. It has been suggested that the symptom develops in stages: first, abnormal cutaneous sensation; then an illusion develops; and finally, the fully formed delusion of infestation occurs. As mentioned earlier, delusional infestation is now viewed as one form of delusional disorder, in particular being a subtype of monosymptomatic hypochondriacal psychosis.

COMMUNICATED INSANITY

Lasègue and Falret (1877) described *la folie à deux* (or *folie communiquée*). Occasionally, a delusion (delusional intuition) is transferred from a psychotic person to one or more others with whom they have been in close association so that the recipient shares the false belief: the principal acquires the delusion first and is dominant, the associate becomes deluded through association with the principal. This situation in which partners accept, support and share each other's beliefs has been called the *psychosis of association*. The associate is usually socially deprived or disadvantaged, mentally or physically.

Gralnick (1942), in a review of the English literature on *folie à deux*, subdivided the condition into four possible relationships between principal and associate.

1. In *folie imposée* the delusions of a mentally ill person are transferred to someone who was not previously mentally ill, although characteristically the victim has some social or psychological disadvantage. Separation of the pair is often followed by remission of symptoms in the associate.
2. *Folie communiquée* occurs when a normal person suffers a contagion of their ideas after resisting them for a long time. Once they acquire these beliefs, they maintain them despite separation.
3. In *folie induite* a person who is already psychotic adds the delusions of a closely associated person to his own.
4. *Folie simultanée* describes a situation in which two or more people become psychotic and share the same delusional system simultaneously. It has been considered that the principal is always psychotic (Soni and Rockley, 1974), but the associate may or may not be psychotic.

However, the validity of this classification has been questioned. It is also not of any particular clinical value, and the psychopathological differences are questionable (Hughes and Sims, 1997).

In a case report of a family affected with *folie à quatre* (Sims et al., 1977), the initially referred patient believed that a large industrial concern had put 'bugging' devices in the walls of his brother's house. He claimed that employees of the firm had been following him everywhere and interfering with his own house. His wife believed this story initially and produced supposedly corroborative evidence. A year later, following his inpatient treatment, she no longer accepted the plot and she believed her husband to be mentally ill. She was a very anxious person who had previously received psychiatric treatment and came from a family in which three members had suffered from Huntington's chorea. When the patient's brother was visited at home, it was found that he, and the sister who lived with him, both believed in the plot and were both currently receiving treatment for a schizophrenic illness in which first-rank symptoms were present.

Folie à deux demonstrates how the content of belief is dictated by social and environmental circumstances, but the precise form of the symptoms varies according to the nature of the illness. Thus the nonpsychotic victim of *folie imposée* will show delusion-like ideas, overvalued ideas or misinterpretations but will not show 'true' delusions or delusional percept.

An interesting variation on *folie imposée* was described by Aldridge and Tagg (1998). This was the case of a 7-year-old boy who had presented with spurious psychotic symptoms induced by living in isolation with his mother, who suffered from schizophrenia. Initially, he was withdrawn, uncommunicative and ritualistic, with delayed development. At school, he was fearful of toys and teachers, crouching under a table, and was ritualistic concerning timekeeping and toileting, during which he would remove all his clothing and walk backwards into the toilet. His only speech was to repeat the clock time in a ritualistic way. Foster placement was made with a single mature woman, experienced with children, and after a year, this abnormal behaviour had disappeared, and he had made progress consistent with his mild degree of learning disability.

Folie à deux presents most often in married couples, in sister-sister dyads, in mother-daughter dyads and in twins. It can form the basis of suicide pacts, even though these are rare. It is not well recognized enough that it can underpin violence and homicide within families.

DELUSIONS OF CONTROL

These delusions, otherwise known as passivity or made experiences, are discussed with disorder of thinking in Chapter 9.

The Reality of Delusions

The degree to which delusions influence the reality of the world inhabited by a patient is most probably best judged by how far patients act on their beliefs. Patients with schizophrenia do not always act on their delusions, but quite frequently they do. A man who believed that American battleships were sailing down the main street of Birmingham, United Kingdom (which is 100 miles from the sea) had the refined social conscience to report this to the police. Persons holding delusions of morbid jealousy are potentially very dangerous: extreme physical violence and murder not uncommonly occur in this context. The patient with depressive delusions of guilt and unworthiness may well act on them by killing themself.

Although there is a growing literature casting doubt on whether delusions are false beliefs (as discussed earlier in the chapter), what is inescapable is that patients do often act on the content of these beliefs. For practical purposes, the content of a delusion is important because it yields information about the likely behaviour of a patient. In other words, the content of delusions acts to motivate behaviour, to give reason to action and to justify conduct; that is, it has predictive power. For this reason alone, the content of delusion is relevant to clinical practice. Hemsley and Garety (1986) have commented on 'the lack of action consequent with apparently sincerely held beliefs', whereas, paradoxically, forensic psychiatric studies have generally found that psychotic symptoms, especially delusions, are frequently a major factor resulting in the offence (Taylor, 1985). Buchanan (1993) has reviewed the descriptions of situations in which patients act on their delusions. He considers that for affective illnesses, both delusional belief and action may be consequent on the abnormal mood state. In other circumstances, action can be seen as being caused by a combination of 'belief' and 'desire' triggered by factors such as 'noticings': belief clearly is influenced by occurrence of delusion; desire corresponds to concepts such as motivation, drive and inclination; noticing is influenced by the perceptual and cognitive changes of the psychotic state. For an investigation into violence in a high-security hospital population, Taylor et al. (1998) concluded, 'as symptoms were usually a factor driving the index offence, treatment appears as important for public safety as for personal health'. The conclusion here is that delusions, like normal beliefs, do not necessarily result in action. They may be expressed yet not influence behaviour in any discernible way. However, like normal beliefs, they may motivate behaviour in a way that is comprehensible given the content of the belief.

In general, violent behaviour in response to delusions is not common; however, in a sample of 83 consecutively admitted deluded subjects, some aspect of the actions of half of them was congruent with the content of their delusions (Wessely et al., 1993). When acting on the delusions was described by the subjects themselves, it was associated with being aware of evidence that supported their belief and with having actively sought out such evidence; with a tendency to reduce the conviction with which a belief was held when that belief was challenged; and with feeling sad, frightened or anxious as a consequence of the delusion (Buchanan et al., 1993).

Erroneous Ideation

OVERVALUED IDEA

An overvalued idea is an acceptable, comprehensible idea pursued by the patient beyond the bounds of reason. It is usually associated with abnormal personality. Disorders associated with overvalued ideas have been reviewed by McKenna (1984), whose definition of overvalued idea 'refers to a solitary, abnormal belief that is neither delusional nor obsessional in nature, but which is preoccupying to the extent of dominating the sufferer's life'. It is *overvalued* in the sense that it causes disturbed functioning or suffering to the person themself or to others. The background on which an

overvalued idea is held is not necessarily unreasonable or false. It becomes so dominant that all other ideas are secondary and relate to it: the patient's whole life comes to revolve around this one idea. It is usually associated with very strong affect that the person, because of his temperament, has great difficulty in expressing.

According to McKenna, the term was introduced by Wernicke (1906), who distinguished it from obsession, in that it was not experienced subjectively as 'senseless', and from delusion. Jaspers considered that delusion is qualitatively different from normal belief, with a radical transformation of the meaning attached to events and incorrigible to an extent quite unlike normal belief. An overvalued idea, on the contrary, is an isolated notion associated with strong affect and abnormal personality and similar in quality to passionate political, religious or ethical conviction. For Jaspers (1959), then, overvalued ideas are 'convictions that are strongly toned by affect which is understandable in terms of the personality and its history'. Furthermore, Jaspers says, 'they are isolated notions that develop comprehensibly out of a given personality and situation'. Fish (1967) considered there was frequently a discrepancy between the degree of conviction and the extent to which the belief directed action. However, the patient with an overvalued idea invariably acted on it, determinedly and repeatedly; it is almost carried out with the drive of an instinct, like nest building. In many respects, these definitions attempt to locate overvalued ideas somewhere between normal beliefs and delusions. Overvalued ideas differ from delusions in that they arise comprehensibly from what we know about the person and his situation. They are more like passionate political, religious or ethical convictions than normal beliefs. This suggests that there is something about the tenacity of the conviction that distinguishes these overvalued ideas from normal beliefs, yet the degree of conviction and incorrigibility is thought to be less than that of delusions. It is obvious, however, that the degree of conviction is not a safe basis for distinguishing between delusions and overvalued ideas. A safer approach is to regard overvalued as comprehensible in the context of the patient's history and life.

McKenna lists the disorders of content commonly associated with the form of overvalued idea. These

TABLE 8.1 Disorders with Overvalued Ideas		
Content of Disorder	**Abnormality of Personality**	**Reference(s)**
Paranoid state: querulous or litigious type		Jaspers (1997), Kraeprlin (1905)
Morbid jealousy		Ey (1954), Shepherd (1961)
Hypochondriasis	Abnormality of personal-	Merskey (1979), Pilowsky (1970)
Dysmorphophobia	ity is usually present with	Hay (1970), Munro (1980)
Parasitophobia (Ekbom's syndrome)	overvalued ideas in all these	Hopkinson (1973)
Anorexia nervosa	conditions	Crisp (1980), Dally (1969)
Transsexualism		Huxley et al. (1981)

After McKenna, 1984, with permission.

are represented in Table 8.1. The psychopathology is not an overvalued idea in all cases of each of these conditions; for instance, morbid jealousy may be delusional and hypochondriasis may occur secondary to depressed mood. However, when an overvalued idea is found, it is usually associated with abnormal personality.

Morbid jealousy is often manifested as an overvalued idea. A husband was terrified that his wife was being unfaithful to him because of her casually flirtatious conduct. He checked on her every movement, interrogated her repeatedly, examined her underwear, employed detectives to follow her and misinterpreted any innocent contact she had with other men. On examination, he was not deluded, but the importance he attached to investigating and maintaining his wife's fidelity and the time taken to do this was so excessive that it destroyed his family life and lost him his job.

The form of the abnormal idea in many of the disturbances of body image, for example, *dysmorphophobia*, is usually an overvalued idea. A person with *paranoid personality* disorder became involved in a protracted lawsuit because a farmer ploughed across a public right of way. It is reasonable that hikers get annoyed when a footpath is destroyed, but this person took reasonable irritation to extreme lengths and constructed a mantrap to eliminate the farmer. His enthusiasm for footpaths had become an overvalued idea.

PARANOID IDEAS AND SYNDROMES

In psychiatry, the word *paranoid* is taken to mean 'self-referent' and is not limited to *persecutory* delusions; all delusions are delusions of reference in that they relate to the patient themself. A person will not form a delusional belief concerning 6-inch men on Mars unless they themself are significantly implicated in some way. So a paranoid delusion is a delusion of self-reference, not necessarily persecutory in nature. A paranoid personality disorder is that type of abnormal personality in which the person's reaction to other people is unduly self-referent; a paranoid state (see Chapter 19) includes those mental states in which self-referent phenomena are conspicuous, that is, *delusion-like ideas of reference* or *overvalued ideas* predominate. A patient, all of whose delusions are grandiose in nature and none of them persecutory, may still be suffering from *paranoid* schizophrenia.

Although primary delusions are characteristic of schizophrenia, secondary delusions (delusion-like ideas) occur in a number of conditions, for example, bipolar mood disorder in both manic and depressive phases, epilepsy and other organic psychosyndromes, acute drug intoxication, various alcoholic states and, of course, schizophrenia. The term *paranoid* originally was synonymous with delusional insanity. Kraepelin (1905) used the term more specifically to describe the condition in which there are delusions but no hallucinations. The personality, mood state and volition of the patient, in Kraepelin's description, are well preserved.

REFERENCES

Aldridge, M.L., Browne, K.D., 2003. Perpetrators of spousal homicide: a review. Trauma Violence Abuse 4 (3), 265–276.

Aldridge, S., Tagg, G., 1998. Spurious childhood psychosis induced by schizophrenia in the parent. Adv. Psychiatr. Treat. 4, 39–43.

Ang, P.C., Weller, M.P.I., 1984. Koro and psychosis. Br. J. Psychiatry 145, 335.

Bayne, T., Fernandez, J., 2009. Delusion and self-deception: mapping the terrain. In: Bayne, T., Fernandez, J. (Eds.), Delusion and

Self-Deception: Affective and Motivational Influences on Belief Formation. Psychology Press, New York.

Bentall, R.P., 1993. Cognitive biases and abnormal beliefs: towards a model of persecutory delusions. In: David, A.S., Cutting, J.C. (Eds.), The Neuropsychology of Schizophrenia. Lawrence Erlbaum, Hove.

Berner, P., 1991. Delusional atmosphere. Br. J. Psychiatry 159, 88–93.

Berrios, G.E., 1985. Delusional parasitosis and physical disease. Compr. Psychiatry 26, 395–403.

Berrios, G.E., 1996. The History of Mental Symptoms: Descriptive Psychopathology since the Nineteenth Century. Cambridge University Press, Cambridge.

Berrios, G.E., Morley, S.J., 1984. Koro-like symptoms in a non-Chinese subject. Br. J. Psychiatry 145, 331–334.

Berson, R.J., 1983. Capgras' syndrome. Am. J. Psychiatry 140, 969–978.

Bortolotti, L., 2010. Delusions and Other Irrational Beliefs. Oxford University Press, Oxford.

Brockington, I., 1991. Factors involved in delusion formation. Br. J. Psychiatry 159, 42–45.

Buchanan, A., 1993. Acting on delusion: a review. Psychol. Med. 23, 123–134.

Buchanan, A., Reed, A., Wessely, S., et al., 1993. Acting on delusions II: the phenomenological correlates of acting on delusions. Br. J. Psychiatry 163, 77–81.

Capgras, J., Reboul-Lachaux, J., 1923. L'illusion des sosies dans un délire systematique chronique. Bulletin de la Société Clinique de Médecine Mentale 11, 6–16.

Catalano, G., Catalano, M.C., Embi, C.S., Frantel, R.L., 1991. Delusions about the Internet. South. Med. J. 92, 609–610.

Christodoulou, G.N., 1978. Syndrome of subjective doubles. Am. J. Psychiatry 135, 249–251.

Christodoulou, G.N., 1991. The delusional misidentification syndromes. Br. J. Psychiatry 159, 65–69.

Colby, K.M., 1977. Appraisal of four psychological theories of paranoid phenomena. J. Abnorm. Psychol. 86, 54–59.

Conrad, K., 1958. Die Beginnende Schizophrenie. Thieme Verlag, Stuttgart.

Cotard, J., 1882. Nihilistic delusions. In: Hirsch, S.R., Shepherd, M. (Eds.), 1974. Themes and Variations in European Psychiatry. (M. Rohde, Trans). John Wright, Bristol, pp. 353–374.

Courbon, P., Fail, G., 1927. Syndrome d'illusion de Frégoli et schizophrenie. Bulletin de la Société Clinique de Médecine Mentale 15, 121–124.

Courbon, P., Tusques, J., 1932. Illusion d'intermétamorphose et de charme. Ann. Med.-Psychol. (Paris) 90, 401–405.

Crisp, A.H., 1980. Anorexia Nervosa: Let Me Be. Academic Press, London.

Cutting, J., 1985. The Psychology of Schizophrenia. Churchill Livingstone, Edinburgh.

Dally, P., 1969. Anorexia Nervosa. Heinemann, London.

Daly, M., Wilson, M., Weghorst, S.J., 1982. Male sexual jealousy. Ethol. Sociobiol. 3 (1), 11–27.

de Clérambault, G.G., 1942. Les psychoses passionelles. In: Fretet, J. (Ed.), Oeuvre Psychiatrique. Presses Universitaire, Paris.

Eagles, J.M., 1983. Delusional depressive in-patients, 1892–1982. Br. J. Psychiatry 143, 558–563.

Edelstyn, N.M.J., Riddoch, M.J., Oyebode, F., 1999. A review of the phenomenology and cognitive neuropsychological origins of the Capgras syndrome. Int. J. Geriatr. Psychiatry 14, 48–59.

Edelstyn, N.M.J., Riddoch, M.J., Oyebode, F., Humphreys, G.W., Forde, E., 1996. Visual processing in patients with Frégoli syndrome. Cognit. Neuropsychiatry 1, 103–124.

Ekbom, K., 1938. Praeseniler Dermat-zooenwahn. Acta Psychiatr. Scand. 13, 227–259.

Ellis, H.D., de Pauw, K.W., Christodoulou, G.N., Papageorgiou, L., Milne, A.B., Joseph, A.B., 1993. Responses to facial and non-facial stimuli presented tachistoscopically in either or both visual fields by patients with the Capgras delusion and paranoid schizophrenics. J. Neurol. Neurosurg. Psychiatry 56, 215–219.

Ellis, P., Mellsop, G., 1985. De Clérambault's syndrome—a nosological entity. Br. J. Psychiatry 146 (1), 90–93.

Enoch, D., 1991. Delusional jealousy and awareness of reality. Br. J. Psychiatry 159, 52–56.

Enoch, M.D., Trethowan, W.H., 1979. Uncommon Psychiatric Syndromes, second ed. John Wright, Bristol.

Ey, H., 1950. Jalousie morbide. In: Etudes Psychiatriques, vol. II. de Bronwen, Paris.

Ey, H., 1954. Etudes Psychiatriques, vol. II. Desclée, Paris.

Fish, F., 1967. Clinical Psychopathology. John Wright, Bristol.

Freud, S., 1907. Delusions and dreams in Jensen's gravida. In: Standard Edition of the Complete Psychological Works, vol. IX (J. Strachey, Trans, 1959). Hogarth Press, London.

Freudenmann, R.W., Lepping, P., 2009. Delusional infestation. Clin. Microbiol. Rev. 22 (4), 690–732.

Garety, P., 1991. Reasoning and delusions. Br. J. Psychiatry 159, 14–18.

Garety, P., Helmsley, D.R., Wessely, S., 1991. Reasoning in deluded schizophrenic and paranoid subjects: biases in performance on a probabilistic inference task. J. Nerv. Ment. Dis. 179, 194–201.

Gogol, N., 1972. Diary of a Madman and Other Stories (R. Wilks, Trans). Penguin, London.

Gralnick, A., 1942. Folie à deux: the psychosis of association. A review of 103 cases and the entire English literature. Psychiatr. Q. 16, 230–263.

Griesinger, W., 1845. Mental Pathology and Therapeutics. (C.L. Robertson, J. Rutherford, Trans, 1882). William Wood and Co, New York.

Gruhle, H.W., 1915. Self-description and empathy. Zeitschrift fuer Gesundheitswesen Neurologie und Psychiatrie 28, 148.

Guirguis, W.R., 1981. Pure erotomania in manic-depressive psychosis. Br. J. Psychiatry 138, 139–140.

Gwee, A.L., 1963. Koro – a cultural disease. Singapore Med. J. 4, 119–122.

Hagen, F.W., 1870. Studien auf dem Geblete der arztlichen seelenhelikunde. Bersold, Erlagen, Germany.

Hamilton, M., 1978. Fish's Outline of Psychiatry, third ed. John Wright, Bristol.

Hart, B., 1921. The Psychology of Insanity. Cambridge University Press, Cambridge.

Hay, G.G., 1970. Dysmorphophobia. Br. J. Psychiatry 116, 399–406.

Hay, G.G., 1983. Feigned psychosis – a review of the simulation of mental illness. Br. J. Psychiatry 143, 8–10.

Hemsley, D.R., Garety, P.A., 1986. The formation and maintenance of delusions: a Bayesian analysis. Br. J. Psychiatry 149, 51–56.

Higgins, J., 1990. Affective psychoses. In: Bluglass, R., Bowden, P. (Eds.), Principles and Practice of Forensic Psychiatry. Churchill Livingstone, Edinburgh.

Hopkinson, G., 1970. Delusions of infestation. Acta Psychiatr. Scand. 46, 111–119.

Hopkinson, G., 1973. The psychiatric syndrome of infestation. Psychiatrica Clinica 6, 330–345.

Hughes, T.A., Sims, A.C.P., 1997. Folie à deux. In: Bhugra, D., Munro, A. (Eds.), Troublesome Disguises: Underdiagnosed Psychiatric Syndromes. Blackwell Scientific, Oxford.

Hunter, R., MacAlpine, I., 1970. Three Hundred Years of Psychiatry 1535-1860. Oxford University Press, Oxford.

Huq, S.F., Garety, P.A., Hemsley, D.R., 1988. Probabilistic judgements in deluded and non-deluded subjects. Q. J. Exp. Psychol. (Hove) 40A, 801–812.

Huxley, P.J., Kenna, J.C., Brandon, S.C., 1981. Partnership in transsexualism, part II. The nature of the partnership. Arch. Sex. Behav. 10, 143–160.

Jaspers, K., 1997. General Psychopathology (J. Hoenig, M.W. Hamilton, Trans). The Johns Hopkins University Press, Baltimore.

Kaney, S., Bentall, R.P., 1989. Persecutory delusions and attributional style. Br. J. Med. Psychol. 62, 191–198.

Kaney, S., Bentall, R.P., 1992. Persecutory delusions and the self-serving bias: evidence from a continuing judgement task. J. Nerv. Ment. Dis. 180, 773–780.

Kendler, K.S., Glaser, W.M., Morgenstern, H., 1983. Dimensions of delusional experience. Am. J. Psychiatry 140, 466–469.

Kinderman, P., Kaney, S., Morley, S., Bentall, R.P., 1992. Paranoia and the defensive attributional style: deluded and depressed patients' attribution about their own attributions. Br. J. Med. Psychol. 65, 371–383.

Klaf, F.S., Hamilton, J.G., 1961. Schizophrenia: a hundred years ago and today. J. Ment. Sci. 107, 819–827.

Kraepelin, E., 1905. Lectures on Clinical Psychiatry, third ed. (T. Johnstone, Trans, 1917). W. Wood, New York.

Kretschmer, E., 1927. The sensitive delusion of reference. In: Hirsch, S.R., Shepherd, M. (Eds.), 1974. Themes and Variations in European Psychiatry. (J. Candy, Trans). John Wright, Bristol.

Laing, R.D., 1961. The Self and Others. Tavistock, London.

Lapierre, Y.D., 1972. Koro in a French Canadian. Can. Psychiatr. Assoc. J. 17, 333–334.

Lasègue, C., 1852. Cited by Cotard, J., 1882. Du délire des négations. Archives de Neurologie 4 (152–170), 282–296.

Laségue, C., Falret, J., 1877. La folie à deux (ou folie communiquée). Ann. Med. Psychol. (Paris) 18, 321 (R. Michaud, Trans, 1964), supplement to Am. J. Psychiatr. 121, 4.

Lyon, H.M., Kaney, S., Bentall, R.P., 1994. The defensive function of persecutory delusions: evidence from attribution tasks. Br. J. Psychiatry 164, 637–646.

Matussek, P., 1953. Untersuchungen uber die Wahnwahrnehmung. 2. Mitteilung. Schwizer. Arch Neurol Psychiatry 71, 189–210.

McGrath, P., 1990. Spider. Penguin, London.

McKenna, P.J., 1984. Disorders with overvalued ideas. Br. J. Psychiatry 145, 579–585.

McLaughlin, J.A., Sims, A.C.P., 1984. Co-existence of Capgras and Ekbom syndromes. Br. J. Psychiatry 145, 439–441.

Mellor, C.S., 1991. Delusional perception. Br. J. Psychiatry 159, 104–107.

Merskey, H., 1979. The Analysis of Hysteria. Baillière Tindall, London.

Morris, M., 1991. Delusional infestation. Br. J. Psychiatry 159, 83–87.

Morrison, A., 1848. Cases of Mental Disease. Longman and S. Highley, London.

Moselhy, H., Oyebode, F., 1997. Delusional misidentification syndromes: a review of the Anglophone literature. Neurol. Psychiatry Brain Res. 5, 21–26.

Mullen, P., 1990. Morbid jealousy and the delusion of infidelity. In: Bluglass, R., Bowden, P. (Eds.), Principles and Practice of Forensic Psychiatry. Churchill Livingstone, Edinburgh.

Mullen, P.E., 1997. Disorders of passion. In: Bhugra, D., Munro, A. (Eds.), Troublesome Disguises: Underdiagnosed Psychiatric Syndromes. Blackwell Scientific, Oxford.

Mullen, P.E., Pathé, M., 1994. The pathological extensions of love. Br. J. Psychiatry 165, 614–623.

Munro, A., 1980. Monosymptomatic hypochondriacal psychosis. Br. J. Hosp. Med. 24, 34–38.

Munro, A., 1988. Monosymptomatic hypochondriacal psychosis. Br. J. Psychiatry 153, 37–40.

Munro, A., 1997. Paranoia or delusional disorder. In: Bhugra, D., Munro, A. (Eds.), Troublesome Disguises: Underdiagnosed Psychiatric Syndromes. Blackwell Scientific, Oxford.

Oyebode, F., Edelstyn, N.M.J., Patel, A., Riddoch, M.J., Humphreys, G.W., 1996. Capgras syndrome in vascular dementia: recognition memory and visual processing. Int. J. Geriatr. Psychiatry 11, 71–73.

Oyebode, F., Jamieson, R., Mullaney, J., Davison, K., 1986. Koro – a psychophysiological dysfunction? Br. J. Psychiatry 148, 212–214.

Parnas, J., 2013. On psychosis: Karl Jaspers and beyond. In: Stanghellini, G., Fuchs, T. (Eds.), One Century of Karl Jaspers' General Psychopathology. Oxford University Press, Oxford.

Pilowsky, I., 1967. Dimensions of hypochondriasis. Br. J. Psychiatry 113, 89–93.

Pilowsky, I., 1970. Primary and secondary hypochondriasis. Acta Psychiatr. Scand. 46, 273–285.

Porter, S., Williams, C., 1997. Psychiatric dilemmas – surgery and the mental health act (1983). J. R. Soc. Med. 90, 327–330.

Pryse-Phillips, W., 1971. An olfactory reference syndrome. Acta Psychiatr. Scand. 47, 485–509.

Reilly, T.M., 1988. Delusional infestation. Br. J. Psychiatry 153, 44–46.

Roberts, G., 1991. Delusional belief systems and meaning in life: a preferred reality. Br. J. Psychiatry 159, 19–28.

Roberts, G., 1992. The origins of delusion. Br. J. Psychiatry 161, 298–308.

Schneider, K., 1920. The stratification of emotional life as the structure of the depressive states. Zentralblatt fuer die Gesamte Neurologie und Psychiatrie 59, 281.

Schneider, K., 1949. The concept of delusion 'Zum Begriff des Wahns'. Fortschritte der Neurologie-Psychiatrie 17, 26–31. In: Hirsch, S.R., Shepherd, M. (Eds.), 1974. Themes and Variations in European Psychiatry (H. Marshall, Trans). John Wright, Bristol.

Schneider, K., 1957. Primary and secondary symptoms in schizophrenia. Fortschritte der Neurologie-Psychiatrie 25. In: Hirsch, S.R., Shepherd, M. (Eds.), 1974. Themes and Variations in European Psychiatry (H. Marshall, Trans). John Wright, Bristol, pp. 487–490.

Serretti, A., Lattuada, E., Cusin, C., Smeraldi, E., 1999. Factor analysis of delusional disorder symptomatology. Compr. Psychiatry 40, 143–147.

Shepherd, M., 1961. Morbid jealousy: some clinical and social aspects of a psychiatric symptom. J. Ment. Sci. 107, 687–753.

Shrestha, K., Rees, D.W., Rix, K.J.B., Hore, B.D., Faraghere, B., 1985. Sexual jealousy in alcoholics. Acta Psychiatr. Scand. 72, 283–290.

Sims, A.C.P., 1972. The English hospital, Tangier 1883–1908. Med. Hist. 16, 285–290.

Sims, A.C.P., 1986. The psychopathology of schizophrenia with special reference to delusional misidentification. In: Christodoulou, G.M. (Ed.), The Delusional Misidentification Syndromes. Karger, Basel.

Sims, A.C.P., 1992. Symptoms and beliefs. J. R. Soc. Health 112, 42–46.

Sims, A.C.P., White, A.C., 1973. Co-existence of the Capgras and de Clerambault syndromes – a case history. Br. J. Psychiatry 123, 635–663.

Sims, A.C.P., Salmons, P.H., Humphreys, P., 1977. Folie à quatre. Br. J. Psychiatry 130, 134–138.

Soni, S.D., Rockley, G.J., 1974. Socio-clinical substrates of folie à deux. Br. J. Psychiatry 125, 230–235.

Spitzer, M., 1994. The basis of psychiatric diagnosis. In: Sadler, J.Z., Wiggins, O.P., Schwartz, M.A. (Eds.), Philosophical Perspectives on Psychiatric Diagnostic Classification. Johns Hopkins University Press, Baltimore.

Stoddart, W.H.B., 1908. Mind and its Disorders. Lewis, London.

Taylor, P.J., 1985. Motives for offending among violent and psychiatric men. Br. J. Psychiatry 147, 491–498.

Taylor, P.J., Leese, M., Williams, D., Butwell, M., Daly, R., Larkin, E., 1998. Mental disorder and violence. Br. J. Psychiatry 172, 218–226.

Todd, J., Dewhurst, K., 1955. The Othello syndrome. J. Nerv. Ment. Dis. 122, 367–374.

Trethowan, W.H., 1967. Erotomania – an old disorder reconsidered. Alta 2, 79–86.

Trollope, A., 1869. He Knew He Was Right. Strahan, London.

Videbech, T., 1966. Chronic olfactory paranoid syndromes. Acta Psychiatr. Scand. 42, 183–212.

Walker, C., 1991. Delusion: what did Jaspers really say? Br. J. Psychiatry 159, 94–103.

Wernicke, C., 1906. Fundamentals of Psychiatry. Thieme, Leipzig.

Wessely, S., Buchanan, A., Reed, A., et al., 1993. Acting on delusion 1: prevalence. Br. J. Psychiatry 163, 69–76.

Winters, K.L., Neale, J.M., 1983. Delusions and delusional thinking in psychotics: a review of the literature. Clin. Psychol. Rev. 3, 227–253.

World Health Organization, 1992. The ICD-10 Classification of Mental and Behavioral Disorders: Clinical Description and Diagnostic Guidelines. World Health Organization, Geneva.

Yap, P.M., 1965. Koro – a culture-bound depersonalization syndrome. Br. J. Psychiatry 3, 43–50.

Chapter 9

Disorder of the Thinking Process

Chapter Outline

KEYWORDS

Formal thought disorder
Circumstantiality
Concrete thinking
Passivity experience

Summary

Thinking and its processes are little understood. This means that abnormalities of thinking cannot be easily related to any clearly described, already established notion of what normal processes are and how abnormal processes depart from these normal processes. In this chapter, fantasy thinking, imaginative thinking and conceptual thinking are described. Against this background, a model of thinking depending on the association of ideas and governed by a determining principle is described. This then provides the basis for a discussion of abnormalities of the form of thinking, a particularly complex area of psychopathology, as it requires the ability both to follow closely what someone is saying and to conclude that the sequence of ideas or the association of ideas may be awry. In the final section, Schneider's first-rank symptoms are described with examples:

With time and years the individual becomes so lazy in public life that he is not even capable of writing any more. On such a sheet of paper, one can squeeze many letters if one is careful not to transgress by one 'square shore'. In such fine weather one should be able to take a walk in the woods. Naturally, not alone, but with a girl. At the end of the year one always renders the annual accounting. The sun is now in the sky yet it is not yet ten o'clock.

Eugene Bleuler (1857–1939)

This chapter is concerned with disorder of thinking and the next chapter with disorders of language. Thinking and thought processes are little understood. Although there is increasing interest in the subject by cognitive neuroscientists, their primary focus of study misses what is of interest to the clinical psychopathologist, namely, the subjective experience of thinking, particularly as it relates to abnormalities of thinking. Cognitive neuroscientists are interested in the nature of problem-solving; in the various kinds of reasoning, including analogic, inductive and deductive; in the nature of logic and belief formation; and in understanding decision-making. These are important subjects and can be impaired in psychiatric disorders. However, the process that makes these aspects of thinking possible; the unique relationship of the subject to their own thoughts, the experience of thoughts flowing coherently and the effortless yet goal-driven dimension of thinking thoughts that underpin problem-solving and reasoning is poorly understood and researched. Admittedly, it is difficult to study the subjective aspects of thinking, and mostly one is concerned with objective phenomena of psychic life—what Jaspers (1997) calls *performance*.

There are two distinct aspects in studying disorder of thinking: the patient's subjective awareness of their own disturbed thinking patterns and the manifestation of abnormal thinking they betray in their speech (see Chapter 10). This latter is the expression of thought and determines what the observer may deduce about the patient's thinking. We need to enquire also about the experience of thinking in the patient's description of their subjective psychological processes. *Formal thought disorder* from the subjective, phenomenological standpoint is abnormality in the mechanism of thinking described by the patient introspecting into their own processes of thought; that is, the patient describes in their own words a process of thinking that is clearly abnormal to the outside observer.

Types of Thinking

The process of thinking was divided by Fish (1967) into the following three types:
- undirected fantasy (dereistic) or autistic thinking;
- imaginative thinking; and
- *rational* or conceptual thinking.

These three types have slightly different implications for psychopathology, the description and categorization of morbid processes. They can be considered as *functions* of thinking; that is, they are the necessary mechanisms for thinking to take place but are not

themselves manifest in the phenomena. We can contrast those phenomena, which are the products of the *performance* of thinking, the percept or the idea, with the functions that do not become explicit.

FANTASY THINKING

This may be of short duration, for example, the daydream before going to sleep, or it may become an established way of life. Jaspers quotes Montaigne: 'Plutarch says of people who waste their feelings on guinea-pigs and pet dogs, that the love element in all of us, if deprived of any adequate object, will seek out something trivial and false rather than let itself stay unengaged. So the psyche in its passions prefers to deceive itself, or even in spite of itself invent some nonsensical object rather than give up all drive or aim'.

Fantasy has an important function in the way we all carry out our everyday activities; for instance, we model our speech and behaviour in imagination before an important encounter or event, and afterwards we rehearse our performance in fantasy to evaluate it and assess whether we could have done better (see Imaginative Thinking later in the chapter). To be able to harness our imagination constructively, we require the capacity for undirected fantasy and the learned skill to structure thoughts. Fantasy also allows a person to escape from or deny reality, or alternatively to convert reality into something more tolerable and less requiring of corrective action. A 20-year-old young woman, who had a very deprived childhood and walked the city streets at night as a prostitute, listened to a vicar broadcasting on local radio. She started to send him and his wife flowers and cards, made contact with them and began to call them 'Mum' and 'Dad'. When questioned by the police one night, she gave their names as next of kin and said they really were her parents.

Shy, reserved people, not suffering from mental illness, may use dereistic thinking to compensate for the disappointments of life. Bleuler (1911) saw this isolation from the real world into autistic thinking as characteristic of schizophrenia: 'The very common preoccupation of young hebephrenics with "the deepest questions" is nothing but an autistic manifestation'. Fantasy, especially in some with neurotic traits, may develop from the stage of being deliberate and sporadic into an established mode; the person comes to believe the contents of their fantasy, which become subjectively real and accepted as fact. Freud, in his later writings, considered that this was so in some of the accounts he received from women of an incestuous relationship with their father during childhood (Jones, 1962). However, in his early writings he had considered that they had experienced actual sexual assault but had used unconscious mechanisms to repress this knowledge (Isräels and Schatzman, 1993; Webster, 1995). Various types of experience come into the category of acting out fantasy, such as *pathologic lying* (pseudologia fantastica) and *factitious disorders*.

Fantasy is usually understood to be the creation of images or ideas that have no external reality. However, fantasy thinking may also reveal itself in the denial of external events. The observations for which the psychodynamic explanation of *ego defence mechanisms* has been described are relevant in this context. The slip of the tongue or the 'forgetting' of the emotionally laden word is not accidental; it is a form of self-deception. The obvious, significant, but unpleasant object of perception may be 'overlooked', and this often reveals fantasy denial. Fantasy thinking denies unpleasant reality, even though the fantasy itself may also be unpleasant. This rearranging or transformation of reality is shown by neurotic patients habitually and all people occasionally. Jonathan Swift commented on it: 'When man's fancy gets astride of his reason; when imagination is at cuffs with the senses; and common understanding, as well as common sense, is kicked out of doors, the first proselyte he makes is himself' (Swift, 1667–1745).

IMAGINATIVE THINKING

The term *imagination* covers psychological states such as fantasy (as just described), the generation of novel ideas and the creative outputs that constitute art or discoveries in science. There are at least three components of imagination: mental imagery, counterfactual thinking and symbolic representation. Mental imagery refers to the ability to create image-based mental representations of the world. Counterfactual thinking refers to the capacity to disengage from reality to think of events and experiences that have not occurred and may never occur. Symbolic representation is the use of concepts or images to represent real-world objects or entities (Roth, 2004). This is, of course, the basis of language, art and mathematics.

A facet of this type of thinking that comes from a psychoanalytic theoretical stance is the concept of *maternal reverie* (Bion, 1962). The mother, while in the situation, both physical and mental, of 'holding the baby' (Winnicott, 1957), has a capacity for reverie or daydreaming on the baby's behalf; this usually concerns the future happiness and achievements of the baby. Wilfred Bion (1897–1979) would regard this as a necessary factor in the healthy development of the self-sensation of the baby; when maternal reverie breaks down—for example, in puerperal depression—the baby experiences this as distress. The process of maternal reverie is clearly analogous in some ways to the prayers of a religious person on another's behalf.

There is a role for imagination in perspective taking. Phrases such as 'putting oneself in someone else's shoes' show how the capacity for imaginative thinking allows us to shift perspective and to free ourselves from the compelling constraints of the immediate and the personal in order to grasp the position and experience of the other person. This skill is essential to clinical practice in psychiatry and of course also to interacting with other people in general. Thomas Fuchs (2018) makes the point that the 'as if' function is fundamental to our capacity to suspend the force of immediate experience and to enter a virtual or fictional world, one that makes metaphor, symbolic expressions and map-making possible.

RATIONAL OR CONCEPTUAL THINKING

Problem-solving and reasoning are two key aspects of rational thinking. Problem-solving is defined as the set of cognitive processes that we apply to reach a goal when we must overcome obstacles to reach that goal, and reasoning is the cognitive process that we use to make inferences from knowledge and to draw conclusions. These aspects of thinking are distinct but related, so that reasoning can be involved in problem-solving (Smith and Kosslyn, 2007). Strategies for problems involve the use of heuristics, that is, rules of thumb that usually give the correct answer. Typically, reasoning involves analogies, induction or deduction. Analogic reasoning involves the application of solutions to already known problems to new problems with similar characteristics. For example, if you lose the keys to your locked briefcase, you can apply the knowledge to this new problem that sharp-ended implements can be used to open padlocks. Inductive reasoning depends on the use of specific known instances to draw an inference about unknown instances. Commonly, this is formulated as generalizing from a single instance to all instances or from some members of a category known to have a given property to other instances of that category. This is known as category-based induction. An example is 'my cat has four legs', therefore 'all cats have four legs'. Deductive reasoning involves an argument in which if the premises are true, the conclusion cannot be false. This is usually studied by way of syllogism: (1) all Martians are green, (2) my father is a Martian and (3) my father is green.

Problem-solving and reasoning both require the capacity to form concepts. This is the capacity for abstraction—the ability to theorize about the world—and it includes the categorization of objects or events in the world and the clarification of the concepts that determine the category or class under investigation.

HEURISTICS AND DECISION-MAKING

There is emerging and robust evidence about the systems underlying decision-making processes. Superficially, these systems do not seem relevant to our understanding of the kinds of problems that are demonstrated in abnormalities of thinking but closer examination shows that they are likely to be important and relevant as they come under scrutiny in psychiatric disorders.

Kahneman (2011) summarizes the evidence for the involvement of two cognitive systems in decision-making: System 1, which operates automatically and quickly with little or no effort and no sense of voluntary control; and System 2, which allocates attention to the effortful mental activities that demand it, including complex computations. The operations of System 2 are said to be associated with subjective experience of agency, choice and concentration. In an earlier paper, Tversky and Kahneman (1974) argued that, in situations where a judgement is made under conditions of uncertainty, certain heuristics are at play and often lead to errors of judgement. These are the *representativeness* heuristic, the *availability* heuristic and the *adjustment and anchoring* heuristic. *Representativeness*, for example, refers to how similarity to a class of objects or events, in the absence of additional information, biases judgements and hence

resulting in errors of judgement. *Availability* refers to the degree to which the probability of an event occurring is determined by the ease with which instances or occurrences can be brought to mind. The risk of heart attacks in middle-aged men might be determined by how many instances can be readily brought to mind, a bias that is determined by the ease of retrievability of instances. Finally, adjustment and anchoring refer to the manner in which initial values are adjusted to yield final answers; the best example of this is our differing responses to terms such as *90% fat free* and *10% fat*. It is obvious that abnormalities in the use of these heuristics probably have a role either in the development of delusions or the maintenance of abnormal beliefs.

Kahneman (2011) concludes, 'The attentive System 2 is who we think we are. System 2 articulates judgements and makes choices, but it often endorses or rationalizes ideas and feelings that were generated by System 1. You may not know that you are optimistic about a project because something about its leader reminds you of your beloved sister or that you dislike a person who looks vaguely like your dentist. If asked for an explanation, however, you will search your memory for presentable reasons and will certainly find some. Moreover, you will believe the story you make up.'

The Processes of Disordered Thinking

A MODEL OF ASSOCIATIONS BASED ON JASPERS

In this model of thinking (psychological performance), thoughts (psychological events) can be seen to flow in an uninterrupted sequence so that one or more *associations*, with resulting further psychological events, may arise from each thought. The sequence of thoughts, with the associations linking them, forms the framework of this model, which is represented diagrammatically in Fig. 9.1.

The mass of possible associations resulting from a psychic event is called a *constellation*. There are an enormous number of possible associations but thinking usually proceeds in a definite direction for various immediate and compelling reasons. This consistent flow of thinking towards its goal is ascribed to the *determining tendency* (Jaspers). The idea of *associations* is not intended to imply that one psychological event evokes another by an automatic, unintelligent, nonverbal reflex but that the thought, which may be

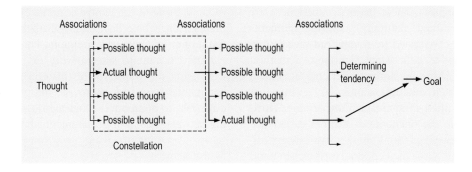

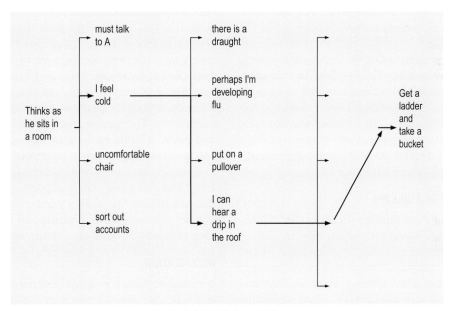

Fig. 9.1 Model of association.

expressed verbally or not, is a concept that results in the formation of a number of other concepts, one of which is given prominence by operation of the determining tendency. This model is conjectural but has some value in allowing description of the abnormalities of thinking and speech that occur in mental illness. In addition to Jaspers' description of his model of associations, a description that has face validity given the cases seen in psychiatry, there are other models. For example, Kahneman's (2011) in which the subject's world is constructed by associations that link ideas of circumstances, events, actions, and outcomes that co-occur with some regularity, either at the same time or within a relatively short interval. As these links

are formed and strengthened, the pattern of associated ideas comes to represent the structure of events in a subject's life and also determines the way in which a subject interprets the present and predicts the future. In other words, the association of ideas is not random but is built on past experiences and is determined by memory functions.

The foregoing discussion about Jaspers' model of association is built on observations of patients' presentations. Russell Hurlburt (2011) investigations of what he terms *pristine inner experience*, in contrast, is an assiduous empirical study of actual inner subjective experience. By inner experience he means thoughts, feelings and sensations that momentarily appear in conscious awareness. These pristine experiences are unscripted, unedited, naturally occurring moments that are usually concealed from view but revealed by use of Descriptive Experience Sampling, a method developed by Hurlburt. Inner experience is shown to be fractionated, multiple momentary events that appear as if unified in a stream. Furthermore, Hurlburt shows that the phenomena of inner experience include unsymbolized thinking, sensory awareness, inner speech and visual perception. Hurlburt's method takes inner experience seriously, avoids presuppositions about the nature of inner experience and documents the actual content of inner experience at the time of recording.

We are subjectively aware of our thought process being a stream or a flow. To develop the metaphor, thoughts are capable of acceleration and slowing, of eddies and calms, of precipitous falls, of increased volume of flow, of blockages. This analogy should not be taken too far because it is without neurophysiologic basis, but it is useful for examining certain abnormalities and is based on subjective experience.

ACCELERATION OF THINKING

Acceleration of flow of thinking occurs as *flight of ideas*. In this, there is a logical connection between each of two sequential ideas expressed. However, the goal of thinking is not maintained for long. It is continuously changing because of the effect of frivolous affect and a very high degree of distractibility. The determining tendency is weakened, but associations are still formed normally. The speed of forming such associations and therefore of the pattern of thought is grossly accelerated. This is demonstrated in Fig. 9.2.

Here is an example of such flight of ideas from a female patient, aged 45, with mania. She said: 'They thought I was in the pantry at home … Peekaboo … there's a magic box. Poor darling Catherine, you know, Catherine the Great, the fire grate, I'm always up the chimney. I want to scream with joy … Hallelujah!' Discussing the transcript of this conversation when her mental state had improved, the patient found it quite easy to point out the logical bridges in her thinking between each pair of statements, but there was no sense of building up an argument from the first to the final statement.

Markedly different from the manic flight of ideas with pressure of speech and multiple but linked association is the *confusion psychosis* described by Fish (1962). In this, thinking is disordered but mood and psychomotor activity are unimpaired. In the excited form of this, incoherent pressure of speech is prominent, the context of which is out of keeping with the situation. There may be transient, almost playful, misidentifications of people; fleeting ideas of reference; and auditory hallucinations. In the inhibited state of confusion psychosis, there is poverty of speech, almost mutism. There may also be perplexity, ideas of reference, ideas of significance, illusions and hallucinations—auditory, visual or somatic. This is usually a cycloid psychosis in its presentation, and other features of manic-depressive psychosis may be present.

RETARDATION

In retardation (such as occurs in depression), thinking, although goal directed, proceeds so slowly with such morbid preoccupation and with gloomy thoughts that the person may fail to achieve those goals. The patient is likely to show little initiative and to begin neither planning nor spontaneous activity. When asked a question, they will ponder it, but as no thought comes to them, they make no response. Eventually, after

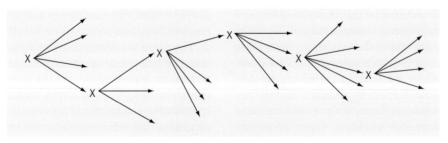

Fig. 9.2 Abnormal flow of thinking: flight of ideas.

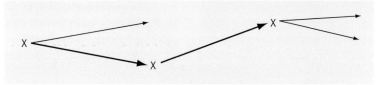

Fig. 9.3 Retardation.

considerable delay, the answer usually comes. They have difficulty making decisions and concentrating; there is loss of clarity of thought and poor registration of those events they need to remember. In terms of the model of the flow of thinking, in retardation there is both poverty and slowness in the formation and progression of associations (Fig. 9.3).

Depression, although usually associated with retardation of thought, may occur with *agitation*; there may be a complex situation with impaired concentration from retardation and a subjective experience of restless, anxious thoughts. Thus Sutherland (1976), a middle-aged psychologist describing his own mental illness, said:

I contemplated throwing myself off the cross-Channel ferry … We arrived in Naples … and my friends … were upset by my condition while feeling powerless to help… whilst the others sat at the table I rolled around moaning in the dust. I revisited many of the places I had once loved: the Museo Nazionale with its magnificent mosaics pillaged from Pompeii, Pompeii itself and Capri. None of them evoked a spark of interest – I stared listlessly and uncomprehendingly at the pictures in the museum with harrowing thoughts still racing in my mind. I could not guide the children round Pompeii, since I could not concentrate sufficiently to follow the plan. Capri had lost its beauty and charm. I could not even giggle at the vulgarity of the interior of Axel Munthe's villa, though the beauty of the formal garden and the magnificent view of the island and the sea from the belvedere evoked a slight response. The phrase 'see Naples and die' echoed through my mind: I was convinced I would never return alive to England, let alone ever revisit Naples.

This possible combination of depressed affect and accelerated activity can be seen to conform quite readily with Kraepelin's (1904) description of *mixed affective states*.

CIRCUMSTANTIAL THINKING

In both flight of ideas and retardation, affect influences the speed of thinking: it dictates which idea takes precedence and can also distort judgement. In *circumstantial thinking*, the slow stream of thought is not impeded by affect but by a defect of intellectual grasp, a failure of differentiation of the *figure* from *ground*. Characteristically, this occurs in patients with epilepsy, and it is seen in other organic states and in learning disability. A somewhat similar process occurs with obsessional personality, but here the excess of detail is introduced anxiously to avoid any possible omissions: *i*'s are dotted, *t*'s crossed to such an extent that the process of reaching a goal is substantially impaired. On being asked a question, circumstantial thought is shown by the patient in a reply that contains a great welter of unnecessary detail, obscuring and impeding the answer to the question. All sorts of unnecessary associations are explored exhaustively before the person returns to the point. Their whole conversation becomes a mass of parentheses and subsidiary clauses. They even have to explain and apologize for these digressions before they can get back to moving towards the goal. However, the determining tendency remains, and they do eventually answer the question. This is a case of not being able to see the wood for the trees. Circumstantial thinking is represented diagrammatically in Fig. 9.4.

INTERRUPTION TO THE FLOW OF THOUGHT

There are many ways in which the continuity of flow of thinking may be disturbed. Carl Schneider (1930) has described some of these abnormalities: *verschmelzung* (fusion, literally 'melting'), *faseln* (muddling), *entgleiten* (snapping off) and *entgleisen* (derailment). These processes (and others) occur together to give the patient a feeling of confusion and bewilderment. They are likely to complain of feeling bemused, to be lacking in

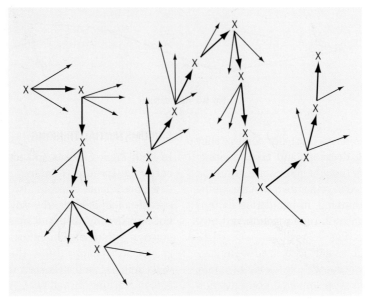

Fig. 9.4 Model of circumstantial thinking.

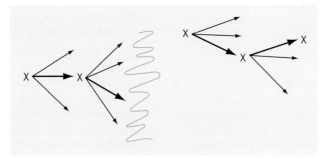

Fig. 9.5 Model of derailment.

concentration and to be slightly apprehensive of they know not what. They cannot precisely describe their altered thinking and consequent changes in speech.

In *derailment* (Fig. 9.5), there is a breakdown in association so that there appears to be an interpolation of thoughts bearing no understandable connection with the chain of thoughts: 'The traffic is rumbling along the main road. They are going to the north. Why do girls always play pantomime heroes?' Such an excerpt from the speech of a patient with schizophrenia contains no meaningful connections, even to the patient themself. With derailment, the subject is unable to link the ideas and describes a change in their direction of thinking.

With *fusion*, there is some preservation of the normal chain of associations, but there is a bringing together of heterogeneous elements. These form links that cannot be seen as a logical progression from their constituent origins towards the goal of thought. A female patient with schizophrenia, aged 38, wrote the following:

Two men are controlling the brain through telethapy [sic] or by means of ways of the spirit who open and closes the back channels of my brain releasing words and holding back the truth, by no means will I speak but will answer only to written questions by means of writing, knowing full well the channels of my brain is filtering and only half

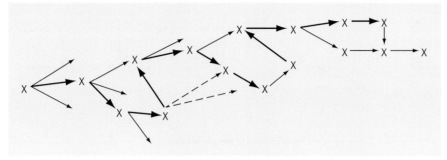

Fig. 9.6 Model of fusion.

of what is the truth, also I knowing I am being read not only by a few but many very clever people but not at all acceptable they make people believe that I am some kind of miracle which I am not, I only hold the name Holyland which came to me by marrying Alfred Holyland, only by doing this do they wish to make some false stories of me coming from some special place which I have not.

Fusion is demonstrated at the beginning of this excerpt, where she says that the brain is controlled 'by means' and then this word becomes associated with 'ways'. 'Telethapy'—not the same as telepathy—is a neologism. There are also examples of passivity. 'Channels' and 'means' are used as stock words, that is, they are used more often in her conversation than their normal meaning could suggest, and they take on for her a greater range of meaning than usual. It is difficult to represent this diagrammatically, and I hope the result in Fig. 9.6 is not misleading.

Schneider's *mixing* or *muddling* implies a grossly disordered amalgam of the constituent parts of a single thought process and represents extreme degrees of fusion and derailment. The resultant speech disorder has been called *drivelling*.

Thought Blocking

Snapping off is the experience a patient with schizophrenia has of their chain of thought, quite unexpectedly and unintentionally, breaking off or ceasing. It may occur in the middle of sorting out a problem or even in midsentence. It is not caused by distraction by other thoughts, and, on introspecting, the patient can give no adequate explanation for it; it simply occurs. It is otherwise described as *thought blocking,* a somewhat misleading term. The patient may explain it as

thought withdrawal: 'My thinking stopped because the thoughts were suddenly taken out of my head'. Fig. 9.7 shows a model of thought blocking.

There is little discussion in the literature about the possibility of patients actually having no thoughts whatsoever, but this possibility is the natural corollary of thought blocking. Hurlburt (1990) described two patients with schizophrenia who using the Descriptive Experience Sampling reported that they were not thinking about anything in the moment that their experiences were sampled. In one, at the moment of sampling, he reported that he was just walking without thought, an experience described as like having a void within. Another, a female patient reported that she was not engaged in any verbalizations, mental images, active listening, observing or anything else she would recognize as a thought or mental experience. Hurlburt concluded that patients with schizophrenia, in general, had reduced amounts of inner verbalizations compared to normal subjects. But, even more unusual, he concluded that patients whose conditions were decompensating may have no inner experience at all.

CHANGES IN THE FLOW OF THINKING

Two further abnormalities of the flow of thought are *crowding of thought* and *perseveration*.

Crowding of thought occurs in schizophrenia. The patient describes their thoughts as being passively concentrated and compressed in their head. The associations are experienced as being excessive in amount, too fast, inexplicable and outside the person's control. The patient may even locate their thinking anatomically as being 'crowded into the back of my head' or elsewhere. It becomes a headlong chase or dance of

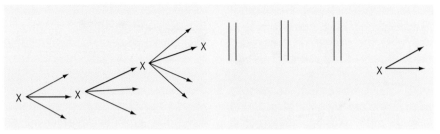

Fig. 9.7 Model of thought blocking.

thoughts and has some of the characteristics of flight of ideas, but it also shows a schizophrenic quality of passivity being controlled from outside.

Perseveration (see Chapter 5) is mentioned here as a disturbance of the flow of thinking. It is characteristically an organic symptom. The patient retains a constellation of ideas long after they have ceased to be appropriate. An idea from that constellation that occurred in a previous sequence of thought is given in answer to a different question. In perseveration, a correct response is given by the patient to the first stimulus, for example, 'Where do you live?'—'Rowley Regis'. However, any subsequent stimuli that demand different responses may get this same, by now inappropriate first response, for instance, 'What is the capital of France?'—'Rowley Regis', 'Who lives at home with you?'—'Rowley … my son and his wife'.

Disturbance of Judgement

A *judgement* is a thought that expresses a view of reality. The word is used here in the sense of 'in my judgement, such and such takes place'. To assess whether it is disturbed or not, one needs to measure it against objective fact. This can be difficult, perhaps requiring consultation with an expert in the same field as the patient. Assessment of faulty judgement is not made solely on the basis of that particular belief or argument but on taking the whole of the person's behaviour and opinions into account. A person's claims to be a figure of royalty persecuted by the Marxists could, in fact, be true. But the opinion that their judgement was disturbed would be confirmed if they had suddenly become convinced about their royalty when a psychiatric nurse had commented to them about the tattoos on their arm, or if they were also found to be hoarding

pebbles and dead spiders in an old tobacco tin. Delusions are, of course, a disturbance of judgement. Various forms of thought disorder and intellectual deficit may also result in disturbance of judgement.

DISTURBANCE OF JUDGEMENT AND DELUSION

The thinking or psychological performance required to produce a delusion is quite independent of intelligence. It occurs in clear consciousness with no signs of organic disturbance of the brain. Judgement in other areas of life apart from the delusion can be preserved, and the very ingeniousness the patient uses to explain and defend their delusional belief demonstrates that their essential capacity to think logically is largely intact; only the falsely held belief, the false premise for subsequent beliefs appears disordered. A delusion in schizophrenia is not a simple defect of reasoning; its development cannot be understood solely in relation to the patient's real-life experience. For instance, not all those with delusions of persecution have any first-hand experience of being persecuted. It is an assumption about the world the patient inhabits, which they do not create by a process of logical conscious thought but from false premises. The mechanism underpinning the often spontaneous development of this false premise is yet to be understood. The starting points of the thinking are already 'deluded', and the patient applies logic to elaborate and support their belief.

We can understand why the belief should be within that particular context (associated with the mother; related to interplanetary travel), but we cannot explain how the *form* of a primary delusion should have occurred. This is a fundamental distinction from delusion-like ideas (secondary delusions), which occur, for example, in affective psychoses. In the latter, we can see the *content* being progressively influenced by the changing mood state so that, eventually, the false belief becomes a logical development from the extreme abnormality of mood.

Although it is usual to describe delusions as disorders of thought content, it is important to be aware that primary delusions are not merely to be understood in this way. The whole process of thought in primary delusion is disordered, not just the content. If an idea were formed on delusional grounds—'I knew that my wife was unfaithful immediately I saw the bulb had gone out' (see Chapter 8)—but the notion itself was not false nor unacceptable to the person's peer group (his wife subsequently admitted to being unfaithful), it would still be a delusion because the notion was formed on delusional evidence. There is a difference between *delusion* and *overvalued ideas* in that, although both may be held with absolute conviction, the latter is a reasonable, possibly even true, belief but is dominating conscious thought to an unreasonable extent.

CONCRETE THINKING

Abnormal processes of thinking in schizophrenia and organic states may result in a literalness of expression and understanding. Abstractions and symbols are interpreted superficially without tact, finesse or any awareness of nuance; the patient is unable to free themselves from what the words literally mean, excluding the more abstract ideas that are also conveyed. This abnormality is described as *concrete thinking*. The term was first introduced by Goldstein (1936). It is usually tested for by proverb interpretation or by other psychological tests, but it is well acknowledged that these tests are unreliable. However, it is recognizable clinically, often quite dramatically. For example, a female patient with schizophrenia came into the room for interview and promptly took her shoes off, saying, 'I always like to keep my feet on the ground when I'm talking'. Another patient with long-term schizophrenia was observed by his doctor walking sideways along the hospital corridor. When asked why he was walking like that, he said that it was 'because of the side effects'. And another patient said, 'I was starting to feel high and I didn't want to fly off, so I've tied these dumb-bell weights round my ankle'.

It is important to emphasize, however, that despite the compelling examples of concrete thinking just described, current thinking is that, if anything,

patients with schizophrenia are more likely to subscribe to a more abstract attitude than control subjects (Weiner, 1966; Shimkunas, 1972; Cutting, 2011) so that, for example, when asked 'In what way is a table and a chair alike?', the patients might answer 'objects in the universe'.

PSYCHOLOGICAL THEORIES OF THINKING IN SCHIZOPHRENIA

A number of psychological theories attempt to explain thinking in patients with schizophrenia. These theories are hampered by the fact that there are no satisfactory general theories of thinking. There are now consistent findings of deficits in attention, working memory, recognition memory and executive functions in schizophrenia. These empirical findings are yet to be integrated into a coherent theory that explains the observed and self-reported thinking abnormalities in this condition.

Over-Inclusive Thinking

The difference between the concrete thinking of organic psychiatric disorders and that occurring in schizophrenia was described by Cameron (1944), who considered that in schizophrenia, the patient is unable to preserve conceptual boundaries. This he called *over-inclusive thinking*: ideas that are only remotely related to the concept under consideration become incorporated within it in the patient's thinking. Thus when asked 'Which of the following are essential parts of a room: walls, chairs, floor, a window?', the over-inclusive person with schizophrenia might include 'chair'. This feature of over-inclusiveness can be seen in many aspects of thinking in schizophrenia, and questionnaires have been devised to test for it, particularly involving sorting tests. The lack of adequate connection between two consecutive thoughts is called *asyndesis*.

The concrete thinking of schizophrenia, however, could not be distinguished from that of other psychotic and neurotic patients (Payne et al., 1970), and it was found to be associated with intelligence. Over-inclusive thinking occurred only in about half of the patients with schizophrenia tested, usually those who were more acutely ill. The other half, usually suffering from more chronic illness, showed much more marked *retardation*. McGhie (1969) found that Payne's tests of over-inclusiveness did not select schizophrenia from some other diagnoses, for example, those with obsessional or manic thought disorder, and Gathercole (1965) considered that these tests demonstrated *fluency of association* rather than over-inclusive thinking.

A young man who had suffered from schizophrenia for several years was known to have recently been abusing drugs. To the doctor's enquiry, 'What drugs have you been using?', he replied 'LSD, health foods and marijuana'. This is an example of over-inclusive thinking. However, it was volunteered spontaneously; he might well have given an entirely correct response to a formal questionnaire that did not touch on significant areas of his experience.

It has been suggested by Chen et al. (1995) that there may be a *broadening of category boundary* (e.g., 'furniture') with preservation of internal category structure in patients with schizophrenia. This results in related issues that are actually outside the category being processed by the patient in a way that is similar to those within it. Cutting (2011) argues that what is most prominent is that patients with schizophrenia overcategorize, finding many more and often needless categories to subsume lists within.

Aggernaes et al. (1976) have taken this theory further from the practical and clinical viewpoint. They consider that patients with schizophrenia have not parted from reality; they seem to experience the real world as being real in the same way as normal people do. However, their defect in reality testing results from a diffuse tendency to experience some fantasy items as being real as well.

Schizophrenic Inattention and Abnormality of Working Memory: Effect on Performance

McGhie (1969) has focused on the disturbance in the function of *attention* in patients with schizophrenia: that they are unable to filter and discount sensory data irrelevant to the task being performed. He showed that the performance of patients with schizophrenia was very poor compared with that of normal subjects, but they were not prone to distraction by auditory or visual external stimuli in the way that normal people were. Hebephrenic patients especially showed less distraction and also poor perception and recall of visual information. Hebephrenic patients were considered to have an inability to sweep out irrelevant extraneous information … especially where the situation

demanded the rapid processing and short-term storage of information. This experience is described subjectively: 'When people talk to me now it's like a different kind of language. It's too much to hold at once. My head is overloaded and I can't understand what they say. It makes you forget what you've just heard because you can't get hearing it long enough. It's all in different bits that you have to put together in your head—just words in the air unless you can figure it out from their faces'.

The effect of this inattention in ordinary social life was well observed by Morgan (1977) in his description of 3 weeks lived in close proximity to two patients with chronic schizophrenia:

In the case of Vine our relationship remained just the same, but I did perhaps come to understand his disabilities a little better, and this helped. He would keep 'losing his thread', to some extent in talk but even more noticeably in action. For example, although we went through the sequence of routine tests over 500 times together, he never once completed a sequence without having to be reminded of what came next and what remained to be done each time. Vine's other main trouble was a curious one. I would say to him, for example, 'Let's do the tests first and then I'd like you to get on with the washing up', and I would be surprised when his response to this was to dash off to the sink and start clattering the plates. Eventually I made out that he had some defect of attention. He would often jump like a startled rabbit when he realized he was being addressed anyway, and I think that by the time he had recovered and collected himself from that, the first half of my sentence had gone and all he heard was the second half. Certainly I found that by inserting a little preliminary padding, I got a more competent response.

Frith (1992) hypothesizes that the mechanism for delusions of control was also responsible for the thought or language abnormality in schizophrenia. In this scheme, it is a failure of self-monitoring that is responsible for thought or language disorder. Thus the patient is unable to edit out irrelevant or perseverating phrases, and this results in poor communication. There is also the related possibility that the fundamental problem is in planning. In this scheme, the coherence of the patient's thought or language is undermined by the absence of an explicit goal and plan, and furthermore there is intrusion of thoughts that do not fit in with the overall goal, resulting in disorganized thought or language. In summary, patients with schizophrenia 'are only able to check the accuracy of an utterance *after* [emphasis in original] they have made it. It is therefore difficult for them to avoid producing a string of faulty utterances, even during attempts at repair' (Frith, 1992).

Liddle (2001) defines the disorganization syndrome as consisting of disjointed thought, emotion and behaviour. However, the cardinal symptoms are formal thought disorder, inappropriate affect and bizarre, erratic behaviour. He concludes that disorganization is associated with slowed performance in neuropsychological tasks that demand selection between competing responses or with errors of commission in tasks that require suppression of an inappropriate response. In his view, this suggests that the disorganization found in schizophrenia derives from impairment of the neural circuits responsible for response selection and inhibition. The circuits involved are the ventrolateral frontal cortex, the left superior temporal gyrus and the adjacent inferior parietal lobule. There is also involvement of the anterior cingulate and thalamus.

Disorder of Control of Thinking

Under this heading, we could discuss three patterns of thinking: passivity of thought, or delusions of control of thinking; obsessions and compulsions in which the unacceptable thoughts are accepted by the patient as being under their control but are resisted; and the rigid control of thought and intolerance for variation that becomes habitual with the anankastic or obsessional personality. The latter two are considered in Chapter 19.

DELUSIONS OF THE CONTROL OF THOUGHT

Control of thinking may be disorganized in that the patient ascribes his own, internal thought processes to outside influences. The subjective disturbance in thinking in schizophrenia is experienced as *passivity*. The patient with schizophrenia experiences their thoughts as foreign or alien, not emanating from themselves and not within their control. There is a breakdown in the way they think of the boundary

between themself and the outside world, so that they can no longer accurately discriminate between the two. They may describe passivity of thought, thought withdrawal, thought insertion and/or thought broadcasting; these are *first-rank symptoms* of *schizophrenia* (Schneider, 1959). In Table 9.1 the first-rank symptoms are listed.

Various forms of thought passivity are described. The patient may describe sharing their thoughts with other people or their thoughts being controlled or

TABLE 9.1 First-Rank Symptoms of Schizophrenia and Symptoms from the Present State Examination	
First-Rank Symptom[a]	**Equivalent Symptom from the Present State Examination[b]**
Delusion	
Delusional percept	Primary delusion
Auditory hallucinations	
Audible thoughts	Thought echo or commentary
Voices arguing or discussing	Voices about the patient
Voices commenting on the patient's action	Voices about the patient
Thought disorder: passivity of thought	
Thought withdrawal	Thought block or withdrawal
Thought insertion	Thought insertion
Thought broadcasting (diffusion of thought)	Thought broadcast or thought sharing
Passivity experiences: delusion of control	
Passivity of affect ('made' feelings)	Delusions of control
Passivity of impulse ('made' drives)	Delusions of control
Passivity of volition ('made' volitional acts)	Delusions of control
Somatic passivity (influence playing on the body)	Delusions of alien penetration

[a]Schneider, K., 1959. Clinical Psychopathology, fifth ed. (M.W. Hamilton, Trans). Grune & Stratton, New York.
[b]Wing, J.K., Cooper, J.E., Sartorius, N., 1974. The Measurement and Classification of Psychiatric Symptoms: An Instruction Manual for the PSE and Catego Program. Cambridge University Press, Cambridge.

influenced from outside themself. These *delusions of control* are often associated with delusional explanations of how their thinking could be controlled, for example, with the use of electronic devices, computers or telepathy. *Thought insertion* is described, in which they believe that their thoughts have been placed there from outside themself. Correspondingly, they may describe their thoughts being taken away from themself against their will: *thought withdrawal.* This may be given as an explanation for thought blocking when the thoughts stop and the mind suddenly goes completely blank. Thought insertion and withdrawal are first-rank symptoms of schizophrenia; *thought blocking* is not because it is difficult to decide whether it is truly thought blocking, some form of retardation or other difficulty with thinking, and blocking is also subjectively similar to epileptic absences. *Thought broadcasting* occurs in schizophrenia when the patient describes their thoughts as leaving themself and being diffused widely out of their control. It also is a passivity experience and of first rank.

A further subjective symptom associated with thought of first-rank importance is the experience of *audible thoughts*, that is, hearing one's own thoughts out loud. The patient knows that they are their thoughts, yet they hear them audibly while they are thinking them or just before or after thinking them. This is, of course, a disorder of perception, an auditory hallucination (see Chapter 7).

Earlier in the chapter, we discussed fusion, mixing, derailment and crowding of thought, all of which occur in schizophrenia. The resultant confusion causes a loss of ability to think clearly, often described in terms of passivity. The patient may feel that their brain is replaced by cotton wool or convoluted rubber. Their thoughts are jumbled, muzzy, vague, blurred: 'I try to part my way through them but they are like treacle and keep on coming back and making me stick'.

First-Rank Symptoms of Schizophrenia

First-rank symptoms of schizophrenia are discussed in this section for convenience because many of them are examples of disorder of control or possession of thoughts. According to Schneider, the presence of one or more first-rank symptoms in the absence of organic disease can be used as positive evidence for schizophrenia. These symptoms of first rank are not a comprehensive list of the clinical features of schizophrenia,

for the changes in affect, volition and motor activity that may occur in the condition are not included, and many other types of delusion, hallucination and disorder of thinking also occur in schizophrenia. For a symptom to be regarded as first rank, it must have the following characteristics.

- It must occur with reasonable frequency in schizophrenia.
- It must generally not occur in conditions other than schizophrenia.
- It must not be too difficult to decide whether the symptom is or is not present.

There are some symptoms that occur only in schizophrenia but occur too rarely to be of practical use as first-rank symptoms. There are many features that are characteristic of schizophrenia but may also occur in other conditions, for example, unspecified auditory hallucinations, poverty of affect and over-inclusive thinking. There are some symptoms that occur only in schizophrenia, but there is too much scope for argument as to whether it is, or is not, this precise symptom for it to be valued as of first rank. An example of this is a *primary delusion*. Some clinicians may regard a particular belief of the patient as primary delusion, whereas others do not.

Although first-rank symptoms are used as a diagnostic checklist, a patient who exhibits seven of them is not more severely ill than someone who shows three. To elicit them requires considerable clinical experience; they cannot be collected quantitatively by riding past the patient on a bicycle! For a psychiatrist to use them clinically, they must first know them. Second, they must know how this person from this social and racial background is likely to describe any particular first-rank symptom ('my thoughts are controlled by television', 'my thoughts are controlled by the spirits of my dead ancestors'). Third, they must ask the appropriate direct questions skilfully without putting words in their patient's mouth. Fourth, they must be able to interpret the patient's answers and decide whether a first-rank symptom is being described. The whole process requires a dextrous use of the phenomenological method as described in Chapter 1.

Many practising psychiatrists' comment at this stage of the discussion of first-rank symptoms would be 'Why bother?' They would also agree that it is often difficult to diagnose schizophrenia, that it is important not to give this label to people who do not suffer from the illness and that it is equally important to treat those who do suffer from it appropriately, effectively and as early in the course of illness as possible.

In clinical practice, the eliciting of first-rank symptoms could best be seen as a means of deciding the degree of certainty that may be attached to the diagnosis. In a patient who shows the general features of schizophrenia (delusion, hallucination, thought disorder, disordered affect, volition, motor activity, behaviour, social relationships, life history), the diagnosis is made, but some doubts remain. If first-rank symptoms are found, then, in the absence of clear organic pathology, one can reckon that the diagnosis has been confirmed. Some of the first-rank symptoms are found to be less reliable at follow-up than others as indicators of schizophrenia, for example, voices heard arguing (Mellor et al., 1981). One of the advantages of first-rank symptoms as a diagnostic tool is that, because of their emphasis on form rather than content, a person who is feigning mental illness is unlikely to produce them. They therefore have a subsidiary use as a method of distinguishing between true and *simulated psychosis*, for example, in prisoners. Despite the value of first-rank symptoms indicating schizophrenia when they are present, there are undoubtedly patients in whom they cannot be elicited; schizophrenia still remains, to some extent, a diagnosis of exclusion (Carpenter and Buchanan, 1994).

Examples of First-Rank Symptoms

The only type of *delusion* that is regarded as of first rank is a *delusional perception,* that is, a normal perception delusionally interpreted and regarded as being highly significant to the patient (see Chapter 8). Examples of delusional percept and of other first-rank symptoms as follows are cited by Mellor (1970, p. 18). Delusional perception is exemplified in the following account:

A young Irishman was at breakfast with two fellow lodgers. He felt a sense of unease, that something frightening was going to happen. One of the lodgers pushed the salt cellar towards him (he appreciated at the same time that this was an ordinary salt cellar and his friend's intention was innocent). Almost before the salt cellar reached him he knew he must return home, 'to greet

the Pope, who is visiting Ireland to see his family and to reward them … because Our Lord is going to be born again to one of the women … And because of this they (all the women) are all born different with their private parts back to front'.

Three types of auditory hallucinations are regarded as being of first rank. These are *audible thoughts, voices heard arguing* and *voices giving a running commentary.* What is meant by *audible thoughts* is the patient's experience of hearing their own thoughts said out loud. In British usage, the symptom sometimes carries its German name, *Gedankenlautwerden,* or its French one, *écho de pensées.* The patient may hear people repeating their thoughts out loud just after they have thought them, answering their thoughts, talking about them having said them audibly or saying aloud what they are about to think so that their thoughts repeat the voices. They often become very upset at the gross intrusion into their privacy and concerned that they cannot maintain control of any part of themselves, not even their thoughts:

A 35-year-old painter heard a quiet voice with 'an Oxford accent', which he attributed to the BBC. The volume was slightly lower than that of normal conversation and could be heard equally well with either ear. He could locate its source at the right mastoid process. The voice would say, 'I can't stand that man, the way he holds his hand he looks like a poof' … He immediately experienced whatever the voice was saying as his own thoughts, to the exclusion of all other thoughts. When he read the newspaper the voice would speak aloud whatever his eyes fell on. He had not time to think of what he was reading before it was uttered aloud.
Mellor (1970, p. 16)

Voices heard arguing with each other implies two or more hallucinatory voices quarrelling or discussing with each other. The patient usually features in the third person in the content of these arguing voices. The symptom is not likely to be volunteered spontaneously in this form; the patient does not actually say, 'I hear voices that argue or discuss with each other'. So the symptom has to be cautiously and subtly enquired for:

A 24-year-old male patient reported hearing voices coming from the nurse's office. One voice, deep in pitch and roughly spoken, repeatedly said, 'G.T. is a bloody paradox', and another, higher in pitch, said, 'He is that, he should be locked up.' A female voice occasionally interrupted, saying 'He is not, he is a lovely man.'

Mellor (1970, p. 16)

Hallucinatory *voices giving a running commentary* on the patient's activities occur and are of first rank. The time sequence of the commentary may be such that it takes place just before, during or after the patient's activities. Again, the symptom is not volunteered spontaneously but may quite often be inferred from the patient's complaints against his voices. For the interviewer, there is always the problem of asking questions in such a way that they are 'let in on the inside'. They are asking questions about perceptions that are quite obvious to the patient. The patient does not know that their particular perception is unique, that other people do not share their perceptual experience. So the interviewer has the difficulty of asking questions about something of which they have no personal experience; the patient has to answer questions that, because of their situation, seem to have no point. The abnormal thing about *voices commenting* is that they should be experienced as perceptions and as coming from outside the self; many normal people have thoughts, recognized as their own and coming from inside themselves, commenting on their actions:

A 41-year-old housewife heard a voice coming from the house across the road … The voice went on incessantly in a flat monotone describing everything she was doing, with an admixture of critical comments. 'She is peeling potatoes, got hold of the peeler, she does not want that potato, she is putting it back, because she thinks it has a knobble like a penis, she has a dirty mind, she is peeling potatoes, now she is washing them.'

Mellor (1970, p. 16)

Passivity experiences are those events in the realm of sensation, feeling, drive and volition that are experienced as *made* or influenced by others. They have been well described as delusions of control, because the patient's experience of the event being made to occur takes the form of a delusion. The terms *disorders of passivity, made experiences, delusions of control* and *disorders of personal activity* are, in practice, synonymous and

interchangeable. The event is experienced as alien by the patient in that it is not experienced by the patient as their own but inserted into the self from outside. Passivity experiences of thinking occur as thought withdrawal, thought insertion or thought broadcasting. In *thought withdrawal,* it is believed by the patient that their thoughts are in some way being taken out of their mind; they have some feeling of loss resulting from this process. It may be coupled with other thought passivity experiences:

A 22-year-old woman said, 'I am thinking about my mother, and suddenly my thoughts are sucked out of my mind by a phrenological vacuum extractor, and there is nothing in my mind, it is empty.'

Mellor (1970, p. 16)

In *thought insertion,* the patient experiences thoughts that do not have the feeling of familiarity, of being their own, but they feel that they have been put in their mind without their volition from outside themself. As in thought withdrawal, there is clearly a disturbance in the self-image and especially in the boundary between what is self and what is not self; thoughts that have in fact arisen inside themself are considered to have been inserted into their thinking from outside:

A 29-year-old housewife said, 'I look out of the window and I think the garden looks nice and the grass looks cool, but the thoughts of Eamonn Andrews come into my mind. There are no other thoughts there, only his … He treats my mind like a screen and flashes his thoughts onto it like you flash a picture.'

Mellor (1970, p. 17)

In *thought broadcasting,* the patient experiences their thoughts withdrawn from their mind and then, in some way, made public and projected over a wide area. The explanation they give for how this can occur will, as usual for the content of a delusion, depend on their background culture and predominant interests:

A 21-year-old student said, 'As I think, my thoughts leave my head on a type of mental ticker-tape. Everyone around has only to pass the tape through their mind and they know my thoughts.'

Mellor (1970, p. 17)

Obviously, careful enquiry must be made about the nature of 'influence' or 'control'. There is a phenomenological world of difference between the statements 'My thinking is influenced by my parents inasmuch as my thoughts are crowded from the back into the front of my head'—a passivity experience, and 'What I do is influenced by my father in that I ponder what he would do in the circumstances and then do the same' (or 'do the opposite')—not passivity. All passivity experiences are regarded as first-rank symptoms. It is not of great significance to decide which type of passivity is described—whether it is, for example, passivity of impulse or of volition—but it is important diagnostically to decide whether it is a passivity experience. *Passivity of emotion* occurs when the affect that the patient experiences does not seem to them to be their own. They believe that they have been *made* to feel it:

A 23-year-old female patient reported, 'I cry, tears roll down my cheeks and I look unhappy, but inside I have a cold anger because they are using me in this way, and it is not me who is unhappy, but they are projecting unhappiness onto my brain. They project upon me laughter, for no reason, and you have no idea how terrible it is to laugh and look happy and know it is not your, but their reaction.'

Mellor (1970, p. 17)

In *passivity of impulse*, the patient experiences a drive, which they feel is alien, to carry out some motor activity. The impulse may be experienced without the subject carrying out the behaviour. A Jewish woman, aged 55, suffering from schizophrenia said, 'I feel my hand going up to salute, and my lips saying "Heil Hitler" … I don't actually say it … I have to try very hard to stop my arm from going up … they put drugs in my food; that is what makes it happen'. If carried out, the *action* is admitted to be the patient's own, but they feel that the *impulse* that precipitated them into doing it was not their own:

A 26-year-old engineer emptied the contents of a urine bottle over the ward dinner trolley. He said, 'The sudden impulse came over me and I must do it. It was not my feeling, it came into me from the X-ray

department, that was why I was sent there for implants yesterday. It was nothing to do with me, they wanted it done. So I picked up the bottle and poured it in. It seemed all I could do.'

Mellor (1970, p. 17)

Similarly, with *passivity of volition* the patient feels that it is not their will that carried out the action:

A 29-year-old shorthand typist described her actions as follows, 'when I reach my hand for the comb it is my hand and arm which move, and my fingers pick up the pen, but I don't control them … I sit there wanting them to move, and they are quite independent, what they do is nothing to do with me … I am just a puppet who is manipulated by cosmic strings. When the strings are pulled my body moves and I can't prevent it.'

Mellor (1970, p. 17)

Somatic passivity is the belief that outside influences are playing on the body. It is not the same as haptic hallucination, but it is a delusional belief that the body is being influenced from outside the self. It may occur in association with various somatic hallucinations. For example, a kinaesthetic hallucination occurred with a passivity experience given as explanation by a patient who felt that their hand was being drawn up to their face. They could feel it moving, although, in fact, it was motionless. Somatic passivity may also occur in association with a normal percept; these experiences are quite common in schizophrenia:

A 38-year-old man had jumped from a bedroom window, injuring his right knee which was very painful. He described his physical experience as, 'The sun-rays are directed by US army satellites in an intense beam which I can feel entering the centre of my knee and then radiating outwards causing the pain.'

Mellor (1970, p. 16)

First-rank symptoms are of general use, diagnostically, in clinical practice, and they have also been adapted for psychiatric research. The method of ascertaining and measuring schizophrenic symptoms, among other symptoms, developed by Wing et al. (1974) in their Present State Examination uses first-rank symptoms as a basis for diagnosing schizophrenia.

The Present State Examination provides the clinician with a means of ascertaining which symptoms and syndromes are present.

Koehler (1979), in a review of the way various authors describe the presence of first-rank symptoms in the English literature, considered that they were sometimes used in a very narrow and sometimes a very wide sense. He makes the distinction between *alienation* of thought and *influence* of thought and makes a plea for clear statements on the boundary criteria for first-rank symptoms and the nosologic bias attached to the phenomena. From the preceding quoted examples of Mellor, alienation is necessary—that is, a delusion of control and not just an experience of influence of thought. Similarly, thought broadcasting would be regarded as first-rank when the patient describes this as having occurred outside their control, irrespective of whether these thoughts are shared with others. Thus this chapter is recommending a narrow use of first-rank symptoms. First-rank symptoms have been employed to establish the diagnosis; they are not necessarily useful prognostically (Bland and Orn, 1980).

This difference between alienation or experience of control and influence can be exemplified by the schizophrenic symptom of *thought insertion*. Thought insertion is more concrete than the insertion of an idea into one's thinking. A normal person may say, 'My mother gave me the idea' or even 'The idea was put into my head by my mother'. Neither of these is thought to be insertion. The patient experiencing passivity believes that, by some concrete process, the boundaries of their self involving thinking are so invaded that their mother is actually placing thoughts inside their head (see Chapter 12) so that they think her thoughts, or perhaps she, is thinking inside them.

REFERENCES

Aggernaes, A., Haugsted, R., Myschetsky, A., Paikin, H., Vitger, J., 1976. A reliable clinical technique for investigation of the experienced reality and unreality qualities connected with everyday life experiences in psychotic and non-psychotic persons. Acta Psychiatr. Scand. 53, 241–257.

Bion, W.R., 1962. The psycho-analytic study of thinking. Intern. J. Psychoanal. 43, 306–310.

Bland, R.C., Orn, H., 1980. Schizophrenia: Schneider's first-rank symptoms and outcome. Br. J. Psychiatry 137, 63–68.

Bleuler, E., 1911. In: Dementia Praecox or the Group of Schizophrenias (J. Zinkin, Trans, 1950). International Universities Press, New York.

Cameron, N., 1944. Experimental analysis of schizophrenic thinking. In: Kasanin, J.J. (Ed.), Language and Thought in Schizophrenia. University of California Press, Berkeley.

Carpenter, W.T., Buchanan, R.W., 1994. Schizophrenia. N. Engl. J. Med 330, 681–690.

Chen, E.Y.H., McKenna, P.J., Wilkins, A., 1995. Semantic processing and categorization in schizophrenia. In: Sims, A. (Ed.), Speech and Language Disorders in Psychiatry. Gaskell, London.

Cutting, J., 2011. A Critique of Psychopathology. The Forest Publishing Company, Forest Row.

Fish, F., 1967. Clinical Psychopathology. John Wright, Bristol.

Fish, F.J., 1962. Schizophrenia. John Wright, Bristol.

Frith, C.D., 1992. The Cognitive Neuropsychology of Schizophrenia. Lawrence Erlbaum Associates, Hove.

Fuchs, T., 2018. The "As-If" function and its loss in schizophrenia. In: Summa, M., Fuchs, T., Vanzago, L. (Eds.), Imagination and Social Perspectives. Routledge, New York, pp. 83–98.

Gathercole, C.E., 1965. A note on some tests of over-inclusive thinking. Br. J. Med. Psychol. 38, 59–62.

Goldstein, K., 1936. The modification of behaviour consequent to cerebral lesions. Psychiatr. Q. 10, 586–610.

Hurlburt, R.T., 1990. Sampling Normal and Schizophrenic Inner Experience. Plenum, New York.

Hurlburt, R.T., 2011. Investigating Pristine Inner Experience: Moments of Truth. Cambridge University Press, Cambridge.

Isräels, H., Schatzman, M., 1993. The seduction theory. Hist. Psychiat. 4, 23–60.

Jaspers, K., 1997. General Psychopathology (J. Hoenig, M.W. Hamilton, Trans). The Johns Hopkins University Press, Baltimore.

Jones, E., 1962. The Life and Work of Sigmund Freud. Penguin, Harmondsworth.

Kahneman, D., 2011. Thinking, Fast and Slow. Penguin Books, London.

Koehler, K., 1979. First rank symptoms of schizophrenia: questions concerning clinical boundaries. Br. J. Psychiatry 134, 236–248.

Kraepelin, E., 1904. Lectures on Clinical Psychiatry (E.T. Johnston, Trans). Hafner, New York.

Liddle, P.F., 2001. Disordered Mind and Brain: The Neural Basis of Mental Symptoms. Gaskell, London.

McGhie, A., 1969. Pathology of Attention. Penguin, Harmondsworth.

Mellor, C.S., 1970. First rank symptoms of schizophrenia. Br. J. Psychiatry 117, 15–23.

Mellor, C.S., Sims, A.C.P, Cope, R.V., 1981. Changes of diagnosis in schizophrenia and first rank symptoms: an eight year follow-up. Compr. Psychiatry 2, 184–188.

Morgan, R., 1977. Three weeks in isolation with two chronic schizophrenic patients. Br. J. Psychiatry 131, 504–513.

Payne, R.W., Hochberg, A.C., Hawks, D.V., 1970. Dichotic stimulation as a method of assessing the disorder of attention of an over-inclusive schizophrenic patient. J. Abnorm. Psychol. 76, 185–193.

Roth, I., 2004. Imagination. In: Gregory, R.L. (Ed.), The Oxford Companion to the Mind. Oxford University Press, Oxford.

Schneider, C., 1930. Psychologie der Schizophrenie. Thieme, Leipzig.

Schneider, K., 1959. Clinical Psychopathology (M.W. Hamilton, Trans), fifth ed. Grune & Stratton, New York.

Shimkunas, A.M., 1972. Conceptual deficit in schizophrenia: a reappraisal. Br. J. Med. Psychol. 45, 149–157.

Smith, E.E., Kosslyn, S.M., 2007. Cognitive Psychology: Mind and Brain. Prentice Hall, Englewood Cliffs, NJ.

Sutherland, N.S., 1976. Breakdown: A Personal Crisis and a Medical Dilemma. Weidenfeld & Nicholson, London.

Tversky, A., Kahneman, D., 1974. Judgment under uncertainty: heuristics and biases. Science 185, 1124–1131.

Webster, R., 1995. Why Freud Was Wrong. HarperCollins, London.

Weiner, L.B., 1966. Psychodiagnosis in Schizophrenia. Wiley, New York.

Wing, J.K., Cooper, J.E., Sartorius, N., 1974. The Measurement and Classification of Psychiatric Symptoms: An Instruction Manual for the PSE and Catego Program. Cambridge University Press, Cambridge.

Winnicott, D.W., 1957. The Child and the Family: First Relationships. Tavistock Publications, London.

Disorder of Speech and Language

KEYWORDS

Language
Speech
Aphasia
Mutism
Alogia

Summary

Speech is the aspect of language that corresponds to the mechanical and articulatory functions that allow language to be vocalized, whereas language is itself a complex system based on a number of elements including phonemes, syntactic structure, semantics, prosody and pragmatics, all designed to aid communication and to encode facts in memory. Abnormalities of speech are common in neurology but rare in psychiatry. Language and thinking disorders are intricately affected in psychiatric disorders, particularly in schizophrenia. The actual relationship between thinking and language is yet to be fully elucidated.

To speak is not only to utter words, it is to propositionize. A proposition is such a relation of words that it makes one new meaning.

J. Hughlings Jackson (1932)

It is very obvious that the functions of thinking and speaking overlap and cannot be readily separated from each other; at the same time, they are clearly different. The contents of this chapter cannot be considered in isolation from its predecessor, although this one considers speech and language from a different perspective.

Maher (1972, p. 3) proposed a model that attempted to demonstrate the link between thinking and the behaviour of speech in language:

conceptualizing the relationship between language and thought. The model might be likened to a typist copying from a script before her. Her copy may appear to be distorted because the script is distorted although the communication channel of the typist's eye and hand are functioning correctly. Alternatively, the original script may be perfect, but the typist may be unskilled, making typing errors in the copy and thus distorting it. Finally, it is possible for an inefficient typist to add errors to an already incoherent script. Unfortunately, the psychopathologist can observe only the copy (language utterances): he cannot examine the script (the thought). In general most theorists concerned with schizophrenic language have accepted the first of the three alternatives, namely that a good typist is transcribing a deviant script. The patient is correctly reporting a set of disordered thoughts. As Critchley put it: 'Any considerable aberration of thought or personality will be mirrored in the various levels of articulate speech – phonetic, phonemic, semantic, syntactic and pragmatic'. The language is a mirror of the thought.

The script is likened to thought and the typist to language. Most clinicians have taken the view that language closely mirrors thought and see the primary abnormality as the thinking disorder (Beveridge, 1985). Disordered language is then seen as merely a reflection of this underlying disturbance with diagnosis of thought disorder only possible on the basis of what the patient says. Some of the more recent linguistic theories used for the analysis of schizophrenic speech contradict the primacy of thinking.

The assumption that language directly mirrors thought can be challenged (Newby, 1995). One tradition argues that language itself structures thinking and concepts and determines how the world is understood. This view derives from the works of Edward Sapir (1884–1939) and Benjamin Whorf (1897–1941). In essence, the Sapir–Whorf hypothesis says that language influences cognition. There is limited empirical support for this view, and Pinker (1994) concludes that 'the representations underlying thinking, on the one hand, and the sentences in a language, on the other, are in many ways at cross-purposes ... People do not think in English or Chinese or Apache; they think in a language of thought. This language of thought probably looks a bit like all these languages; presumably it has symbols for concepts, and arrangements of symbols that correspond to who did what to whom'. This radical view contradicts the point-to-point relationship

between language and thought implicit in Maher's proposition noted earlier and the linguistic determinism of the Sapir–Whorf hypothesis.

The relationship between thinking and language is as complicated for organic disorders as it is for schizophrenia: there can be quite marked disturbance in the use of language with no apparent thought disorder. This is revealed in the rare isolated abnormalities of specific function of language described in this chapter. An understanding of how the healthy person expresses thoughts in language can be achieved only by study of the normal development of language. This is outside the scope of this book but is discussed in relation to perception in Carterette and Friedman (1976).

Language is built of a number of elements. *Phonemes* are the most basic sounds that are available for use in language, and any particular language, such as English, uses only a limited repertoire of phonemes. The repertoire used in English may share only a limited overlap with that used, for example, in Yoruba. *Morphemes* are produced from phonemes and are the smallest meaningful unit of a word, and combinations of morphemes make up words. A morpheme may be a word such as 'do' or 'un'. *Syntax* (grammar) is the allowable combination of words in phrases and sentences and includes the rules that determine word order. *Semantics* are the meanings that correspond to the words and include the meaning of all possible sentences. *Prosody* refers to the modulation of vocal intonation that influences accents, and also the literal and emotional meanings of words and sentences. The *pragmatics* of language is the study of the ways that language is used in practice. This is a relatively new area of study. It refers to the multiple potential meanings of any utterance, which requires knowledge of context and of the speakers for full interpretation. For example, the sentence 'this room is cold' can have any of several meanings depending on the identity of the speaker, the context of the utterance and who is being addressed, that is the social or relative distance of the addressee. It is perhaps important to distinguish between language and speech for our purpose. Speech is the aspect of language that corresponds to the mechanical and articulatory functions that allow language to be vocalized. Thus for language to become speech the vocal cords, the palate, the lips and the tongue need to perform a complex and synchronized dance of intricate steps. The dissociation between poorly articulated speech and intact language indicates that these two functions are separate.

Chomsky's (1986) theory of language is the most influential. Essentially, Chomsky argued that language is like an instinct, and furthermore that 'every sentence that a person utters or understands is a brand new combination of words, appearing for the first time in the history of the universe. Therefore a language cannot be a repertoire of responses; the brain must contain a recipe or programme that can build an unlimited set of sentences out of a finite list of words. The programme may be called a mental grammar' (Pinker, 1994). In addition to this, children rapidly develop these complex grammars without formal instruction. This suggests that they must be innately endowed with a plan common to the grammars of all languages, a universal grammar. How language develops, how word meaning is learned and the neuropsychology of language are all areas of increasing study.

Speech Disturbances

This subject is dealt with in textbooks of neurology and has been reviewed by Critchley (1995); it is only summarized here. Many abnormalities, such as paraphasia, have both organic and psychogenic causes (as described earlier); diagnosis will require full medical and psychiatric history and neurologic and mental state examination.

APHONIA AND DYSPHONIA

Aphonia is the loss of the ability to vocalize; the patient talks only in a whisper. *Dysphonia* denotes impairment with hoarseness but without complete loss of function. It occurs with paralysis of the ninth cranial nerve or with disease of the vocal cords.

Aphonia may also occur without organic disease in *dissociative aphonia*, not uncommon as a presentation among ear, nose and throat outpatients. Such a patient may speak in a 'stage whisper'; phonation may fluctuate according to the response of those the person is addressing.

DYSARTHRIA

Disorders of articulation may be caused by lesions of the brainstem such as bulbar and pseudobulbar palsy.

It may also occur with structural or muscular disorders of the mouth, pharynx, larynx and thorax. Idiosyncratic disorders of articulation are sometimes seen in schizophrenia and, perhaps, with personality disorders consciously produced.

STUTTERING AND STAMMERING

These have in the past been enquired about in the psychiatric history under neurotic disturbances of childhood along with behaviours such as nail biting. However, psychogenic aetiology has certainly now been disproved, and any association with neuroticism may well be secondary to the barriers in communication that stuttering causes.

LOGOCLONIA

This describes the spastic repetition of syllables that occurs with parkinsonism (Scharfetter, 1980). The patient may get stuck using a particular word.

ECHOLALIA

The patient repeats words or parts of sentences that are spoken to them or in their presence. There is usually no understanding of the meaning of the words. It is most often demonstrated in excited schizophrenic states with learning disability and with organic states such as dementia, especially if dysphasia is also present.

CHANGES IN THE VOLUME AND INTONATION OF SPEECH

Many depressed patients speak quietly with a monotonous voice. Manic patients often speak loudly and excitably with much variation in pitch. Excited patients with schizophrenia may also speak loudly; intonation and stresses on words may be idiosyncratic and inappropriate. None of these modes of behaviour has diagnostic significance. The speed and flow of talk mirrors that of thought and is dealt with in Chapter 9.

UNINTELLIGIBLE SPEECH

Speech may be unintelligible for several reasons, and most of the abnormalities described here, if taken to extremes, will result in incomprehensibility.

- *Dysphasia* may be so profound that, although syllables are produced, speech is unintelligible.

- *Paragrammatism* (disorder of grammatical construction) and *incoherence of syntax* may occur in several disorders. Recognizable words may be so deranged in their sentences as to be meaningless—*word salad,* as occurs in schizophrenia. In mania, the speed of association may be so rapid as to disrupt sentence structure completely and render it meaningless, whereas in depression retardation may so inhibit speech that only unintelligible syllables, often of a moaning nature, are produced.
- Private meaning may occur in schizophrenia with the use of (1) new words with an idiosyncratic, personal meaning—*neologisms*; (2) *stock words* and *phrases* in which existing words are used with special individual symbolic meaning; or (3) a private language that may be spoken (*cryptolalia*), or written (*cryptographia*).

Organic Disorders of Language

Dysphasic symptoms are probably more useful clinically than any other cognitive defect in indicating the approximate site of brain pathology (David et al., 2007). However, the auditory, visual and motor mechanisms of speech are spread through several parts of the brain; often several functions are affected and lesions are usually diffuse, and thus precise brain localization is often not possible. Ninety percent of right-handed people without any brain damage have speech located in the left hemisphere, and 10% have right hemisphere speech. Among those who are left-handed or ambidextrous, 64% have left hemisphere speech, 20% right hemisphere and 16% bilateral speech representation.

SENSORY DYSPHASIA

The terms *aphasia* and *dysphasia* are often used interchangeably. However, aphasia implies the loss of language altogether, and dysphasia implies impairment of, or difficulty with, language. Dysphasia is conventionally divided for classification purposes into *sensory* (receptive) and *motor* (expressive) types. Frequently, there is a global impairment of language with evidence of impairment of both elements. Table 10.1 summarizes some of the abnormalities that occur with the different aspects of language that are impaired.

Pure Word Deafness (Subcortical Auditory Dysphasia)

In *pure word deafness,* the patient can speak, read and write fluently, correctly and with comprehension. They cannot understand speech, even though hearing

TABLE 10.1 Impairment of Language Function with Different Types of Dysphasia						
Type	Spontaneous Speech-Fluent	Comprehension	Repetition	Naming	Reading	Writing
Pure word deafness	+	–	–	+	+	+ (not to dictation)
Pure word blindness					–	+
Primary sensory dysphasia		–	–		–	–
Conduction dysphasia			–		Aloud –, compr.n +	–
Nominal dysphasia				–		
Pure word dumbness	–		–			
Pure agraphia					+	–
Primary motor dysphasia		–		–	±, aloud –, compr.n ±	–
Alexia with agraphia				–	–	–
Isolated speech area	–	–		–	–	–
Transcortical motor dysphasia	–			–	Aloud –, compr.n +	
Transcortical sensory dysphasia		–		–	–	–

Compr.n, Comprehension.
After Lishman (1997), with permission of Blackwell Scientific.

is unimpaired for other sounds; they hear words as sounds but cannot recognize the meaning even though they know that they are words. This is therefore a form of agnosia (lack of recognition) for the spoken word.

Pure Word Blindness (Subcortical Visual Aphasia)

The patient with *pure word blindness* can speak normally and understand the spoken word; they can write spontaneously and to dictation but cannot read with understanding (*alexia*). The condition is therefore *agnosic alexia without dysgraphia*. They may have more difficulty with printed than handwritten script. Such a patient will also suffer a right homonymous hemianopia (loss of the right half of the field of vision in both eyes) and an inability to *name* colours even though colour can be perceived.

Primary Sensory Dysphasia (Receptive Dysphasia)

Patients with *primary sensory dysphasia* are unable to understand spoken speech, with loss of comprehension of the meaning of words and of the significance of grammar. Hearing otherwise is not impaired. Consequent on this deficit in the auditory association cortex (*Wernicke's area*), there is also impairment of speech, writing and reading. Speech is fluent, with no appreciation of the many errors in the use of words, syntax and grammar.

Conduction dysphasia could be considered to be a type of sensory dysphasia in which sensory reception of speech and writing are impaired in that the patient cannot repeat the message although they can speak and write it. If they are questioned on the message, they are able to give 'yes' or 'no' answers correctly, thus demonstrating comprehension. There are marked errors of grammar and syntax (*syntactical dysphasia*).

Nominal Dysphasia

The patient with *nominal dysphasia* is unable to produce names and sounds at will. They may be able to describe the object and its function and to recognize the name when presented: a patient described a watch as a 'clock vessel'. Typically, 'empty' nouns such as 'thing' and 'object' are used frequently, and 'distinguishing' nouns rarely. Speech is flat, the structure of sentences generally correct and understanding unimpaired.

Jargon Dysphasia

In *jargon dysphasia* speech is fluent, but there is such gross disturbance for words and syntax that speech is unintelligible. The intonation and rhythm of speech are retained. This is considered a severe type of sensory dysphasia; there is failure to evaluate the patients' own speech, in that patients are not emotionally disturbed when listening to recordings of their own grossly impaired speech.

MOTOR APHASIA
Pure Word Dumbness

The patient with *pure word dumbness* understands spoken speech and writing and can respond to comments. Writing is preserved but speech is indistinct and cannot be produced at will. There is no local disturbance of muscles required in speaking, and the disability is an apraxia limited to movements required for speech.

Pure Agraphia

Pure agraphia is an isolated inability to write that may also occur with unimpaired speech (*agraphia without alexia*); there is normal understanding of written and spoken material. This is the equivalent for writing of pure word dumbness in speech.

Primary Motor Dysphasia

In *primary motor dysphasia* there is disturbance to the processes of selecting words, constructing sentences and expressing them. Speech and writing are both affected, and there is difficulty in carrying out complex instructions, even though understanding for both speech and writing may be preserved. The patient finds it difficult to choose and pronounce words, and speech is hesitant and slow; they recognize their errors, try to correct them and are clearly upset. Gesture may be used to replace verbal communication. Speech is attempted and recognized as spoken words, but words are omitted and sentences shortened, and perseveration occurs.

Alexia with Agraphia

Visual aspects of language are construed as being more complex than auditory in that visual schemata are required—'seeing the written word inside his head', *in addition* to auditory—'hearing the words in one's head'. In *alexia with agraphia,* the patient is unable to read or write, but speaking and understanding speech are preserved. Alexia in this condition is similar to that of pure word blindness: the patient cannot understand words that are spelt out aloud, showing that they are effectively illiterate because of disturbance of the visual symbolism of language.

Isolated Speech Area

Impaired comprehension may occur with slow, hesitant speech in an abnormality in which it is assumed that the anatomic Wernicke's and Broca's areas and the connections between them are intact but connections from other parts of the cortex with this language system are disturbed. Two types, expressive and receptive, are described: *transcortical motor dysphasia* and *transcortical sensory dysphasia.*

Most frequently, of course, with dysphasia, there is a mixture of expressive and receptive elements and the clear syndromes cannot be demonstrated, but their significance is partly theoretical in demonstrating the range of anatomic lesions and the specificity of resultant symptoms. This description has been exclusively concerned with the symptoms; precise description of the anatomic lesions and of associated neurologic symptoms is outside our scope. It is important to distinguish the phenomena of dysphasia, perhaps with neologisms and defects of syntax, from the *word salad* of schizophrenia with superficially similar defects of language. *Verbigeration* describes the repetition of words or syllables that expressive aphasic patients may use while desperately searching for the correct word. In psychosis, most often in catatonia, verbigeration is an example of mannerisms or stereotypy of speech in which words or phrases are either spontaneously repeated or provoked by questions that result in repetition of words or phrases. Hamilton (1974) describes repetition of one or several sentences or strings of fragmented words, going on for hours at a time. Sometimes the string is of incomprehensible jargon in a monotonous voice. The example is from Kraepelin (1919): 'Dear Emily, give me a kiss; we want to get well, a greeting and it would be nothing. We want to be brave and beautiful, follow, follow, mother, so that we can come home soon. The letter was for me; take care, that I get it', and the patient repeated this for 3 hours without stop.

MUTISM

Mutism, refraining from speech during consciousness, is an important sign in psychiatric illness with an extensive differential diagnosis. Eliciting the history and mental state becomes impossible in a mute patient. All the major categories of psychiatric disorder may manifest mutism: learning disability, organic brain disease (sometimes drug related), functional psychosis and neurosis and personality disorder. Some more specific causes include depressive illness, catatonic schizophrenia and dissociative disorder. Mutism occurs as an essential element of stupor (Chapter 3), and it is necessary to assess the level of consciousness as part of a full neurologic examination for all patients with this sign. If there is no lowering of consciousness as in functional psychoses and neuroses, it is likely that the mute patient understands everything that is said around them. As well as specific brain disorders, the causes of stupor include general metabolic disorders that also affect the brain, such as hepatic failure, uraemia, hypothyroidism and hypoglycaemia.

Schizophrenic Language Disorder

Defective communication in language is the defining characteristic of schizophrenia according to Crow (1997), and it is associated with genetic variation at the time language was acquired by *Homo sapiens.* The use of language by people with schizophrenia can differ from that in normal people, and this difference can be subtle and unrelated to positive symptoms such as delusions and hallucinations. There is good reason to believe that the abnormalities of language use are associated with thought disorder. The precise nature of the language abnormality has so far defied clarification, and this account is provisional; it describes the way some of the phenomena have been viewed and conceptualized. There is no single explanatory theory that unifies the disparate abnormalities that have been observed and described. Investigation into language disorder may be ascribed to one of the four models shown in Table 10.2.

CLINICAL DESCRIPTION AND THOUGHT DISORDER

The only unequivocal demonstration of disorder of thinking can be through language. Thought disorder may be revealed in the flow of talk (as in Chapter 9), disturbed content and use of words and grammar, and

TABLE 10.2 Models for Investigating Language Disorder in Schizophrenia	
Model of Language	**Technique Employed**
Concept of thought disorder	Psychiatric: clinical description of schizophrenic speech
Behavioural learning theory	Word association test, multiple choice vocabulary test
Statistical model	
Linguistic model	The Cloze technique, type:token ratio
	Analysis of syntax, cohesion or propositions

After Beveridge (1985), with permission.

TABLE 10.3 Categorization of Thought Disorder in Speech	
Clinician	**Categorization**
Kraepelin	Akataphasia
Bleuler	Loosening of associations
Gardner	Form of regression
Cameron	Asyndesis
Goldstein	Concrete thinking
Von Domarus	Defect of deductive reasoning
Schneider	Derailment, substitution, omission, fusion and drivelling

in the inability to conceptualize appropriately. Critchley (1964) considered that the 'causation of schizophrenic speech affection lies in an underlying thought disorder, rather than in a linguistic inaccessibility'. Some of the ways in which clinicians have categorized schizophrenic thought disorder manifesting in speech are linked in Table 10.3.

The German psychopathologic literature on schizophrenic language and speech disorders was concerned with the rules of language dysfunction; it consistently reported the patient's uncertainty in choosing the correct metaphorical level in communication (Mundt, 1995). Kraepelin (1919) defined *akataphasia* as a disorder in the expression of thought in speech. *Loss of the continuity of associations*, which implied incompleteness in the development of ideas, was the first of the functions included among the fundamental symptoms of schizophrenia by Bleuler (1911).

Gardner (1931) considered thought disorder to be a form of *regression*. Cameron (1944), in describing *asyndesis*, considered there to be an inability to preserve conceptual boundaries and a marked paucity of genuinely causal links. He gave the example of a patient who, given these alternatives, completed the sentence 'I get warm when I run because …' with *all* the words: 'quickness, blood, heart of deer, length, driven power, motorized cylinder, strength'. The patient was prone to use imprecise expressions—*metonyms*, for example, a patient said he was alive:

Because you really live physically, because you have menu three times a day; that's the physical [What else is there beside the physical?] Then you are alive mostly to serve a work from the standpoint of methodical business.

He also demonstrated *over-inclusive thinking* in which a loose association of concepts that were related in some way to the dominant theme became interwoven into responses, for example:

[The wind blows] Due to velocity. [Question repeated] Due to loss of air, evaporation of water. [What gives the velocity?] the contact of trees, of air in the trees.

Concrete thinking, a term denoting an inability to think abstractly was proposed by Goldstein (1944), but the validity of this was challenged by Payne et al. (1959). Allen (1984) considers that speech-disordered patients with schizophrenia produce evidence of concrete thinking, thinking without inferring and restricted to what is explicitly stated, whereas nonspeech-disordered patients with schizophrenia do not. When the thematic organization of speech was analysed for patients with positive speech disorder (incoherence of speech) or negative speech disorder (poverty of speech), there was no difference found: speech-disordered patients, positive as well as negative, showed cognitive restriction and produced fewer inferences than nonspeech-disordered patients.

A deficiency in the logic of *deductive reasoning* in schizophrenia was suggested by Von Domarus (1944). Some of the abnormalities of thinking expressed in speech observed by Schneider are discussed in Chapter 9.

An attempt has been made by Andreasen (1979) to classify the description of patients' cognitive and linguistic behaviour on the phenomena demonstrated without making inferences about concepts of 'global' thought disorder; these abnormalities occur in both mania and schizophrenia. Some types of thought disorder, such as *neologism* and *blocking*, occurred too infrequently to have diagnostic significance. However, she found high reliability between raters with many types of thought disorder and also discrimination between different psychotic illnesses. Derailment, loss of goal, poverty of content of speech, tangentiality and illogicality were particularly characteristic of schizophrenia. *Derailment* implies loosening of association so that ideas slip on to either an obliquely related, or totally unrelated, theme. *Loss of goal* is the failure to follow a chain of thought through to its natural conclusion. *Poverty of content of speech* includes poverty of thought, empty speech, alogia, verbigeration and negative formal thought disorder; patients' statements convey little information and tend to be vague, over-abstract, overconcrete, repetitive and stereotyped. *Tangentiality* means replying to a question in an oblique or even irrelevant manner. *Illogicality* implies drawing conclusions from a premise by inference that cannot be seen as logical.

Misuse of Words and Phrases

The patient with schizophrenia sometimes shows misuse of words in that they have, in the terminology of Kleist (1914), a defect of word storage. They have a restricted vocabulary and so use words idiosyncratically to cover a greater range of meaning than they usually encompass. These are called *stock words or phrases,* and their use will sometimes become obvious in a longer conversation in which an unusual word or expression may be used several times. For example, a patient used 'dispassionate' as a stock word, and used it frequently with a bizarre and idiosyncratic meaning in the course of a few minutes' speech. A woman who was delusionally concerned that the police were intruding into her private affairs interspersed her conversation, often bizarrely, with the expression 'confidentially speaking'.

This abnormality appears partly to reflect a poverty of words and syntax and also an active tendency for words or syllables by association to *intrude* into thoughts and therefore speech soon after utterance. In the sample of speech in Chapter 9, the following words could be seen as stimuli and responses by

intrusion: 'means'—'ways', 'opens'—'closed', 'holding back the truth'—'by no means will I speak', 'written questions'—'by means of writing', 'miracle'—'Holyland'. They also appear to be stock words or phrases in that they are used with greater frequency and with a greater range of meaning than is normal and correct.

Words carry a *semantic halo*, that is, their constellation of associations is greater than just the dictionary meaning of the word. A boy aged 16 steals an apple. If I call him 'a trespasser', it has biblical associations; 'a criminal' suggests a greater degree of viciousness than the action merits; 'a delinquent' is readily associated with his youthfulness because of the phrase 'juvenile delinquent'. The constellations of associations in patients are disordered in that they often make apparently irrelevant associations. These may be explained by misperception of auditory stimuli with specific inattention; the actual mediation of associations in patients with schizophrenia may be similar to that in healthy people. This comes some way to explaining why the associations seem appropriate subjectively to the patient themselves, as they do not realize that they have misperceived the cue: it seems reasonable to them but is quite irrelevant to the interviewer. To quote Maher, 'What seems to be bizarre is not the nature of the associations that intrude into the utterance, but the fact that they intrude at all' (Maher, 1972).

Among the disorders of words, *neologism* is well recognized. A patient believed that their thoughts were influenced from outside themself by a process of 'telegony'. Although such a word does actually exist, the patient had no notion of this nor what it meant. They created the word to describe a unique experience of his for which no adequate word existed. A 47-year-old male patient with schizophrenia and expansive mood described himself thus: 'I am the triplicate actimetric kilophilic telepathic multibillion million genius'— which does suggest a certain grandiosity!

The unintentional puns of schizophrenia have been explained by Chapman et al. (1964). If a word has more than one meaning, it is likely that one usage is *dominant*. For example, the majority of people, in most contexts, would be more likely to use the word 'bay' to refer to an inlet of the sea than to a tree, the noise a hound makes, the colour of a horse, an opening in a wall, the second branch of a stag's horn, an uncomfortable place at which to stand or even, phonetically, a Turkish governor! There is a marked tendency in schizophrenia to show *intrusion* of the dominant meaning when the context demands the use of a less common meaning. Chapman et al. (1964) used a sentence such as 'the tennis player left the court because he was tired' and asked patients with schizophrenia to interpret its meaning with one of three explanations: one referring to a tennis court, one to a court of law and one altogether irrelevant. An analysis of responses shows that dominant meanings, here a court of law, intrude into the responses quite frequently, but intrusion of minor meanings is less frequent.

Maher (1972) has described disorder of language in schizophrenia in which intrusion occurs through *clang associations* with the initial syllable of a previous word: 'the subterfuge and the mistaken planned *sub*stitutions'. This is unlike the clang associations that occur normally in poetry, in humour and in manic speech in which the *clang* occurs in terminal syllables. The repetitiveness of speech disorder is also thought to be associated with the intrusion of associations: the normal process of eliminating irrelevant associations does not take place so that a word in a clause will provoke associations by pun, clang and ideational similarity. When that clause is completed, a syntactically correct clause may then be inserted, disrupting meaning but demonstrably associated with that previous word or idea.

Maher considers that an inability to maintain attention may account for the language disturbances seen in some patients. Disturbed attention allows irrelevant associations to intrude into speech, similarly to the disturbance affecting the filtering of sensory input. In this theory, normal coherent speech is seen as the progressive and instantaneous inhibition of irrelevant associations to each utterance, and so the determining tendency proceeds with the active elimination of those associations that are not goal directed. This is but one of many potential explanations for the observed abnormalities.

Destruction of Words and Grammar

Alogia is a term used to describe negative thought disorder, or poverty of thoughts as expressed in words. Correspondingly, *paralogia* is used to describe positive thought disorder, or the intrusion of irrelevant or

bizarre thought. *Paraphasia* is a destruction of words with interpolation of more or less garbled sounds. Although the patient is only able to produce this nonverbal sound, it clearly has significance or meaning to them. *Literal paraphasia* is gross misuse of the meaning of words to such an extent that statements no longer make any sense. *Verbal paraphasia* describes the loss of the appropriate word but the statements are still meaningful, for example a patient described a chair as 'a four-legged sit-up'.

Disturbances in words and their meanings are much more common in schizophrenia than disturbance of grammar and syntax. However, grammar is also sometimes altered; the loss of parts of speech is described as *agrammatism*. Adverbs are occasionally lost, resulting in coarsening and poverty of sentences, a form of *telegramese*. For example, 'rich table is worn; the woman is rich to write; son is also lamentation'. This, as well as showing *stock words* (rich—lamentation), shows loss of parts of speech, for example, the indefinite article. The meaning is more disjointed than the grammar. *Paragrammatism* occurs when there is a mass of complicated clauses that make no sense in achieving the goal of thought. However, the individual phrases are, in themselves, quite comprehensible.

It seems probable that the rules of syntax are preserved in schizophrenia long after a marked disturbance in the use of words, so that, if in the preceding clause an intrusive association were to replace the word 'rules', the word used would probably, correctly, be a noun. For instance, the patient just discussed might have said in this context 'the *lamentations* of syntax are …'

In addition to the observed abnormalities already described, there are suggestions that patients with schizophrenia demonstrate lack of use of cohesive ties in discourse (for a full discussion, see McKenna and Oh, 2005). Cohesive ties in discourse are devices that are utilized to link sentences together, so that speech is not merely a collection of unrelated sentences. There are four main types of cohesive ties: *reference, conjunction, lexical cohesion* and *ellipsis*. *References* in English are personal pronouns such as 'he', 'she', 'they', 'it'; demonstratives are such words as 'this' and 'that'; and comparatives such terms as 'smaller than', 'equal to', etc. In the following sentences, 'He' is a reference tie: '*I met Peter yesterday.* **He** *was wearing a dark suit*'. In the sentence *'She went to the High Street this morning* **and** *bought some cakes from the supermarket'*, 'and' is a conjunction tie. A lack of use of cohesive ties means that the listener in dialogue with a patient with schizophrenia can have difficulty following the speech of the patient.

PSYCHOGENIC ABNORMALITIES

Andreasen (1979) showed that the abnormalities of language present in schizophrenia were also present in mania. Furthermore, McKenna and Oh (2005) make the case that there is a continuum of language or thought disturbance from schizophrenia through mood disorder to organic disorders such as epilepsy and frontotemporal dementia. The point that McKenna and Oh want to emphasize is that language abnormalities in schizophrenia have a neurologic substrate, linking the observed disturbances to aphasia, a return to the ideas that originated with Kleist in the 20th century.

Manic speech has been analysed, and the speech and number of associations demonstrated in *flight of ideas* and *pressure of talk* is seen in the greater number of *cohesive links* occurring in manic speech. The content of depressive speech is, of course, influenced by the mood state, and so also is the choice of words. Sentences tend to be short and have fewer and simpler associations, with *retardation*.

Hysterical mutism may occur as an abnormal reaction to stress. A man aged 35 had been unable to tolerate the continual nagging from his wife and her two sisters who lived with them. One day, after heavy drinking the previous evening, he smashed his wife's furniture at home and then became mute for 24 hours. He was eventually referred from the accident and emergency department to the psychiatric ward, and speech returned gradually over the next 2 to 3 days without other treatment.

With the phenomenon of *approximate answers* (Chapter 5), the patient gives an incorrect answer to a simple question: 'How many legs has a sheep?'—'Five'. This is, according to Anderson and Mallinson (1941), 'a false response to the examiner's question where the answer, although wrong, indicates that the question had been grasped'. This symptom may occur in a number of conditions, including schizophrenia in which it is often associated with fatuous mood; dissociative

disorder, previously designated hysterical pseudodementia (before making such a diagnosis, the wise psychiatrist thoroughly excludes an organic cause); Ganser's syndrome; and other organic conditions.

Eccentric and pedantic use of words may sometimes be seen in those with *anankastic personality;* obsessionality obtrudes into the choice of words and construction of sentences.

STATISTICAL MODEL OF LANGUAGE

The *Cloze* procedure involves deleting words from the transcripts of speech and assessing whether the omitted word can be predicted. Maher considered that, in schizophrenia, the greater the severity of the illness, the greater is the degree of unpredictability of the utterance of language. In normal speech, *a* large *part* of every sentence *could be* omitted without losing *the* meaning. For example, if the words 'a ... part ... could be ... the' were omitted from the last sentence, the meaning would still be obvious; if letters were omitted from words, for instance *nrml spech,* the meaning is still clear. *Predictability* is the ability to predict the missing words accurately; in this sense, patients with schizophrenia are unpredictable in their speech. They are likely to use unexpected words and phrases. In the perception of language, the patient with schizophrenia is less able to gain information from the redundancies, both semantic and syntactic, in everyday speech.

A sophistication of the *Cloze procedure* has been investigated by Newby (1998). This involves the following:

- The modified Cloze procedure in which the nature of the inserted word is noted, such as its part of speech.
- In the reverse Cloze procedure, thought-disordered patients were asked to make sense of a script that had been mutilated by instituting the Cloze procedure, for example, by deleting every fourth or fifth word. Patients with schizophrenia performed significantly worse than a control group of orthopaedic patients, with manic-depressive patients intermediate on both modified and reverse Cloze procedures.

Schizophrenic speech is considered less predictable than normal speech, and lack of predictability is more marked with clinically manifest thought disorder (Manschreck et al., 1979). An experiment was carried out using the Cloze procedure in which raters were asked to assess passages of schizophrenic or normal speech with the fourth or fifth word deleted. With fifth word deletion, thought-disordered schizophrenic speech was significantly less predictable than normal or nonthought-disordered schizophrenic speech; this latter was no less predictable than normal speech.

Whether schizophrenic speech is really less redundant than normal has been questioned by Rutter (1979), who was able to demonstrate no difference. The view that schizophrenic language can be reduced to such simple mathematical rules has been rejected by Mandelbrot (1968). But studies using this technique continue, even if sporadically, and demonstrate that the speech and language of patients with psychosis may be less predictable than that of controls (Adewuya and Adewuya, 2006).

The *type:token ratio* is a measure of the number of different words compared with the total number of words used by a speaker (Zipf, 1935). Maher concluded that the type:token ratio of schizophrenic patients was lower than for normal subjects. The tendency of schizophrenic patients to repeat certain words and use them in an idiosyncratic way is referred to as the use of *stock words*.

LINGUISTIC APPROACHES TO SCHIZOPHRENIA

Various linguistic theories have been applied to schizophrenia (for a full discussion, see McKenna and Oh, 2005). These methods of analysis of schizophrenic language are tentative and do not yet cover the range of abnormalities occurring in the condition. Chomsky (1959) proposed that humans are able to use strings and combinations of words they have never heard before through use of a limited set of integrative processes and generalized patterns. However, Moore and Carling (1982) have labelled Chomskyan linguistics a *container* view of language, separated from the real way users of language apply it to their own meanings and contexts. Individual case studies have used tape-recorded interviews with patients with schizophrenia to demonstrate distinctive abnormalities. However, on closer analysis, such abnormalities are often found to occur in the speech of normal people, although less frequently. A further study of bilingual patients showed psychotic symptoms to be present in their native language but absent in their second language.

The problem of individual studies is, of course, the extent to which they can be generalized to all patients with schizophrenia.

Syntactical Analysis

In studies of speech analysed for syntax, compared with manic and normal controls, patients with schizophrenia showed less complex speech, fewer well-formed sentences, more semantic and syntactic errors and less fluency. There were also marked use of paraphrasias, agrammatisms, anomia, pronoun word problems, circumlocutions, etc. These problems seemed to be associated with a general intellectual impairment (McKenna and Oh, 2005). Such studies do not, of course, justify the conclusion that differences are due directly to the disease or to thought disorder, nor does it take into account the social context or emotional aspects. However, marked differences are of interest when one considers that the majority of patients with schizophrenia do not show overt disorder of language.

Propositional Analysis

This is a form of textual analysis in which the text is broken down into its component propositions, and these are then represented diagrammatically to show the 'mental geometry' (Hoffman et al., 1982). Normal speech is considered to proceed as in a single tree diagram with all branches leading from a single key proposition, but psychotic speech more often breaks the 'rules' of propositional relationships.

Observers, listening to the speech of patients with schizophrenia, are often struck with its oddity and deviance. It has been considered by Chaika (1995) that this is not purely a deficit of syntax but more a phenomenon like severe and repeated slips of the tongue, in which the error is a lapse of executive control, a lapse of volition. It has been shown by Morice (1995) that with increasing complexity of syntax there is an increase in the number of errors in the speech of patients with schizophrenia; speakers expressing very simple sentences made relatively few errors. One of his patients expressed this: 'and communicating ordinarily I can get lost in the chaos of the language'.

This finding was confirmed by Thomas and Leudar (1995) using the Hunt test, a written test in which subjects produce syntactically complex sentences from simple input phrases. Communication-disordered patients with schizophrenia made more errors than noncommunication-disordered patients with schizophrenia or normal controls, and these errors were more likely to occur with more complex syntactic structures. The patients were therefore thought to have a discrete failure of language processing that was distinct from the more general cognitive disorders of the condition.

Although these methods are still experimental, the patient's use of language and syntax does enable a quantitative method of evaluating the mental state and subjective experience to be developed. Study of language disorder should be an area in which descriptive psychopathology can contribute to psychiatric research.

REFERENCES

Adewuya, O.A., Adewuya, A.O., 2006. Predictability of speech and language in Nigerian patients with psychosis: a controlled study. Psychiatry Res. 143, 199–204.

Allen, H.A., 1984. Positive and negative symptoms and the thematic organisation of schizophrenic speech. Br. J. Psychiatry 144, 611–617.

Anderson, W.E., Mallinson, W.P., 1941. Psychogenic episodes in the course of major psychoses. J. Ment. Sci. 87, 383–396.

Andreasen, N.C., 1979. Thought, language and communication disorder. Arch. Gen. Psychiatry 36, 1315–1330.

Beveridge, A., 1985. Language Disorder in Schizophrenia. MPhil Thesis. University of Edinburgh.

Bleuler, E., 1911. Dementia Praecox: Or the Group of Schizophrenias. International University Press, New York.

Cameron, N., 1944. Experimental analysis of schizophrenic thinking. In: Kasanin, J. (Ed.), Language and Thought in Schizophrenia. University of California Press, Berkeley.

Carterette, G., Friedman, M.P., 1976. Handbook of Perception. Language and Speech, vol. VII. Academic Press, New York.

Chaika, E., 1995. On analyzing schizophrenic speech: what model should we use? In: Sims, A.C.P. (Ed.), Speech and Language Disorders in Psychiatry. Gaskell, London.

Chapman, L.J., Chapman, J.P., Miller, G.A., 1964. A theory of verbal behaviour in schizophrenia. In: Maher, B.A. (Ed.), Progress in Experimental Personality Research, vol. 1. Academic Press, New York.

Chomsky, N., 1959. Review of Skinner. Language 35, 26–58.

Chomsky, N., 1986. Knowledge of Language: Its Nature, Origin and Use. Praeger, New York.

Critchley, E.M.R., 1995. Growth points in the neurology of speed and language. In: Sims, A.C.P. (Ed.), Speech and Language Disorders in Psychiatry. Gaskell, London.

Critchley, M., 1964. The neurology of psychotic speech. Br. J. Psychiatry 110, 353–364.

Crow, T.J., 1997. Is schizophrenia the price that *Homo sapiens* pays for language? Schizophr. Res. 28, 127–141.

David, A.S., Fleminger, S., Kopelman, M.D., Lovestone, S., Mellers, J.D.C., 2007. Lishman's Organic Psychiatry: A Textbook of Neuropsychiatry. Wiley-Blackwell, Chichester.

Gardner, G.E., 1931. The measurement of psychotic age: a preliminary report. Am. J. Psychiatry 10, 963–975.

Goldstein, K., 1944. Methodological approach to the study of schizophrenic thought disorder. In: Kasanin, J.S. (Ed.), Language and Thought in Schizophrenia. University of California Press, Berkeley.

Hamilton, M., 1974. Fish's Clinical Psychopathology: Signs and Symptoms in Psychiatry. John Wright, Bristol.

Hoffman, R.E., Kirstein, L., Stopek, S., Cicchetti, D.V., 1982. Apprehending schizophrenic discourse: a structural analysis of the listener's task. Brain Lang. 15, 207–233.

Jackson, J.H., 1932. Selected Writings of John Hughlings Jackson. Hodder and Stoughton, London.

Kleist, K., 1914. Aphasie und Geisteskrankheit. Munch Med. Wochenschr. 61, 8.

Kraepelin, E., 1919. Dementia Praecox and Paraphasia (B.M. Barclay, Trans). Livingstone, Edinburgh.

Lishman, W.A., 1997. Organic Psychiatry: The Psychological Consequences of Cerebral Disorder, third ed. Blackwell, Oxford.

Maher, B.A., 1972. The language of schizophrenia: a review and interpretation. Br. J. Psychiatry 120, 3–17.

Mandelbrot, B., 1968. Information theory and psycholinguistics. In: Oldfield, R.C., Marshall, J.C. (Eds.), Language. Penguin Books, London. 1968.

Manschreck, T.C., Maher, B.A., Rucklos, M.E., White, M.T., 1979. The predictability of thought-disordered speech in schizophrenic patients. Br. J. Psychiatry 134, 595–601.

McKenna, P., Oh, T., 2005. Schizophrenia Speech: Making Sense of Bathroots and Ponds that Fall in Doorways. Cambridge University Press, Cambridge.

Moore, T., Carling, C., 1982. Understanding Language: Towards a Post-Chomskyan Linguistics. Macmillan, London.

Morice, R., 1995. Language impairments and executive dysfunction in schizophrenia. In: Sims, A.C.P. (Ed.), Speech and Language Disorders in Psychiatry. Gaskell, London.

Mundt, C., 1995. Concepts of schizophrenic language disorder and reality assessment in German psychopathology. In: Sims, A.C.P. (Ed.), Speech and Language Disorders in Psychiatry. Gaskell, London.

Newby, D., 1998. 'Cloze' procedure refined and modified: 'modified Cloze', 'reverse Cloze' and the use of predictability as a measure of communication problems in psychosis. Br. J. Psychiatry 172, 136–141.

Newby, D.A., 1995. Analysis of language: terminology and techniques. In: Sims, A.C.P. (Ed.), Speech and Language Disorders in Psychiatry. Gaskell, London.

Payne, R.W., Matussek, P., George, E.I., 1959. An experimental study of schizophrenic thought disorder. J. Ment. Sci. 105, 627–652.

Pinker, S., 1994. The Language Instinct. Penguin Books, London.

Rutter, D.R., 1979. The reconstruction of schizophrenic speech. Br. J. Psychiatry 134, 356–359.

Scharfetter, C., 1980. General Psychopathology: An Introduction. Cambridge University Press, Cambridge.

Thomas, P., Leudar, I., 1995. Syntactic processing and communication disorder in first onset schizophrenia. In: Sims, A.C.P. (Ed.), Speech and Language Disorders in Psychiatry. Gaskell, London.

Von Domarus, E., 1944. The specific laws of logic in schizophrenia. In: Kasanin, J.S. (Ed.), Language and Thought in Schizophrenia. University of California Press, Berkeley.

Zipf, G.K., 1935. The Psychobiology of Language. Houghton Mifflin, Boston.

Insight

Chapter Outline

KEYWORDS

Insight
Self-awareness
Self-monitoring
Theory of mind

Summary

Insight, in psychiatry, refers to the capacity of the patient to recognize that their mental symptoms are indicative of mental illness and that these symptoms require treatment. It is now known to be associated with impaired cognitive function and predicts poor compliance with treatment, compulsory admission and coercive treatment in hospital. The underlying neural mechanism of poor insight is starting to be illuminated and is linked more widely to deficits in self-awareness, self-monitoring, empathy and theory of mind:

A man who knows who and what he is, his position in the world, and what the persons and things are around him; who judges according to known, or intelligible rules; and who, if he has singular ideas or singular habits, can give a reason for his opinions and his conduct; a man who, however wrong he may act, is not misled by any uncontrollable impulse or passion; who does not idly squander his means; who knows the legal consequences of his actions; who can distinguish between unseemly and seemly behaviour, who feels that which is proper and that which is improper to utter, according to the circumstances in which he is placed; and who reverences the subject and the ministers of religion; a man who, if he cannot always regulate his thoughts and his temper and his actions, is not continually in the extremes, and if he errs, errs as much from benevolence and hesitation, as from passion and excitement, and more frequently: lastly, a man who can receive reproof, and acknowledge when he has needed correction.

John Perceval (1840)

Self-awareness is a basic human ability. It refers to the ability to recognize one's own existence and experience and the existence and experience of others. It includes the facility for monitoring the events in one's own life and the ability to make decisions about the future on the basis of that knowledge. Furthermore, it involves the ability to communicate this awareness of self and others to other human beings (Marková, 1987). This characteristically human ability is partly the subject of Sophocles' (496–406 BCE) *Oedipus the King*, in which Oedipus' quest for self-knowledge resulted in his discovery that he had killed his own father and fathered children by his own mother. The aphorism 'Know Thyself' is said to have been inscribed at the forecourt of the Temple to Apollo at Delphi and in *The Apology*, Socrates (470–399 BCE) says, 'The unexamined life is not worth living for a human being'. These references to self-knowledge in antiquity underline the place of this notion in human life.

Self-awareness obviously takes in much more than an awareness of illness, but it is plain that the psychiatric notion of *insight* is a subset of the general concept of self-awareness or self-knowledge. *Insight,* as a notion, is much wider than just knowing whether one is ill, and if so, having a sensible view regarding treatment. It involves our capacities for introspection, empathy and communication; not only is it glimpsing ourselves as we really are but also ourselves as others see us, and therefore others as they really are because they go through the same repertoire of mental mechanisms that we do. Even for the most private and internal of insights, what might be termed our *social awareness*, the capacity for relationships, for empathy, and knowing and understanding how our behaviour will affect the emotions and experience of other people is important. Insight is the direct product of knowing ourselves. It is a quality that has been highly valued by most mental health clinicians, because a strong link is assumed between having insight and have better quality of life and a more fulfilling life (McGorry and McConville, 1999).

Although, in psychiatry, we concentrate mostly on the narrow meaning of insight with regard to mental illness, we need to retain this broader concept. Often, our work with patients involves us having insight into their thinking and behaviour because of our capacity for empathy as fellow human beings and also helping them gain insight into themselves and the roots of their problems.

The relationship between this capacity for insight in a general sense and the practical issues of treatment is close. A physician suffering from delusional disorder advertised and sold magnets for the medical treatment of arthritis and hay fever. They strongly believed that this form of treatment was of unequalled value for virtually all medical conditions, and they had physically assaulted a pharmacist who had tried to persuade them otherwise. They decried the validity of the whole of psychiatry, 'because I am a scientist and everything has to be proved with evidence'. Because of their lack of insight into their own condition and the nature of their beliefs, it was impossible to initiate treatment. Their symptoms persisted long term.

Jaspers (1997) has written about the patient's attitude to their illness under the following headings:

1. Understandable attitudes to the sudden onset of acute psychosis (perplexity, awareness of change)
2. Working through the effects of acute psychoses
3. Working through the illness in chronic states
4. The patient's judgement of their illness
5. The determination to fall ill
6. The attitude to one's own illness: its meaning and possible implications

All these points, and especially 3, 4 and 6, involve the process of insight, the knowledge of oneself with particular reference to illness. A person who becomes seriously and suddenly ill, whatever the nature of the illness, after previously having been fit for many years, is astonished by their change of health status. Such a person is likely to undergo a profound change in self and body image. They have become a person who, from being healthy and seeing illness as something that happens to other people, now sees themself as potentially frail and vulnerable. This can be personally enriching and is not necessarily a wholly negative experience.

Insight in Clinical Practice

So that they can better help their patient with a possible mental illness, the psychiatrist asks specific questions about the patient's opinions concerning their illness. These include their degree of acknowledgement of illness, their attitudes to illness, their understanding of the effects of their illness on their current capabilities and future prospects. All this adds up to the assessment of *insight* into their condition. Insight is not an absolute; it can vary in its impairment with different facets of the condition; for example, a patient could have some limited understanding concerning their unlikelihood to obtain a job compatible with their qualifications but virtually no understanding as to how their psychotic symptoms interfere with relationships. Thus insight is now not considered to be an all-or-none phenomenon in either clinical evaluation or measurement, but rather a dimensional one so that subjects can have different levels of awareness of their illness (Surguladze and David, 1999).

All mental illnesses will alter the patient's worldview and capacity to cope with circumstances. Assessment of insight measures the awareness of this change by the patient and their ability to adapt to the change. Insight is highly complex as a function. It is the understanding of the individual about their own state of health, capacity and worth; it also relates this assessment of internal state to other people and the world outside. In other words, insight requires both inner and outer orientation. This aspect of insight becomes more apparent later in this chapter, in the discussion of the contribution of Gestalt psychology to the conceptualization of insight. Insight in Gestalt psychology is oriented towards problem solving in the external world, whereas insight in clinical practice is inner-directed.

David (1990) regards insight as composed of three distinct, overlapping dimensions: the recognition of morbid psychological change, the labelling of this change as deriving from mental illness and the understanding that this change requires treatment that needs to be complied with. An assessment schedule was constructed for determining the nature of insight and quantitative loss of insight correlated with the degree of psychopathology (David et al., 1992).

One of the most frustrating aspects of practising psychiatry is, from the point of view of the treating professional, the apparent inability of patients to recognize and/or admit that they are mentally ill. Patients, especially those with schizophrenia, often deny that their experiences are abnormal and that they are unwell. Daniel Schreber (1842–1911) described his attitude towards his auditory verbal hallucinations

in his book *Memoirs of My Nervous Illness* (Schreber, 1955) as follows:

I noticed therefore with interest that according to Kraepelin's TEXTBOOK OF PSYCHIATRY (5th edition, Leipzig, 1896, p. 110 ff) which had been lent to me, the phenomenon of being in some supernatural communication with voices had frequently been observed before in human beings whose nerves were in a state of morbid excitation. I do not dispute that in many of these cases one may be dealing with mere hallucinations, as which they are treated in the mentioned textbook. In my opinion science would go very wrong to designate as 'hallucinations' all such phenomena that lack objective reality, and to throw them into the lumber room of things that do not exist.

Furthermore, Schreber continues:

Science seems to deny any reality background for hallucinations … In my opinion this is definitely erroneous, at least if so generalized.

These quotations from Daniel Schreber demonstrate one of the most complex aspects of the nature of insight. This is the capacity to have an attitude towards abnormal experiences in others where one can recognize them as pathologic, but to deny the abnormality of the experience in oneself and to designate it as not being evidence of mental illness. This is the so-called *double book-keeping.*

The resulting refusal to cooperate with treatment and rehabilitation causes long-term suffering for the patients and their carers. It is this capacity of patients to understand their own illness that is evaluated clinically in *insight.* Like many other concepts, terminological confusion exists, with textbooks describing insight as the patient's capacity to form judgements about their own illness and mental state. In recent years, there has been a resurgence of interest in the concept with attempts to define it reliably and quantifiably and to study its correlates (Kumar and Sims, 1998).

Overview of the Concept

The attitude of the patient towards their illness has obvious clinical implications, and insight tries to assess the awareness of the patient concerning the impact their illness has had on their life and their capacity to adapt to the changes brought about by it. As a function, it is highly complex and has to do with an individual's evaluation of their self and nonself and their relatedness (see Chapter 12). In clinical practice, only certain aspects are given importance, such as the patient's awareness of illness and compliance with prescribed treatment. The assessment of insight assumes more importance in psychosis, as the incongruence between the patient's and others' view of their illness often leads to difficulties with treatment. The convention in psychiatry is that insight is unimpaired in nonpsychotic conditions, but it can be seen that a broader view nearer to the lexical definition is relevant when neurotic symptoms hamper the full realization of a person's potential.

DEVELOPMENT OF THE CONCEPT

Contributions to the development of the concept of insight derive from psychopathology, Gestalt psychology and psychoanalysis. In Gestalt psychology, insight is conceived as a sudden, unexpected solution to a problem. According to Marková (2005), the 'suddenness' specifies an abrupt solution to a problem, the 'unexpectedness' refers to the surprise element of the event and the term *solution to a problem* signals the discreteness of the event in time. In essence, in Gestalt psychology, insight is by definition related to a specific task, a problem that stands in need of solution in the external world. Furthermore, there has been extensive debate within Gestalt psychology about the nature of insight, whether it is a unique human facility that is also a specific cognitive skill. The fact that, in Gestalt psychology, insight refers to a problem in the external world distinguishes it from the concept of insight in clinical practice. In clinical practice, insight focuses on understanding of changes or happenings within an individual.

For Jaspers (1997), typically the patient's attitude to their illness involves 'an awareness of illness' in which the patient 'expresses a feeling of being ill and changed, but there is no extension of this awareness to all his symptoms nor to the illness as a whole. It does not involve any objectively correct estimate of the severity of the illness nor any objectively correct judgement of its particular type'. For Jaspers, 'only when all this is present and there has been a correct judgement of all the symptoms and the illness as a whole according to type and severity, can we speak of *insight* [emphasis in original]'. Thus for Jaspers, insight becomes manifest only when the patient is able to turn away from the content of their psychic experiences towards making a judgement about it and inquiring into its causes and reasons. Lewis' (1934) definition of insight as 'a correct attitude to morbid change in oneself' is a restatement of Jaspers' description of insight. Freud (1981) used the term *insight* to denote knowledge of illness but, on the whole, in psychoanalytic therapy the development of a deeper awareness of self is considered to be the goal of treatment. This is another way of saying that in psychoanalysis, insight refers to knowledge and understanding of one's unconscious mental processes. This is a more complex notion of insight because it involves the patient acquiring understanding of the unconscious motivations of their behaviour and, in the light of Freud's structure of the mind, it suggests a degree of depth of understanding.

David (1990) has proposed that insight is composed of the three overlapping dimensions described earlier. It has been suggested that parallels can be drawn between the loss of insight in psychiatric patients and the loss of awareness of disease of parts of the body in certain neurologic conditions. In cortical blindness, left-sided hemiplegia after stroke and amnesic syndrome, lack of awareness of disease is well recognized. The term *anosognosia* was coined by Babinski (1857–1932) to refer to the unawareness or denial of hemiplegia seen in patients after a stroke. There is a difference, however, between the lack of insight seen in psychiatry and the lack of awareness seen in neurologic disease. In psychiatry, lack of insight is often attended by a wider loss of judgement beyond merely the symptoms or their implications for the patient. In neurologic cases, the lack of awareness is focused on a discrete disability. Nonetheless, even though the lack of insight in psychiatry and lack of awareness of disease in neurology are not identical, it may be that comparisons may point to possible neurobiological bases that they share in common.

There is increasing interest in *cognitive insight* as opposed to clinical insight. *Cognitive insight* is a term derived from the work of Beck et al. (2004) and refers to a combination of self-reflection and the ability to question one's own conclusions. Cognitive insight is a core feature of metacognition, an aspect of cognition, which enables the ability to reflect on one's own thoughts, intentions, emotions and beliefs. It is an aspect of cognition that is fundamental to critical self-appraisal. Thus concepts of cognitive insight and metacognition are related to clinical insight, but wider. On the face of it, these ought to be predictably related, but empirical evidence of significant association is inconsistent (Pijnenborg et al., 2020).

There are certain philosophic problems when we consider insight in patients with psychosis. People without any psychiatric illness vary in their ability to know themselves and the consequences of their personalities. Because at least some conceptualizations of psychosis rely on the lack of insight as a defining feature, discussion concerning the concept can become circular. Added to this is the fact that varying degrees of insight can occur and that nonverbalization of insight may be different from the lack of it. Yet another problem is that a possibly specious model in which a 'normal' part of the mind is capable of passing judgement on the 'abnormality' of another part has to be entertained. This works for as long as the clinician recognizes that it is merely a way of speaking, not necessarily an accurate representation of how self-monitoring takes place. As David (2020) has suggested, the notion of cognitive insight, at least, makes it possible to start to conceive of clinical insight in the context of normal psychological processes, thereby expanding our comprehension of how impaired insight arises in the context of illness.

MEASUREMENT OF INSIGHT

Earlier attempts to measure insight centred on its role in psychodynamic therapies. Tolor and Reznikoff (1960) developed a test using hypothetical situations based on common defence mechanisms and found a correlation with intelligence. This test was used by Roback and Abramowitz (1979), who found a correlation in those with schizophrenia between greater subjective distress and better behavioural adjustment. The validity of this test for general clinical work is affected by the concept of insight being based on psychodynamic rather than psychopathologic features.

Any reliable and valid measure of insight in clinical practice should be based on the following four assumptions:

- insight is complex and multidimensional,
- cultural factors need to be taken into account,
- the level of insight can vary across the many manifestations of mental illnesses, and
- information about the nature of a person's illness from situations other than the interview should be taken into account (McGorry and McConville, 1999).

McEvoy et al. (1989a) developed a questionnaire to measure insight, defined as the patient's awareness of the pathologic nature of their experiences and also their agreement with the treating professionals about the need for treatment. The Insight and Treatment Attitudes Questionnaire (ITAQ) is a validated 11-item, semi-structured interview that generates a score from 0 (no insight) to 22 (maximum insight). Using this questionnaire, they found no correlation with aspects of acute psychopathology.

The Schedule for Assessment of Insight in Psychosis was published in 1992 (David et al., 1992) in which, apart from the recognition of mental illness and compliance with treatment, the ability to re-label unusual mental events as pathologic was also included. There were seven items with a maximum possible score of 14 and an additional item on hypothetical contradiction.

The Scale to Assess Unawareness of Mental Disorder (Amador and Strauss, 1993) is a much more comprehensive scale with six general items and four subscales, from which 10 summary scores can be calculated. Other scales available are the Global Insight Scale (Greenfield et al., 1989) and the self-reported Insight Scale for Psychosis (Birchwood et al., 1994). The scale by Marková and Berrios (1991) is more directed to evaluating aspects of self-awareness and less to clinical definition of insight with regard to illness. This is also true for the Beck Cognitive Insight Scale (Beck et al., 2004) that measures a wider notion of insight, encompassing patients' capacity for evaluating their anomalous experiences and their erroneous inferences. The scale is composed of two subscales: self-reflectiveness and self-certainty.

Other approaches have been to use the 'lack of insight and judgement' item of the Positive and Negative Syndrome Scale (PANSS; Kay et al., 1987) as a single global measure of insight, and the use of psychopathology vignettes. McEvoy et al. (1993) used vignettes that cast specific psychopathologic features in everyday language to judge whether patients demonstrated these features and the degree to which they attributed them to mental illness. They found that patients failed to acknowledge negative symptoms and failed to view positive symptoms as evidence of mental illness.

From earlier impressionistic assessments of a global nature, measurement of insight has more recently progressed to the use of operationalized definitions and standardized instruments. Although the different instruments might be measuring different aspects of a complex phenomenon, there is at least the freedom to choose one to suit specific clinical or research aims. There is an inverse correlation between insight, the severity of psychopathology and positive affective disturbance (Sanz et al., 1998).

SCHIZOPHRENIA

It is not really surprising that most of the research work on the clinical correlates of insight has been on patients with schizophrenia. McEvoy et al. (1989a) reported that insight as measured by the ITAQ did not correlate with either the severity of acute psychopathology or the changes in psychopathology with treatment. They speculated whether the mechanisms underlying the production of positive symptoms and disturbed insight were independent and whether the latter was more resistant to the effective use of neuroleptic medication. David et al. (1992) found that the 'total insight score' in their study had a moderate inverse correlation with the Present State Examination (Wing et al., 1974) total score, which was an indication of the global severity of the illness. Both David et al. (1992) and McEvoy et al. (1989b) found that, as a group, involuntary (that is compulsorily admitted) patients have less insight. Overall, it does appear that the relationship between poor insight and aspects of psychopathology is not linear but complicated by other factors, including compliance with treatment.

Another approach to investigating clinical insight in psychosis is to study help-seeking behaviour, which is construed as involving five steps, namely (1) the recognition that one has a problem, (2) acting on the recognition of the problem, (3) choosing where

to access help, (4) making contact and (5) disclosing the nature of the problem (Nordgaard et al., 2020). In this approach, the first step in help-seeking behaviour involves symptom perception, symptom evaluation and symptom interpretation. It is obvious that help-seeking behaviour overlaps with aspects of clinical insight. Nordgaard et al. (2020) report a qualitative study that demonstrates that our current notions of clinical insight are far too narrow as it ignores contextual factors. For example, in their study often patients recognize and identify that there is a problem 'I worried about some of the experiences that I have had, and I wanted to find an explanation? Is it because I'm a human being and some human beings just have some semi-experiences [sic]?' The decision on what to do about the experiences was often determined by the results of inquiries from others 'I asked my close friend how often he had such experiences- but he never did. That was unfortunate. then I asked about other experiences, but he also didn't recognize those. It made me sad to hear. Then I asked him if he thought I should see a doctor and he said it was probably a good idea'. And the decision about making contact with the identified source of help was influenced by fear of the consequences of disclosing the recognized aberrant experiences 'I was scared that I was going to end up in a, well, a crazy place, where people are just yelling and screaming'. The setting of clinical insight in the wider context of the literature on health beliefs and illness behaviour allows for a more comprehensive account of clinical insight, one that recognize the roles of society and culture in determining self-awareness and action. As Jacob (2020) argues, our notions of clinical insight need not devalue patients' beliefs and explanations as these are often consistent with local and culturally accepted explanations.

Insight and Cognitive Impairment

It has often been speculated that poor insight may have a neurologic basis. Lysaker and Bell (1994) found that subjects with impaired insight performed more poorly than subjects with unimpaired insight on the Wisconsin Card Sorting Test (WCST). They used the PANSS item of 'lack of insight and judgement' to measure insight. This item had been shown by factor analytical studies to be a member of the component composed of symptoms of cognitive impairment such as cognitive disorganization, poor attention, stereotyped thinking and poor abstract thinking. However, using a different methodology, Kemp and David (1996) failed to show a relationship between insight and neuropsychological deficits. It is possible that chronicity of the illness could be an additional variable, which predisposes to cognitive impairment. David et al. (1992) had found a relationship between aspects of insight and intellectual performance. Cuesta et al. (1995) failed to show any relationship between insight and poor performance on the WCST. However, the study did not use any of the standard rating scales to measure insight. In another study, Upthegrove et al. (2002) showed that impaired digit span as a measure of working memory was significantly associated with insight as measured by a standardized measure. Additionally, it is becoming clearer that insight correlates with indices of cognitive functions including measures of error monitoring, empathy and theory of mind (Pegaro et al., 2013; Pijnenborg et al., 2013; Kao et al., 2013). However, on balance, the exact nature and extent of these relationships is still unresolved. As in other clinical situations, the relationship may not be a straightforward one, as other variables, such as the chronicity of illness, treatment factors and gender may be involved.

OUTCOME

The relationship between insight and outcome is complex. First, greater insight seems to predict hopelessness, depression and suicide (Ampalam et al., 2012; Balhara and Verma, 2012; Schrank et al., 2014). Awareness of the adverse social implications of mental illness may be the mediating factor between insight and depression (Thomas et al., 2014). But definitely the relationships are complex. It has been shown that cognitive insight as opposed to merely clinical insight has a role in mediating between distress and depression in psychosis. Clinical insight is associated with less psychotic symptoms and better social functioning but paradoxically associated with depression, psychological distress and poorer subjective outcome. Cognitive insight, in particular the domain of self-reflexivity, on the other hand in the initial stages leads to increased awareness of sadness and grief about the experience of psychosis but ultimately may lead to reduced distress (García-Mieres et al., 2020).

Second, McEvoy et al. (1989c) found that patients with good insight were significantly less likely to be rehospitalized and tended to be more compliant with treatment 30 days after discharge; the overall relationship between insight and outcome closely approached statistical significance. Their measure of 'after-care environment', which aimed to reflect the degree to which others' efforts were helpfully invested in maintaining the patient in treatment, was not related to insight. Amador and Strauss (1993) also found their measures of insight to be correlated with the course of the illness.

Related to the issue of prognosis and outcome is compliance with treatment. The relationship between poor insight and poor compliance with treatment has been shown by Bartko et al. (1988), Lin et al. (1979) and McEvoy et al. (1989c).

The balance of evidence seems to be that higher levels of awareness of having an illness are associated with better medication compliance and clinical outcome (Amador et al., 1991) in schizophrenia. However, there is a risk of circularity of logic, in that some of the measures of insight are based on definitions of insight that include noncompliance. Moreover, compliance with prescribed treatment is a much more complex phenomenon affected by social factors and beliefs about health and sickness (Bebbington, 1995). It is also possible that the relationship between compliance and different aspects of insight may be different. David et al. (1992) found that treatment compliance was not strongly related to the ability to recognize one's own delusions and hallucinations and to re-label them as abnormal.

It is interesting that patients may comply with treatment, even though they do not believe themselves to be ill, if the social milieu is conducive (McEvoy et al., 1989b, 1989c). The role of health beliefs and illness representation in determining compliance with treatment is recognized, but how these interact with insight to influence treatment compliance has yet to be extensively studied. The domains of illness representation are identity (the label of the disease), causes (explanatory models), timeline (onset and anticipated duration), control (belief that self can influence outcome) and consequences (functional as well as other consequences) (Brownlee et al., 2000). What is obvious is that insight is not the only determinant of care-seeking and treatment adherence (see Nordgaard et al., 2020). McEvoy et al. (1993) proposed that insight would improve with attempts at psychosocial rehabilitation. This was further studied by Lysaker and Bell (1995) on a sample of patients with a diagnosis of schizophrenia or schizoaffective disorder. Earlier, Lysaker et al. (1994) had found insight as measured by the item on PANSS to be correlated with poor levels of work quality and participation in rehabilitative programmes. In their study reported in 1995, patients enrolled in vocational rehabilitative programmes were found to have improved insight after 5 months. This improvement was greater for patients with comparatively few cognitive deficits, echoing their earlier findings regarding a relationship with cognitive impairments. However, the lack of a control group limits the generalizability of the findings. It does seem an interesting suggestion that vocational rehabilitation can favourably affect insight in the absence of cognitive impairment. McEvoy et al. (1993) have proposed that enhanced self-esteem from rehabilitation may underlie improvement in insight.

So far, the discussion has centred on the role and influence of clinical or cognitive insight in determining the nature and quality of outcome. Thirioux et al. (2020) have suggested that empathy, which they conceptualize as the capacity to internally experience the other's thoughts through a process incorporating hetero-centred visuospatial perspective-taking and embodiment, is involved alongside cognitive insight in determining the quality of insight. This goes to show that a concept such as clinical insight that is simple and serviceable within the clinic may be a composite of several different cognitive skills that is complex and irreducible to simple notions.

BIPOLAR DISORDERS

Ghaemi et al. (1995) studied insight in patients in acute mania using the ITAQ and found that improvement in insight did not correlate with recovery from other symptoms. However, as in schizophrenia, poor insight was correlated with involuntary admission. Swanson et al. (1995) used the case vignette method to study insight in two groups of patients with schizophrenia and mania. They found a qualitative difference between mania and schizophrenia in that patients with schizophrenia but not mania had reduced awareness of features of their illness. However, although the

manic patients were aware of their symptoms, they did not agree that these emanated from a mental illness. Amador et al. (1994) and Michalakes et al. (1994), on the other hand, found no significant difference between patients with schizophrenia and mania on measures of insight. The former found that severely manic patients were similar to patients with schizophrenia on scores of insight, whereas depressed and schizoaffective patients had more insight. In conclusion, it seems to be that both schizophrenia and bipolar disorder patients have impaired insight, and the mediating factors may be severity of symptoms and cognitive impairment, especially working memory impairment (Varga et al., 2007).

CRITICISMS OF THE CONCEPT

The recent resurgence of interest in insight has had its share of criticism. Medical anthropologists have criticized the concept of insight for failing to recognize that people can have various culturally shaped frameworks to explain their illnesses, all possibly valid. From this point of view, the concept of insight is 'Eurocentric and essentially arrogant' (Perkins and Moodley, 1993), as it dictates that patients should, apart from agreeing that they are mentally ill and requiring treatment, also agree to reconstruct their experiences within the terms and concepts of Western psychiatry. Johnson and Orrell (1995) have reviewed work by social scientists on cultural and social variations in lay perceptions of mental illness and argue that these would influence insight. Social and cultural backgrounds influence perceptions of stigma from mental illness and the congruence of the patients with Western medical views of mental illness. The ability to re-label mental phenomena as abnormal may be less influenced by social factors compared with beliefs about the causation of mental illness. Although there are few studies in this area, evidence seems to be emerging that social and cultural factors are important in the diagnosis of poor insight. For example, differences in the ethnic background of the psychiatrist and the patient appear to influence the judgement of the former about insight (Johnson and Orrell, 1996).

AETIOLOGY OF IMPAIRED INSIGHT

Attempts to explain the causation of poor insight have focused on three hypotheses (Amador et al.,

1991; Lysaker and Bell, 1994). The first two focus on putative psychological mechanisms. It has been suggested that refusal to take prescribed medication, implying poor insight, is a wilful preference for the experience of psychotic phenomenology over drug-induced normality. The second formulation suggests that patients deny illness at a psychological level to help them cope with normal life as they recover from a psychosis. A third explanation has suggested that poor insight may have something to do with cognitive impairment, drawing on similarities with neurologic conditions such as anosognosia. As mentioned earlier, studies have found a significant correlation between impaired performance on the WCST and poor insight, suggesting that cognitive impairments resulting from frontal lobe deficits may underlie poor insight in schizophrenia. A fourth explanation is that disruption of neural mechanisms and networks underlying self- and other-monitoring are involved. In a 2012 study, patients with schizophrenia demonstrated less activation in the posterior cingulate cortex in the self- and other-reflection conditions and less activation in the precuneus in the other-reflection condition compared with healthy controls. Better insight was associated with greater response in the inferior frontal gyrus, anterior insula and inferior parietal lobule during self-reflection. In addition, better cognitive insight was associated with higher activation in ventromedial prefrontal cortex during self-reflection (van der Meer et al., 2013). More recently, there is the suggestion that symptom unawareness may be distinct from symptom misattribution and that this distinction may be underpinned by differing neurobiology as demonstrated by functional magnetic resonance imaging investigation (Shad and Keshavan, 2015). Clearly, there is still much to learn about the true nature of insight.

In the advent of the distinction between clinical and cognitive insight, there has been increasing interest in determining the underlying neural substrate for these distinct types of insight in psychosis. Pijnenborg et al. (2020) report from their systematic review and meta-analysis that poorer clinical insight was related to smaller whole brain grey matter and white matter volume and grey matter volume of the frontal gyri. Cognitive insight, on the other hand, was positively correlated with structure and function of the hippocampus and ventrolateral prefrontal cortex. In

essence, clinical insight is a reflection of spatially diffuse global and frontal abnormalities suggesting that clinical insight relies not on simple or discrete brain regions, but on a range of cognitive processes. They conclude that clinical insight is a complex construct with several partly overlapping dimensions that may be associated with functioning over several overlapping brain areas. These may involve error monitoring and correction, working memory and cognitive flexibility, and the ability to use explicit feedback of others to improve task performance. Finally, higher order social cognitive and self-oriented processes such as self-reflectiveness, affective mentalizing and empathy may be involved.

REFERENCES

Amador, X.F., Strauss, D.H., Yale, S.A., 1991. Awareness of illness in schizophrenia. Schizophr. Bull. 17, 113–132.

Amador, X.F., Strauss, D.H., 1993. Assessment of insight in psychosis. Am. J. Psychiatry. 150, 873–879.

Amador, X.F., Flum, M., Andreasen, N.C., 1994. Awareness of illness in schizophrenia and schizoaffective and mood disorders. Arch. Gen. Psychiatry. 51, 826–836.

Ampalam, P., Deepthi, R., Vadaparty, P., 2012. Schizophrenia—insight, depression: a correlation study. Ind. J. Psychol. Med. 34, 44–48.

Balhara, Y.P., Verma, R., 2012. Schizophrenia and suicide. East Asia Arch. Psychiatry. 22, 126–133.

Bartko, G., Herzog, I., Zador, G., 1988. Clinical symptomatology and drug compliance in schizophrenic patients. Acta Psychiatr. Scand. 77, 74–76.

Bebbington, P.E., 1995. The context of compliance. Int. Clin. Psychopharmacol. 9 (Suppl. 5), 45–50.

Beck, A.T., Baruch, E., Balter, J.M., Steer, R.A., Warman, D.M., 2004. A new instrument for measuring insight: the Beck Cognitive Insight Scale. Schizophr. Res. 68, 319–329.

Birchwood, M., Smith, J., Drury, V., 1994. A self-report insight scale for psychosis; reliability, validity, and sensitivity to change. Acta Psychiatr. Scand. 89, 62–67.

Brownlee, S., Leventhal, H., Leventhal, E.A., 2000. Regulation, self-regulation, and construction of the self in the maintenance of physical health. In: Boekartz, M., Pintrich, P.R., Zeidner, M. (Eds.), Handbook of Self-Regulation. Academic Press, San Diego.

Cuesta, M.J., Peralta, V., Caro, F., 1995. Is poor insight in psychotic disorders associated with poor performance on the Wisconsin card sorting test? Am. J. Psychiatry. 152, 1380–1382.

David, A.S., 1990. Insight and psychosis. Br. J. Psychiatry. 156, 798–808.

David, A.S., 2020. Insight and psychosis: the next 30 years. Br. J. Psychiatry. 217 (3), 521–523.

David, A.S., Buchanan, A., Reed, A., Almeida, O., 1992. The assessment of insight in psychosis. Br. J. Psychiatry. 161, 599–602.

Freud, A., 1981. Insight: its presence and absence as a factor in normal development. In: Solint, A.J., Eissler, R.S., Freud, A. (Eds.), The Psychoanalytic Study of the Child, vol. 36. Yale University Press, New Haven, CT.

García-Mieres, H., De Jesús-Romero, R., IDENTITY group, Ochoa, S., Feixas, G., 2020. Beyond the cognitive insight paradox: self-reflectivity moderates the relationship between depressive symptoms and general psychological distress in psychosis. Schizophr. Res. 8 (222), 297–303.

Ghaemi, S.N., Stoll, A.L., Pope, H.G., 1995. Lack of insight in bipolar disorder: the acute manic episode. J. Nerv. Ment. Dis. 183, 464–467.

Greenfield, D., Strauss, J.S., Bowers, M.B., 1989. Insight and interpretation of illness in recovery from psychosis. Schizophr. Bull. 15, 245–252.

Jacob, K.S., 2020. Insight in psychosis: a critical review of the contemporary confusion. Asian J. Psychiatr. 48, 101921.

Jaspers, K., 1997. General Psychopathology. J. Hoenig, M.W. Hamilton, Trans. The Johns Hopkins University Press, Baltimore.

Johnson, S., Orrell, M., 1995. Insight and psychosis: a social perspective. Psychol. Med. 25, 515–520.

Johnson, S., Orrell, M., 1996. Insight, psychosis and ethnicity: a case-note study. Psychol. Med. 26, 1081–1084.

Kao, Y.C., Liu, Y.P., Lien, Y.J., et al., 2013. The influence of sex on cognitive insight and neurocognitive functioning in schizophrenia. Prog. Neuro-Psychopharmacol. Biol. Psychiatry. 44, 193–200.

Kay, S., Fiszbein, A., Opler, L., 1987. The positive and negative syndrome scale (PANSS) for schizophrenia. Schizophr. Bull. 13, 261–276.

Kemp, R., David, A., 1996. Psychological predictors of insight and compliance in psychotic patients. Br. J. Psychiatry. 169, 444–450.

Kumar, T.M., Sims, A.C.P., 1998. Insight and its measurement in relation to psychosis. Psychiatry Update. 1, 13–18.

Lewis, A., 1934. The psychopathology of insight. Br. J. Med. Psychol. 14, 332–348.

Lin, I.F., Spiga, R., Fortsch, W., 1979. Insight and adherence to medication in chronic schizophrenics. J. Clin. Psychiatry. 40, 430–432.

Lysaker, P., Bell, M., 1994. Insight and cognitive impairment in schizophrenia: performance on repeated administrations of the Wisconsin card sorting test. J. Nerv. Ment. Dis. 182, 656–660.

Lysaker, P., Bell, M., 1995. Work rehabilitation and improvements in insight in schizophrenia. J. Nerv. Ment. Dis. 183, 103–106.

Lysaker, P., Bell, M., Milstein, R.M., 1994. Insight and treatment compliance in schizophrenia. Psychiatry 57, 289–293.

Marková, I., 1987. Human Awareness: Its Social Development. Hutchinson, London.

Marková, I.S., 2005. Insight in Psychiatry. Cambridge University Press, Cambridge.

Marková, I.S., Berrios, G.E., 1991. The assessment of insight in clinical psychiatry: a new scale. Acta Psychiatr. Scand. 86, 159–164.

McEvoy, J.P., Apperson, L.J., Appelbaum, P.S., 1989a. Insight in schizophrenia: its relationship to acute psychopathology. J. Nerv. Ment. Dis. 177, 43–47.

McEvoy, J.P., Applebaum, P.S., Apperson, L.J., 1989b. Why must some schizophrenic patients be involuntarily committed? The role of insight. Compr. Psychiatry. 30, 13–17.

McEvoy, J.P., Freter, S., Everett, G., 1989c. Insight and the clinical outcome in schizophrenia. J. Nerv. Ment. Dis. 177, 48–51.

McEvoy, J.P., Freter, S., Merritt, M., Apperson, L.J., 1993. Insight about psychosis among outpatients with schizophrenia. Hosp. Community Psychiatry. 44, 883–884.

McGorry, P.D., McConville, S.B., 1999. Insight in psychosis: an elusive target. Compr. Psychiatry. 40, 131–142.

Michalakeas, A., Skoutas, C., Charalambous, A., 1994. Insight in schizophrenia and mood disorders and its relation to psychopathology. Acta Psychiatr. Scand. 190, 46–49.

Nordgaard, J., Nilsson, L.S., Gulstad, K., Buch-Pedersen, M., 2020. The paradox of help- seeking behaviour in psychosis. Psychiatr. Q. 92 (2), 549–559. https://doi.org/10.1007/s11126-020-09833-3.

Pegaro, L.F., Dantas, C.R., Banzato, C.E., Fuentes, D., 2013. Correlation between insight dimensions and cognitive functions in patients with deficit or non-deficit schizophrenia. Schizophr. Res. 147, 91–94.

Perceval, J., 1840. A narrative of the treatment experienced by a gentleman during a state of mental derangement to explain the causes and the nature of insanity. In: Bateson, G. (Ed.), Perceval's Narrative: A Patient's Account of His Psychosis. Hogarth Press, London, pp. 1830–1832.

Perkins, R., Moodley, P., 1993. The arrogance of insight? Psychiatr. Bull. 17, 233–234.

Pijnenborg, G.H., Spikman, J.M., Jeronimus, B.F., Aleman, A., 2013. Insight in schizophrenia. Eur. Arch. Psychiatry Clin. Neurosci. 263, 299–307.

Pijnenborg, G.H.M., Larabi, D.I., Xu, P., et al., 2020. Brain areas associated with clinical and cognitive insight in psychotic disorders: a systematic review and meta-analysis. Neurosci. Biobehav. Rev. 9 (116), 301–336.

Roback, H.B., Abramowitz, S.I., 1979. Insight and hospital adjustment. Can. J. Psychiatry. 24, 233–236.

Sanz, M., Constable, G., Lopez-Ibor, I., Kemp, R., David, A.S., 1998. A comparative study of insight scales and their relationship to psychopathological and clinical variables. Psychol. Med. 28, 437–446.

Schrank, B., Amering, M., Hay, A.G., Weber, M., Sibitz, I., 2014. Insight, positive and negative symptoms, hope, depression and self-stigma: a comprehensive model of mutual influences in schizophrenia spectrum disorders. Epidemiol. Psychiatr. Sci. 23, 271–279.

Schreber, D., 1955. In: Memoirs of My Nervous Illness (I. MacAlpine, R.A. Hunter, Trans, Edited with Introduction, Notes and Discussion). Wm. Dawson and Sons Ltd, London.

Shad, M.U., Keshavan, M.S., 2015. Neurobiology of insight deficits in schizophrenia: an fMRI study. Schizophr. Res. 165, 220–226.

Surguladze, S., David, A., 1999. Insight and major mental illness: an update for clinicians. Adv. Psychiat. Treat. 5, 163–170.

Swanson, C.L., Freudenreich, O., McEvoy, J.P., 1995. Insight in schizophrenia and mania. J. Nerv. Ment. Dis. 193, 752–755.

Thirioux, B., Harika-Germaneau, G., Langbour, N., Jaafari, N., 2020. The relationship between empathy and insight in psychiatric disorders: phenomenological, aetiological, and neurofunctional mechanism. Front. Psychiatry. 10, 966.

Thomas, N., Ribaux, D., Phillips, L.J., 2014. Rumination, depressive symptoms and awareness of illness in schizophrenia. Behav. Cogn. Psychother. 42, 143–155.

Tolor, A., Reznikoff, M., 1960. A new approach to insight: a preliminary report. J. Nerv. Ment. Dis. 130, 286–296.

Upthegrove, R., Oyebode, F., George, M., Haque, M.S., 2002. Insight, social knowledge and working memory in schizophrenia. Psychopathology 35, 341–346.

van der Meer, L., de Vos, A.E., Stiekem, A.P., et al., 2013. Insight in schizophrenia: involvement of self-reflection networks? Schizophr. Bull. 39, 1288–1295.

Varga, M., Magnusson, A., Flekkoy, K., David, A.S., Opjordsmoen, S., 2007. Clinical and neuropsychological correlates of insight in schizophrenia and bipolar 1 disorder: does diagnosis matter? Compr. Psychiatry. 48, 583–591.

Wing, J.K., Cooper, J.E., Sartorius, N., 1974. Measurement and Classification of Psychiatric Symptoms. Cambridge University Press, Cambridge.

SELF AND BODY

The Disordered Self

Chapter Outline

KEYWORDS

Ego
Body image
Self-image
Autoscopy
Possession state

Summary

The *self* is a construct that has changed in meaning and significance over the years. There are five putative, formal characteristics of the self: ego vitality, ego activity, unity of the self over time, self-identity and boundary of the self. These formal aspects of the self can be impaired by psychiatric disorders. The sense of vitality can be impaired to produce a feeling of deadness, the extreme example being nihilistic delusions. In disorder of activity the 'my-ness' of actions, the sense of being an agent enacting one's will in the world, can be disrupted as occurs in passivity experiences. The unity of the self over time is markedly affected in autoscopy and dissociative identity disorders. Additionally, disorder of self-identity is illustrated by possession states and phenomena such as lycanthropy. Finally, abnormalities of the distinction between self and nonself (disturbance of boundary) are central to our understanding of such diverse experiences in schizophrenia as passivity experiences, thought insertion and thought withdrawal.

Often, when I was alone, I sat down on this stone, and then began an imaginary game that went something like this: 'I am sitting on top of this stone and it is underneath'. But the stone also could say 'I' and think: 'I am lying here on this slope and he is sitting on top of me'. The question then arose: 'Am I the one who is sitting on the stone, or am I the stone on which he is sitting?' This question always perplexed me, and I would stand up, wondering who was what now.

Jung (1963)

181

The self was never meant to be a solid object like a stone, a horse, or a weed, nor even a concept to be considered as semantically tantamount to changes in blood flow or test scores. Of course, patients with disordered minds do sport hurting, afflicted and cursing selves but not as they do carcinomas or broken legs. Their selves live in the same realm as do their virtues, vices, beliefs and aspirations, and that is where they should remain.

Berrios and Marková (2003)

Ego and Self

The *self* is a construct that has changed in meaning and significance since the inception of Hellenistic philosophy (Berrios and Marková, 2003). From the mid-19th century onwards, various concepts about the self have found their way into psychiatry such that, in contemporary psychiatry, there is reckoned to be some disturbance in the way one thinks about and estimates oneself; this, of course, differs according to the nature of the illness. There is, however, no consensus on what exactly it means to be a self. There is a plurality of conceptions, including the ecological self, the inter-personal self, the extended self, the private self and the conceptual self among many (Zahavi, 2003). In this chapter, the terms *ego* and *self* are used more or less interchangeably. *Ego* has the advantage of being a technical term and therefore more circumscribed in its meaning; this is also a disadvantage when it is simply oneself, as is usually understood and subjectively experienced, that is being referred to.

Freud's use of the word *ego* echoes Nietzsche (1901):

It is this which sees everywhere deed and doer; this which believes in will as cause in general; this which believes in the 'ego' as being, in the ego as substance, and which projects its belief in the ego-substance on to all things.

Freud (1933) described ego as standing 'for reason and good sense while the id stands for the untamed passions'. The ego:

has been modified by the proximity of the external world with its threat of danger… The poor ego has to serve three severe masters and does what it can to bring their claims and demands into harmony with one another.

These demands are always divergent and often seem incompatible. No wonder that the ego so often fails in this task. Its three tyrannical masters are the external world, the super-ego and the id.

Freud (1933)

Embodiment and the Self

There is a convention that separates out the body from the self. This approach dates back at least to Descartes' (1596–1650) dualism in which the body is regarded as distinct from the thinking immaterial self. More recently, there has been a growing body of work both empirical and philosophic that makes the case for a complex interaction between the fact we as persons are embodied, that is that our experiences as a physical being permeates and influences all the central features of consciousness such as thinking, memory, language and of course, the nature of self.

Gibbs (2005) put it like this:

People's subjective, felt experiences of their bodies in action provide part of the fundamental grounding for language and thought. Cognition is what occurs when the body engages the physical, cultural world and must be studied in terms of the dynamical interactions between people and the environment. Human language and thought emerge from recurring patterns of embodied activity that constrain ongoing intelligent behaviour. We must not assume cognition to be purely internal, symbolic, computational, and disembodied, but seek out the gross and detailed ways that language and thought are inextricably shaped by embodied action.

This approach has profound implications not only for how we conceive of the self but also for our understanding of perception, abstract concepts, language and cognitive processes, among other things. There is a natural link between a first person bodily perspective and the self in the brute sense that there can be no self without a body. Again as Gibbs (2005) puts it, 'I know who I am, and that I am, in part, because I see my body … as I move and experience specific sensations as a result of action'. And, the distinction that is drawn between self and nonself is, at least in part, shaped and influenced by the distinction between our body and the physical environment.

In summary, despite the deeply set convention to treat the self and the body as separate entities, it is important to keep in focus the fact the self and the body are truly inseparable and that the conceptual distinction is for convenience only.

Self-Concept and Body Image

The body is unique in that it is experienced by a person both as *subject* of experience and as an *object* with the same materiality as any other physical object in the world. There is a way in which I am subjectively aware of my own body that is different from how I experience a block of wood. But I am also aware that my body is an object in the world, to be viewed and even acted on by others. For most of the time, we are not aware of our body but, for example, in extreme anxiety, traumatic pain and sexual excitement, there is an awareness of the body as an object: 'my heart banging, my finger throbbing'. For the rest of the time, we assume the parts of the body to be integrated, and this integrated body, for practical purposes, coincides with and is coterminous with the 'self' of which we are not separately aware and which we take for granted. In other words it is mostly in times of distress or pain that we become aware of our bodies as distinct from 'ourselves'. It is through our body that we have contact with the world outside our self: movements of the body relate us to external space; our hands have a prehensile tool-like aspect to them that allow us to grasp objects in the world; and our bodies have a physicality about them that occupies space, gives us presence, locating us as objects in the world. One of Eugene Minkowski's (1970) patients said:

I don't want to attach so much attention to my movements, but I am only grub and defaecation. I am only a sort of animal function, and one that injures himself. I have the feeling of being nothing but living tripe. I have neither sensations nor precise ideas. I have the feeling of being nothing but vegetative functions, of being nothing but a mass.

Another said:

One day out of two, my body is hard as wood. Today my body is thick like this wall (points to the wall).

Minkowski referred to these experiences as exaggerated materiality in which the patients demonstrate an increased awareness of the 'objectified' aspect of the body and rendering salient for the clinician an attitude to the body that is not manifest in day-to-day life.

Many terms are used to describe the way a person conceptualizes themselves. Neurologists, neuropsychiatrists, psychoanalysts and psychologists have used variously the terms *body schema, body concept, body cathexis, body image* and *perceived body*. They describe approximately the same thing but with different nuances. For example, *self-concept* tends to refer to the fully conscious and abstract awareness of oneself, whereas *body image* is more concerned with unconscious and physical matters and includes experiential aspects of body awareness. Sometimes self-concept is the same as body concept, and at other times, conscious self is conceptualized as being independent of its 'cage', the body. The *body schema* implies a spatial element and is more than, and usually bigger than, the body itself. For instance, if you imagine yourself on your way to work, automatically included within your schema of yourself are your clothes and your spectacles, if worn. The body schema changes with changing circumstances. When I drive my car, I incorporate within my concept of my physical size the width of my car, so that I am unlikely to attempt to drive through a doorway or up a flight of steps. Spectacles, a cigar, the carpenter's screwdriver and the blind man's stick all contribute to that person's concept of their *self* in a particular situation. *Cathexis* implies the notion of power, force, libido—perhaps analogous to electrical charge: the self that makes things happen!

Social aspects are obviously important. A man with shoulder-length hair is not usually so endowed through neglect; more likely, it represents a deliberate choice—how he sees himself in his social setting. It accords with his chosen peer group and also distinguishes him from those from whom he would wish to be disassociated. Critchley (1950) has commented on 'that curious emotional state usually known as being in love', in which there is 'a compulsive trend in two body images of opposite sex towards propinquity and contiguity, eventually culminating in a total fusion or merger'. As a phenomenologist, one could take exception to Critchley's misuse of the term *compulsive*. According to Schilder (1935), body images are never isolated; they are always encircled by the body images of others. Body images are more closely bound together in the erogenous zones and are social in nature. Our body image and the way other people see us are not exclusively dependent on each other. A person sees themselves and forms their self-image in a social setting. They see themselves in relation to other people; their view of themselves is not totally dependent on, but importantly influenced by, how another individual sees them. It is also determined by how they *believe* that people might see them.

The development of body image has been neatly summarized diagrammatically by Bahnson (1969). He considers that self-image is changeable and amorphous. At any one time, the individual perceives only a small sample from a gallery of possible self-images. In Fig. 12.1 the manner in which '*phenomenological selves* are superimposed on each other like the layers of an onion' is demonstrated. Different aspects of self-image develop as the person increases the scope and complexity of his relationships. The term *ego* is not phenomenologically describable, and there has been argument that the self cannot observe itself; that is, a thing and what observes that thing cannot be the same. However, it is the nature of *self* and *ego* to be experienced as either subject or object: a small nuisance like a mouth ulcer can make me feel uncomfortable (subjectively); I can describe what a person with a mouth ulcer experiences (objectively).

Self-Image and Nonverbal Communication

In a social relationship, a person expresses views they have about themself: their words, and the way they say them, convey how they view their relationship with the other person and also how they see themself, for example, the shopkeeper 'talking down' to a child. Probably more important than this verbal manner of expressing, often unconscious, views on how we see ourselves is *nonverbal communication*. All gestures and postures, movements of the face and pauses in our conversation convey meaning to the person we are talking to; partly, this is also a comment on the way we see ourselves.

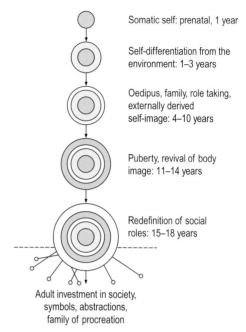

Somatic self: prenatal, 1 year

Self-differentiation from the environment: 1–3 years

Oedipus, family, role taking, externally derived self-image: 4–10 years

Puberty, revival of body image: 11–14 years

Redefinition of social roles: 15–18 years

Adult investment in society, symbols, abstractions, family of procreation

Fig. 12.1 Developmental phases of the self-image.

'The central core of self-image consists for a person of their name, their bodily feelings, body image, sex and age. For a man the job will be central – unless he is suffering from job alienation. For a woman, her family and her husband's job may also be important' (Argyle, 1975). The gender discrimination of that statement is now dated, but it emphasizes that for different people, there are varying aspects that form the essential concept of self. Nonverbal aspects of communication are important in sending and receiving information about the personality. The role in society one has adopted and the group with which one identifies are intentionally conveyed and therefore display self-image. These include 'age, sex, race, social class, rank, occupation, school or college attended, nationality, regional origins, religious group and family connections' (Argyle, 1975). These attributes of the person are often deliberately displayed, but there are other characteristics that will be received nonverbally by observers even when the person has no intention of revealing them, for example, temperament, personality traits such as introversion, intellect, beliefs and values and past experiences.

Nonverbal communication expresses the attitudes of a person, according to Argyle, for the following reasons:

- There is, in some areas of human concern, a lack of language or 'verbal coding'; for example, shape is more readily expressed with the hands than verbally. Describing personality, our own or another's, or commenting on personal relationships is more easily done nonverbally. A person will attempt to communicate nonverbally their own physical attractiveness, role and attitude towards the other person.
- Nonverbal signals are more powerful: actions speak louder than words. For a schoolteacher, beckoning may be more likely to result in action than a verbal order.
- Nonverbal signals are less censored and therefore more likely to be genuine. If conflicting messages are given verbally and nonverbally, the nonverbal signal is accepted as truthful.
- Some messages, because of social censorship, cannot be made explicit in a social setting and therefore cannot be verbalized but can be conveyed nonverbally by appropriate posture, gesture and movement in space. For example, by facial expression and turning away, a person might suggest without making it explicit 'I do not like you and am bored with speaking to you'.
- Verbal messages are punctuated and emphasized nonverbally, for example, the pause at the end of a phrase or the cadence of voice used. These embellishments add meaning to the actual words used.

A person interacts with others by the use of language. However, nonverbal signals are also important in expressing meaning and conveying feelings. The *ego* talks with the body as well as with words.

Awareness of the Body

We have an awareness of our self and an awareness, which overlaps with this but is slightly different, of our bodies. What is this sense of body image or awareness? According to Head and Holmes (1911), the *body schema* is formed as the composite experience of sensations. Schilder (1935) developed further the importance of perceiving sensations in forming the body schema: 'the picture of our own body which we form in our mind, that is to say, the way in which the body appears to ourselves'. Freud (1933) also was concerned with body image in the development of personality: 'the ego is firstly the body ego'. Clearly, abnormality of body image may be the result of abnormal sensations, but this is not always so. For instance, the abnormality of body image of an amputee is directly because of the physical damage, but a hypochondriacal patient may have no abnormal sensations yet believe they have cancer. In transsexualism, a man may have a normal sensory experience of his body but say that he hates his body and especially his penis; he may feel that he is actually a woman trapped inside a male body (Morris, 1974). His disturbed body image is not a result of disturbed sensation; there is a conflict between ego (the way he experiences himself and the gender he ascribes to it) and body image. The distinction made for convenience between this chapter and Chapter 14, between self-awareness and awareness of the body, is artificial.

The body image can be altered through enhancement, diminution (or ablation) or distortion. It incorporates more than just the body, except perhaps for those few occasions when a person is both unclothed and conceptualizing themself as naked: tailors have long tried to persuade us that 'clothes make the man'. Certainly, they are an effective means of nonverbal communication. Clothes give us some insight into the way a person sees themself and also in the way they propose to interact with other people. A person complements their mood and their social role of the moment in their choice of clothes. They wear clothes, as a ship hoists a flag, for signalling, and particular clothes are worn to convey a message to someone who can read it. A medical student wears a suit for an oral examination, a person undoes their collar button on leaving the office for lunch. As the patient comes into a doctor's consulting room, they start to give information about themself from their appearance before either of them utters a word. A person whose clothes are chosen for them, as in mental hospitals in the past, presents a peculiarly bleak and meaningless appearance;

this aspect of their body image is expressionless and conveys nothing of themselves.

🅢 Disorders of Self

In descriptive psychopathology, one uses the term *ego disorders* or *disorders of self* to describe the abnormal inner experiences of *I-ness* and *my-ness* that occur in psychiatric illness. These may occur in the patient's state of *inner awareness* irrespective of any changes they may show in their attitude to, or experience of, the world outside themself. Jaspers (1997), with characteristic clarity, described self-awareness—that is, the ability to distinguish I from *not I*—as having four formal characteristics. Scharfetter (1981, 1995, 2003) added a fifth dimension of *ego vitality* to the list and has made a case for its inclusion based on factor analysis. Previously, this characteristic was incorporated within the awareness of activity, which subsumed 'being' and 'existing' with other present participles. Thus we now have the following characteristics of self-awareness:

- *The feeling of awareness of being or existing* (ego vitality): I know that I am alive and exist, and this is fundamental to awareness of self.
- *The feeling of awareness of activity* (ego activity): I know that I am an agent who initiates and executes my thoughts and actions.
- *An awareness of unity* (ego consistency and coherence): at any given moment, I know that I am one person.
- *Awareness of identity* (ego identity): there is continuity in my biography, physiognomy, gender, genealogic origin, etc.; I have been the same person all the time.
- *Awareness of the boundaries of self* (ego demarcation): I am distinct from other things and beings and can distinguish what is *myself* from the *outside world,* and I am aware of the boundary between self and nonself.

The disorders of inner experience in which these characteristics are disturbed are now explored in more detail. We will deal with these five functions described by Jaspers and Scharfetter in order.

DISORDER OF BEING OR EGO VITALITY

I never have to ask myself the question as to whether I exist. It is an assumption that I make with unquestioning certainty. I am so sure of this that it does not even come on to the agenda of doubts and uncertainties.

My only knowledge that everything else exists is based on the premise that I do.

Being: the patient's experience of their very existence may be altered: 'I do not exist; there is nothing here' or 'I am not alive any more' or 'I am rotting'. This is the core experience of *nihilistic delusions,* which may occur in affective psychoses (see Chapters 8 and 16). See below for an example:

I do not sense myself anymore. I do not exist anymore. When someone speaks to me, I feel as if he were speaking to a dead person. I have to look at myself to be sure that it is I. I have the feeling of being an absent person. In sum, I am a walking shadow.

Minkowski (1970)

Less pronounced nihilistic ideas (not delusions) are experienced as *depersonalization,* an alteration of the way one experiences oneself, which is accompanied by a feeling of an alteration or loss of significance for self: 'I feel unreal, a bit woozy, as though I can't be quite certain of myself any more'.

DISORDER OF ACTIVITY

I do something and know that I am doing it. Everything I do, in everything I experience, through every event that impinges on me, I am aware that the experience has the unique quality of *being mine.* 'It was incredible. I pinched myself to make sure it was really happening to me' expresses the relationship we experience between awareness of reality and activity. It is in our actions, including our thinking, that we reinforce ourselves concerning our existence.

Moving may show abnormality—for example, in the passivity experience or delusions of control of patients with schizophrenia. Schreber described several examples of this experience:

The difficulties which were put in my way defy description. My fingers are paralysed, the direction of my gaze is changed in order to prevent my finding the correct keys, the tempo is quickened by making the muscles of my fingers move prematurely: all these were and still are daily occurrences.

and

the bellowing-miracle when my muscles serving the processes of respiration are set in motion by the lower

God (Ariman) in such a way that I am forced to emit the bellowing noises.

Memorizing and *imagining* may be changed in that the patient with depression feels they are unable to initiate the act of memory or fantasy, or, alternatively, a patient with schizophrenia feels that this activity when it occurs is not initiated by them but from outside themself. A depressed patient said, 'my memory has gone, I have no thoughts, I cannot think at all'.

Willing may be altered—for example, the patient with schizophrenia who no longer experiences their will as being their own. Commonly, neurotic patients describe an inability to initiate activity, a feeling of powerlessness, of being ground down in the face of life's vicissitudes.

Some of these abnormalities of experience of one's own activities are closely associated with mood—for example, the feeling of the depressed patient who believes that they are incapable of doing anything at all: the alteration of self-concept is directly linked to the mood state. Sometimes, however, it is not the affect associated with the change of activity but the belief about the initiation of the activity that is changed. These are the passivity experiences (made experiences), which are discussed in more detail with other first-rank symptoms of schizophrenia in Chapter 9.

DISORDER OF SINGLENESS OR EGO CONSISTENCY AND COHERENCE

In health, a person is integrated in their thinking and behaviour so that they are not aware of their feeling of unity. There is an implicit assumption that they are one person, and they know their limitations and capabilities. This assumption of unity may be lost in some conditions. In *dreams,* one sometimes sees oneself, even perhaps with some surprise, in the drama. In some forms of transcendental meditation, by carrying out repetitive monotonous acts the subject enters a *self-induced* trance in which they can observe themself carrying out the behaviour. 'Self' is both the observer and also the object of observation (Box 12.1).

Autoscopy (Heautoscopy)

Autoscopy is a profoundly conceptually challenging phenomenon in which the usual indivisibility of the self appears to be compromised. According to

---

BOX 12.1 DISORDERS OF SINGLENESS

- There are six types of autoscopy: feeling of presence, negative autoscopy, inner autoscopy, autoscopic hallucination, out-of-body experience, heautoscopy proper.
- Feeling of presence is a distinct feeling of the physical presence of another person.
- Negative autoscopy refers to the failure to perceive one's own body either in a mirror or when looked at directly.
- Inner autoscopy refers to the experience of visual hallucinations of internal organs in extra corporeal space.
- Out-of-body experience is characterized by the projection of an observing (psychological) self in extra personal space seemingly totally dissociated from the physical body.
- Heautoscopy designates a condition in which an individual sees his double, or doppelgänger.

Fish (1967), 'in this strange experience the patient sees himself and knows that it is he. It is not just a visual hallucination because kinaesthetic and somatic sensation must also be present to give the subject the impression that the hallucination is he'. More recently, Brugger and Regard (1997) have identified six types of autoscopy: the *feeling of presence*, *negative heautoscopy*, *inner heautoscopy*, *autoscopic hallucination*, *out-of-body experience* and *heautoscopy proper*.

In the *feeling of presence,* the patient has a distinct feeling of the physical presence of another person. No visual perception is usually reported. The feeling of presence may be confined to one hemispace especially when the experience occurs in association with a seizure.

Negative heautoscopy refers to the failure to perceive one's own body either in a mirror or when looked at directly. This phenomenon is often associated with depersonalization. *Inner heautoscopy* refers to the experience of visual hallucinations of internal organs in extra-corporeal space (Sollier, 1903). *Autoscopic hallucination* is said to occur when a patient sees an exact mirror image of themself, or of their face or trunk. This experience is distinct from *heautoscopy proper* because the patient does not localize themself in the position of the mirror image. These hallucinatory experiences are usually brief, lasting seconds to minutes and followed by flash-like recurrences (Lhermitte, 1951; Dewhurst and Pearson, 1955; Brugger, 2002).

Out-of-body experiences are characterized by the projection of an observing (psychological) self in extra-personal space seemingly totally dissociated from the physical body. In this phenomenon, the patient sees themself and the world from a location distinct from their physical body. There are three phenomenological characteristics here: disembodiment, the impression of seeing the body from a distant and elevated visuo-spatial perspective (the so-called *extra corporeal egocentric perspective*) and the impression of seeing one's own body from this elevated position (Anzellotti et al., 2011).

Heautosocpy proper designates a condition in which an individual sees their double or *doppelgänger*. The double usually appears colourless, can behave independently and may or may not mirror the patient's appearance. There is strong self-identification with the second body, often associated with the experience of existing at and perceiving the world from two places at the same time (Heydrich and Blanke, 2013). There may be vestibular sensations such as extreme lightness of the body, sensation of flying, elevation, rotation and vertigo (Anzellotti et al., 2011; Blanke et al., 2004). There is a North European myth, shared by several countries, that someone may see their *double* ('wraith', 'fetch') shortly before their death, and it has therefore become a sinister omen (Todd and Dewhurst, 1962). These authors present interesting historical material to substantiate the link between perceptual doppelgänger and death. The usual legend is that, as the person lies dying, their wraith floats before their eyes, and they see themself performing all the most disreputable and reprehensible actions of their life; they are paraded before them as they expire.

There is continuing popular interest in the concept of the double. It is the subject of diverse fiction as in *The Double* by Fyodor Dostoevsky (1846), Robert Louis Stevenson's *The Master of Ballantrae* (1889) and Shusaku Endo's *Scandal* (1986). The very worst feature of the double for the subject themself is well illustrated in William Styron's *Darkness Visible* (1991). The terrible, inextricable involvement of the double with the subject in trying to mortify them, goad them, provoke them to destroy the double and/or destroy themself;

the sense of being accompanied by a second self – a wraith-like observer, able to watch with dispassionate curiosity as his companion struggles against the oncoming disaster, or

decides to embrace it … I, the victim-to-be of self-murder, was both the solitary actor and lone member of the audience … I watched myself in mingled terror and fascination.

There is growing evidence that autoscopic phenomena occur in association with seizures (Anzellotti et al., 2011). Furthermore, it has been postulated that autoscopy derives from a failure of integration of proprioceptive, tactile and visual information about the body accompanied by vestibular dysfunction (Blanke et al., 2004; Heydrich and Blanke, 2013). The anatomic basis and mechanism of autoscopy is yet to be clarified, but there is tentative evidence that the left posterior insular is involved in heautoscopy and right occipital cortex in autoscopic hallucination (Heydrich and Blanke, 2013). Because of the hypothesis that autoscopy is a failure of integration, the multimodal junctions between the parietal and temporal lobes and between the parietal and occipital lobes have been implicated. There is experimental work deriving from the application of transmagnetic stimulation of the left temporoparietal junction to produce heautoscopy (*doppelgänger*) (Blanke and Arzy, 2005).

In practice, these phenomena can be extremely difficult to identify and delineate. The following description by a 37-year-old, intelligent man with a history of epilepsy, receiving treatment with phenobarbitone, is considered an example of autoscopic hallucination, but analysis demonstrates features of heautoscopy as well as out-of-the-body experience. The patient held his head rigidly with apparent torticollis to the right. If he rotated it to the left, there was marked head nodding, but not if he turned it further to the right.

I'm standing outside myself on the left hand side but only when I'm sitting down … it comes in short episodes for about 30 seconds … my true self loses all its senses as all the senses are in my hallucinatory self … the true self is just a shell without any senses … the hallucinatory self can see the true self and the whole surroundings, and it seems to me as though the hallucinatory self is looking at me and at other things in the room from a position standing to the left hand side of me, and everything is in the right perspective. If it was occurring now, the hallucinatory self would see you more full face and from higher up than I see you now because it is standing … I can't see it or hear it but it can see the side of my head.

It seems to be there. I know that it isn't me as such. It's like having a dream and you know that it is a dream. I thought it was a dream but it has occurred when I am fully waking. It seems as clear as a nightmare at the time but I know afterwards that it is a figment like a very vivid dream but more real than a dream. I would not see a fleck of dust on my cheek or something like that. The other one is not a different personality.
When this experience occurred, the patient felt all sensation was in the 'hallucinatory self', including hearing, seeing and feeling cold: 'I felt cold on the back of the hallucinatory self'. There had been no experience of taste or smell but there had been an experience of affect. I was talking to a representative. The hallucinatory self felt sorry for this man because he looked abnormal. It had no feelings for the real self. He looked abnormal because I had stopped talking and a glazed expression had come into my eye.

A bizarre example of autoscopy was reported by Ames (1984): the self-shooting of a phantom head. This patient was suffering from schizophrenia. He described seeing and hearing a voice from another head that was set on his own shoulders, attached to his body and trying to dominate his own head. He described himself as having two heads but believed that the other head was actually that of his wife's gynaecologist, whom he believed to be having an affair with her. The voice from the second head was that of the gynaecologist, and there were also the voices of Jesus and Abraham around him, conversing with each other and talking about his having two heads. The patient tried to remove the other head by shooting six shots at it and through his own palate, causing extensive damage to his brain. Ames labelled this condition the *phenomenon of perceptual delusional bicephaly*.

Multiple Personality (Dissociative Identity Disorder)

In dissociative (hysterical) states, so-called dual and multiple personalities have been described (McDougall, 1911; Abse, 1982; Prince, 1905). Slater and Roth (1969) comment:

A girl who is by turns 'May' and 'Margaret', may be quiet, studious and obedient as May, and unaware of Margaret's existence. When she becomes Margaret,

however, she may be gay, headstrong and wilful, and refer to May in contemptuous terms. It seems that these multiple personalities are always artificial productions, the product of the medical attention that they arouse.

The essence of multiple personality is the embodiment of at least two personalities (identities). This phenomenon raises doubts about our natural intuition that an individual human being is indivisible and is an embodied singular person. Prince's account gave a vivid description:

Miss Christine L Beauchamp, the subject of this study, is a person in whom several personalities have become developed; that is to say, she may change personality from time to time, often from hour to hour, and with each change her character becomes transformed and her memories altered. In addition to the real, original or normal self, the self that was born and which was intended by nature to be, she may be anyone of the three persons. I say three different, because, although making use of the same body, each nevertheless, has distinctly different character: a difference manifested by different trains of thought, by different views, and temperament, and by different acquisitive tastes, habits, experiences, and memories.

In a characteristic case study of multiple personality before the conditions for medical practice in the United States resulted in a proliferation of cases of so-called multiple personality disorder, Larmore et al. (1977) described 'a 35-year-old white woman of rural Kentucky background' who had made seven suicide attempts of which she claimed to have no memory. 'Shortly after admission a hypnotic interview was conducted, during which one of the personalities spontaneously revealed herself and gave hints of the existence of other personalities'. Four distinct personalities were identified: *Faith*, 'the primary personality ... known as "the little angel" by personality Alicia ... kind, loving and helpful ... has difficulty in expression ... anger, and in dealing with criticism'; *Alicia*, 'a Satanic agent ... claims control over most of Faith's physiological functions ... manifesting either assaultive or self-destructive behaviour'; *Alicia–Faith*, under the influence of Alicia, 'has only peripheral awareness of Alicia and no knowledge of Faith or Guardian Angel'; *Guardian Angel,* 'first made its appearance following the grandfather's death … claims to be the protector of Faith'.

There has been a vast output of psychiatric literature on the subject of multiple personality disorder based initially on the diagnostic criteria of the third revision, revised, of the Diagnostic and Statistical Manual of Mental Disorders (DSM) (American Psychiatric Association, 1987) and renamed Dissociative Identity Disorder in DSM-5 (American Psychiatric Association, 2013) but often lacking in psychopathologic precision. This has been well summarized by Fahy (1988):

Recently there has been a dramatic rise in the number of case reports of multiple personality disorder (MPD) … A review of the recent literature reveals a poverty of information on reliability of diagnosis, prognosis, or the role of selection bias. It is argued that iatrogenic factors may contribute to the development of the syndrome. There is little evidence from genetic or physiological studies to suggest that MPD represents a distinct psychiatric disorder.

Abse states that 'one-way amnesia' is usual for multiple personality; that is, personality A is amnesic for the other personality B, but the second, B, can discuss the experiences of A. Usually, A is inhibited and depressed and B is freer and more elated. The forms of multiple personality seen in practice are usually:

- simultaneous partial personalities,
- successive well-defined partial personalities, or
- clustered multiple partial personalities.

When such patients have been treated in psychotherapy, ingenious explanations are often given by patient and by therapist for the appearance of the additional personalities. Although this remains a disputed area, an authoritative opinion from Merskey (2000) states:

In this author's view there is no place for the diagnosis of multiple personality disorder in psychiatry, and the important question is how such a diagnosis managed to achieve so much prominence in professional circles in North America, although generally not elsewhere.

Lability in the Awareness of Personality

The loss of unity of self in schizophrenia was exemplified by a patient who described how, every night, he became a horse and trotted down Whitehall. At the same time as this was happening in his mind, he also believed he was in Whitehall watching the horse. This type of symptom has been called *lability in the awareness of personality* and was described by Bonhoeffer (1907) as occurring in paranoid psychosis.

DISORDER OF IDENTITY

I am who I was last week or 30 years ago; I am who I will be next week or in 10 years' time. This truism, which we can claim without hesitation, is by no means certain for some people suffering from schizophrenia or organic states, from neuroses or from depression, or even for some healthy people in abnormal situations (see possession state later in the chapter). This disorder of self-awareness is characterized by changes in the identity of self *over time.*

A person who feels threatened in their job and is afraid of redundancy is not likely to function well because of their feeling of impermanence. A *feeling of continuity* for oneself and one's role is a fundamental assumption of life, without which competent behaviour cannot take place. In health, we have no doubts about the continuity of oneself from our past into our present. However, patients with schizophrenia sometimes deny that they have always been the same person. Characteristically, this takes the form of a *passivity experience,* and the patient claims that at some time in the past they *have been* completely changed from being one person to another, whom they now are. Jaspers (1997) gives an account of one patient who said:

When telling my story I am aware that only part of my present self experienced all this. Up to 23rd December 1901, I cannot call myself my present self; the past self now seems like a little dwarf inside me. It is an unpleasant feeling; it upsets my feelings of existence if I describe my previous experiences in the first person. I can do it if I use an image and recall that the dwarf reigned up to that date, but since then his past has ended.

This complete alteration in the sense of identity is exclusively psychotic; there is a break in the sense of identity of self, and there is a subjective experience of someone completely different, although still described as oneself, 'taking over'.

A feeling of loss of continuity, which is, however, of lesser intensity than the psychotic change described earlier and without its element of passivity, may be experienced in health and in neuroses and personality disorders. The person knows that both people, before and after, are truly them, but they feel very altered from what they were. This may occur after an overwhelmingly important life situation or during emotional development without an outside event. For example, an adolescent may quite suddenly feel in the course of a week 'as if' they are quite a different person. It should be stressed that the sense of reality is never lost to the extent that they actually believe themself to be a different person. In the nonpsychotic, it is more that thoughts and feelings do not seem to be in keeping with their previous self as they have come to accept themself.

In the next chapter, a man is described as developing long-term depersonalization after experiencing massive stress at work, culminating in an extremely harassing journey in which he was the car driver. Afterwards, his wife said that he was never again like the man she had married, 'but like his (nonexistent) twin brother'. She said that, whereas previously he was incisive, was quick thinking and made the decisions in the family, now he lacked self-confidence and she had to do everything. Neither partner was in any doubt that he was the same person, but his whole demeanour had changed *as if* he had become someone similar but not identical.

The feeling of loss of continuity contributes to the inertia of the person with schizophrenia and the apathy of the depressive. Lack of a clear sense of identity from the past continuing into the future is a strong disincentive to concerted activity. The patient with schizophrenia, as part of disturbance of passivity, may have doubts about his continuity from the past to the present; the depressive, secondary to disorder of mood, often sees no continuation into the future: 'everything is bleak, there is nothing to look forward to'.

A part of the sense of continuity of self is accepting that the changes in one's total state at present are *due to illness*. This is the characteristic usually described in the mental state examination under the term *insight* (David, 1990). The individual recognizes that he is still the same person but that his current change in subjectivity is due to the intervening process of illness.

Possession State

This is classified in the 10th revision of the *International Classification of Disease* under dissociative (conversion) disorders (F44)—trance and possession disorders (F44.3) (World Health Organization, 1992). However, although the trance or altered state of conscious awareness is a prerequisite, possession state does not necessarily occur in the context of dissociative or hysterical disorder. It can occur in normal, healthy people in unusual situations, either as a group phenomenon (mass hypnosis) or individually; such a case is described subsequently. There is a *temporary* loss of both the sense of personal identity and full awareness of the surroundings. The person acts as if they have, and believes themself to have been, taken over by another—a spirit, a force, a deity or even another person. The difference between those conditions that constitute disorder and those that may be considered as being within a cultural or religious context alone is that the former are unwanted, cause distress to the individual and those around and may be prolonged beyond the immediate event or ceremony at which it was induced.

Possession of a young, entirely healthy woman with a husband and three children by two 'goddesses' was witnessed in Sri Lanka. The woman had become a *varama,* a healer with special powers, about 2 years previously, when she 'saw' her deceased father-in-law, who came to her and said that she would have supernatural power to help other people and her own family. Her husband had become addicted to *arak,* a local spirit, and his drinking had by then brought the family into extreme economic hardship. After this experience, she offered her services as a healer and solver of domestic difficulties to her village, and several people consulted her each day at home, where she had devoted one tiny room to a sanctuary and another to a waiting room. With her husband blowing a buffalo horn repeatedly and herself chanting, she induced a trance in herself in which she spoke with different voices as either one of two female deities giving advice to her clients, which her husband interpreted. The villagers had found her ministrations to be helpful, it gave useful occupation to her delinquent husband and she had completely solved her own family's financial problems through the gifts she received for services rendered.

A different case, with psychiatric disorder present, was that of a 37-year-old Sri Lankan housewife who believed herself to be possessed by her long-dead grandmother; on three occasions she had gone into a trance, lost contact with the outside world and seen the image of her grandmother coming close to her and trying to squeeze her neck. These episodes were described with fear and distress. She showed symptoms of depressive illness, with poor sleep, early morning wakening, loss of appetite and weight, anergia, fatigue and feeling low in mood; she had been abandoned by her mother when she was 7 years old.

Wijesinghe et al. (1976) surveyed a semiurban population of 7653 people in Sri Lanka and identified 37 subjects, 9 male and 28 female, with 'possession trance states', showing altered state of conscious awareness, behaviour for which the subject did not acknowledge responsibility, and had amnesia for the period of the trance. Episodes, often lasting about 30 minutes, were usually precipitated either by emotional stress or culture-bound stimuli such as witnessing an exorcism ceremony. During trance, subjects were most often restless with rhythmic trembling of the trunk and exaggerated gesturing, speech was aggressive and commanding and, typically, mood was angry; most often, the possessing spirit was that of a close but dead relative. In females especially as the condition continued they were increasingly likely to become permanent adepts. These authors regarded only one of their subjects as suffering from schizophrenia, although 17 of 37 manifested active psychiatric disorder, mostly neurotic in nature.

Possession and trance states straddle the boundary between normative behaviour and abnormal behaviour indicative of a disorder. Moreira-Almeida and Cardeña (2011) argue that lack of personal suffering, absence of social or functional impairment, absence of psychiatric comorbidity, self-control over the experience and personal growth all point in the direction of a nonpathological spiritual experience. It is clear, however, that possession and trance states can occur in the setting of indubitable neurologic disease such as lesions in the basal ganglia and frontoparietal lobes (Basu et al., 2002), hence the need to have an integrative model that is grounded in neuroscience but admits sociocultural processes informed by aspects of how the self is socially constructed (Seligman and Kirmayer, 2008).

Jaspers (1997), in writing about disorders of self-awareness, concerned himself with disorder of content as well as of form. In discussing states of possession, he commented on the rare condition of *lycanthropy*, the patient believing that he has been transformed into an animal, literally a wolf. *Lycanthropy* has a long history in Western societies and identical beliefs of transformation into other feared animals such as the fox in Japan, the tiger, hyena and crocodile in China, Malaysia and India are documented (Fahy, 1989). In antiquity there was belief in the possibility of radical physical transformation of the human body into that of a wolf. However, recent case reports have adopted a robust phenomenological approach and identify the belief of transformation as a delusion of nonspecific value but principally associated with mood disorders, schizophrenia and occasionally organic brain disease (Keck et al., 1988; Fahy, 1989; Kulick et al., 1990). Lycanthropy is usually a transient belief but occasionally the belief can be enduring, lasting for many years (Keck et al., 1988). Koehler et al. (1990) reviewed Jaspers' work in relation to lycanthropy and showed that Jaspers differentiated between states of possession presenting with an altered consciousness and states of possession in which consciousness remains clear; the former were usually dissociative (hysterical) in origin, whereas the latter were more often associated with schizophrenia. This emphasizes the importance for psychiatric diagnosis in assessing psychopathologic form.

DISORDER OF THE BOUNDARIES OF SELF OR EGO DEMARCATION

Disorder of the boundaries of the self refers to the disturbance in knowing where *I* ends and *not I* begins. Abnormality is not confined to schizophrenia. For example, in lysergic acid diethylamide intoxication, the feeling of impending ego dissolution associated with the feeling of self 'slipping away' with considerable anxiety has been described (Anderson and Rawnsley, 1954). One subject put this as:

I was being disorganized … the world around was looking very distorted indeed … things were pretty rocky so I decided to sit back quietly for a moment and reassure myself by returning to my own private inner world. As soon as I introspected in this manner I felt to my dismay that 'I' myself was somehow disturbed. The central core of the personality, the ego, the sense of personal identity, was itself fluctuating and, for want of a better phrase, dissolving.

Another subject said, 'If anyone present went out of the room it felt as though I were being deprived of something. I became smaller—definitely felt vulnerable'.

Boundaries of Self in Schizophrenia

In schizophrenia, the sense of invasion of self appears to be fundamental to the nature of the condition as it is experienced; many but not all *first-rank symptoms* have in common permeability of the barrier between the individual and their environment, loss of ego boundaries (Sims, 1993). There is a merging between *self* and *not self*; this is clearly portrayed in Fig. 12.2, painted by a young patient with schizophrenia. The patient is not aware of the disturbance being one of ego boundaries; he describes a problem only inasmuch as 'other people are doing things to me; events are taking place outside myself'. The external observer finds a blurring or loss of the boundaries of self that is not apparent to the patient himself.

All *passivity experiences* falsely attribute functions to *not self* influences from outside, which are actually coming from inside the self. This is also true for disorders of the possession of thought, such as thought insertion and thought withdrawal. Thought broadcasting obviously involves private thoughts becoming public without the consent or action of the patient. This is another example of a breakdown in the normal boundaries of what is self and nonself. Other experiences, such as *auditory hallucinations*, rely on the patient ascribing internally generated activity, that is, internal speech, to external agencies.

Passivity, *delusion of control*, is discussed in Chapter 9. The subjective experience of passivity is a disorder of the distinction between what is and what is *not self*. Sensations, emotions, impulses and actions that in objective reality come from inside the self are ascribed to *not self*.

Other Alterations to Boundaries

In states of *ecstasy*, there are also disturbances in the boundaries of self (Chapter 16). The participant might describe feeling at one with the universe, merging with

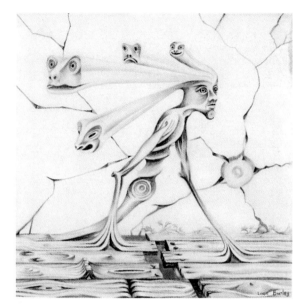

Fig. 12.2 Picture by a young schizophrenic patient.

nirvana, experiencing unity with the saints, identifying with the trees and flowers or a oneness with God. Ecstasy states occur in normal people and in those with personality disorder, as well as in sufferers from psychoses and in epilepsy. In epilepsy it is part of the aura and is characterized by intense feelings of well-being and heightened self-awareness. It is thought to emanate from hyperactivation of the anterior insula rather than the temporal lobe (Picard and Craig, 2009). This alteration in awareness of the boundaries of self is different from that of schizophrenia described earlier. In ecstasy, it is an *as if experience,* and it is mediated affectively.

The phenomenon described by Jung in himself with which this chapter begins is a lack of definition of the boundaries of self. However, there was no loss of reality judgement; it was a game, and Jung did in fact know what was himself and what was the stone. In psychosis, this ability to discriminate is lost. A patient with schizophrenia said, 'I am invaded day and night. I have no more privacy since television came inside me'. Another patient believed that while he was in a hospital ward he was helping other patients because he permeated the medical staff and thereby assisted them in their work.

REFERENCES

Abse, W., 1982. Multiple personality. In: Roy, A. (Ed.), Hysteria. John Wiley, Chichester.

American Psychiatric Association, 1987. Diagnostic and Statistical Manual of Mental Disorders, third ed., revised. American Psychiatric Association, Washington, DC.

American Psychiatric Association, 2013. Diagnostic and Statistical Manual of Mental Disorders, fifth ed., revised. American Psychiatric Association, Washington, DC.

Ames, D., 1984. Self-shooting of a phantom head. Br. J. Psychiatry 145, 193–194.

Anderson, E.W., Rawnsley, K., 1954. Clinical studies of lysergic diethylamide. Monatsschr. Psychiatr. Neurol. 128, 38–55.

Anzellotti, F., Onofrj, V., Maruotti, V., et al., 2011. Autoscopic phenomena: case report and review of literature. Behav. Brain Funct. 7, 2.

Argyle, M., 1975. Bodily Communication. Methuen, London.

Bahnson, C.B., 1969. Body and self-images associated with audiovisual self-confrontation. J. Nerv. Ment. Dis. 148, 262–280.

Basu, S., Gupta, S.C., Akhtar, S., 2002. Trance and possession like symptoms in a case of CNS lesion: a case report. Indian J. Psychiatry 44, 65–67.

Berrios, G.E., Marková, I.S., 2003. The self and psychiatry: a conceptual history. In: Kircher, T., David, A. (Eds.), The Self in Neuroscience and Psychiatry. Cambridge University Press, Cambridge.

Blanke, O., Arzy, S., 2005. The out-of-body experience: disturbed self-processing at the temporo-parietal junction. Neuroscientist 11, 16–24.

Blanke, O., Landis, T., Spinelli, L., Seeck, M., 2004. Out-of-body experience and autoscopy of neurological origin. Brain 127, 243–258.

Bonhoeffer, K., 1907. Klinische Beiträge zur Lehre von den Degenerationspsychosen. Alt's Samml, vol. 7. Marhold, Halle.

Brugger, P., 2002. Reflective mirrors: perspective-taking in autoscopic phenomena. Cognit. Neuropsychiatry 7, 179–194.

Brugger, P., Regard, M., 1997. Illusory reduplication of one's own body: phenomenology and classification of autoscopic phenomena. Cogn. Neuropsychiatry 2, 19–38.

Critchley, M., 1950. The body image in neurology. Lancet 1, 335–341.

David, A.S., 1990. Insight and psychosis. Br. J. Psychiatry 156, 798–808.

Dewhurst, K., Pearson, J., 1955. Visual hallucinations of the self in organic disease. J. Neurol. Neurosurg. Psychiatry 18, 53–57.

Dostoevsky, F., 1846. The Double (C. Garnett, Trans, 1913). Heinemann, London.

Endo, S., 1986. Scandal. Penguin Books, London.

Fahy, T.A., 1988. The diagnosis of multiple personality disorder: a critical review. Br. J. Psychiatry 153, 597–606.

Fahy, T.A., 1989. Lycanthropy: a review. J. R. Soc. Med. 82, 37–39.

Fish, F.J., 1967. Clinical Psychopathology. John Wright, Bristol.

Freud, S., 1933. New introductory lectures on psychoanalysis. Standard Edition of the Complete Works of Sigmund Freud, vol. 22 (J. Strachey, Trans, 1964). Hogarth Press, London.

Gibbs, R.W., 2005. Embodiment and Cognitive Science. Cambridge University Press, Cambridge.

Head, H., Holmes, G., 1911. Sensory disturbances from cerebral lesions. Brain 34, 102–254.

Heydrich, L., Blanke, O., 2013. Distinct illusory own-body perceptions caused by damage to posterior insula and extrastriate cortex. Brain 136, 790–803.

Jaspers, K., 1997. General Psychopathology (J. Hoenig, M.W. Hamilton, Trans). The Johns Hopkins University Press, Baltimore.

Jung, C.G., 1963. Memories, Dreams, Reflections. Collins Routledge and Kegan Paul, London.

Keck Jr., P.E., Pope, H.G., Hudson, J.I., McElroy, S.L., Kulick, A.R., 1988. Lycanthropy: alive and well in the twentieth century. Psychol. Med. 18, 113–120.

Koehler, K., Ebel, H., Vartzopoulos, D., 1990. Lycanthropy and demonomania: some psychopathological issues. Psychol. Med. 20, 629–633.

Kulick, A.R., Pope, H.G., Keck Jr., P.E., 1990. Lycanthropy and self-identification. J. Nerv. Ment. Dis. 178, 134–137.

Larmore, K., Ludwig, A.M., Cain, R.L., 1977. Multiple personality – an objective case study. Br. J. Psychiatry 131, 35–40.

Lhermitte, J., 1951. Visual hallucination of the self. Br. Med. J. 1, 431–434.

McDougall, W., 1911. Suggestion in Encyclopaedia Britannica, eleventh ed. University Press, Cambridge.

Merskey, H., 2000. Conversion and dissociation. In: Gelder, M.G., López-Ibor, J.J., Andreasen, N.C. (Eds.), New Oxford Textbook of Psychiatry. Oxford University Press, Oxford.

Minkowski, E., 1970. Lived Time: Phenomenological and Psychopathological Studies. Northwestern University Press, Evanston, IL.

Moreira-Almeida, A., Cardeña, E., 2011. Differential diagnosis between non-pathological psychotic and spiritual experiences and mental disorders: a contribution from Latin American studies to the ICD-11. Rev. Bras. Psiquiatr. 33 (Suppl. 1), S21–S36.

Morris, J., 1974. Connundrum. Faber and Faber, London.

Nietzsche, F., 1901. In: The Will to Power (W. Kaufmann, R.J. Hollingdale, Trans, 1968). Vintage Books, New York.

Picard, F., Craig, A.D., 2009. Ecstatic epileptic seizures: a potential window on the neural basis for human self-awareness. Epilepsy Behav. 16, 539–546.

Prince, M., 1905. The Dissociation of a Personality. Longman, New York.

Scharfetter, C., 1981. Ego-psychopathology: the concept and its empirical evaluation. Psychol. Med. 11, 273–280.

Scharfetter, C., 1995. The Self-Experience of Schizophrenics: Empirical Studies of the Ego/Self in Schizophrenia, Borderline Disorders and Depression. Private publication, Zurich.

Scharfetter, C., 2003. The self-experience of schizophrenics. In: Kircher, T., David, A. (Eds.), The Self in Neuroscience and Psychiatry. Cambridge University Press, Cambridge.

Schilder, P., 1935. The Image and Appearance of the Human Body: Studies in the Constructive Energies of the Psyche. Kegan Paul, London.

Seligman, R., Kirmayer, L.J., 2008. Dissociative experience and cultural neuroscience: narrative, metaphor and mechanism. Cult. Med. Psychiatry 32, 31–64.

Sims, A.C.P., 1993. Schizophrenia and permeability of self. Neurol. Psychiatry Brain Res. 1, 133–135.

Slater, E., Roth, M., 1969. Personality deviations and neurotic reactions. In: Mayer-Gross, W., Slater, E., Roth, M. (Eds.), Clinical Psychiatry, third ed. Baillière Tindall and Cassell, London.

Sollier, P., 1903. L'autoscopie interne. Revue Philosophique 55, 1–41.

Stevenson, R.L.B., 1889. The Master of Ballantrae. Collins, London.

Styron, W., 1991. Darkness Visible. Jonathan Cape, London.

Todd, J., Dewhurst, K., 1962. The significance of the Doppelgänger (hallucinatory double) in folk-lore and neuropsychiatry. Practitioner 188, 377–382.

Wijesinghe, C.P., Dissanayake, S.A.W., Mendis, N., 1976. Possession trance in a semi-urban community in Sri Lanka. Aust. N. Z. J. Psychiatry 10, 135–139.

World Health Organization, 1992. The ICD-10 Classification of Mental and Behavioural Disorders: Clinical Description and Diagnostic Guidelines. World Health Organization, Geneva.

Zahavi, D., 2003. Phenomenology of self. In: Kircher, T., David, A. (Eds.), The Self in Neuroscience and Psychiatry. Cambridge University Press, Cambridge.

Depersonalization

Chapter Outline

KEYWORDS

Depersonalization
Derealization

Summary

Depersonalization is a subjective state of unreality in which there is a feeling of estrangement, either from a sense of self or from the external environment. Frequently, it is accompanied by the symptom of *derealization*, a term denoting a similar feeling of unreality with regard to awareness of the external world. The localization of this feeling of unreality to a selected part of the body is called desomatization. There may be experience of changes of size or quality, for example, appearing large or small, empty, detached or filled with water or foam. Deaffectualization has been used to describe the consistent loss of the capacity to feel emotion, so that the person seems unable to cry, love or hate. These experiences are associated with anxiety and mood disorders and organic disease such as epilepsy and traumatic brain injury. Depersonalization can also be triggered by the use of cannabis, hallucinogens, ecstasy and alcohol. It can be a brief or long-lasting experience. It is invariably distressing to the patient:

I may be looking with some degree of attentiveness at a tumbler. As long as I say to myself that this tumbler is a glass or metal vessel made for the purpose of putting liquid into it and carrying it into one's lips without upsetting it – as long as I am able to represent the tumbler to myself in a convincing manner – so long shall I feel that I have some sort of relationship with it, a relationship close enough to make me believe in its existence and also, on a subordinate level, in my own. But once the tumbler withers away and loses its vitality … reveals itself to me as something with which I have no relationship, once it appears to me as an absurd object – then from that very absurdity springs boredom, which when all is said and done is simply a kind of incommunicability and the capacity to disengage oneself from it.

Alberto Moravia (1960)

Definitions and Descriptions

Depersonalization is the term used to designate a peculiar change in the awareness of self, in which the individual feels *as if* they are unreal (Sedman, 1972). It is best to reserve the use of the word to this *as if* feeling rather than the experience of unreality that occurs in psychosis. The *as if* prefix is used by the patient, to denote that they are not using words literally (how could they know what it would be like not 'fitting into the world', as all their experience has been in the world?). They are expressing uncertainty and painting a picture, and 'as if' is the best way they can do it. It has been considered that, after depression and anxiety, depersonalization is the most frequent symptom to occur in psychiatry (Stewart, 1964), and 12-month prevalence estimates for depersonalization and derealization in a rural population are put at 19.1% and 14.4% (Aderibigbe et al., 2001).

Schilder (1928), whose classic monograph in 1914 was a turning point in the study of depersonalization, wrote:

To the depersonalized individual, the world appears strange, peculiar, foreign, dream-like. Objects appear at times strangely diminished in size, at times flat. Sounds appear to come from a distance. The tactile characteristics of objects likewise seem strangely altered. Patients characterize their imagery as pale, colourless and some complain that they have altogether lost the power of imagination. The emotions likewise undergo marked alteration. Patients complain they are capable of experiencing neither pain nor pleasure; love and hate have perished with them. They experience a fundamental change in their personality, and the climax is reached with their complaints that they have become strangers to themselves. It is as though they were dead, lifeless, mere automatons. The objective examination of such patients reveals not only an intact sensory apparatus, but also an intact emotional apparatus. All these patients exhibit natural affective reactions in their facial expressions, attitudes, etc.; so that it is impossible to assume that they are incapable of emotional response.

BOX 13.1 COMPONENTS OF DEPERSONALIZATION

- Emotional numbing
- Changes in body experience
- Changes in visual experience
- Changes in auditory experience
- Changes in tactile experience
- Changes in gustatory experience
- Changes in olfactory experience
- Loss of feelings of agency
- Distortions in the experiencing of time
- Changes in the subjective experience of memory
- Feelings of thought emptiness
- Subjective feelings of an inability to evoke images
- Heightened self-observation

After Sierra, M., Berrios, G.E., 2001. The phenomenological stability of depersonalization: comparing the old with the new. J. Nerv. Ment. Dis. 189, 629–636, with permission.

Depersonalization has been defined by Fewtrell (1986) as a subjective state of unreality in which there is a feeling of estrangement either from a sense of self or from the external environment.

A more comprehensive definition has been given by Ackner (1954a). Definitive features are as follows:

- Depersonalization is always subjective; it is a disorder of experience.
- The experience is that of an internal or external change characterized by a feeling of strangeness or unreality.
- The experience is unpleasant.
- Any mental functions may be the subject of this change, but affect is invariably involved.
- Insight is preserved.

Excluded from depersonalization are:

- the experience of unreality of self when there is delusional elaboration,
- the ego boundary disorders of schizophrenia, and
- the loss or attenuation of personal identity.

An even more comprehensive description is given in Sierra and Berrios (2001). The symptoms are listed in Box 13.1. There is consensus that there are four or five principal domains including (1) anomalous body experience, (2) emotional numbing, (3) anomalous subjective recall, (4) alienation from surrounding and (5) body distortion (Sierra, 2009).

The relationship between depersonalization and various theoretical aspects of self-perception in phenomenology has been reviewed by Mellor (1988), who discusses the influences of Jaspers (1997), Mayer-Gross (1935), Schilder (1920) and Schneider (1958) on the concept. Mellor comments on the frequency of the condition and the variety of different psychiatric illnesses with which it may be associated. It may occur with organic psychosyndromes including traumatic brain damage (Grigsby and Kaye, 1993), epilepsy and migraine (Lambert et al., 2002), cannabis, hallucinogens and ecstasy (Matthew et al., 1993; Simeon et al., 2009). It is associated with mood disorders and anxiety disorders including social anxiety (Simeon et al., 1997; Michal et al., 2005). The depth of depression is positively correlated with depersonalization, and in depressed patients with anhedonia, depersonalization was present in 75% of cases (Zikić et al., 2009).

Although the symptom has been described for longer, the term was used by Heymans (1904) and by Dugas and Moutier (1911). The earliest theories implicate the sensory system, but loss of mood and loss of feelings were also prominent in early descriptions (Sierra and Berrios, 1997). Frequently, depersonalization is accompanied by the symptom of *derealization*, a term used by Mapother (1935) to denote a similar change in the awareness of the external world. Depersonalization and derealization often go together, because the ego and its environment are experienced as one continuous whole. However, in Mayer-Gross' cases, about a quarter of patients had depersonalization without derealization, and 15% had only derealization. This relationship between depersonalization and derealization is confirmed in the study by Baker et al. (2003), namely that depersonalization occurs as a primary condition in 71% and is associated with derealization in 73% of cases such that both can effectively be regarded as a single condition. Pure derealization does occur too but is rare. The less a patient takes himself for granted, the more unfamiliar and alien the world around them becomes (Scharfetter, 1980). A young female patient said:

I felt as if I didn't fit into the world … When I saw the moon, I felt I couldn't cope. One day it wasn't there and the next it was. I saw it and it upset me and I went to pieces … I felt I did not want to be alive because I was not related to anything. I just seemed totally out of everything and I started to cry. I couldn't cope with the hurt and the pain. I felt I never would feel part of anything.

It is important to realize that depersonalization, the experience, like other nonpsychotic phenomena, occurs in healthy, normal people. Some people may have feelings of 'not being quite themselves … looking in on themselves from the outside' and so on, without provocation. Others may have such experiences at times of powerful emotional stimuli or life crisis of any valence: extreme happiness, falling in love, the loss of bereavement or intense fear or anger. The actual self-description of depersonalization is similar irrespective of context. Dixon (1963), for example, showed that 46% of college students had experienced symptoms of depersonalization over a 12-month period, and Sedman (1966) reported that 70% of medical students had experienced symptoms of depersonalization in a lifetime. These reports go to show that it is not only that symptoms of depersonalization occur in normal populations but that they are quite common.

There is one particular feature described by patients and not occurring in the depersonalization that healthy people, especially children, may experience spontaneously in states of fatigue, after prolonged sleep deprivation or under sensory deprivation. This is the patient's description of the experience being intensely unpleasant and distressing (Ackner, 1954a). It may subjectively be much the worst symptom in an affective, reactive illness. A young married woman said:

I feel very weird in my head. I have a great deal of torment. My mind will not leave me alone. It's the surroundings; I cannot get my mind to myself. I felt as though I was going to fall over. I feel as if I'm lost in a fog. I just feel as if I'm not in my head. I feel numb.

The symptom is described in a number of ways, and it is often impossible to make a distinction between depersonalization and derealization: 'everything seemed to be going away from me'. The five qualities of the experience of self described in Chapter 12 may each be involved in the description of symptoms, although always with this *as if* character: vitality, activity, singleness, identity (continuity) and boundaries or definition. There is virtually always other evidence of disturbance of mood present: depression or anxiety or both. Coupled with this is a feeling of loss of self-esteem as a very prominent symptom: 'I feel unreal, flat, not properly there, less of a person, as though I can't go and get stuck in'; that is, the feeling of unreality about oneself or one's environment has implications for lack of competence in relationships. The patient not only feels unreal but also 'detached'; there is a barrier to normal communication.

At this point, it is important to emphasize the distinction between depersonalization as a symptom, occurring associated with many psychiatric conditions or no disorder at all, and depersonalization as a syndrome. In their detailed description of the symptoms of depersonalization disorder, based on classic descriptions from authors in the 19th and early 20th centuries, Sierra and Berrios (2001) have listed the following four symptoms as most prevalent for diagnosis: emotional numbing, changes in visual perception, changes in the experience of the body and loss of feelings of agency. In a more recent study, Simeon et al. (2008) demonstrated that the Cambridge Depersonalization Scale (Sierra and Berrios, 2000) yielded five factors: numbing, unreality of self, perceptual alterations, unreality of surroundings and temporal disintegration. In addition, patients with depersonalization appear to have impaired ability to generate visual imagery compared with normal control subjects. However in these individuals with impaired imagery, there was no associated abnormality of perceptual processes as measured by a battery of visual perception tests (Lambert et al., 2001).

These symptoms are sometimes included with a description of depersonalization but, for the sake of clarity, should be separated and regarded as different psychopathologic phenomena. Disturbances of body image or schema, disorder of subjective time sense, hypochondriacal preoccupation, *déjà vu* phenomena or metamorphopsia (the distortion of visually perceived objects) may be described by the same individual and may occur as symptoms of depersonalization syndrome. Langfeldt's (1960) inclusion of schizophrenic passivity experiences within the term *depersonalization* is confusing, and these experiences should be excluded from depersonalization, both as a symptom and as a disorder.

SUBJECTIVE EXPERIENCE OF DEPERSONALIZATION

Depersonalization is difficult for the doctor to portray; more important, it is also extraordinarily difficult for the patient to describe. They often preface their attempts at description by embarrassed statements such as 'sometimes I think I must be going mad' or 'you will think me very peculiar when I tell you this doctor, but …' Then follows a halting and perplexed list of disjointed, unpleasant experiences that the patient feels to be unique and for which they are unable to construe metaphors that satisfy them. Because of their failure in description, they believe that others will find these symptoms either bogus or clear evidence of imminent madness, so they omit them from their initial account even though such symptoms are common among psychiatric patients and cause enormous suffering. Depersonalization is the symptom the patient has when they experience themself as being altered or deficient in some manner; derealization is its equivalent with regard to their experience of things outside themself, that is, of the external world. Because there is no definite and easily ascertained boundary containing self, it is not always easy to decide whether the disorder is depersonalization or derealization. Neither is this important: they merge and overlap and are often simply included within the term *depersonalization*. The hallmark of depersonalization is the 'as if' quality of the experience. This is best understood as the patient's attempt at describing an anomalous experience that is difficult, if not impossible, to capture in language such that the patient is forced to use tentative terms such as *seem like*, *feel like* and *as if* to introduce some analogy to best represent the experience.

There is always a change in mood with depersonalization: the patient loses the *feeling* of familiarity they have for themself or for the world outside themself. They may describe themself as feeling like a puppet: hollow, detached and strange; on the outside; uninvolved with life; not themself; like a ghost, not solid; a stranger to themself. They experience a loss of emotion. Similarly, with derealization they may describe their environment as flat, dim in colour, smaller, distant, cloudy, dream-like, still, 'nothing to do with me' and also lacking in emotional significance.

Depersonalization is common but yet to the patient so obscure and unpleasant that, whenever the description of symptoms is interrupted by the patient's baffled hesitancy, they should be questioned with possible depersonalization symptoms in mind. Their relief at finding someone prepared to listen, and even perhaps understand, is often enormous. Schilder (1935) has described these symptoms as follows:

In a case of depersonalization the individual feels completely changed from what he was previously. This change is present in the ego (self) as well as in the outside world and the individual does not recognize himself as a personality. His actions appear to him as automatic. He observes his actions and behaviour from the point of view of a spectator. The outside world is foreign and new to him and is not as real as before.

Schilder is using the word *personality* here to refer to the whole person, not only personality in the modern sense of the word. This changed awareness of self and its relationships with the environment is always experienced as being intensely unpleasant.

The localization of this symptom to an individual organ is called *desomatization*. There are many different possible parameters in the awareness of different organs: changes of size or quality—for example, appearing large or tiny, empty, detached or filled with water or foam. Sometimes the body or parts of it may be experienced as nonexistent: 'I do not feel I have a body'. The patient may have a feeling of their legs being weightless, of floating or of simply being unfamiliar. Koro, a culture-bound disorder described by Yap (1965) (see also Chapter 8 of this volume), is sometimes described as an example of depersonalization. It is probably best to regard this condition as a culture-specific manifestation of acute anxiety in which the patient believes their penis is shrinking and fears that it will ultimately disappear. Although there may be associated feelings of unreality and watching the drama as a spectator, the primary underlying abnormality is one of intense anxiety. There are reports of a loss of the feeling of agency, that is, as if actions occur as a mechanical process unrelated to the patient. In some patients there are also reports of heightened self-scrutiny (Sierra, 2009).

Change of feeling concerning the body or depersonalization may be associated with distortion of time sense, when the passage of time appears altered in some way: 'time, both past and present, seems quite unreal to me, as if it had never happened and was never going to happen'. Sometimes, the complaint is that memories of events seem to have happened

to somebody else. *Deaffectualization* has been used to describe the consistent loss of the capacity to feel emotion, so that the person seems unable to cry, love or hate (Anonymous, 1972). Indeed, some patients are unable to have an emotional response to music or retain empathy for the suffering of others.

A patient says, 'I am going mad inside my head'; on further questioning, they are describing finding their own mental processes to be strange. The feeling of familiarity that occurs when a person perceives previously known objects (opening the front door at home and looking inside) also occurs when one introspects into one's own thinking (remembering or *fantasizing* my front hall). I know what is there in my thoughts; I know what I will think about any particular object, because it is unlikely to be very different from what I thought about it last time. I also know, in general terms, what I will think about myself because of past experience. It is this assumed certainty that disappears; the loss of familiarity of oneself occurring in depersonalization, or of outside self in derealization, is similar to the abnormality of the feeling of familiarity occurring in *jamais vu* (when there is no sense of previously having seen a well-known object) and its opposite, *déjà vu* (when an unfamiliar object or experience seems to be familiar). This association between the subjective experiences in depersonalization and *déjà vu* phenomena (including *jamais vu*) and commonality in alteration in the feeling of familiarity has been known since the work of Heymans at the beginning of the 20th century (Sno and Draaisma, 1993).

Like other aspects of self-experience, depersonalization has social and situational aspects. Frequently, the person feels that they are less able to accept themself, their personality, their behaviour than other people accept their own. They consider that their feelings about themself, their loss of reality, is unique. This is a barrier to their giving an account of their symptoms, and this in its turn is a barrier to communication in all areas of life. They feel themself to be different, isolated and estranged from others. Depersonalization is an experience within an individual, but it has considerable social consequences.

It frequently occurs in attacks that may be of any duration, from seconds to months. Typically, in depersonalization disorder the altered state lasts for a few hours, in temporal lobe epilepsy for a few minutes and in anxiety disorder for a few seconds. Improvement is usually first manifested in a gradual increase in time free from symptoms rather than a reduction in the symptoms themselves when present. However, it can present as with a chronic nonremitting course.

Onset may be insidious and with no known initiating cause, or it may be in response to a trigger. The most common immediate precipitants are severe stress, depression, panic and marijuana ingestion (Simeon et al., 2003). A middle-aged man who described his depersonalization 'like something supernatural—my body separated from me—a lost feeling' vividly recalled his first attack at the age of 11, when undergoing anaesthesia for the reduction of a fracture. Subsequent attacks felt similar despite the absence of provocation. He had also experienced attacks of sleep paralysis since age 25 and had discovered that by keeping himself awake until very tired, he would fall asleep more quickly and thus avoid it. Another man was severely stressed by his quite unreasonable working conditions, hours of work, unsympathetic employer and difficult car journeys in the course of his work. Early one winter morning, he had an appalling journey through fog along crowded motorways blocked by accidents, and ultimately suffered a lapse of recall for 24 hours in which he remembered nothing of driving to another town, registering himself into a hotel, ordering a meal, hanging up his clothes tidily and going to bed. His next memory was arriving at a local hospital the next day. He remained depersonalized for years subsequently, and his wife described this as 'he's not the man I married; it's like his twin brother'.

Depersonalization is frequently situational, both in its original context and in its repeated occurrences. Factors commonly associated with symptom exacerbation are negative affects, stress, perceived threatening social interaction and unfamiliar environments (Simeon et al., 2003). Many policemen who were involved in a major disaster at a football ground described depersonalization among other symptoms of post-traumatic stress disorder, sometimes lasting for years subsequently (Sims and Sims, 1998). One man described feeling 'switched off … I felt I wasn't on this planet any more'. Because depersonalization occurs at times of great stress, it may occur in the perpetrator of antisocial behaviour (e.g., violent crime), as well as in the victim. Rix and Clarkson (1994) give an account of a man who savagely assaulted his wife with a large spanner: 'It was as if it was a dream or a nightmare. I realized later what I had done but at the time it was as if I wasn't there'. It was considered that depersonalization in this case was linked to dissociation, that although it represented a change in the individual's self-experience it did not affect his volition or intent.

Although in the two preceding cases depersonalization was associated with dissociation, it is important to regard these experiences as distinct phenomena. Empirical evidence also suggests that these experiences, even when associated, are different and do not lie on a continuum (Putnam et al., 1996; Simeon et al., 1998). Neither does depersonalization occur with any greater frequency in chronic dissociative disorders such as dissociative identity disorder (Ross, 1997).

Self-induced episodes of depersonalization, as an unpleasant symptom, have been recorded after particular patterns of behaviour. Thus Kennedy (1976) described self-induced depersonalization persisting as a complaint after transcendental meditation and yoga.

Organic and Psychological Theories

Theories accounting for the occurrence of depersonalization, including organic, psychological, psychoanalytical and those linking it with schizophrenia, were reviewed by Sedman (1970). Depersonalization is regularly cited as a common symptom associated with organic states, especially temporal lobe epilepsy (Sedman and Kenna, 1965). This is based on the contention of Mayer-Gross (1935) that depersonalization is a *preformed functional response* of the brain, that is, a nonspecific mechanism resulting from many influences on the brain, occurring in an idiosyncratic way in individuals in a similar manner to epileptic fits or delirium. He was, in this, following the neurophysiologic hierarchical concepts of Hughlings Jackson (1884), who considered that the highest levels of cerebral function were lost first, leaving uninterrupted the activity of lower levels.

Organic theories purporting to account for depersonalization would suggest that alteration of consciousness acts as a release mechanism. However, Sedman (1970), in reviewing the literature, showed that, even in various forms of organic psychosyndromes, the incidence of depersonalization phenomena was similar to that found in the general population, at between 25% and 50%; in more severe chronic organic psychosis, the rate was lower. From a variety of studies, no quantitative relationship had been demonstrated between the degree of *torpor* (i.e., the stage on the continuum from full alertness to unconsciousness) and the development of depersonalization. On studying the performance of depersonalized subjects on psychosomatic tests, there did not appear to be evidence to support a specific relationship between clouding of consciousness and depersonalization. There appeared to be many individuals who, despite various types of assault on their brains, never developed depersonalization.

From this information, Sedman (1970) concluded that:

there may well be a built in preformed mechanism in approximately 40 per cent of the population to exhibit depersonalization; that the factors which initiate such a response are not specifically those associated with clouding of consciousness; or where clouding of consciousness appears to be playing a part, it may well be the presence of another common factor that is more relevant.

Thus the relationship between depersonalization and brain pathology remains unclear. Depersonalization is certainly not pathognomonic of organic diseases; in fact, there is no organic or psychotic abnormality in the vast majority of sufferers.

The state of increased alertness observed in depersonalization is considered by Sierra and Berrios (1998) to result from activation of prefrontal attentional systems and reciprocal inhibition of the anterior cingulate, leading to experiences of 'mind emptiness' and 'indifference to pain'. The lack of emotional colouring, reported as feelings of unreality, would be accounted for by a left-sided prefrontal mechanism with inhibition of the amygdala. Some authorities describe left-hemispheric frontotemporal activation coupled with decreased left caudate perfusion (Hollander et al., 1992; Phillips and Sierra, 2003), while others' reports emphasize the role of anxiety and the consequent downregulation of emotional processing in the limbic system (Sierra and David, 2011). There are reports of functional imaging abnormalities in regions involved in integration of sensory perception such as the inferior temporal sulcus and right posterior cingulate (Sierra et al., 2014), which align contemporary developments with Ackner's (1954b) original hypothesis that depersonalization is a problem of integration of experience rather than one of perception.

Depersonalization is sometimes associated with self-induced organic states. Thus it occurs after the ingestion of alcohol or drugs, especially psychomimetics such as lysergic acid diethylamide (Sedman and Kenna, 1964), mescaline, marijuana or cannabis (Szymanski, 1981; Carney et al., 1984; Simeon et al., 2009) and with sensory deprivation. It is also described as a side effect with prescribed psychotropic drugs such as the tricyclic antidepressants, but because of the common association between depersonalization and depression, it may be difficult to attribute causation.

Neurochemical findings have identified possible involvement of serotonergic, endogenous opioid and glutamatergic N-methyl-D-aspartic acid pathways. Additionally, there is evidence of widespread metabolic alterations in the sensory association cortex as well as prefrontal hyperactivation and limbic inhibition in response to aversive stimuli (Simeon, 2004). Furthermore, there is association with childhood interpersonal trauma, particularly emotional maltreatment (Simeon et al., 2001; Simeon, 2004).

Depersonalization: Further Considerations

Sometimes there has been considerable confusion over whether depersonalization can be distinguished from the disorders of self-image described in Chapter 12 as occurring in schizophrenia. In fact, passivity experiences have even been described as a variant of depersonalization. However, Meyer (1956), as cited by Sedman (1970), has distinguished schizophrenic ego disturbances from depersonalization on phenomenological grounds, that is, on the description by the patient of their own internal experience. It is of course well recognized that true depersonalization symptoms do occur in patients with schizophrenia, especially in the early stages of the illness, alongside definite schizophrenic psychopathology.

Depersonalization is commonly described in bipolar affective disorder; however, the symptoms occur only in the depressive phase and there are no references to depersonalization occurring in mania (Sedman, 1970).

Anderson (1938) considered that *ecstasy states* occurring in bipolar affective disorders were the obverse of *depersonalization* and that, although the former occurred in mania, the latter occurred in depression. Sedman (1972), in an investigation of three matched groups, each of 18 subjects with depersonalization and depressive and anxiety symptoms, considered that the results stressed the importance of depressed mood in depersonalization, whereas anxiety seemed to carry no significant relationship.

Many other authors have stressed the close association between the symptoms of depersonalization and anxiety. For instance, Roth (1959, 1960) described the *phobic anxiety depersonalization syndrome* as a separate nosologic entity, but saw it as a form of anxiety on which the additional symptoms are superimposed in a particular group of individuals. He considered depersonalization to be more common with anxiety than with other affective disorders, for example, depression. The phobic symptoms are usually agoraphobic in nature. The patient, most often female, married and often in the third decade of life, has a great fear of being conspicuous in an embarrassing way in public, for example, fainting or being taken ill suddenly on a bus or in a supermarket. Fear of leaving the house unaccompanied develops from this, so that the patient is frightened of being at a distance from familiar surroundings without some supporting figure to whom she can turn. She may be unable to go out of the house at all, even with her husband. She may feel panicky on her own at home and so keeps her child off school, a potential precipitating factor in subsequent school refusal.

The symptom of dizziness is a very common complaint and frequently results in referral to ear, nose and throat departments. Fewtrell and O'Connor (1989) discuss two possible models for the relationship of this condition to depersonalization: one that dizziness and depersonalization are the same experience described differently; the other, a bipolar hypothesis, proposes that the two experiences form opposite ends of a dimension describing disturbed *self–outside world* relationships.

Although depersonalization is commonly described in association with agoraphobia, other phobic states, panic disorder, various types of depressive condition, post-traumatic stress disorder and other nonpsychotic conditions, it may also appear as a pure depersonalization syndrome, and Davison (1964) has described episodic depersonalization in which other aetiologic factors or comorbid disorders are not prominent.

In psychoanalytic theory, depersonalization has taken on a rather different meaning, and therefore there are different explanations for its origin. Psychoanalysts have been less concerned with describing the phenomena than the underlying concept of the alienation of the ego. For example, in the work of the existentialist school, as typified by Binswanger (1963), there is discussion of the *depersonalization of man*.

The distressing experience of depersonalization with a feeling of unreality remains central to the description of the disordered self. The disturbance that causes this may be organic or environmental, psychotic or existential. Concern about the experience of self and of the environment most commonly occur together.

REFERENCES

Ackner, B., 1954a. Depersonalization I. Aetiology and phenomenology II. Clinical syndromes. J. Ment. Sci. 100, 838–872.

Ackner, B., 1954b. Depersonalization: II. Clinical syndromes. J. Ment. Sci. 100, 853–872.

Aderibigbe, Y.A., Bloch, R.M., Walker, W.R., 2001. Prevalence of depersonalization and derealization experiences in a rural population. Soc. Psychiatry Psychiatr. Epidemiol. 36, 63–69.

Anderson, E.W., 1938. A clinical study of states of 'ecstasy' occurring in affective disorders. J. Neurol. Psychiatry 1, 1–20.

[Anonymous], 1972. Depersonalisation syndromes [leading article]. Br. Med. J. 4, 378.

Baker, D., Hunter, E., Lawrence, E., et al., 2003. Depersonalisation disorder: clinical features of 204 cases. Br. J. Psychiatry 182, 428–433.

Binswanger, L., 1963. Being-in-the-world. In: Selected Papers of Ludwig Binswanger (J. Needleman, Trans, 1975). Basic Books, London.

Carney, M.W.P., Bacelle, L., Robinson, B., 1984. Psychosis after cannabis abuse. Br. Med. J. 288, 1047.

Davison, K., 1964. Episodic depersonalisation: observations on seven patients. Br. J. Psychiatry 110, 505–513.

Dixon, J.C., 1963. Depersonalization phenomena in a sample population of college students. Br. J. Psychiatry 109, 371–375.

Dugas, L., Moutier, F., 1911. La Depersonalisation. Felix Alcon, Paris.

Fewtrell, W.D., 1986. Depersonalization: a description and suggested strategies. Br. J. Guid. Counc. 14, 263–269.

Fewtrell, W.D., O'Connor, K.P., 1989. Dizziness and depersonalization. Adv. Behav. Res. Ther. 10, 201–218.

Grigsby, J., Kaye, K., 1993. Incidence and correlates of depersonalization following head trauma. Brain Inj. 7, 507–513.

Heymans, G., 1904. Eine Enquête über Depersonalisation und 'Fausse Reconnaisance. Z. Psychol. 36, 321–343.

Hollander, E., Carrasco, J.L., Mullen, L.S., Trungold, S., DeCaria, C.M., Towey, J., 1992. Left hemispheric activation in depersonalization disorder: a case report. Biol. Psychiatry 31, 1157–1162.

Hughlings Jackson, J., 1884. Croonian lectures on evolution and dissolution of the nervous system. In: Taylor, J. (Ed.), 1958, Selected Writings of John Hughlings Jackson, vol. 2. Staples Press, London, pp. 3–120.

Jaspers, K., 1997. General Psychopathology (J. Hoenig, M.W. Hamilton, Trans). The Johns Hopkins University Press, Baltimore.

Kennedy, R.B., 1976. Self-induced depersonalization syndrome. Am. J. Psychiatry 133, 1326–1328.

Lambert, M.V., Sierra, M., Phillips, M.L., David, A.S., 2002. The spectrum of organic depersonalization: a review plus four new cases. J. Neuropsychiatry Clin. Neurosci. 14, 141–154.

Lambert, M.V., Senior, C., Phillips, M.L., Sierra, M., Hunter, E., David, A.S., 2001. Visual imagery and depersonalization. Psychopathology 34, 259–264.

Langfeldt, G., 1960. Diagnosis and prognosis of schizophrenia. Proc. R. Soc. Med. 52, 595–596.

Mapother, E., 1935. Cited by Mayer-Gross. 1935.

Matthew, R.J., Wilson, W.H., Humphreys, D., Lowe, J.V., Weithe, K.E., 1993. Depersonalization after marijuana smoking. Biol. Psychiatry 33, 431–441.

Mayer-Gross, W., 1935. On depersonalisation. Br. J. Med. Psychol. 15, 103–122.

Mellor, C.S., 1988. Depersonalisation and self-perception. Br. J. Psychiatry 153 (Suppl. 2), 15–19.

Meyer, J.E., 1956. Studien zur Depersonalisation. Monatsschr. Psychiatr. Neurol. 132, 221–232.

Michal, M., Kaufhold, J., Grabhorn, R., Krakow, K., Overbeck, G., Heidenreich, T., 2005. Depersonalization and social anxiety. J. Nerv. Ment. Dis. 193, 629–632.

Moravia, A., 1960. Boredom (A. Davidson, Trans). New York Review Books, New York.

Phillips, M.L., Sierra, M., 2003. Depersonalization disorder: a functional neuroanatomical perspective. Stress 6, 157–165.

Putnam, F.W., Carlson, E.B., Ross, C.A., et al., 1996. Patterns of dissociation in clinical and non-clinical samples. J. Nerv. Ment. Dis. 184, 673–679.

Rix, K.J.B., Clarkson, A., 1994. Depersonalisation and intent. J. Forens. Psychiatry 5, 409–419.

Ross, C., 1997. Dissociative Identity Disorder: Diagnosis, Clinical Features and Treatment of Multiple Personality. John Wiley, New York.

Roth, M., 1959. The phobic anxiety–depersonalization syndrome. Proc. R. Soc. Med. 52, 587–595.

Roth, M., 1960. The phobic anxiety–depersonalization syndrome and some general aetiological problems in psychiatry J. Neuropsychiatr. 1, 292–306.

Scharfetter, C., 1980. General Psychopathology: An Introduction. Cambridge University Press, Cambridge.

Schilder, P., 1920. Medizinische Psychologie (D. Rapaport, Trans, 1953, as *Medical Psychologie*). International Universities Press, New York.

Schilder, P., 1928. Depersonalisation. In: Introduction to Psychoanalytic Psychiatry Nervous and Mental Disease Monograph, Series 50. W.W. Norton, New York.

Schilder, P., 1935. The Image and Appearance of the Human Body: Studies in the Constructive Energies of the Psyche. Kegan Paul, London.

Schneider, K., 1958. Clinical Psychopathology, fifth ed. (M.W. Hamilton, Trans). Grune and Stratton, New York.

Sedman, G., 1966. Depersonalization in a group of normal subjects. Br. J. Psychiatry 112 (490), 907–912.

Sedman, G., 1970. Theories of depersonalisation: a reappraisal. Br. J. Psychiatry 117, 1–14.

Sedman, G., 1972. An investigation of certain factors concerned in the aetiology of depersonalisation. Acta Psychiatr. Scand. 48, 191–219.

Sedman, G., Kenna, J.C., 1964. The occurrence of depersonalisation phenomena under LSD. Psychiatr. Neurol (Basel). 147, 129–137.

Sedman, G., Kenna, J.C., 1965. Depersonalisation in temporal lobe epilepsy and the organic psychoses. Br. J. Psychiatry 111, 293–299.

Sierra, M., 2009. Depersonalization: A New Look at a Neglected Syndrome. Cambridge University Press, Cambridge.

Sierra, M., Berrios, G.E., 1997. Depersonalization: a conceptual history. Hist. Psychiat. 8, 213–229.

Sierra, M., Berrios, G.E., 1998. Depersonalization: neurobiological perspectives. Biol. Psychiatry 44, 898–908.

Sierra, M., Berrios, G.E., 2000. The Cambridge Depersonalization Scale: a new instrument for the measurement of depersonalization. Psychiatry Res. 93, 153–164.

Sierra, M., Berrios, G.E., 2001. The phenomenological stability of depersonalization: comparing the old with the new. J. Nerv. Ment. Dis. 189, 629–636.

Sierra, M., David, A.S., 2011. Depersonalization: a selective impairment of self-awareness. Conscious Cog. 20 (1), 99–108.

Sierra, M., Nestler, S., Jay, E.L., Ecker, C., Feng, Y., David, A.S., 2014. A structural MRI study of cortical thickness in depersonalisation disorder. Psychiatry Res. 30, 224 (1),1–7.

Simeon, D., 2004. Depersonalisation disorder: a contemporary overview. CNS Drugs 18, 343–354.

Simeon, D., Knutelska, M., Nelson, D., Guralnik, O., 2003. Feeling unreal: a depersonalization disorder update of 117 cases. J. Clin. Psychiatry 64, 990–997.

Simeon, D., Kozin, D.S., Segal, K., Lerch, B., 2009. Is depersonalization disorder initiated by illicit drug use any different? A survey of 394 adults. J. Clin. Psychiatry 70, 1358–1364.

Simeon, D., Guralnik, O., Schmeidler, J., Sirof, B., Knutelska, M., 2001. The role of childhood interpersonal trauma in depersonalization disorder. Am. J. Psychiatry 158, 1027–1033.

Simeon, D., Gross, S., Guralnik, O., Stein, D.J., Schmeidler, J., Hollander, E., 1997. Feeling unreal: 30 cases of DSM-IIIR depersonalization disorder. Am. J. Psychiatry 154, 1107–1113.

Simeon, D., Guralnik, O., Gross, S., Stein, D.J., Schmeidler, J., Hollander, E., 1998. The detection and measurement of depersonalization disorder. J. Nerv. Ment. Dis. 186, 536–542.

Simeon, D., Kozin, D.S., Segal, K., Lerch, B., Dujour, R., Giesbrecht, T., 2008. De-constructing depersonalization: further evidence for symptom clusters. Psychiatry Res 157, 303–306.

Sims, A., Sims, D., 1998. The phenomenology of post-traumatic stress disorder: a symptomatic study of 70 victims of psychological trauma. Psychopathology 31, 96–112.

Sno, H.M., Draaisma, D., 1993. An early Dutch study of *déjà vu* experiences. Psychol. Med. 23, 17–26.

Stewart, W.A., 1964. Panel on depersonalization. J. Am. Psychoanal. Assoc. 12, 171–186.

Szymanski, H.V., 1981. Prolonged depersonalization after marijuana use. Am. J. Psychiatry 138, 231–233.

Yap, P.M., 1965. Koro—a culture-bound depersonalisation syndrome. Br. J. Psychiatry 111, 43–50.

Zikić, O., Cirić, S., Mitković, M., 2009. Depressive phenomenology in regard to depersonalization level. Psychiatr. Danub. 21, 320–326.

Disorder of the Awareness of the Body

KEYWORDS

Hypochondriasis
Disgust
Dysmorphophobia
Body integrity identity disorder
Anorexia nervosa
Muscle dysmorphia

Summary

The body is the physical manifestation of the individual being. It is the material, corporeal interface with the external world. The world is experienced through the body's senses. The body, also, is itself experienced as an object in the world. In this chapter, we examine the following:

- disorders of beliefs about the body including beliefs of illness, disease and death,
- disorders of bodily function, including the loss of sensory, motor or cognitive function that occur in the conversion and dissociative disorders,
- disorders of the experience of the physical characteristics of the body and of the emotional and aesthetic value, and
- complex disorders of the sensory awareness of the body that almost exclusively derive from neurologic lesions.

Even though these abnormal experiences are disparate, what binds them together into a coherent aspect of psychopathology is that the body as experienced is at their heart.

Beside fear and sorrow, 'sharp belchings, fulsome crudities, heat in the bowels, wind and rumblings in the guts, vehement gripings, pain in the belly and stomach sometimes after meat that is hard of concoction, much watering of the stomach, and moist spittle, cold sweat.'

Robert Burton (1577–1640), The Anatomy of Melancholia *(1628)*

*To some, ill health is
a way to be important,
Others are stoics,
a few fanatics,
who won't feel happy until
they are cut open.*

W.H. Auden (1969)

The physicality of the body is ever present: there is density, mass, movement, action, speed, position, heat, cold and various degrees of touch, pain and so on. Since Descartes (1596–1650), the relationship between mind and body has stimulated much investigation and discussion. Descartes' original claim was that the mind and body are distinct and different; furthermore, that the mind can exist without the body. There are other theories that attempt to account for the nature of mind and body. Materialist theories propose that the body is all there is, and variations of these theories account for mind in different ways, whereas idealist theories make the opposite claim that the mind is all that exists. The fact that many descriptions of mood, cognition, volition and other psychological functions are expressed in physical terms—*a heavy heart, bone-headed, guts and determination, a pain in the neck*—underlines the inextricable relationship between mind and body and emphasizes the degree to which the body can become a means of communicating distress and bodily metaphors used to consciously or unconsciously express feelings. Whether these metaphors originally derive from the physical manifestations of emotional distress or whether the language, that is, the metaphor, structures the experience is a moot point. What is clear is that there is no ready division between the subjective experience of self and body. A 10-year-old girl put this relationship thus: 'You feel better if you've done your homework; if you haven't you get a horrible pain in your stomach'. Finally, because the body is itself an object in the world, it inhabits a world of values and norms such that there are 'good' and 'bad' bodies, 'desirable' and 'undesirable' bodies. In addition, a subset of values is aesthetics, so that there are 'beautiful' and 'ugly' bodies. This means that individuals approach both their own and other people's bodies with an attitude: they appraise bodies with a set of beliefs and expectations, form judgements and act towards bodies with approval or disapproval.

The Body in Psychopathology

Our bodies have an objective physicality like all other material objects in the world. However, there is also the subjective, animated body that is alive and with which we deeply identify. These two aspects of our bodies have different words in German that denote them: *Körper* refers to the body as an object and *Leib* to the subjectively experienced body. Pollio et al. (2008) conducted a phenomenological investigation of adults' intuitions of their daily-embodied experiences. The participants' responses focused on eight situations:

1. Awareness of the body when engaged in an activity;
2. Awareness of the body when experiencing aches, pains, illness and fatigue;
3. Awareness of the body as presented to other people in posture and dress;
4. Awareness of the body during pregnancy and during sexual intimacy and arousal;
5. Awareness of changes in the body over time;
6. Awareness of the body as an aspect of identity, for example, as a Christian;
7. Awareness of the presence or absence of others; and
8. Awareness of strong emotions.

In addition to awareness of the body in these situations, the respondents also had three unique modes of experiencing their bodies. These modes include the experience of engagement, corporeality and interpersonal meaning. Experience of engagement was subdivided into (1) body in vitality during episodes the person is fully engaged in the world with no sense of the body as physical, but there is a consciousness of well-being and (2) body in activity during activities when the person experiences the concrete movements as central to the experience, for example, during running. Experience of corporeality includes (1) the body as instrument, that is, as a tool, and (2) as an object that has limits and that can be impaired by illness. Finally, experiences of interpersonal meaning refer to the social and symbolic meaning of our bodies.

The experience of interpersonal meaning of our bodies is dealt with in studies of the sociology of the body. We engage with others and interact with them from the first-person perspective of a person who is embodied. The physical characteristics of our bodies including size, shape, mannerisms, gait and so on significantly influence our relationships, perceptions of others and how we too are perceived. Furthermore, our bodily conduct, how we control our bodily urges, the quality and standard of self-grooming and personal hygiene contribute to our identity and personal characteristics and define how others appraise us. In short, the body in society has profound implications for issues relating to health, gender, sexual preference, ethnicity, disability, social status and politics. It is therefore self-evident that any description of abnormalities of body awareness will have implications far beyond the scope of medicine or psychiatry. For a detailed examination of these matters, see Howson (2013).

Finally, the body is central to Merleau-Ponty's (1962) phenomenology. His claim is that although the body is an object, it is like no other object because it is the medium by which we experience all other objects. He writes, 'I observe external objects with my body, I handle them, examine them, walk round them, but my body itself is a thing which I do not observe: in order to be able to do so, I should need the use of a second body which itself would be unobservable'. These ideas have been further developed in more modern studies—and the suggestion is not merely that our bodies are central to our experience of the material world but that such brain functions such as perception, memory, concept formation, language and so forth are influenced by the configuration and activities of our bodies. Gibbs (2005) exemplifies this point:

Perception cannot be understood without reference to action. People do not perceive the world statically, but by actively exploring the environment. For instance, if I move closer to the table in front of me, I see the textured lines in the wood surface better. If I turn my head, I distinctly hear the music playing softly on the stereo behind me. If I move to the steaming cup of coffee on the counter, and lean over close by, I clearly smell the scent of coffee beans. Each bodily movement enables my sensory organs to do their work depending on my motivations and goals.

It is obvious from the foregoing that the body and self are conceptually linked and that brain functions depend on the body in action. The separation of abnormalities of self and of body in distinct chapters are merely for convenience and by convention.

To form a cohesive framework for conceptualizing the disorders of self and the diverse abnormalities of body image, one needs to apply the methods of descriptive psychopathology. In Chapter 12, the nature of self and the pathology of the experience of self were discussed. In this chapter, disorders of the awareness of body are discussed.

Classification

Cutting (1997) gives a good outline of the classification of disorders of awareness of the body, which has been adapted for this chapter (Table 14.1). There are disorders of beliefs about the body, including beliefs of illness, disease and death (discussed subsequently). In this group are also the disorders of dissatisfaction with the body, which occur in eating disorders. These dissatisfactions with the body are best understood as arising from negative cognitive evaluations, that is, beliefs about the body. Next, there are disorders of bodily function, including the loss of sensory, motor or cognitive function that occurs in the dissociative disorders. There are disorders of the experience of the physical characteristics of the body. These include disorders of the experience of the size, shape, structure or weight of the body. Finally, there are complex disorders of the sensory experience of the body that almost exclusively derive from neurologic lesions.

Disorders of Beliefs About the Body (Bodily Complaint Without Organic Cause)

Classification of these disorders is difficult, partly because the symptoms are obscure in origin and

TABLE 14.1   Classification of Disorders of Awareness of the Body

Classification	Details
Beliefs About the Body	
Illness and disease	Hypochondriacal symptoms
Body dissatisfaction	Real and ideal body weight discrepancy
Function of the Body	
Sensory deficits	For example, dissociative sensory loss (blindness)
Experience of Physical Characteristics of the Body	
Size	Microsomatognosia, macrosomatognosia and body image disturbance
Shape	'My jaws are misshapen'
Colour	Skin colour may be experienced as lighter
Structure	'My lungs are connected to my abdomen'
Weight	Feelings of lightness or heaviness
Experience of Emotional Value of the Body	
Anosognosic overestimation	Exaggeration of body's strength
Misoplegia	Hatred of body part
Dysmorphophobia	Feeling of ugliness or defect of body or one of its parts
Experience of Sensory Awareness of the Body and the World	
Palinaptia	Persistence of sensation beyond the duration of contact with stimuli
Exosomesthesia	Cutaneous sensation in extrapersonal space
Alloaesthesia	Experience of sensation on contralateral side to stimulation

After Cutting, J., 1997. Principles of Psychopathology. Oxford University Press, Oxford., p. 317, with permission of Oxford University Press.

partly because there are different theoretical bases for the words used. For example, *conversion hysteria* was used as a term that referred to the presumed unconscious conversion of an unacceptable affect into a physical symptom. *Hypochondriasis* refers to a concern with symptoms and with illness that the outside observer regards as excessive; the same amount of concern or complaint associated with pathology that the doctor regards as justifying it would not be deemed hypochondriacal. *Dysmorphophobia* is a phenomenological term and refers to the subjective experience of dissatisfaction with bodily shape or form (Fig. 14.1).

HYPOCHONDRIASIS

Hypochondriasis describes the subjective and undue awareness of physical symptoms, which are interpreted as signalling serious illness. It is a symptom and not a disease. There are many different modes of expression: minor pain and discomfort dominate the person's life and occupy their attention; they may have unreasonable fears about the likelihood of developing serious illness and feel a need to take excessive precautions; they may misinterpret benign blemishes as having sinister pathologic significance. These expressions of dissatisfaction may occur on their own or in any combination, and they can affect any bodily system or psychological process. Hypochondriacal symptoms are common and usually transient. Only a minority come to medical attention, and only a selected atypical proportion of these are seen by psychiatrists.

There is a distinction between illness fears, when there are no bodily symptoms, and the fears and distress, which are not associated with bodily symptoms but merely arise out of the possibility of serious illness. This shows the overlap between illness phobias (unreasonable fear of developing illness) and hypochondriasis (preoccupation with symptoms). There is often difficulty in diagnosis when a person with demonstrable physical pathology complains excessively about their symptoms; their complaints appear to be out of proportion to the anticipated suffering and disability of the illness. Necessary and entirely routine medical examination and investigation tend to reinforce the patient's symptoms. Somatic symptoms without organic pathology are extremely common and may result from misunderstanding the nature and significance of physiologic activity aggravated by emotion (Kellner, 1985). The mechanisms underlying hypochondriacal symptoms include misinterpretation of normal bodily sensations; conversion of unpleasant affect, especially depression, into physical symptoms; and the

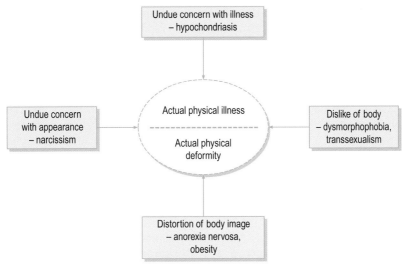

Fig. 14.1 Disorders of bodily complaint.

experience of autonomic symptoms directly caused by disorder of mood.

Explicit in the identification of hypochondriasis is the condition of the patient themselves. Implicit, however, is the doctor who labels their patient *hypochondriacal* and deems them *sick*. In a society that is so conscious of physical health and external physical appearance, the patient may have to shout 'hypochondriacally' because the doctor will only listen out for physical complaints. What the symptoms communicate to other people is an important component of all disorders of bodily awareness; concentration on the subjective aspects of symptoms should not detract from their social implications. Hypochondriasis is not uncommonly an iatrogenic condition induced by the doctor's failure to listen to their patient's story and inability to give appropriate weight to psychological aspects contributing to symptoms.

What Is Hypochondriasis?

By derivation, the word *hypochondrium* refers to the anatomic area below the rib cage (Fig. 14.2) and hence dysfunction of the liver or spleen. Such words as *atrabilious* or *melancholia* refer to the black bile that was considered to be associated with hypochondriacal complaint and depressed mood. Kenyon (1965) has defined hypochondriasis as morbid preoccupation with the body or state of health.

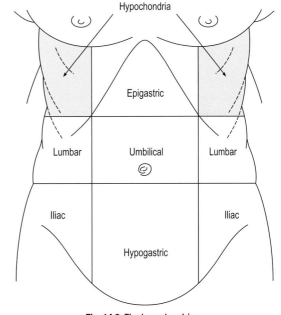

Fig. 14.2 The hypochondrium.

Is hypochondriasis a separate condition—a symptom or a syndrome, a noun or an adjective? It is best to regard hypochondriasis as a symptom rather than a distinct condition. It is not unitary as a condition but a disorder of content rather than of form. The content is the excessive concern with health, either physical or mental, and the interpretation of subjective experience as deriving from serious illness. The form of the condition may be quite variable. Even though the term *hypochondriacal* is best retained as description rather than as a discrete disease entity (Kenyon, 1976), current classification systems have a purely hypochondriacal disorder.

Barsky and Klerman (1983) have considered that the word hypochondriasis is used to describe four quite distinct concepts:

1. It describes a psychiatric syndrome characterized by physical symptoms disproportionate to demonstrable organic disease, fear of disease and the conviction that one is sick, preoccupation with one's body and pursuit of medical care.
2. Hypochondriasis is seen psychodynamically as a derivative of aggressive or oral drives or as a defence against guilt or low self-esteem.
3. It results from a perceptual amplification and augmentation and a cognitive misinterpretation of normal bodily sensations.
4. It is a socially learned illness behaviour to which the philosophy and practice of the medical profession lends support.

Only the first of these is psychopathologic in nature. These concepts are not alternatives but are all present to a different extent in the individual sufferer. Some individuals use a *somatic style* to describe their perception of internal discomfort. Appleby (1987) points out that closer examination reveals a descriptive triad of the patient being convinced that they have a disease, fearing the disease and being preoccupied with their body. He emphasizes that the patient needs to understand their symptoms before any improvement can be expected.

Bridges and Goldberg (1985) have assessed somatic presentation of psychiatric disorder in primary care in a series of 500 inceptions to illness among 2500 attendees. Their operational criteria for *somatization* were as follows:

- *Consulting behaviour:* Seeking medical help for somatic manifestations and not presenting psychological symptoms.
- *Attribution:* The patient considers somatic manifestations to be caused physically.
- *Psychiatric illness:* Psychiatric diagnosis justified by psychiatrists.

- *Response to intervention:* The research psychiatrist is of the opinion that treatment of the psychiatric disorder would benefit somatic symptoms.

These authors consider that somatization is a common mode of presentation of psychiatric illness and partly explains the failure of family doctors to detect psychiatric disorders in primary care.

Trying to distinguish between organic and psychological elements of disease or between mental and physical illness is a fruitless task based on an outmoded and misleading linguistic distinction (Kendell, 2001). Psychological conflict may be mediated via physical illness, and a physical illness results in psychosocial sequelae. Both somatic and psychological symptoms occur, and it is perfectly possible for a patient to have a hypochondriacal reaction to a clearly defined organic illness.

A patient who regards themself as having symptoms of illness communicates this to relatives and also to the doctor in a tacit request for both help and labelling (Parsons, 1951). To come to medical attention, the person has to carry out a particular set of actions, that is, undertake illness behaviour (Mechanic, 1962, 1986). Illness behaviour includes the manner in which symptoms are differentially perceived, evaluated and acted upon by different kinds of people and in different social situations. Whereas some people may be able to make light of symptoms, shrug them off and avoid seeking medical attention, others may respond to trivial pain and discomfort by readily seeking care. It is clear, therefore, that individual characteristics as well as social cultural ones determine how any one individual will respond to symptoms.

Individual determinants of hypochondriasis seem to include preoccupation with bodily functions or with the idea of harbouring an illness, rumination about illness, suggestibility, unrealistic fear of infection, fascination with medical information and fear of prescribed medication (Fink et al., 2004). Fear of death also seems to be an integral aspect of hypochondriasis (Noyes et al., 2002b), and childhood adversity (including traumatic events and serious illness and injury) and parental modelling of illness behaviour in childhood are vulnerability factors (Noyes et al., 2002a; Kirmayer and Looper, 2006). Anxiety (Olatunji et al., 2009) and disgust (Davey, 2011) also appear to underlie hypochondriasis. Disgust, in this context, is conceived of as a disease-avoidant emotion, and disgust propensity and sensitivity are regarded as vulnerability factors for a number of disorders including blood-injection-injury phobia and hypochondriasis. *Cyberchondriasis*, a term referring to excessive and repeated health-related searches on the Internet, reveals aspects of hypochondriasis that may have remained covert, namely, that behavioural aspects include searching for health information on diagnosed and undiagnosed disorders, seeking out descriptions of other people's experience of illness and using message boards and support groups. However, these behaviours only provoke more distress and anxiety (Muse et al., 2012; Starcevic and Berle, 2013).

There are very marked cultural differences in the presentation of symptoms of disordered mood; somatization of emotional distress applies to both anxiety and depression (Rack, 1982). The predominance of description of somatic over mood symptoms in depressive illness has been reported from India, Pakistan, Bangladesh, Hong Kong, the West Indies and various African countries. The reasons for this include the expectations the patient has of what the doctor can do, the use of somatic symptoms as metaphor for distress and the social unacceptability of psychological symptoms. The Bradford Somatic Inventory has been devised for a multiethnic comparison of the frequency of somatic symptoms, their anatomic localization and their association with psychiatric disorder (Mumford et al., 1991). Immigrant populations from Pakistan in the United Kingdom demonstrate more somatic symptoms on the Bradford Somatic Inventory compared with the native population. These symptoms are associated with recognizable anxiety and depression as measured by validated questionnaires (Farooq et al., 1995).

Psychopathology of the Hypochondriacal Patient

The *content* of hypochondriasis is the excessive concern with health, either physical or mental. Possible *forms* of the condition are listed below. These forms of the *content* of concern about cancer can include the following:

- A *hallucinatory* voice may say to the patient, 'You have cancer, you are moribund'.
- A *secondary delusion* associated with affective illness may occur in which the patient unreasonably

believes they have cancer; they are quite unable to accept their doctor's reassurance. The belief is understandable in relation to the patient's overall depressed mood state. That such secondary delusions could be associated with affective psychoses was clearly described by Cotard (1882): 'she blamed herself and felt guilty. After some months she entertained hypochondriacal delusions, believing that she had no stomach and that her organs had been destroyed; she attributed these beliefs to the effects of an emetic which she had, in fact, been given'. This association of hypochondriacal and nihilistic delusions with depressive psychosis in the elderly has been called Cotard's syndrome.

- The *delusion* may be *primary* in nature. A patient with schizophrenia believed that he had been inoculated under a general anaesthetic with a transmissible cancer because others believed him to be homosexual.
- Hypochondriasis often manifests as an *overvalued idea*. Such a person is constantly worried and concerned about the risk of illness and the need to take precautions in ways that their friends find ridiculous, for instance, in the lengths that they will go to avoid a possible carcinogen. They consider it perfectly reasonable that they should take due care to maintain their health, but they agree that their measures are excessive. They cannot stop themself, night or day, from thinking, worrying and trying to prevent illness. Such an overvalued idea is found reasonable or at least not alien to the person's nature but preoccupies the mind to an unreasonable extent in that the whole energy and being becomes directed towards this single idea.
- The hypochondriacal idea may take the form of an *obsessional rumination* in which the possibility of a particular illness or a form of words, as 'I have cancer', may recur. This is recognized as being both 'alien to my nature' but also 'coming from inside myself'. It is resisted yet occurs repetitively.
- Without its amounting to a delusion, patients may often have hypochondriacal symptoms of a nonspecific nature in the course of a *depressive* illness. It may be possible to reassure them

concerning any particular symptom, but this does not make them feel better in their mood nor does it prevent the occurrence of further hypochondriacal symptoms in the form of depressive ruminations.

- In the context of acute or chronic *anxiety,* the patient may be prone to multitudinous worries concerning illness and fears of illness. The normal sensorium is interpreted as symptoms; symptoms are interpreted as serious illness. Most hypochondriacal symptoms occur in relation to anxiety and depression; the other forms of disorder are much less frequent.

The commonest bodily symptoms implicated in hypochondriasis are musculoskeletal; gastrointestinal, including indigestion, constipation and other preoccupation with malfunction; and central nervous system, including headache (Kenyon, 1964). The most commonly affected parts of the body are head and neck, abdomen and chest. In 16% of patients, symptoms are predominantly unilateral, and of these, 73%, according to Kenyon, were left-sided. There was no significant physical abnormality found in 47% of those admitted to a psychiatric ward for hypochondriasis. Pain was prominent in 70% of patients.

Hypochondriasis may be associated with smell; bodily appearance; sexual hypochondria; ear, nose and throat symptoms; and ophthalmologic abnormalities (Karseras, 1976) such as *asthenopia,* which includes such complaints as ocular discomfort, aching eyes, soreness, pressure in or around the eyes, tiredness of eyes, grittiness, chronic redness, feelings that the eyes are pushed out on stalks, tightness of the skin across the bridge of the nose or pricking of the skin around the eyes. Photophobia is a common hypochondriacal complaint, as are 'floaters'—muscae volitantes, photopsia and sometimes diplopia.

Hypochondriacal complaints may relate to psychological symptoms and the fear of mental illness. In this context, sleep is often involved, with subjective feelings of sleep not occurring at all, not occurring in sufficient amount or not being of satisfactory quality. Fear of madness and inevitable psychiatric deterioration is commonly associated with acute anxiety disorders and with depressive illness.

Disorders of Bodily Function— Conversion and Dissociation

Psychopathology has, as its subject matter, actual conscious psychological phenomena. Although our main concern is with pathologic phenomena, it is also necessary to know what people experience in general and how they experience it; in short, psychopathology is interested in the full range of conscious psychological phenomena. The foregoing raises the question of whether experiences that are not in conscious awareness, such as those that are the subject of this section, can ever be the proper subject of psychopathology because these experiences are not in conscious awareness. These experiences and behaviours have an antique pedigree and were, until recently, described by the term *hysteria.*

The meaning and validity of the term *hysteria* has been argued about for centuries (Veith, 1965). Slater (1965) wished to reject the diagnosis of hysteria while retaining the word as an adjective to describe certain types of symptoms and personality. Lewis (1975) summarized this controversy: 'The majority of psychiatrists would be hard put to it if they could no longer make a diagnosis of 'hysteria' or 'hysterical reaction'; and in any case a tough old word like hysteria dies very hard. It tends to outlive its obituarists.' Classically, physical symptoms, usually mimicking neurologic disturbances such as seizures, paralysis, tremors, blindness and gait abnormalities occur in the setting of psychological distress without accompanying expected physical findings on examination. The term *conversion* was used to denote the fact that emotional distress or psychological conflict had been converted into physical complaints. A related term is *dissociation,* referring to the disturbance of the basic unity of the self, resulting in the apparent separation of aspects of the self from one another. For example, a seemingly conscious individual may report that they are unable to recall vital aspects of their biography despite having no demonstrable abnormalities of memory. It is obvious that the term *dissociation* is merely a descriptive concept for something factually experienced and encountered in clinical practice, as well as a theory for what happens in the particular state, and thus it provides the hypothesis for explaining an observed clinical fact. It is a concept that does not describe anything uniform but touches on modes of extra-conscious explanatory mechanism.

The implications that may be drawn from the conceptualization of conversion and dissociation are as follows:

1. The presenting symptoms are psychologically determined despite being physical in nature;
2. Causation is thought to be unconscious and hence the patient is not aware of the psychological determinants;
3. Symptoms may carry some sort of advantage to the patient, the so-called primary or secondary gain; and
4. The symptoms occur by the mediation of the putative explanatory but ill-defined processes of *conversion* or *dissociation*.

At 10-year follow-up of patients diagnosed with hysteria at a neurologic hospital, many were found to have subsequently developed a serious physical or psychiatric illness, and for this reason, the existence of hysteria as a diagnostic category was questioned (Slater and Glithero, 1965). Follow-up of 113 patients diagnosed as hysterical by psychiatrists revealed 60% with evidence of affective disorder and only 13% with a consistent picture of hysteria (Reed, 1975). However, Merskey and Buhrich (1975) carried out a follow-up on patients diagnosed as having motor conversion symptoms at a neurologic hospital and a control group of other patients from the same clinical setting. They found a higher rate of organic symptoms at follow-up in the control group. From follow-up studies of neurologic or psychiatric patients, when the diagnosis of hysteria has been highly inclusive, other organic and psychiatric conditions have commonly manifested, but 15% to 20% still retain the diagnosis of hysteria.

For a diagnosis of dissociative disorder or functional neurological symptom disorder to be made, positive psychological features must be present and characteristic organic features should be absent. It is important to emphasize the danger of misidentifying genuine physical illness as functional disturbance. Thus for *astasia-abasia* (Fig. 14.3) for example to be considered dissociative, the symptoms should have psychogenic aetiology; the patient is unaware of this, and the symptoms can be seen to be a way of dealing with stress. If symptoms are clearly consciously produced, deliberate disability, malingering or artefactual illness is present.

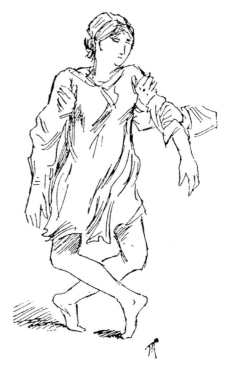

Fig. 14.3 Astasia-abasia. (From Merskey, H., Buhrich, N.A., 1975. Hysteria and organic brain disease. Br. J. Med. Psychol. 48, 359–366.)

One may have to distinguish between the symptoms of the original illness—for example, head injury—and a secondary hysterical reaction (Sims, 1985).

Epidemic, communicated or *mass* hysteria now commonly termed *mass psychogenic illness* or *mass sociogenic illness* has been known and described from earliest times, for example, the physical symptoms of conversion type associated with the millennialist movements of the Middle Ages (Cohn, 1958), in a closed female community in a French 17th-century convent (Huxley, 1952), and among Lancashire mill girls (St Clare, 1787). A rather similar epidemic spread through a school in Blackburn 180 years later, with symptoms of overbreathing, dizziness, fainting, headache, shivering, pins and needles, nausea, pain in the back or abdomen, hot feelings and general weakness (Moss and McEvedy, 1966). The spread of such epidemics has been described: they almost always occur in young females; they often start with a girl of high status in her peer group who is unhappy; they tend to occur in largest numbers in the younger children in a secondary school, that is, just after the

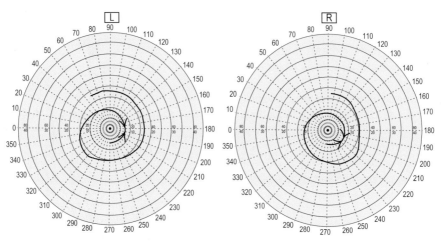

Fig. 14.4 Visual fields of a hysterical patient.

age of puberty; they appear to affect most severely those who on subsequent testing are found to be the most unstable. What seems to characterize these outbreaks are symptoms occurring among people with shared beliefs about the relevant symptoms in the absence of identifiable environmental cause and little clinical or laboratory evidence of disease. Often symptoms spread by 'line-of-sight' transmission and may escalate with vigorous or prolonged emergency or media response (Jones, 2000). The outbreaks also seem to mirror prominent social concerns, changing in relation to context and circumstance. From the late 20th-century onwards, symptoms appear to be triggered by sudden exposure to an anxiety-generating agent, most commonly an innocuous odour or food poisoning rumours or chemical and biological terrorism themes (Bartholomew and Wessely, 2002). Reports continue to be published (Aldous et al., 1994; Chowdhury and Brahma, 2005; Kharabsheh et al., 2001; Kokota, 2011).

It would be unrewarding to list all the possible symptoms that may be of conversion or dissociative origin: motor, sensory, pain and alterations in consciousness. With the use of skilled examination and additional neurophysiologic techniques, for example, in the investigation of dissociative blindness, it is often possible to demonstrate discrepancy between the severity of symptoms and physiologic dysfunction, which may be minimal or absent. The physiologic impossibility of these symptoms is well demonstrated

in Fig. 14.4, which shows the visual field of a patient complaining of impaired vision.

It is important to take into account the effect these symptoms have on other aspects of a patient's behaviour and social relationships. Symptoms result in the patient being regarded as *ill* or *disabled,* and this alters the way they are perceived both by relatives and friends and by the medical and related professions. There may be long-term physical consequences of motor symptoms, for example, contractures; this is the ultimate mimicry that conversion symptoms show of organic conditions.

Classically, mood in these conditions is described as *belle indifference.* Such a mood occurred in a girl aged 20 with severe disability that had entailed her using crutches for the previous 2 years. She smiled with sublime resignation at her unfortunate situation, and everyone around her was relieved that she accepted her symptom so stoically! However, some patients with conversion symptoms show higher autonomic arousal than do anxious and phobic patients (Lader and Sartorius, 1968).

Disorders of the Physical Characteristics and Emotional Value of the Body (Dislike of the Body)

This section deals with how the body is subjectively experienced as a physical object that has both symbolic and aesthetic value to the individual. These two aspects of a person's attitude towards their own body are distinct but interrelated. A distorted subjective experience of the body, the so-called distortion of body image, may occur independently of approval or disapproval or indeed of dislike of the body. Furthermore, the body can be appraised as ugly, that is, as aesthetically unattractive, in the absence of demonstrable abnormality of body image. Firstly, there are those abnormalities that derive from psychiatric disorders and are discrete but yet not pure as they are transdiagnostic in nature. Then there are the conditions such as dysmorphophobia and anorexia nervosa that are treated as disorders in their own right.

Disorders of the Physical Characteristics of the Body

DISTURBANCE OF SHAPE EXPERIENCE

Luckianowicz (1967) described a number of conditions including zoophilic and sexual metamorphosis, and loss of bodily shape. Zoophilic metamorphosis is often based on a combination of bodily sensations and hallucinatory experiences.

A labourer of 53, suffered from recurrent depression. He complained: 'For some weeks… I felt that my face was getting smaller and pointed, like in a dog. I also noticed that my children and wife had their faces slowly changing into dog's faces.' He further detected the smell of a dog from his body and 'my urine smelt like dog's water'.

Sexual metamorphosis entails complex sensory experience of transformation into the other sex:

A 30-year-old, single clerk, complained: 'For some time I had a feeling that my breasts became large and full, and my buttocks became plum, like in a woman. I can see in a mirror that it is not so, but still I have this strange sensation in the corresponding parts of my body. I don't know how to describe it. It is a sort of pressure from the inside upon my skin, pushing it out, and stretching. The feeling you have when your body becomes swollen […]'

Loss of bodily sensation is akin to Cotard syndrome but distinct and is often associated with epilepsy and is described in a case recovering from insulin coma therapy:

It is most frightening and distressing. Each time I come around it's the same: there is vast black ocean of nothingness, from which I, a tiny speck of light emerge. Slowly I become aware of myself. But I have no shape, no weight, no mass. I am just a spot of light floating in the vast ocean of darkness. It is a most frightening experience and I always lose consciousness again. I just can't stand this distressing feeling of formless and timeless existence for long. I may have this awful experience several times before I regain my shape and become myself again.

REDUPLICATION OF THE BODY OR ITS PARTS

In addition to the abnormalities of shape experience Luckianowicz (1967) also described experiences of body reduplication. These experiences involve reduplication of the body and its part. Often these conditions are described in the context of migraine left-sided hemispheric lesions but can also be seen in schizophrenia:

I often feel that I have two bodies, one outside the other, only a little larger than my actual body. I feel that the 'inner' body is the real one, and the 'outer' is more like something artificial, a sort of shell over a hermit crab although it has the shape and appearance of my 'real' body.

In some cases, the body is experienced as split into two halves:

A married woman of 58, when depressed, often had the feeling 'as if my body was split into two halves, like a stem of a tree struck by lightning. They both feel a few inches apart and there is nothing between them, but a black, empty hole; black and empty and dead.'

Some patients describe additional body parts. A patient with a diagnosis of schizophrenia described the following:

Every night I have intercourse with the Devil. Sometimes he forgets his penis in my privates and then I feel it there all day long. It is like a stiff piece of wood. Sometimes it burns and feels like hot iron. I always feel two small horns on my head and my feet feel like a goat's hooves.

DYSMORPHOPHOBIA (BODY DYSMORPHIC DISORDER)

Many people are dissatisfied with the way they look and, of course, this does not of itself constitute a psychiatric symptom. However, unreasonable loathing or excessive preoccupation with a disliked feature may result in psychiatric referral. Such people may show generalized disapproval of their appearance, or it may be concentrated on one feature. Dysmorphophobia was first defined by Morselli (1886) as 'a subjective feeling of ugliness or physical defect which the patient feels is noticeable to others, although his appearance is within normal limits'. As the meaning of the term *phobia* has changed in the past century, Berrios (1996) considers that *dysmorphophobia* is at least as satisfactory a term as modern equivalents such as *body dysmorphic disorder*. According to Andreasen and Bardach (1977), the primary symptom of dysmorphophobia is the patient's belief that they are unattractive.

Dysmorphophobia has been defined, more inclusively, as the primary complaint of some external physical defect thought to be noticeable to other people, but, objectively, its appearance lies within normal limits (Hay, 1970). Patients presenting to a plastic surgeon for cosmetic rhinoplasty were examined psychiatrically. They were, as a group, more disfigured than a control group, and they showed some psychological disturbance in that 40% showed disorder of personality. There was, however, no relationship between the degree of deformity and the amount of psychological disturbance. Hay and Heather (1973) commented that when surgery was carried out, those patients with minimal disfigurement did as well as those with more marked defects, both subjectively in description of their self-image and on psychological testing. They considered that the degree of deformity was not of major importance in coming to a decision with regard to operation. Patients reported marked improvement in their appearance 6 months after rhinoplasty, and this was associated with reduction of psychiatric symptom scores (Robin et al., 1988).

Body dysmorphic disorder occurs most frequently in late adolescence; three-quarters of patients are female, and most are either single or divorced (Veale et al., 1996). There is frequent comorbidity with mood disorder, social phobia and obsessive compulsive disorder, and 72% of cases manifested personality disorder, usually of paranoid, avoidant or obsessive compulsive type. Twenty-four percent of this group of patients had attempted suicide. In a similar American study, 73% of patients reported excessive mirror checking, 63% reported attempts to camouflage their 'deformities' and others reported grooming or skin picking (Phillips et al., 1993, 2005). Almost all had severe limitations of their social activities. Most patients had suffered from a major mood disorder, and 17% had made suicide attempts. The most frequently reported body parts, in order of concern, are skin, hair, nose, stomach, teeth, weight, breasts, buttocks, eyes, thighs, eyebrows, legs, face size or shape, chin, lips, arms, hips, cheeks and ears (Phillips et al., 2005).

Those complaining about their face, and especially their nose, do so in extreme and exaggerated terms despite the deformity often being relatively slight. The dissatisfaction with their appearance and the extent to which they feel others are aware of their disfigurement are quite out of proportion, as are the discomfort and disturbance in function: 'agonising pain' and 'total inability to breathe'. At the same time, the actual description is often quite imprecise: 'the skin under my eyes joins my nose in a funny way' (Birchnell, 1988). Because of the extreme degree of reaction they show, they may contemplate radical remedies, for example, wishing to have their nose amputated or threatening to kill themselves. Dysmorphophobia is a relatively common disturbance of self and usually takes the psychopathologic *form* of an *overvalued idea*.

The complaint of dysmorphophobia is made by the subject in relation to others but is not usually based on the opinion of others. So a patient complains of his nose, or the small size of her breasts, and considers that others will regard them as ugly or unattractive. Often the appearance is well within normal limits, with no deformity, but the patient is convinced that surgery will be beneficial. Patients often present in their late teens or early 20s. There is quite often underlying personality disorder of anankastic or dependent types; there may be depressed mood disturbance as a reaction to the complaint, and such patients not infrequently talk of, and attempt, suicide.

A female student, aged 20, was referred to the psychiatric clinic after self-poisoning. When asked her problem, she burst into tears and said, describing the small size of her breasts:

Basically there is a big difference between me and other girls. I've always been self-conscious. I used to pad myself. Even my mother made fun of me. I've tried to convince myself I would change physically. I don't feel like a total woman. I have to buy clothes that look ridiculous on top. My present boyfriend I have been going out with for over a year always talks about other girls he has. He went to a dance and danced with another girl, I knew that it was because she was bigger-busted than me. I was always aware of my figure, that I am not attractive ... I detest myself, I hate my body ... I don't like my boyfriend touching me there, I can't wear nice clothes, I can't make the best of what I already have ... even my little sister of 16 has more than I have ever had.

It is of interest to note that surgery can result in restitution of normal body image. In a study of 11 young women with no other disease and breast size not grossly inappropriate for body size requesting reduction mammoplasty, Hollyman et al. (1986) found that, after surgery, body image had returned to normal; self-confidence, feelings about femininity and sexual attractiveness were also enhanced.

Symptoms of dysmorphophobia are sometimes described by patients with schizophrenia. It may occur as the first symptom as the condition develops, and the clinician should therefore look carefully for suggestive symptoms. It may also be present in the established case and will then show characteristic schizophrenic symptomatology. A 19-year-old African-Caribbean girl, previously diagnosed with schizophrenia, said:

The Spirit is a man, he feels warm and moves in me. I can't feel yet. I've got to pray for my new body. I'll have it in March. I will have to look beautiful, I don't feel beautiful at the moment, I don't look nice enough. I'll have a nice face, nice teeth, red eyebrows, red eyes, pupils red and smooth red lips. My skin will be light and I'll have long fair thick hair down to my knees. My voice will be different and I'll have a new tongue. I'll speak many languages. I'll sing too. My brain and my mind will be the same. I'll have long fingernails, a smaller waist, bigger breasts and my legs will be a bit

shapelier. My figure will change from 33" 24" 35" to 38" 18" 36".

There is emerging evidence that visual processing of faces and objects may be impaired in individuals with body dysmorphic disorder. Abnormalities include inability to identify faces with emotional expressions under experimental conditions (Feusner et al., 2010a) and the use of greater detail-orientated and piecemeal processing of faces compared with controls (Feusner et al., 2010b). Impairments of face processing appear to correlate with demonstrable abnormalities in frontostriatal systems (Feusner et al., 2010c), and regional brain volumes of the left inferior frontal gyrus and amygdala are positively correlated with severity scores of dysmorphic disorder (Feusner et al., 2009). These findings suggest that, despite the absence of gross abnormalities of perception, face and visual object processing impairments may underlie the negative evaluations of the body that are characteristic of dysmorphophobia.

BODY INTEGRITY IDENTITY DISORDER

This is a rare condition in which there is an apparent mismatch between the body image and the physical body. Patients have a strong desire to change the physical body so that it coincides with the body image. The most common desire is to amputate a major limb or to sever the spinal cord to become paralysed. Patients are reported as saying, 'I can feel exactly where my leg should end and my stump should begin. Sometimes this line hurts or feels numb' or 'my limbs do not feel like they belong to me, and should not be there' (Blom et al., 2012). Reports suggest that surgery is followed by a feeling of completeness, wholeness and satisfaction. It is perhaps significant that approximately half of a cohort of patients studied said that they felt sexually aroused when they saw a disabled person resembling their own desired disability or felt sexually aroused when imagining themselves being disabled (Blom et al., 2012).

DISTURBANCE OF EATING AND BODY SIZE

Disturbance of eating occurs with various conditions in which alteration of body image either causes eating disorder or results from it. Two conditions are discussed: anorexia nervosa and bulimia nervosa. Once again, it is the subjective aspects, the effect on self-image, that concerns us here and not the physical aspects.

Anorexia Nervosa

This is a condition that in the past was misplaced diagnostically; initially, sufferers were usually thought to be physically ill. Marcé (1860), however, considered it to be one form of hypochondriasis. Anorexia nervosa is an illness that occurs mainly in young women; the proportion of male cases seen ranges from 1 in 20 to about 1 in 10 in different series (Dally and Gomez, 1979), and the proportion of boys is higher in childhood. There is a failure to eat, low body weight and amenorrhoea. It has been considered by Crisp (1975) that the disorder is primarily a *weight phobia*, a fear of increasing body weight, and not only a feeding disorder similar to those of childhood. Prominent is the fear of loss of control; if one eats normally, one will be unable to stop and therefore become fat. As well as an abnormal self-image, there are also abnormal attitudes towards food, gender and sex. How does the patient with anorexia nervosa see herself? It is in part a narcissistic disorder according to Bruch (1965), who has called it 'the pursuit of thinness'. In the definition in *International Classification of Diseases* (10th revision), body image distortion is one of five essential features: 'There is body image distortion in the form of a specific psychopathology whereby a dread of fatness persists as an intrusive, overvalued idea and the patient imposes a low weight threshold on himself or herself' (World Health Organization, 1992, p. 177). The other features are:

- body weight at least 15% below that expected,
- weight loss is self-induced,
- amenorrhoea, and
- delayed or arrested puberty.

Anorexia nervosa became more common in the United Kingdom in the latter part of the 20th century (Kendell et al., 1973). It is much rarer in, for example, India and other developing countries. This apparent difference in prevalence suggests that it may well be linked to social attitudes towards thinness, dieting and slimming. In the Western world, slimness is regarded as beautiful, and dieting may become a social norm that acts as a persuasive pressure on an impressionable adolescent female whose body weight has increased a little more than average at puberty. If there are other psychological difficulties and social conflicts, the slimming may get out of control. In other parts of the world where the aesthetic norms of feminine beauty are based on a fulsome body, the pressure towards thinness is less but the pressure towards obesity may be greater. Even in Western society, the prevalence of anorexia nervosa is not uniform within society but rather is determined by gender, age, socioeconomic class and ethnicity.

Patients with anorexia nervosa often deny their thinness and sometimes claim to be too fat. Because of their extreme concern over their physical size and weight, a technique was devised by Slade and Russell (1973) to investigate bodily perception in anorexics. This involved comparing real size in subjects (measured by an anthropometer) and perceived size, which was measured by the observer moving horizontal lights to a distance that the subject estimated as the width across four body regions: face, chest, waist and hips. Compared with an age-matched normal control group, anorexic patients significantly overestimated their own perceived width at all regions, with the face being overestimated by more than 50%. Although actually thinner at the chest, waist and hips, anorexic patients saw themselves as fatter than normal women. The body image disturbance could not be accounted for by a general perceptual disorder because anorexics were fairly accurate at the measurement of width of wooden blocks and also extremely accurate at measuring physical height. They tended to overestimate the width of other people, but not by as much as themselves. The body image distortion tended to lessen as patients put on weight, especially if they did so slowly. It was shown that a greater degree of body image disorder held a worse prognosis. Slade and Russell (1973) considered that 'patients with anorexia nervosa show a faulty appreciation of their own body image in the sense that they perceive their bodies as possessing an exaggerated girth'. It was found by Garfinkel et al. (1979) that some anorexic subjects tend to overestimate body size and that this overestimate was stable over a year and not affected by weight change.

Experimental work by Button et al. (1977) called into doubt the findings that anorexics alone overestimate their size and normal females are more accurate and that disturbance of body perception is variable among anorexic patients. This finding has now been confirmed in a large meta-analysis by Cash and Deagle (1997). Body image disturbance does not appear to be associated with other features of either anorexia nervosa or bulimia nervosa and does not help to differentiate normal women from patients with eating disorder. Furthermore, attitudinal body dissatisfaction as measured by questionnaires or self: ideal discrepancy best differentiated the patients from the normal control subjects. Thus the role of perceptual size estimation inaccuracy, the formal measure of body image distortion, as a diagnostic criterion of anorexia nervosa has to be called into question.

Slade (1988) has also shown that nonanorexic subjects overestimate the dimensions of their body, especially normal females, neurotic subjects, those who are pregnant and patients with secondary amenorrhoea. He has contrasted the use of *full body* techniques (with distorting mirrors, photographs, television images) for investigating this with *part of body* methods (visual size estimation, callipers) and has shown that relatively fixed cognitive attitudes towards body size with the former demonstrate irrational beliefs about body shape, whereas a more fluid state of the estimation of body size depends more on emotional factors that change over time. He has also shown that the more 'overfat' the individual considers herself to be, the more dissatisfied she will be.

Many recent studies have been carried out in supposedly normal populations. Strauman et al. (1991) studied the views of self in a large number of female undergraduates for the factors they described as 'actual:ideal self-discrepancy' and 'actual:ought discrepancy'. They showed that the actual:ideal discrepancy correlated with body shape dissatisfaction. The actual:ought discrepancy was associated with what they described as anorexic-related attitudes and behaviours and actual:ideal discrepancy with bulimic-related attitudes and behaviours. Gustavson et al. (1990) investigated body image distortion and showed differences between normal students and those suffering from eating disorders. Moore (1988) surveyed 854 females aged between 12 and 23 years from outpatient clinics; 67% were found to be dissatisfied with their weight and 54% with their shape.

Zellner et al. (1989) studied the effects of eating abnormalities and gender on the perception of desirable body shape, using figure drawings by their subjects. They found that women desire to be thinner than they think they are and that women with eating disorders desire to be thinner than that degree of thinness that they think that men will find attractive. Steiger et al. (1989) found that anorexics, but not bulimics, exhibited body image distortion and that body weight predicted the degree of body image disturbance. Dolan et al. (1990) demonstrated differences between white, African-Caribbean and Asian British women for some of the symptoms of eating disorders but no differences for body image disorder.

Supported by these studies is the finding of a clear association between body image disturbance and eating disorder. This is related inversely to weight—that is, the lower the weight, the greater the degree of body image abnormality. Thus, in general, those with anorexia are more affected than those with bulimia nervosa.

A perpetual question is the degree to which culture influences body image and to what extent the social environment has a significant impact on body image. There is evidence that body dissatisfaction is prevalent in females across ethnic groups in the same country and across national boundaries (Angelova and Utermohlen, 2013; Baillie and Copeland, 2013; Demuth et al., 2013; Santana et al., 2013). There are factors unique to particular settings. So in the Bulgarian context, faith and traditional fasting differentially affected the behaviours of women depending on their pre-existing predisposition to disordered eating. For vulnerable women, fasting acted via reinforcement of asceticism and dietary restraint to induce weight management to achieve a desired thin figure consistent with sociocultural norms (Angelova and Utermohlen, 2013). In the United States, European American women endorsed 'a curvy-thin or athletic ideal body', whereas African American women 'resisted notions of a singular ideal body' (Webb et al., 2013). In an elegant study, Bagrowicz et al (2013) investigated a sample of Japanese students who had recently arrived in New York City to see what the influence of endemic obesity was. After 2 months in New York, the Japanese students had thinner self-image but 'a fatter ideal-image' and consequently less body dissatisfaction. This study suggests that social environment rapidly influences ideal body size.

It does seem that abnormality of self and body image is universal in eating disorders: 'I eat therefore I am'. There are associations between abnormal eating, especially in anorexia nervosa, and low body weight, with a belief or fear that 'I am too fat' and with a more pervasive denial of self. In attempting to investigate the factors that influence this overestimation of their body size by anorexic and bulimic women, Hamilton and Waller (1993) studied the influence of media portrayal of idealized female bodies. They concluded that women with eating disorders overestimated themselves substantially more after seeing such images than after seeing photographs of neutral objects. Such images in the media do appear to influence female behaviour, at least in some vulnerable people.

Strober et al. (1979) assessed perception of body size, subjective experience of body image distortions and differentiation of body concepts by asking adolescent anorexic patients and controls to draw the human figure soon after their hospital admission and 6 months later. Both groups tended to overestimate size at both times, but experiences denoting estrangement from the body, insensitivity to body sensations and weakness of body boundaries were more prevalent in anorexics, and they persisted at high levels after frank symptoms of weight and eating disorder had subsided. There was a greater degree of a more persistent body image distortion in those who vomited. These authors considered that 'defects in body image formation render the anorexic vulnerable to their manifest pathology, which is itself activated by maturational conflicts unique to adolescence'.

The underlying fear of loss of control and the incessant need for vigilance concerning any calorie that enters the mouth influence all other areas of the patient's life. Obsessional tidiness and cleanliness may be manifested, as well as attempts to control the behaviour of other people at home. An anorexic patient controlled the behaviour of her parents and twin sister by threatening to starve herself yet further if they would not cooperate. She weighed not only her own food but that of all the other members of the family. Before her illness, she and her sister both weighed about 57 kg, but as her anorexia progressed, she insisted on her twin eating her food also, which the patient cooked.

As a result, the patient dropped in weight to about 32 kg, while her sister reached 83 kg.

The role of chemosensory function in eating disorders and in anorexia nervosa in particular is only starting to be investigated and explored (Leland et al., 2021). There is a growing body of evidence that patients with anorexia nervosa salivate less than controls in response to olfactory stimuli, whereas patients with bulimia salivate more. Furthermore, patients with anorexia nervosa have impaired identification and threshold functions for taste compared to controls, and this was also true for patients with bulimia nervosa. These changes improved with treatment, but there remained residual impairment. Impairment of olfaction was equivocal.

Bulimia Nervosa

This condition was first described by Russell in 1979. Although the patient is currently of normal or near-normal weight, there is often a history of anorexia nervosa with weight loss (Fairburn and Cooper, 1984). Body image distortion is also a feature of the condition, with the patient believing herself to be too fat and too heavy.

The characteristic eating disorder is of gross preoccupation with food, with episodic binge eating or gorging. This is frequently countered with self-induced vomiting and other methods of weight reduction such as abuse of drugs, such as laxatives or amphetamine-like drugs, or voluntary starvation. Weight is thus maintained with a fragile stability; sometimes weight loss may reach anorexic proportions, and sometimes there may be mild obesity that is associated with feelings of guilt. The fear of putting on weight and the dominating preoccupation with food is an *overvalued idea*.

There is marked dissatisfaction with the body in bulimia nervosa that is similar to that in anorexia nervosa (Cash and Deagle, 1997). There is evidence that the dissatisfaction with the body derives from cognitive evaluative dissatisfaction and is not dependent on sensory perception, although it may be influenced by mood (Gardner and Bockenkamp, 1996). Various abnormal behaviours may occur, including alcohol abuse, shoplifting (especially involving stealing food) and deliberate self-harm. A variety of serious physical complications may result from rigorous self-induced vomiting or purging.

Underlying factors are particularly centred on doubts concerning femininity (Lacey et al., 1986). Poor relationships with parents, academic striving, parental marital conflict and poor relationships with the patients' own peers also occur. These patients described major life events in the areas of sexual conflict, major changes in life circumstances and experience of loss.

Muscle Dysmorphia

Muscle dysmorphia is a term used to describe the pathologic preoccupation with muscularity. It is characterized by preoccupation with (1) muscle size and build, (2) the belief that one's muscles are too small, (3) excessive time spent in the gymnasium weightlifting, (4) use of anabolic steroids and bulking diets and (5) in extreme form, cosmetic surgery including pectoral implants. It is sometimes referred to as *reverse anorexia* or *bigorexia* (Pope et al., 1997; Choi et al., 2002). The exact nosologic status of muscle dysmorphia is uncertain. Some authors have described it as a variant of body dysmorphic disorder (Choi et al., 2002), others as a male variant of anorexia nervosa (Murray et al., 2010), and others have commented on the relationship with obsessive compulsive disorder (Chung, 2001). It is probably best in the current state of knowledge to regard it as a phenomenon that can occur in a variety of psychiatric disorders rather than as a disorder in its own right.

Mitchison et al. (2021) report a point prevalence of muscle dysmorphia of 2.2% in adolescent boys and 1.4% in adolescent girls and conclude that the condition is relatively common in early to late adolescence. In boys it is associated weightlifting regime that interferes with life, whereas in girls they are more likely to report discomfort with body exposure.

There is consistent evidence that men with muscle dysmorphia have disturbed body image, disordered eating and excessive exercising (Murray et al., 2012). In weightlifters, its prevalence has been reported as 13.6% (Behar and Molinari, 2010). Body checking, which can be construed as evidence of body dissatisfaction, is common in muscle dysmorphia (Cafri et al., 2008; Walker et al., 2009). In comparison to weightlifters without muscle dysmorphia, patients with muscle dysmorphia were more likely to have body dissatisfaction, abnormal eating attitudes, use anabolic

steroids and have a history of anxiety or depression. They also complained of shame and embarrassment, poorer quality of life and previous attempted suicide, and there was evidence of impaired occupational and social functioning (Olivardia et al., 2000; Pope et al., 2005). There is evidence that men with muscle dysmorphia have attentional biases towards subjectively negative areas of their own bodies and towards positive areas of hypermuscular bodies of others accompanying with significant deterioration in their body image and affect. It is thought that these attentional biases may serve to maintain severe muscularity dissatisfaction (Waldorf et al., 2019).

Disorders of the Sensory Awareness of the Body (Organic Changes in Body Image)

Disease of, and trauma to, the brain alter the body image in a variety of ways. This is either because of damage of the conceptualized object, for example, amputation with phantom limb or blindness necessarily altering the way one perceives oneself, or damage to the process of conceptualization itself, for example, damage to a section of the corpus callosum. Often, of course, there is scattered damage, as with arteriopathy or multiple sclerosis, and these two features cannot be separated.

The expression *body image* as used in neurology was defined by Critchley (1950) as the mental idea that an individual possesses about his own body and its physical and aesthetic attributes. Visual sensation, tactile impulses and proprioceptive stimuli contribute to the formation of body image but are not essential; after the amputation of a limb, a phantom limb retaining the integrity of the body image occurs in the majority of cases. The body image 'lives on the fringe of awareness and is by no means obtrusive in ordinary circumstances. It is however available and can be brought into consciousness as soon as the stream of attention voluntarily or involuntarily focuses upon it' (Critchley, 1950). Morbid changes in the body image may show enhancement, diminution (or ablation) or distortion. In neurology, the term *body schema* is used for the awareness of spatial characteristics of one's own body, involving current and previous sensory information, whereas *body experience* is more comprehensive, including psychological and situational factors also (Cumming, 1988). The parietal lobes play a major role, but the somatoaesthetic afferent system and the thalamus are also involved.

PATHOLOGIC ACCENTUATION OF BODY IMAGE (HYPERSCHEMAZIA)

Pain or discomfort causes the affected part of the body to loom large. After dropping a heavy weight on his great toe, a man felt his body to be 'an insubstantial shell around a huge throbbing toe'. Such a description of the painful organ seeming larger in size is frequent after surgery and traumatic injury. When size is affected, the body may feel larger (*macrosomatognosia*). Critchley gives several examples of neurologic lesions causing enhancement of an organ.

- With partial paralysis of a limb, the affected segment gives the impression of being too heavy and too big; for example, with Brown-Séquard paralysis (unilateral lesion of the spinal cord), the side with the pyramidal signs is hyperschematic, whereas the other side, with loss of pain and temperature sensation, is perceived as normal in body schema.
- Unilaterally, after thrombosis of the posterior inferior cerebellar artery.
- In multiple sclerosis, again unilaterally.

Hyperschemazia may also occur with peripheral vascular disease when the affected limb feels larger and heavier. It may also occur in acute toxic states. Nonorganic cases occur with hypochondriasis, in depersonalization states, with dissociation (conversion disorder, e.g., pseudocyesis) and, occasionally, in dreams.

DIMINISHED OR ABSENT BODY IMAGE (HYPOSCHEMAZIA, ASCHEMAZIA)

This may occur when afferent and efferent innervation is lost; for example, with transection of the spinal cord, the patient may feel sawn off at the waist.

Hyposchemazia or *microsomatognosia* may accompany the sensory deprivation of weightlessness, for instance, under water. With vertigo, the patient may feel excessively light, as if floating in the air.

Parietal lobe lesions may result in complicated states of diminution of the body image. Critchley

(1950) cites a patient with embolism of the right middle cerebral artery:

It felt as if I was missing one side of my body (the left), but it also felt as if the dummy side was lined with a piece of iron so heavy that I could not move it … I even fancied my head to be narrow, but the left side from the centre felt heavy, as if filled with bricks.

At one time he thought that his paralyzed leg belonged to the man in the next bed. His body felt to him half as wide as it should have done. Lying on the left side gave him the sensation that he was 'lying on a void', that he was at the extreme edge of the bed and would presently fall off. In the early days he also felt that he had no penis at all. On this account he was clumsy with the urinal and the bed was frequently soiled. His sensations of owning a penis returned quite suddenly one morning in association with an erection, and it afterwards felt quite normal.

In *hemisomatognosia* (hemidepersonalization), which was described by L'Hermitte (1939) and is a unilateral misperception of one's own body, the patient behaves as though the limbs on one side are missing; this may occur as part of an epileptic aura or migraine. *Anosognosia* describes the lack of awareness of disability, which may, for instance, occur with neglect of a hemiplegic limb. *Hemispatial neglect* describes those patients who, when asked to perform a variety of behavioural tasks in space, neglect the hemispace contralateral to their lesion (Cumming, 1988). Gerstmann's syndrome (Gerstmann, 1930) comprises finger agnosia, acalculia, agraphia and right–left disorientation.

The most severe example of an absent body image is that of Ian Waterman, who at the age of 19 years suffered a total deafferentation of his body from the neck down, resulting in damage to the sensory nerves underpinning touch, the sense of movement and position (proprioception) but sparing sensations of temperature, pain and the motor nerves involved in movement. As Jonathan Cole describes it, 'At that point unable to feel or move, he felt completely disembodied, he had lost touch – literally – with his own body; if he did not look, he did not know it [his body] was there. He was without body in the sense that he could no longer make use of it

... He was terrified' (Cole, 2016). It took tremendous effort to move his limbs under visual guidance, every movement was a performance: 'I rarely touch on why I put so much effort into "performing", because I don't want to be perceived as artificial or false'. This rare case emphasizes the marked distinction between the body as experienced and the self that does the experiencing. In Ian Waterman's case, he continued to be a self even when he could not feel his body. Although, strictly speaking, this is not the whole story because he could visualise his body but not feel it.

Again, nonorganic conditions such as depersonalization may also show diminution of body image. An anxious and depersonalized patient said, 'I don't feel at all the same person. Sometimes my head feels so numb when I walk to the shops. I feel I've left half my body behind'. This was clearly an *as if* experience.

DISTORTION OF THE BODY IMAGE (PARASCHEMAZIA)

This may occur with enhancement or diminution of the body image. It may occur with the use of hallucinogenic drugs such as mescaline, marijuana and lysergic acid diethylamide. Parts of the body may feel distorted, twisted, separated from the rest of the body or merged with the external environment. These experiences can affect either the whole body or part of it, such as the limbs or head. The shape can be experienced as misshapen: 'my lower jaw is twisted and my teeth no longer close properly' or 'my left arm is shrunken and gnarled, a bit like a tree trunk'. When the structure of the body is affected, often it is the internal organs that are the focus of concern:

I assert therefore that on my body, particularly on my bosom, there are present the properties of a nervous system corresponding to a female body and I am certain that a physical examination would confirm this.

and

Food and drink taken simply poured into the abdominal cavity and into the thighs, a process which however unbelievable it may sound, was beyond all doubt for me as I distinctly remember the sensation.

Schreber (1955)

Changes in the experience of weight can involve a sense of either heaviness or lightness. With hashish:

the sensations produced were those of exquisite lightness and airiness ... I expected to be lifted up and carried away by the first breeze ... the walls of my frame were burst outward and tumbled into ruin, and without thinking what form I wore... I felt that I existed throughout a vast extent of space. The blood pulsed from my head, sped through uncounted leagues before it reached my extremities; the air drawn into my lungs expanded into seas of limpid ether, and the arch of my skull was broader than the vault of heaven. I was a mass of transparent jelly, and a confectioner poured me into a twisted mould.

Taylor (1856)

The value attached to the body can be disturbed. This disturbance can vary from strong, positive overvaluation of the body or its parts to a devaluation of the body extending to dislike or hatred of it. In right-sided hemiparesis, patients can sometimes maintain that their weak arm is in fact stronger and more useful than before. This is referred to as *anosognosic overestimation* (Cutting, 1997). *Misoplegia* is the hatred of a limb and is associated with left-sided parietal lesions (Cutting, 1997).

Distortion of body image may occur with epileptic aura and, rarely, with migraine.

Phantom Limb

This occurs immediately after the loss of a limb in virtually all patients, and it is particularly common after the traumatic loss of a limb or if there had been a pre-existing painful condition of the limb. The onset appears immediately as the anaesthesia wears off in the majority of cases but may be delayed for up to a few weeks in about 25% of cases. The phantom may last for a few days or weeks then gradually fades from consciousness. There are, however, cases that have persisted for decades. As well as occurring with the loss of a limb, this type of distortion of body image is relatively common after surgical removal of an eye, parts of the face, breasts, the rectum or the larynx. There are reports of phantom ulcer pains after partial gastrectomy and of menstrual cramp after hysterectomy. If an amputee experiences a generalized peripheral neuritis involving sensation, paraesthesia will also occur in the phantom limb. The amputee is aware of the phantom limb in space and also experiences pain in the space conceived as being occupied by the limb.

With time, the limb appears to change in size. The image shrinks, but unevenly, distal joints shrinking more slowly than proximal; this is the so-called telescoping phenomenon. There are several postulated explanations for *telescoping*. In loss of the upper limb, telescoping is thought to occur because there is over-representation of the hand in the sensory cortex, hence this is the area from which sensation survives longest. There is also the possibility that telescoping occurs because the representation of the limb in the primary somatosensory map changes progressively. The posture of the phantom is often said to be 'habitual', for example, partially flexed at the elbow, with forearm pronated. The limb can sometimes feel fixed in an awkward position, and this can cause the patient difficulty, for instance, in walking upstairs. The limb may feel twisted and painful.

There is increasing literature on the plasticity of the somatosensory system, using phantom limb as a natural experiment to demonstrate deafferentation after loss of a limb and corresponding reorganization of the somatosensory map (Ramachandran and Hirstein, 1998). After loss of the upper limb, sensory input from the face and upper arm have been shown to invade the hand territory, such that sensory stimulus to the face can be mislocalized in the phantom limb.

Orbach and Tallent (1965) described the body concepts of patients 5 to 10 years after the construction of a colostomy. These patients had a conviction that they had been seriously damaged.

They believed that their bodily intactness and integrity had been violated. In common with such beliefs many patients on a fantasy level perceived the operation as a physical or sexual assault. Patients who fantasized the surgery as a sexual assault were supported in this belief by the colostomy stoma, a new opening in the front of the body. Most men regarded this opening as evidence of having been feminized, whereas women often interpreted it as the addition of a second vagina. The bleeding from the stoma reinforced the fantasy of a second vagina because it was interpreted as comparable to menstruation.

In one-fifth of patients, preoccupation about the bodily processes concerned food intake and elimination was embodied in a replacement concept, which attempted to establish equality between intake and evacuation by eating approximately as much as had recently been evacuated. A majority of the remaining patients communicated a sense of confusion about the machinery and functioning of their bodies.

When colostomy patients were initially studied and the reports published, the constriction of activity and of the life space were emphasized. It is now apparent that the constriction is paralleled by a body concept of being damaged and fragile as a consequence of the injury.

Mastectomy also results in relatively severe disturbance in self-concept and body image. A patient described this as 'I will never be like before ... it is like a hole, like a gap ... When I lie on that side, it's like being a man' (Hopwood and Maguire, 1988). Body image problems result not only from the loss of body part or disfigurement but also from the loss of bodily function. The disorder of self-image is frequently associated with depressive symptoms.

Phantom limb pain may be psychologically determined (Parkes, 1976). Forty-six amputees were studied 4 to 8 weeks and 13 months after amputation; a third to a half showed moderate disturbance tending to persist a year later.

Body image disturbance is not necessarily associated with abnormal sensation or perception. The hypochondriac may believe they have cancer although they have no physical symptoms. The transsexual experiences their body normally, but they believe that they are in the wrong body. The narcissist is inordinately concerned with their body; nevertheless, they are quite accurate in their objective quantitative perception of self, that is, they know how long their nose is or how far they can throw a cricket ball. When sensation is abnormal or even deficient altogether in some modality, for example, with blindness or deafness, body image is undoubtedly altered, but this alteration does not in any way imply mental illness; the alteration of body image is usually appropriate to the disability.

Culture-Bound Disorders of Body Image

Various culturally determined 'hysterical' conditions have been described by Langness (1967). These

TABLE 14.2	Culture-Bound Disorders of Body Image		
Disorder	**Diagnostic Equivalent**	**Location**	**Key Symptom(s)**
Koro	Anxiety state	Southeast Asia	Belief that the penis will retract into the abdomen and cause death
Frigophobia	Obsessive compulsive neurosis	East Asia	Morbid fear of the cold, preoccupation with loss of vitality, compulsive wearing of layers of clothes
Latah	Hysteria	Malaysia	Hyper suggestibility, automatic obedience, coprolalia, echolalia, echopraxia, echomimia, altered consciousness, disorganization, depression and anxiety
Evil eye	Phobic neurosis	Mexico, North Africa	Strong glances are harmful; precautions taken to avoid or counteract evil eye
Voodoo	Phobic neurosis	Haiti	Violation of taboo may result in death
Windigo	Depressive reaction	Canada, First Nations	Fear of engaging in cannibalism and of becoming a sorcerer, depression of mood
Amok	Dissociative state	Malaysia	Neurasthenia, depersonalization, rage, automatism and violent acts

After Kiev, A., 1972. Transcultural Psychiatry. Penguin, Harmondsworth, with permission of Penguin.

conditions have in common a sudden, dramatic onset related in time to a psychosocial upset. Manifestations of these conditions are grossly unusual behaviour, volatile mood, transient occurrences of alterations of speech, depersonalization with altered body awareness and symptoms somewhat similar to delusions and hallucinations. The course of these conditions is usually limited to 1 to 3 weeks, but they may recur with further episodes. They appear to be more likely in those predisposed with histrionic (hysterical) personalities. The precise symptoms are often localized to that particular culture and demonstrate how neurotic symptoms in their content comply with the expectations of the society in which they occur. For instance, Adair, writing from Bath in 1786, described how fashion influenced the great and opulent in the choice of their diseases and considered that Queen Anne's nervousness resulted in the transfer of similar symptoms 'to all who had the least pretensions to rank with persons of fashion'.

Some of the culturally localized disorders of awareness of the body are summarized in Table 14.2 (Kiev, 1972). The variability of such syndromes is immense, but the preoccupation with bodily organs and functions is common to many of them. The bizarre nature of symptoms—for example, koro in which there is fear of the penis shrinking into the abdomen—is often explained by a faulty knowledge of human anatomy and physiology that seems naive to doctors practising in Europe. However, it is not generally known how ignorant British patients are concerning the organization and functions of the organs they cannot see. Hospital outpatients were compared with doctors by Boyle (1970) in their understanding of commonly used medical terms. As might be expected, the doctors were consistent in their use of terms, but patients had enormous variation in their understanding of such terms as *piles, least starchy food, palpitation jaundice* and *flatulence*. When asked to detail the surface anatomy of internal organs—for example, bladder, kidneys and thyroid gland—the patients showed great variation and were generally quite inaccurate. There are also bizarre anomalies of body image and function occurring in practice in the United Kingdom. A young Lancashire woman working in a mill complained of migrainous headaches and ascribed these to insufficiently heavy periods. This explanation was found to be culturally acceptable to her peers.

REFERENCES

Adair, J.M., 1786. Medical Cautions for the Consideration of Invalids, Those Especially Who Resort to Bath. Dodsley and Dilly, Bath.

Aldous, J.C., Ellam, G.A., Murray, V., Pike, G., 1994. An outbreak of illness among schoolchildren in London: toxic poisoning not mass hysteria. J. Epidemiol. Community Health 48, 41–45.

Andreasen, N.C., Bardach, J., 1977. Dysmorphophobia: symptom or disease? Am. J. Psychiatry 134, 673–675.

Angelova, R.A., Utermohlen, V., 2013. Culture-specific influences on body image and eating distress in a sample of urban Bulgarian women: the roles of faith and traditional fasting. Eat. Behav. 14, 386–389.

Appleby, L., 1987. Hypochondriasis: an acceptable diagnosis? Br. Med. J. 294, 857.

Auden, W.H., 1969. The art of healing: in Memoriam David Protech, MD. In: Epistle to a Godson. Collected Poems, 1976. Faber and Faber, London, p. 626.

Bagrowicz, R., Watanabe, C., Umezaki, M., 2013. Is obesity contagious by way of body image? A study of Japanese female students in the United States. J. Community Health 38, 834–837.

Baillie, L.E., Copeland, A.L., 2013. Disordered eating and body image in Chinese and Caucasian students in the United States. Eat. Beyond Behav. 14, 314–319.

Barsky, A.J., Klerman, G.L., 1983. Overview: hypochondriasis, bodily complaints and somatic styles. Am. J. Psychiatry 140, 273–283.

Bartholomew, R.E., Wessely, S., 2002. Protean nature of mass sociogenic illness. Br. J. Psychiatry 180, 300–306.

Behar, R., Molinari, D., 2010. Muscle dysmorphia, body image and eating behaviours in two male populations. Rev. Med. Chil. 138, 1386–1394.

Berrios, G.E., 1996. The History of Mental Symptoms: Descriptive Psychopathology since the Nineteenth Century. Cambridge University Press, Cambridge.

Birtchnell, S.A., 1988. Dysmorphophobia – a centenary discussion. Br. J. Psychiatry 153, 41–43.

Blom, R.M., Heenekam, R.C., Denys, D., 2012. Body integrity identity disorder. PLoS One 7, e34702.

Boyle, C.M., 1970. Difference between patients' and doctors' interpretation of some common medical terms. Br. Med. J. 2, 286–289.

Bridges, K.W., Goldberg, D.P., 1985. Somatic presentation of DSM-III psychiatric disorders in primary care. J. Psychosom. Res. 29, 563–569.

Bruch, H., 1965. Anorexia nervosa and its differential diagnosis. J. Nerv. Ment. Dis. 141, 555–566.

Burton, R., 1628. The Anatomy of Melancholia. Cripps, Oxford.

Button, E.J., Fransella, F., Slade, P.D., 1977. A reappraisal of body perception disturbance in anorexia nervosa. Psychol. Med. 7, 235–243.

Cafri, G., Olivardia, R., Thompson, J.K., 2008. Symptom characteristics and psychiatric comorbidity among males with muscle dysmorphia. Compr. Psychiatry 49, 374–379.

Cash, T.F., Deagle, E.A., 1997. The nature and extent of body-image disturbances in anorexia nervosa and bulimia nervosa: a meta-analysis. Int. J. Eat. Disord. 22, 107–125.

Choi, P.Y.L., Pope Jr, H.G., Olivardia, R., 2002. Muscle dysmorphia: a new syndrome in weightlifters. Br. J. Sports Med. 36, 375–377.

Chowdhury, A.N., Brahma, A., 2005. An epidemic of mass hysteria in a village in West Bengal. Indian J. Psychiatry 47, 106–108.

Chung, B., 2001. Muscle dysmorphia: a critical review of the proposed criteria. Perspect. Biol. Med. 44, 565–574.

Cohn, N., 1958. The Pursuit of the Millennium. Secker and Warburg, London.

Cole, J., 2016. Losing Touch – A Man without His Body. Oxford University Press, Oxford.

Cotard, M., 1882. Nihilistic delusions. Reprinted. In: Hirsch, S.R., Shepherd, M. (Eds.), Themes and Variations in European Psychiatry. John Wright, Bristol, p. 1974.

Crisp, A.H., 1975. Anorexia nervosa. In: Silverstone, T., Barraclough, B. (Eds.), Contemporary Psychiatry. Headley Brothers, Ashford, pp. 150–158.

Critchley, M., 1950. The body image in neurology. Lancet 1, 335–341.

Cumming, W.J.K., 1988. The neurobiology of the body schema. Br. J. Psychiatry 153, 7–11.

Cutting, J., 1997. Principles of Psychopathology. Oxford University Press, Oxford.

Dally, P., Gomez, J., 1979. Anorexia Nervosa. Heinemann, London.

Davey, G.C., 2011. Disgust: the disease-avoidance emotion and its dysfunctions. Philosophical Transactions of the Royal Society London. Series B. Biological Sciences 366, 3453–3465.

Demuth, A., Czerniak, U., Ziółkowska-Łajp, E., 2013. A comparison of a subjective body assessment of men and women of the Polish social elite. Homo 64, 398–409.

Dolan, B., Lacey, J.H., Evans, C., 1990. Eating behaviour and attitudes to weight and shape in British women from three ethnic groups. Br. J. Psychiatry 157, 523–528.

Fairburn, C.G., Cooper, P.J., 1984. The clinical features of bulimia nervosa. Br. J. Psychiatry 144, 238–246.

Farooq, S., Gahir, S.M., Okyere, E., Sheikh, A.J., Oyebode, F., 1995. Somatization: a transcultural study. J. Psychosom. Res. 39, 883–888.

Feusner, J.D., Bystritsky, A., Hellemann, G., Bookheimer, S., 2010a. Impaired identity recognition of faces with emotional expressions in body dysmorphic disorder. Psychiatry Res. 179, 318–323.

Feusner, J.D., Moller, H., Altstein, L., et al., 2010b. Inverted face processing in body dysmorphic disorder. J. Psychiatr. Res. 44, 1088–1094.

Feusner, J.D., Moody, T., Hembacher, E., et al., 2010c. Abnormalities of visual processing and frontostriatal systems in body dysmorphic disorder. Arch. Gen. Psychiatry 67, 197–205.

Feusner, J.D., Townsend, J., Bystrisky, A., Moller, H., Bookheimer, S., 2009. Regional brain volumes and symptom severity in body dysmorphic disorder. Psychiatry Res. 172, 161–167.

Fink, P., Ørnbøl, E., Toft, T., Sparle, K.C., Frostholm, L., Olesen, F., 2004. A new, empirically established hypochondriasis diagnosis. Am. J. Psychiatry 161, 1680–1691.

Gardner, R.M., Bockenkamp, E.D., 1996. The role of sensory and nonsensory factors in body size estimations of eating disorder subjects. J. Clin. Psychol. 52, 3–15.

Garfinkel, P.E., Moldofsky, H., Garner, D., 1979. The stability of perceptual disturbances in anorexia nervosa. Psychol. Med. 9, 703–708.

Gerstmann, J., 1930. The symptoms produced by lesions of the transitional area between the inferior parietal and middle occipital gyri. Reprinted. In: Rottenberg, D.A., Hochberg, F.H. (Eds.), Neurological Classics in Modern Translation. Hafner Press, New York, p. 1977.

Gibbs, R.W., 2005. Embodiment and Cognitive Science. Cambridge University Press, Cambridge.

Gustavson, C.R., Gustavson, J.C., Pumariega, A.J., et al., 1990. Body-image distortion among male and female college and high school students, and eating-disordered patients. Percept. Mot. Skills 71 (Pt 1), 1003–1010.

Hamilton, K., Waller, G., 1993. Media influences on body size estimation in anorexia and bulimia: an experimental study. Br. J. Psychiatry 162, 837–840.

Hay, G.G., 1970. Dysmorphophobia. Br. J. Psychiatry 116, 399–406.

Hay, G.G., Heather, B.B., 1973. Changes in psychometric test results following cosmetic nasal operations. Brit. J. Psychol. 122, 89–90.

Hollyman, J.A., Lacey, J.H., Whitfield, P.J., Wilson, J.S.P., 1986. Surgery for the psyche: a longitudinal study of women undergoing reduction mammoplasty. Br. J. Plast. Surg. 39, 222–224.

Hopwood, P., Maguire, G.P., 1988. Body image problems in cancer patients. Br. J. Psychiatry 153, 47–50.

Howson, A., 2013. The Body in Society – an Introduction, second ed. Polity Press, Cambridge.

Huxley, A., 1952. The Devils of Loudon. Penguin, Harmondsworth.

Jones, T.F., 2000. Mass psychogenic illness: role of the individual physician. Am. Fam. Physician 15, 2649–2653.

Karseras, A.G., 1976. Psychiatric aspects of ophthalmology. In: Howells, J.G. (Ed.), Modern Perspectives in the Psychiatric Aspects of Surgery. Macmillan, London.

Kellner, R., 1985. Functional somatic symptoms and hypochondriasis. Arch. Gen. Psychiatry 42, 821–833.

Kendell, R.E., 2001. The distinction between mental and physical illness. Br. J. Psychiatry 178, 490–493.

Kendell, R.E., Hall, D.J., Hailey, A., Babigian, H.M., 1973. The epidemiology of anorexia nervosa. Psychol. Med. 3, 200–203.

Kenyon, F.E., 1964. Hypochondriasis: a clinical study. Br. J. Psychiatry 110, 478–488.

Kenyon, F.E., 1965. Hypochondriasis: a survey of some historical, clinical and social aspects. Br. J. Med. Psychol. 38, 117–133.

Kenyon, F.E., 1976. Hypochondriacal states. Br. J. Psychiatry 129, 1–14.

Kharabsheh, S., Al-Otoum, H., Clements, J., et al., 2001. Mass psychogenic illness following tetanus-diphtheria toxoid vaccination in Jordan. Bull. World Health Organ. 79, 764–770.

Kiev, A., 1972. Transcultural Psychiatry. Penguin, Harmondsworth.

Kirmayer, L.J., Looper, K.J., 2006. Abnormal illness behaviour: physiological, psychological and social dimensions of coping with distress. Curr. Opin. Psychiatry 19, 54–60.

Kokota, D., 2011. View point: episodes of mass hysteria in African schools – study of literature. Malawi Med. J. 23, 74–77.

Lacey, J.H., Coker, S., Birtchnell, S.A., 1986. Bulimia: factors associated with its aetiology and maintenance. Int. J. Eat. Disord. 5, 475–487.

Lader, M., Sartorius, N., 1968. Anxiety in patients with hysterical conversion symptoms. J. Neurol. Neurosurg. Psychiatry 13, 490–495.

Langness, L.L., 1967. Hysterical psychosis: the cross-cultural evidence. Am. J. Psychiatry 124, 143–152.

Leland, E.M., Xie, D.X., Kamath, V., Seal, S.M., Lin, S.Y., Rowan, N.R., 2022. Psychophysical chemosensory dysfunction in eating disorders: a qualitative systematic review. Eat. Weight Disord. 27 (2), 429–447. https://doi.org/10.1007/s40519-021-01189-2.

Lewis, A.J., 1975. The survival of hysteria. Psychol. Med. 5, 9–12.

L'Hermitte, J., 1939. L'image de Notre Corps. Revue Nouvelle Critique, Paris.

Luckianowicz, A., 1967. Body Image" disturbances in psychiatric disorders. Brit. J. Psychiat. 113, 31–47.

Marcé, L.V., 1860. Note on a form of hypochondriacal delusion consecutive to the dyspepsias and principally characterized by refusal of food (A. Blewett, A. Bottéro, Trans. 1994). Hist. Psychiat. 5, 273–283.

Mechanic, D., 1962. Students under Stress: A Study in the Social Psychology of Adaption. Free Press, New York.

Mechanic, D., 1986. The concept of illness behaviour: culture, situation and personal predisposition. Psychol. Med. 16, 1–7.

Merleau-Ponty, M., 1962. Phenomenology of Perception. Routledge, London.

Merskey, H., 1979. The Analysis of Hysteria. Baillière Tindall, London.

Merskey, H., Buhrich, N.A., 1975. Hysteria and organic brain disease. Br. J. Med. Psychol. 48, 359–366.

Mitchison, D., Mond, J., Griffiths, S., Hay, P., Nagata, J.M., Bussey, K., 2021. Prevalence of muscle dysmorphia in adolescents: findings from the EveryBODY study. Psychol. Med. 1–8.

Moore, D.C., 1988. Body image and eating behaviour in adolescent girls. Am. J. Dis. Child. 142, 1114–1118.

Morselli, E., 1886. Sulla dismorfofobia e sulla tafefobia. Bolletino Accademia delle Scienze Mediche di Genova VI, 100–119.

Moss, P.D., McEvedy, C.P., 1966. An epidemic of over-breathing among schoolgirls. Br. Med. J. 2, 1295–1300.

Mumford, D.B., Davington, J.T., Bhatnagar, J.S., Hussain, Y., Mirza, S., Naraghi, M.M., 1991. The Bradford Somatic Inventory: a multi-ethnic inventory of somatic symptoms reported by the Indo-Pakistan Subcontinent. Br. J. Psychiatry 158, 379–386.

Murray, S.B., Rieger, E., Touyz, S.W., De La Garza Garcia, Y., 2010. Muscle dysmorphia and the DSM-V Conundrum: where does it belong? A review paper. Int. J. Eat. Disord. 43, 483–491.

Murray, S.B., Rieger, E., Hildebrandt, T., et al., 2012. A comparison of eating, exercise, shape, and weight related symptomatology in males with muscle dysmorphia and anorexia nervosa. Body Image 9, 193–200.

Muse, K., McManus, F., Leung, C., Mehrebian, B., Williams, J.M., 2012. Cyberchondriasis: fact or fiction? A preliminary examination of the relationship between health anxiety and searching for health information on the Internet. J. Anxiety Disord. 26, 189–196.

Noyes Jr., R., Stuart, S., Longley, S.L., Langbehn, D.R., Happel, R.L., 2002b. Hypochondriasis and fear of death. J. Nerv. Ment. Dis. 190, 503–509.

Noyes Jr., R., Stuart, S., Langbehn, D.R., Happel, R.L., Longley, S.L., Yagla, S.J., 2002a. Childhood antecedents of hypochondriasis. Psychosomatics 43, 282–289.

Olatunji, B.O., Deacon, B.J., Abramowitz, J.S., 2009. Is hypochondriasis an anxiety disorder? Br. J. Psychiatry 194, 481–482.

Olivardia, R., Pope Jr., H.G., Hudson, J.L., 2000. Muscle dysmorphia in male weightlifters: a case control study. Am. J. Psychiatry 157, 1291–1296.

Orbach, C.E., Tallent, N., 1965. Modification of perceived body and of body concept. Arch. Gen. Psychiatry 12, 126–135.

Parkes, C.M., 1976. The psychological reaction to loss of a limb: the first year after amputation. In: Howells, J.G. (Ed.), Modern Perspectives in the Psychiatric Aspects of Surgery. Macmillan, London.

Parsons, T., 1951. Illness and the role of the physician: a sociological perspective. Am. J. Orthopsychiatry 21, 452–460.

Phillips, K.A., Menard, W., Fav, C., Weisberd, R., 2005. Demographic characteristics, phenomenology, comorbidity, and family history in 200 individuals with body dysmorphic disorder. Psychosomatics 46, 317–325.

Phillips, K.A., McElroy, S.L., Kerk, P.E., Pope, H.G., Hudson, J.I., 1993. Body dysmorphic disorder: 30 cases of imagined ugliness. Am. J. Psychiatry 150, 302–308.

Pollio, H., Henley, T., Thompson, C., 2008. The Phenomenology of Everyday Life: Empirical Investigations of Human Experience. Cambridge University Press, Cambridge.

Pope, C.G., Pope, H.G., Menard, W., Fay, C., Olivardia, R., Phillips, K.A., 2005. Clinical features of muscle dysmorphia among males with body dysmorphic disorder. Body Image 2, 395–400.

Pope Jr., H.G., Griber, A.J., Choi, P., Olivardia, R., Phillips, K.A., 1997. Muscle dysmorphia: an under-recognized form of body dysmorphic disorder. Psychosomatics 38, 548–557.

Rack, P., 1982. Race, Culture and Mental Disorder. Tavistock, London.

Ramachandran, V.S., Hirstein, W., 1998. The perception of phantom limbs. The DO Hebb lecture. Brain 121, 1603–1630.

Reed, J.L., 1975. The diagnosis of 'hysteria. Psychol. Med. 5, 13–17.

Robin, A.A., Copas, J.B., Jack, A.B., Kaesar, A.C., Thomas, P.J., 1988. Reshaping the psyche: the concurrent improvement in appearance and mental state after rhinoplasty. Br. J. Psychiatry 152, 539–543.

Russell, G.F.M., 1979. Bulimia nervosa: an ominous form of anorexia nervosa. Psychol. Med. 9, 429–448.

Santana, M.L., Silva Rde, C., Assis, A.M., Raich, R.M., Machado, M.E., de Júnor Pinto, E., 2013. Factors associated with body image dissatisfaction among adolescents in public schools in Salvador, Brazil. Nutr. Hosp. 28, 747–755.

Schreber, D., 1955. Memoirs of My Nervous Illness. Dawson, London.

Sims, A.C.P., 1985. Head injury, neurosis and accident proneness. In: Trimble, M.R. (Ed.), Advances in Psychosomatic Medicine: Neuropsychiatry. Karger, Basel.

Slade, P.D., 1988. Body image in anorexia nervosa. Br. J. Psychiatry 153, 20–22.

Slade, P.D., Russell, G.F.M., 1973. Awareness of body dimension in anorexia nervosa: cross-sectional and longitudinal studies. Psychol. Med. 3, 188–199.

Slater, E., 1965. Diagnosis of hysteria. Br. Med. J. 1, 1395–1399.

Slater, E., Glithero, E., 1965. A follow-up of patients diagnosed as suffering from hysteria. J. Psychosom. Res. 9, 9–13.

St Clare, W., 1787. Country News. *The Gentleman's Magazine* 57, 1268. Cited by Hunter, R., Macalpine, I., 1963. Three Hundred Years of Psychiatry. Oxford University Press, London.

Starcevic, V., Berle, D., 2013. Cyberchondria: towards a better understanding of excessive health-related Internet use. Expert Rev. Neurother. 13, 205–213.

Steiger, H., Fraenkel, L., Leichner, P.P., 1989. Relationship of body-image distortion to sex-role identifications, irrational cognitions, and body weight in eating-disordered females. J. Clin. Psychol. 45, 61–65.

Strauman, T.J., Vookles, J., Berenstein, V., Chaiken, S., Higgins, E.T., 1991. Self-discrepancies and vulnerability to body dissatisfaction and disordered eating. J. Pers. Soc. Psychol. 61, 946–956.

Strober, M., Goldenberg, I., Green, J., Saxon, J., 1979. Body image disturbance in anorexia nervosa during the acute and recuperative phase. Psychol. Med. 9, 695–701.

Taylor, B., 1856. The hasheesh eater. Putnam's Monthly Magazine of American Literature. Science and Art 8, 233–239.

Veale, D., Boocock, A., Gournay, K., et al., 1996. Body dysmorphic disorder: a survey of 50 cases. Br. J. Psychiatry 169, 196–201.

Veith, I., 1965. Hysteria: The History of a Disease. University of Chicago Press, Chicago.

Waldorf, M., Vocks, S., Düsing, R., Bauer, A., Cordes, M., 2019. Body-oriented gaze behaviours in men with muscle dysmorphia diagnoses. J. Abnorm. Psychol. 128 (2), 140–150.

Walker, D.C., Anderson, D.A., Hildebrandt, T., 2009. Body checking behaviours in men. Body Image 6, 164–170.

Webb, J.B., Warren-Findlow, J., Chou, Y., Adams, L., 2013. Do you see what I see?: an exploration of inter-ethnic ideal body size comparisons among college women. Body Image 10, 369–379.

World Health Organization, 1992. The ICD-10 Classification of Mental and Behavioural Disorders: Clinical Description and Diagnostic Guidelines. World Health Organization, Geneva.

Zellner, D.A., Harner, D.E., Adler, R.L., 1989. Effects of eating abnormalities and gender on perceptions of desirable body shape. J. Abnorm. Psychol. 98, 93–96.

The Psychopathology of Pain

Chapter Outline

KEYWORDS

Pain asymbolia
Phantom pain
Burning mouth syndrome
Vulvodynia

Summary

Pain is an unpleasant experience that involves the conscious awareness of noxious sensations, hurting and aversive feelings associated with actual or potential tissue damage (International Association for the Study of Pain, 1994). It is often conceptualized as a mood state. In psychiatry, pain can present as being heightened, markedly diminished or occurring in the absence of demonstrable cause. The most problematic cases are those in which pain is the focus of presentation but there is an absence of identifiable physical cause. Facial pain, burning mouth syndrome, vulvodynia and psychogenic itch are illustrative examples of this problem.

'You want to hear of me, my dear? That's something new, I am sure, when anybody wants to hear of me. Not at all well, Louisa. Very faint and giddy.' 'Are you in pain, dear mother?'

'I think there's a pain somewhere in the room,' said Mrs Gradgrind, 'but I couldn't positively say that I have got it.'
               ***Charles Dickens (1854),* Hard Times**

Since Aristotle, pain has been classified not as a perception but as a mood state, and so excluded from the five senses. It is conceptually a most difficult topic, hard to describe and to categorize; the only aspect that is clear is that it represents a state of subjective suffering of the patient. But what does he mean by 'my pain'? Where is it and what is it? Certainly, the *meaning* of the pain is more than the pain itself, and often it is the reason for the sensation being interpreted as suffering. A patient with soreness of the throat believed themself to have cancer of the throat; their mother had died of that condition. The relation between symptoms and their meaning is not straightforward. Another person believed themselves to be suffering from venereal disease without having been exposed to the risk. But they had previously been successfully treated for Hodgkin's disease. They had no fears concerning their factual and potentially lethal illness but only admitted consciously to fearing the impossible.

Phenomenological aspects of the experience of pain are not well charted, although in general medicine this is, above all others, the area in which phenomenology could be most helpful: pain is a subjective experience that occurs only in consciousness (Bond, 1976). The psychiatrist is often confronted with the problem of whether the pain is *physical* or *mental*, *organic* or *functional*, *medical* or *psychiatric*, and, of course, the answer for each contrasted pair is often both. We may then be requested to assess how much of the pain is psychogenic, although this is virtually impossible because, following Aristotle, pain is a state of mind, even when there is such an obvious cause as a haematoma under the fingernail.

Organic or Psychogenic Pain?

The transmission of pain results in a subjective, conscious experience. For an account of the anatomic basis for pain and also the physiologic and biochemical mechanisms, the reader is referred to Wall and Melzack (1999). There is a threshold for pain: light pressure is perceived as touch, heavy pressure as pain. An explanation for this has been suggested in the *gate control theory* of Melzack and Wall (1965), who considered that painful stimulation through the thin myelinated and unmyelinated fibres results in positive feedback in the substantia gelatinosa; this is transmitted in the lateral spinothalamic tract. However, this gate is under the influence of the higher centres, which can override the local input, as demonstrated by the effect of *attention*: sometimes pain is not felt when attention is directed away from the affected site. Current biochemical theories are also important in accounting for the mediation of pain.

Other theories involve the study of presynaptic and postsynaptic mechanisms in the central nervous system (Nathan, 1980). Electrical stimulation in various sites in the brainstem, including the medulla oblongata, the periaqueductal grey matter and the hypothalamus around the third ventricle, may produce analgesia. Endogenous opiate substances (endorphins) have been discovered to inhibit nerve fibres reporting noxious events. This was initially discovered after electrical stimulation in the periaqueductal grey matter of the brainstem in rats but has subsequently been demonstrated in humans (Bond, 1976). Central nervous system mechanisms for the modulation of pain include descending modulatory control and an increasing number of neurotransmitters, especially serotonin and endogenous opioids; it is almost certainly the interaction of these different systems that is effective in pain modulation (Fields and Basbaum, 1994). There is also increasing understanding of the molecular basis of pain. The role of sodium channels after nerve injury and the genes encoding for the expression of particular sodium channels in primary sensory neurons is gradually being elucidated (Waxman, 1999; Waxman et al., 1999).

The temptation to regard pain simply as any other sensation creates certain dilemmas. For example, what is the subjective experience of the person who complains of severe pain with no organic pathology detectable or the person with mild pathology who complains of excruciating pain? How does one assess the person with an apparently painful injury who claims they did not notice any pain at the time?

Purely organic, physiologic terms, and also psychological, emotional words have been used. Beecher (1959) believed that pain could be defined and listed many distinguished physiologists and psychiatrists to support his case. However, Merskey (1976) considers that pain is a psychological experience, private to the individual but tending to be described in terms of damage to the body, and so defined pain as 'an unpleasant experience which we primarily associate with tissue damage or describe in terms of such damage, or both'.

Clearly, irrespective of the physical stimulus, psychological factors are enormously important in the appreciation of pain. For example, *psychological analgesia* in obstetric care, using psychological preparation, explanation and sometimes hypnosis, will result in 5% to 10% of subjects experiencing little or no pain, 15% to 20% experiencing only moderate pain and in the rest, pain is not modified, but fear and anxiety are diminished (Bonica, 1994). Doctors have frequently, through neglecting subjective evaluation, missed the important distinction between the experience of pain and its physical causes (Noordenbos, 1959). The patient assumes that their pain indicates the presence of physical illness, but pain of various types is a common symptom in many psychiatric conditions without there being physical pathology.

The experience of psychogenic pain has been associated with particular personality types (Engel, 1959). The most important traits of personality associated with pain are those of anxiousness, depressiveness and the cyclothymic personality at its depressive pole—hysterical, hypochondriacal and obsessional traits (Bond, 1976). Subjects with such personality traits developed to abnormal extent are especially likely to respond to life stresses with pain. Complaints of pain are common in neurotic disorder, especially with chronic anxiety or hysterical traits (Merskey, 1965).

It is important to be careful in attempting to distinguish pain of physical origin from that which is largely psychogenic: generalizations can be dangerous. However, Trethowan (1988) considers that there are certain important differences between pain of psychiatric and organic origin. These are as follows:

- Pain associated with psychiatric illness tends to be more diffuse and less well localized than pain due to a physical lesion. It spreads with a non-anatomic distribution.
- Pain is complained of as a constant feature. It may become more severe at times, but it persists unremittingly. Physical pains usually have more definite provocative agents and are relieved by specific measures.
- Psychogenic pain is clearly seen to be associated with an underlying disturbance of mood that appears to be primary in both time and causation.
- It seems to be much more difficult to accurately describe the quality of psychogenic pain. The patient is in no doubt that they are suffering, that the pain is very unpleasant and that they feel they cannot bear it. But in contrast to painful damage to a defined organ, when pain may be described as burning (skin), shooting (nerve) or gripping (heart muscle), the patient with nonorganic pain can find no adequate words for description.

- A further addition to this list is the finding of progression of the severity and extent of the pain over time—unusual for a purely physically mediated pain without increased tissue damage (Tyrer, 1986).

Pain and Heightened Sensation

Generalized increase in sensory input may be experienced as pain. This is exemplified by hyperacousia: the patient complains of noises being uncomfortably loud. There is no objective improvement in their capacity to hear, but the threshold at which sound is perceived as unpleasantly loud is lowered. Noises, even a normal speaking voice, are described as painful to listen to.

With lysergic acid diethylamide, intense pain may be experienced in the limbs, which seem to the sufferer to be twisted or contorted. Similarly, in the early stages of thiamine deficiency, there may be increased sensitivity to pain. In these situations, there is an alteration to perception of sensations so that they are experienced as pain.

During consciousness, the person receives countless sensations from all over their body, such as itching, distension, pressure, borborygmi, mild aching, thumping, warmth and so on. These form the *sensorium* of the body image; they make possible the location of self in space. Most of these sensations escape attention for most of the time. However, occasionally the person concentrates and may take action to eliminate the sensation—scratch their ear or cross their legs. Attention to such sensations, especially if linked to an unpleasant emotion, may occasion the experience of pain. Noticing the sensation results in fear, and the distress of this emotion is perceived as pain.

This would appear to be the explanation for the *vital feelings* of depression described in Chapter 16. Vital feelings are the localization of depression in a bodily organ, complained of, perhaps as pain, in the head or chest or elsewhere. On further questioning, symptoms are described as being unpleasant, painful pressure or even a feeling of misery and depression in that organ: morbid interpretations of ordinary bodily sensations. The sensation is unpleasant but normal and would be ignored in health. With disorder of affect, the sensation may be morbidly interpreted as being due to cancer, tuberculosis or venereal disease. There are, of course, also actual physical changes in depression, for example, slowing of peristalsis and decreased gastrointestinal secretions, and these may also provoke unpleasant sensations such as spasm and constipation.

Central pain (thalamic syndrome) is experienced as a spontaneous burning sensation that can be activated by cutaneous stimulation or temperature changes. It can also present as tactile allodynia, cold allodynia or ongoing pain (Greenspan et al., 2004). It is usually intractable and occurs in the setting of cerebrovascular accident, multiple sclerosis, syringomyelia and spinal cord injury. The current hypothesis is that it arises as a result of disruption in the spinothalamic pathways associated with ectopic neuronal discharges and potentially involves adrenergic, GABAergic, glycine and other neurotransmitters (Devulde et al., 2002).

Diminished Pain Sensation and Pain Craving

In certain situations, there is a decrease in the perception of pain. *Pain asymbolia* is a condition in which situations that should give rise to pain do not (Schilder and Stengel, 1931). This condition can occur as a congenital or an acquired disorder. There are at present five recognized hereditary varieties, usually associated with autonomic neuropathies including anhidrosis (Butler et al., 2006). Several mutations of nerve growth factor have been identified (Einarsdottir et al., 2004). Acquired pain asymbolia has also been described in patients with vascular lesions, predominantly left-sided and involving the insular (Berthier et al., 1988). Patients with pain asymbolia show an absent or inadequate response to painful stimuli over the entire body and an inability to learn appropriate escape or protective responses. Other features include anhidrosis, lack of thermal sensitivity, self-mutilation, intellectual disability, recurrent fever secondary to anhidrosis and failure to thrive (Dias and Charki, 2012). In patients with schizophrenia and their relatives, there is evidence of elevated pain thresholds and pain tolerance demonstrated by relative insensitivity to finger pressure (Hooley and Delgado, 2001). Self-damage of a gross nature also occurs sometimes in schizophrenia, for example, self-castration. In other situations, such as acute drunkenness, there is diminished appreciation due to the central depressant action of alcohol,

and opiates similarly are analgesic through their action on the central appreciation of pain.

Attention is also an important factor in the perception of pain. Excitement or aggression, as in footballers or soldiers, may render the subject oblivious to serious injury. When a wound has advantages to the patient—for example, enabling a soldier to leave the battlefield—it causes less pain than when the injury is seen as wholly disadvantageous. Various psychological techniques can reduce the experience of pain, including hypnosis, various stratagems in childbirth, placebo medication and, possibly, acupuncture. In dissociation (conversion), there may be localized anaesthesia and analgesia for the affected limb; for example, the patient may describe no perception of pinprick sensation.

A blunting and perverting of pain perception is described in severe learning disability, resulting occasionally in gross self-damage. The patient may bang their head so that there is chronic haematoma formation, bite themselves or otherwise harm themselves repeatedly, causing permanent damage. Meanwhile, they appear to experience no pain or even discomfort. Self-application of constricting bands has been described in schizophrenia and organically disordered patients (Dawson-Butterworth et al., 1969). These are most often applied to the left arm; despite extensive tissue damage, the patient does not complain of pain.

Self-inflicted harm occurs also in those of disturbed personality without intellectual disability. Such behaviour may include skin cutting, wrist slashing, skin burning, self-hitting, severe skin scratching and bone breaking (McElroy et al., 2000). These patients are usually female (Graff and Mallin, 1967), and the behaviour appears to be linked with the desire to relieve tension and alleviate negative emotions. There is empirical evidence that it does relieve negative emotions (Klonsky, 2007). There is also limited evidence that the self-injurious behaviour has several possible goals: as self-punishment, to influence personal relationships, to reduce tendency to dissociation and also to induce intense sensory stimulation (Box 15.1).

Pain Without Organic Cause

Unfortunately, pain is an unpleasant feature common to almost all medical settings; it is a frequent complaint in medical, surgical, gynaecologic and psychiatric

BOX 15.1   EXAMPLES OF SELF-INJURIOUS BEHAVIOUR

When SHE's home alone, she cuts herself, slicing off her nose to spite other people's faces. She always waits and waits for the moment when she can cut herself unobserved. No sooner does the sound of the closing door die down than she takes out her little talisman, the paternal all-purpose razor. SHE peels the blade out of its Sunday coat of five layers of virginal plastic. She is very skilled in the use of blades; after all, she has to shave her father, shave that soft paternal cheek under the completely empty paternal brow, which is now undimmed by any thought, unwrinkled by any will. This blade is destined for HER flesh. This thin, elegant foil of bluish steel, pliable, elastic. SHE sits down in front of the magnifying side of the shaving mirror; spreading her legs, she makes a cut, magnifying the aperture that is the doorway into her body. She knows from experience that such a razor cut doesn't hurt, for her arms, hands, and legs have often served as guinea pigs. Her hobby is cutting her own body.

   (From Jelinek, E., 1988. The Piano Teacher (J. Neugroschel, Trans). Weidenfeld and Nicholson, New York).

Late at night I went into the bathroom and took the broken pieces of a razor blade which I had kept. I slashed my wrist again and again, as deeply as I could. I knew perfectly well that it would not kill me, not like the times before. They have been something quite different. As my writing to you comes to a close, the pain is so unbearable inside me that a force of such strength has driven me to inflict a physical pain on myself in the hope of appeasing the other.

   (From Ferguson, S., 1973. A Guard Within. Chatto and Windus, London).

practice. Recalcitrant cases may be referred to a pain clinic, and prominent among such referrals are those in whom no organic basis can be found to account for the complaint of pain (Tyrer, 1985). Pain in the back and in the head and face, particularly, is often found not to be associated with organic lesions. From 3% to 5% of patients, depending on how referrals are made, have measurable psychiatric disturbance.

There are various possible mechanisms to explain the presence of pain without physical disease: autonomic nervous activity may be interpreted and elaborated through fear of possible consequences, normal sensations may be experienced as painful in situations of stress or in fear, relatively minor pain and discomfort of benign cause may be misinterpreted as being more ominous than it really is.

Classification of nonorganic pain is complex. As well as occurring as a primary disturbance, pain also may be conspicuous with hypochondriasis, with somatization disorder and, especially, with depression in mood disorder. In Tyrer's series, two-thirds of those patients without organic cause and with measurable psychiatric disturbance were diagnosed as suffering from major depressive disorder. The remainder had personality disorders, anxiety state, hysteria (dissociative disorder) and drug dependence; paraphrenia and organic brain syndrome also occurred, but rarely (Tyrer, 1985).

Pain without adequate organic explanation is one of the most difficult problems psychiatrists are called on to treat. In a study of patients with pain referred to psychiatrists in a general hospital, the head and neck was the most common site, followed by the back, abdomen, arm or leg, rectum or genitalia and chest (Pilling et al., 1967). In 32% of these medical and surgical patients, pain was the presenting complaint, and it was considered that these patients 'spoke to their physicians in terms of pain or other organic symptoms rather than anxiety, depression and the like'. In the evaluation of the significance of emotional factors in chronic pain, adequate history and examination, including the assessment of attribution and the relationship with mood state, was found to be most helpful (Tyrer, 1992); the most useful questionnaires were the Hospital Anxiety and Depression Scale (Zigmond and Snaith, 1983) and the West Haven-Yale Multidimensional Pain Inventory (Kerns et al., 1985).

It is, of course, wholly understandable that someone suffering pain should be miserable and that chronic pain or the anticipation of recurrent pain should provoke depression of mood. This is often so much taken for granted that no steps are taken to alleviate the depressed mood if the cause of the pain is obvious. However, if the perception of pain is considered to have two separate contributions—the sensory perception and the investing affect—efforts to relieve the latter, if successful, will produce a global diminution of pain. Pain can be a cause of depression, and in this situation treatment for the depression is appropriate. The role and place of depression in chronic pain is exemplified in the report by Roughan et al. (2021) which showed that chronic pain is associated with an increased risk of depression, increased risk of recent suicide attempt, higher use of tobacco and misuse of painkillers. Furthermore, increased pain severity was associated with increased number of depressive episodes. Pain response to antidepressants in this sample of patients with chronic pain was negligible.

PAIN AND LOSS

The best known model for this topic is the *phantom limb* pain so often experienced in amputees (see Chapter 14). Pain is experienced within a limb that is not there; that is, spatially, pain is located outside the patient. However, this is not a hallucination. The person knows full well that they have lost their leg and that the *feeling* of pain is inside themselves. The body image takes a long time to adjust to a change such as an amputation, and it may never do so fully. Ramachandran and Hirstein (1998) provide a thorough review of the subject. The phantom limb experience occurs almost immediately after the loss of a limb in the vast majority of cases, and the incidence may be even higher after a traumatic loss. In the case of surgical amputations, phantoms appear as soon as the anaesthetic wears off. The phantom is present for a few days or weeks and gradually fades but may persist for years or even decades in some people. Indeed, some people are able to recall a phantom limb at will after its disappearance.

Phantoms are most common after amputation of an arm or a leg but have been reported after mastectomies or removal of parts of the face; even phantom internal viscera can produce sensations of bowel movements and flatus. The posture of the limb can become habitual, as with the arm, often partially flexed at the elbow with forearm pronated, and when the phantom fades from consciousness, especially with the forearm, it becomes progressively shorter until the patient is left with just the phantom hand. Perhaps most surprisingly, children with congenitally missing limbs can experience phantoms. Originally, it was thought that phantom pain was due to stump neuromas but given that people born without limbs (amelia) can have phantom pain, neuromas do not seem necessary for phantom pain to occur. The persistence of central representation of the amputated limb is largely responsible for the phantom illusion and associated pain and provides some understanding of the influence of the body schema on subjective experience. In amputees, the body schema continues to exist irrespective of the absence of sensory input from an actual limb and as for amelia, the experience of phantom limbs, points to

existence of neural systems ready to respond to sensory inflows from limbs. Phantom limbs in amelia and following amputation point to the likely correctness of Melzack's notion of neuromatrix, a widespread network of thalamocortical and limbic loops that is basically innate and responds and adapts to sensory inputs and motor commands during a person's life .

PSYCHOGENIC FACIAL PAIN

It has been known for a long time that many patients with chronic pain at a variety of sites do not have abnormal physical signs and do not manifest serious organic illness. *Atypical facial pain* is an especially frequent and intractable example, manifesting no organic signs but causing great suffering; the patient is referred from surgeon to dentist to pain clinic physician to psychiatrist, often without benefit. It tends to occur in the nonmuscular areas of the face, either unilaterally or bilaterally. It is poorly localized and does not tend to follow any definable nerve distribution. It is described as a throbbing, deep, diffuse, boring or nagging pain. It can last for years and can be continuous or episodic in nature (Zakrzewska, 2002, 2013). Such pain has often been associated with depression. Lascelles (1966) described a series of 93 patients suffering from prolonged facial pain, of whom the majority suffered from *atypical depression* with intense fatigue, tension and sleep disorder superimposed on 'obsessive' personality; 53 of these patients responded well to antidepressant therapy. Blumer and Heilbronn (1982) have seen chronic, intractable pain without organic cause as being a variant of depressive illness. Garvey et al. (1983) investigated the association between headache and depression in 116 patients suffering from major depressive disorder. During a nondepressed period, these patients experienced a similar rate for headache to that of nondepressive control subjects, but they had a markedly increased rate during depressive episodes. Feinmann et al. (1984) investigated the efficacy of an antidepressant, dosulepin (dothiepin), in the treatment of psychogenic facial pain. Seventy-one percent of patients were free of symptoms at 9 weeks, compared with 47% in a placebo group; at a 12-month follow-up, 81% of patients were pain-free. Good prognostic indicators for successful treatment included pain after an adverse life event, minimal previous surgical intervention and freedom from pain after 9 weeks' treatment. Such studies would suggest an association between facial pain without physical signs and depressive illness.

BURNING MOUTH SYNDROME

A group of heterogeneous skin conditions that present with unpleasant skin sensations including itching, burning, stinging or numbness are well recognized as liable to affect face, scalp and perineum. These conditions are poorly understood but demonstrate an interplay among neuropathic pain, neuropathic itch, neurology and psychiatric disorders (Gupta and Gupta, 2013). When these conditions affect the oral cavity, it is referred to as *burning mouth syndrome*, a condition characterized by intraoral burning for which no medical or dental cause can be identified (Ducasse et al., 2013). The abnormal oral sensations include burning, pricking (pins and needles), allodynia (pain on brushing the teeth and gums), tingling, numbness, itching and sensation of electrical discharges (Braud et al., 2013). These sensations occur principally on the tip of the tongue, the lateral aspects of the tongue, lips, hard and soft palate (Sun et al., 2013) and may involve pain radiating to the lower and upper jaws, the inner aspects of the cheeks and the gums. Despite normal salivation, patients often complain of xerostomia and dysgeusia. Burning mouth syndrome seems to occur most frequently in perimenopausal females (Dahiya et al., 2013). There is evidence of elevated rates of depression and anxiety in burning mouth syndrome compared to control groups. Moura et al., (2018) report moderate or severe depression in 25% of their sample. It is still too early to determine how far burning mouth syndrome is down to neuralgic pain or nociceptive dysfunction.

VULVODYNIA

Vulvodynia can be defined as persistent, spontaneous, unwelcomed, intrusive and distressing vulval sensation (Markos and Dinsmore, 2013). It is a little-understood condition. A frequent subtype is termed *provoked vestibulodynia* in which the experienced pain or discomfort is provoked by sexual intercourse rather than merely occurring spontaneously (Bois et al., 2013). There is some evidence that vulvodynia is associated with generalized hyperalgesia and that there are augmented brain responses to thumb pressure, that is, stimulation of an area remote from the vulva demonstrable within the insula, dorsal midcingulate, posterior cingulate and thalamus compared with normal control subjects. This is interpreted as showing augmented central pain processing in vulvodynia (Hampson et al., 2013). In focal as opposed to diffuse vulvodynia, when the pain is localized at 1 and 11 o'clock, it tends to be experienced as deep pain within the vestibule, and the pain is provoked by sexual intercourse or the insertion of a tampon. Pain at 5 and 7 o'clock is less severe (Donders and Bellen, 2012). There are considerable associated adverse effects on quality of life and on intimate relationships with sexual partners (Ponte et al., 2009; Xie et al., 2012; Bois et al., 2013; Smith et al., 2013).

Male patients can also present with a condition similar to vulvodynia. The patients present with burning sensation in the penis and scrotum, and this condition is termed *penoscrotodynia*. The current proposed classification is generalized, focal, provoked, unprovoked and mixed types (Markos, 2011).

PSYCHOGENIC ITCH

Itch and the desire to scratch is a normal response to skin sensations. Pruritogenic itch (physiologic itch) is transmitted by dedicated afferent neurons much as is pain. Mediators of itch include the 'cross-talk' between dermal Mast cells and adjacent cutaneous afferents. In addition, there are a number of neuropeptides (neurotensin and substance P, for example) involved in the process (Greaves, 2010). Some cases, which are considered to be neuropathic in origin, are thought to be related to damage to the peripheral nervous system, such as in postherpetic neuralgia, brachioradial pruritus, notalgia paresthetica, central nervous damage to the spinal cord by tumours and demyelinating disease such as multiple sclerosis (Yosipovitch and Samuel, 2008). The itch sensation in these conditions is analogous to neuropathic pain and overlaps with burning, aching and stinging sensations. Psychogenic itch, on the other hand, occurs in the absence of a physical cause and is unrelated to demonstrable nerve damage. It can be associated with depression and obsessive compulsive disorder (Calikuşu et al., 2003), anxiety and delusions of parasitosis. The French psychodermatology group has proposed diagnostic criteria to include the following three: localized or generalized pruritus sine materia, chronic pruritus lasting longer than 6 weeks and the absence of a somatic cause. In addition, there should be three additional criteria from the following seven: chronological relationship of pruritus with one or several life events that could have psychological repercussions, variations in intensity associated with stress, nocturnal variations, predominance during rest or inaction, associated psychiatric disorders, improvement in response to psychotropic agents and improvement in response to psychotherapy (Misery et al., 2007). There is continuing debate about how best to classify and conceive of psychogenic itch. Misery (2021) further proposed three distinct ways of thinking of an itch: pruriceptive that arises from actual or threatened damage to non-neural tissue; neuropathic that is analogous to neuropathic pain and arises from a lesion or disease of the somatosensory nervous system; and a new category termed *pruriplastic itch* that arises from altered pruriception and best construed as a dysfunction of itch processing systems. In this schema, psychogenic itch would be classified as pruriplastic itch.

Pain and Suffering

Pain is an appropriate study for the phenomenologist, in that the external signs may be irrelevant and the subjective experience all-important. The chief problem in assessing pain is the extraordinary difficulty a patient has in describing the quality of their pain: the greater the psychogenic component of the pain, the more difficult it is to find the right words to describe it. Sometimes, it seems that pain may be needed as a neurotic solution to a neurotic conflict: for the equilibrium to remain, it is necessary for the pain to be retained. It has been considered by Trethowan (1988) that such a patient 'is not suffering from pain at all. What they are suffering from is suffering'.

There are differences between the person suffering from organically determined pain and the chronic sufferer with multiple symptoms whose pain is considered psychogenic. The latter truly suffers but does not show the physical correlates of severe pain. It seems that the state of suffering in which this person exists finds expression, dons respectability and can only be communicated when it is transformed peripherally into a specific pain. Pain may occur with little

suffering, as in the injection of local anaesthetic that, after the small prick, brings relief from a worse pain. Suffering may also occur without pain, but it may also be described as pain, and this may be the nature of many neurotic complaints of pain. This transposition of affect is wholly understandable when one considers the semantics of suffering. Suffering of all nonphysical kinds—indignation, humiliation, disappointment—finds expression in pain terms: taking pains, feeling crushed, bruised self-esteem, rubbing salt in the wound, getting one's fingers burnt, searing remarks. It is not just that pain is a metaphor for suffering, but in many situations suffering can be experienced and explained by the sufferer only in terms of *pain*.

So the use of pain words can be construed metaphorically, and the neurotic patient may follow this to its logical conclusion and describe concretely the unbearable and humiliating suffering of their daily existence as complaints of localized physical pain. The experience of pain is a physical sensation that takes on an affective component for its expression and interpretation. This affective component—suffering—may occur without physical perception and sometimes still be experienced by the person themself as pain.

REFERENCES

Beecher, H.K., 1959. Measurement of Subjective Responses, Quantitative Effects of Drugs. Oxford University Press, New York.

Berthier, M., Starktein, S., Leiguarda, R., 1988. Asymbolia for pain: a sensory–limbic disconnection syndrome. Ann. Neurol. 24, 41–49.

Blumer, D., Heilbronn, M., 1982. Chronic pain as a variant of depressive disease: the pain-prone disorder. J. Nerv. Ment. Dis. 70, 381–406.

Bois, K., Bergeron, S., Rosen, N.O., McDuff, P., Gregoire, C., 2013. Sexual and relationship intimacy among women with provoked vestibulodynia and their partners: associations with sexual satisfaction, sexual function, and pain self-efficacy. J. Sex. Med. 10, 2024–2035.

Bond, M.R., 1976. Psychological and psychiatric aspects of pain. In: Howells, J.G. (Ed.), Modern Perspectives in the Psychiatric Aspects of Surgery. Macmillan, London, pp. 109–139.

Bonica, J.J., 1994. Labour pain. In: Wall, P.D., Melzack, R. (Eds.), Textbook of Pain, third ed. Churchill Livingstone, Edinburgh.

Braud, A., Touré, B., Agbo-Godeau, S., Descroix, V., Boucher, Y., 2013. Characteristics of pain assessed with visual analogue scale and questionnaire in burning mouth syndrome: a pilot study. J. Orofac. Pain 27, 235–242.

Butler, J., Fleming, P., Webb, D., 2006. Congenital insensitivity to pain—review of a case with dental implications. Oral Surg. Oral Med. Oral Pathol. Oral Radiol. Endod. 101, 58–62.

Calikuşu, C., Yücel, B., Polat, A., Baykal, C., 2003. The relation of psychogenic excoriation with psychiatric disorders: a comparative study. Compr. Psychiatry 44, 256–261.

Dahiya, P., Kamal, R., Kumar, M., Niti, M., Gupta, R., Chaudhary, K., 2013. Burning mouth syndrome and menopause. Int. J. Prev. Med. 4, 15–20.

Dawson-Butterworth, K., Wallen, G.D.P., Gittleson, N.L., 1969. Self-applied constricting bands. Br. J. Psychiatry 115, 1255–1259.

Devulde, R., Crombez, E., Mortier, E., 2002. Central pain: an overview. Acta Neurol. Belg. 102, 97–103.

Dias, E., Charki, S., 2012. Congenital insensitivity to pain with anhidrosis. J. Pediatr. Neurosci. 7, 156–157.

Dickens, C., 1854. Hard Times. Penguin, London.

Donders, G., Bellen, G., 2012. Characteristics of the pain observed in the focal vulvodynia syndrome. Med. Hypotheses 78, 11–14.

Ducasse, D., Courtet, P., Olie, E., 2013. Burning mouth syndrome: current clinical, physiopathologic, and therapeutic data. Reg. Anesth. Pain Med. 38, 380–390.

Einarsdottir, E., Carlsson, A., Minde, J., et al., 2004. A mutation in the nerve growth factor beta gene (NGB) causes loss of pain perception. Hum. Mol. Genet. 13, 799–805.

Engel, G.L., 1959. 'Psychogenic' pain and the pain prone patient. Am. J. Med. 26, 899.

Feinmann, C., Harris, M., Cawley, R., 1984. Psychogenic facial pain: presentation and treatment. Br. Med. J. 288, 436–438.

Ferguson, S., 1973. A Guard within. Chatto and Windus, London.

Fields, H.L., Basbaum, A.I., 1994. Central nervous system mechanisms of pain modulation. In: Wall, P.D., Melzack, R. (Eds.), Textbook of Pain, third ed. Churchill Livingstone, Edinburgh.

Garvey, M.J., Schaffer, C.B., Tuason, V.B., 1983. Relationship of headaches to depression. Br. J. Psychiatry 143, 544–547.

Graff, H., Mallin, R., 1967. The syndrome of the wrist-cutter. Am. J. Psychiatry 124, 36–42.

Greaves, M.W., 2010. Pathogenesis and treatment of pruritus. Curr. Allergy Asthma Rep. 10, 236–242.

Greenspan, J.D., Ohara, J., Sarlani, E., Lenz, F.A., 2004. Allodynia in patients with post-stroke pain (CPSP) studied by statistical quantitative sensory testing within individuals. Pain 109, 357–366.

Gupta, M.A., Gupta, A.K., 2013. Cutaneous sensory disorder. Semin. Cutan. Med. Surg. 32, 110–118.

Hampson, J.P., Reed, B.D., Clauw, D.J., et al., 2013. Augmented central pain processing in vulvodynia. J. Pain 14, 579–589.

Hooley, J.M., Delgado, M.L., 2001. Pain insensitivity in the relatives of schizophrenic patients. Schizophr. Res. 47, 265–273.

International Association for the Study of Pain, 1994. Classification of chronic pain: descriptions of chronic pain syndromes and definitions of pain terms. In: Task Force on Taxonomy (Suppl. 3). IASP Press, Seattle.

Jelinek, E., 1988. The Piano Teacher (J. Neugroschel, Trans). Weidenfeld and Nicholson, New York.

Kerns, R.D., Turk, D.C., Rudy, T.F., 1985. The West Haven–Yale Multidimensional Pain Inventory (WHYMPI). Pain 23, 345–356.

Klonsky, E.D., 2007. The functions of deliberate self-injury: a review of the evidence. Clin. Psychol. Rev. 27, 226–239.

Lascelles, R.G., 1966. Atypical facial pain and depression. Br. J. Psychiatry 112, 651–659.

Markos, A.R., 2011. Dysaesthetic penoscrotodynia: nomenclature, classification, diagnosis and treatment. Int. J. STD AIDS 22, 483–487.

Markos, A.R., Dinsmore, W., 2013. Persistent genital arousal and restless genitalia: sexual dysfunction or subtype of vulvodynia? Int. J. STD AIDS 24, 852–858.

McElroy, S.L., Arnold, L.M., Beckman, D.A., 2000. Habit and impulse control disorders. In: Gelder, M.G., López-Ibor, J.J., An-

dreasen, N.C. (Eds.), New Oxford Textbook of Psychiatry. Oxford University Press, Oxford.

Melzack, R., 1990. Phantom limbs and the concept of a neuromatrix. Trends Neurosci. 13 (3), 88–92.

Melzack, R., Wall, P.D., 1965. Pain mechanisms: a new theory. Science 150, 971.

Merskey, H., 1965. The characteristics of persistent pain in psychological illness. J. Psychosom. Res. 9, 291.

Merskey, H., 1976. The status of pain. In: Hill, O. (Ed.), Modern Trends in Psychosomatic Medicine 3. Butterworth, London, pp. 166–186.

Misery, L., 2021. Pruriplastic itch—a novel pathogenic concept in chronic pruritus. Front. Med. 7, 615118. https://doi.org/10.3389/fmed.2020.615118.

Misery, L., Alexandre, S., Dutray, S., et al., 2007. Functional itch disorder or psychogenic pruritus: suggested diagnosis criteria from the French psychodermatology group. Acta Derm. Venereol. 87, 341–344.

Moura, B.S., Ferreira, N., DosSantos, M.F., Janini, M., 2018. Changes in the vibration sensitivity and pressure pain thresholds in patients with burning mouth syndrome. PloS one, 13 (5), e0197834.

Nathan, P., 1980. Recent advances in understanding pain. Br. J. Psychiatry 136, 509–512.

Noordenbos, W., 1959. Pain: Problems Pertaining to the Transmission of Nerve Impulses Which Give Rise to Pain. Elsevier, London.

Pilling, L.F., Bannick, T.L., Swenson, W.M., 1967. Psychological characteristics of patients having pain as a presenting symptom. Can. Med. Assoc. J. 97, 387.

Ponte, M., Klemperer, E., Sahay, A., Chren, M.M., 2009. Effects of vulvodynia on quality of life. J. Am. Acad. Dermatol. 60, 70–76.

Ramachandran, V.S., Hirstein, W., 1998. The perception of phantom limbs. The DO Hebb lecture. Brain 121, 1603–1630.

Roughan, W.H., Campos, A.I., García-Marín, L.M., et al., 2021. Comorbid chronic pain and depression: shared risk factors and differential antidepressant effectiveness. Front. Psychiatry 12, 643609.

Schilder, P., Stengel, E., 1931. Asymbolia for pain. Arch. Neurol. Psychiatry 25, 598–600.

Smith, K.B., Pukall, C.F., Chamberlain, S.M., 2013. Sexual and relationship satisfaction and vestibular pain sensitivity among women with provoked vestibulodynia. J. Sex. Med. 10, 2009–2023.

Sun, A., Wu, K.M., Wang, Y.P., Lin, H.P., Chen, H.M., Chiang, C.P., 2013. Burning mouth syndrome: a review and update. J. Sex. Med. 42, 649–655.

Trethowan, W.H., 1988. Pain as a psychiatric symptom. In: Hall, P., Stonier, P.D. (Eds.), Perspectives in Psychiatry. John Wiley, Chichester.

Tyrer, S., 1985. The role of the psychiatrist in the pain clinic. Psychiatr. Bull. 9, 135–136.

Tyrer, S., 1986. Learned pain behaviour. Br. Med. J. 292, 1–2.

Tyrer, S., 1992. Psychiatric assessment of chronic pain. Br. J. Psychiatry 160, 733–741.

Wall, P.D., Melzack, R., 1999. Textbook of Pain, fourth ed. Churchill Livingstone, Edinburgh.

Waxman, S.G., 1999. The molecular pathophysiology of pain: abnormal expression of sodium channel genes and its contributions to hyperexcitability of primary sensory neurons. (Pain Suppl.), 6 S133–S140.

Waxman, S.G., Dib-Hajj, S., Cummins, T.R., Black, J.A., 1999. Sodium channels and pain. Proc. Natl. Acad. Sci. U.S.A. 96, 7635–7639.

Xie, Y., Shi, L., Xiong, X., Wu, E., Veasley, C., Dade, C., 2012. Economic burden and quality of life of vulvodynia in the United States. Curr. Med. Res. Opin. 28, 601–608.

Yosipovitch, G., Samuel, L.S., 2008. Neuropathic and psychogenic itch. Dermatol. Ther. 1, 32–41.

Zakrzewska, J.M., 2002. Facial pain: neurological and non-neurological. J Neurol Neurosurg Psychiatry. 6; 72. Suppl 2(Suppl 2): ii27–ii32.

Zakrzewska, J.M., 2013. Differential diagnosis of facial pain and guidelines for management. Br. J. Anaesth. 111, 95–104.

Zigmond, A.S., Snaith, R.P., 1983. The hospital anxiety and depression scale. Acta Psychiatr. Scand. 67, 361–370.

EMOTIONS AND ACTION

Chapter 16

Affect and Emotional Disorders

Chapter Outline

KEYWORDS

Emotion

Ecstasy

Anhedonia

Alexithymia

Prosody

Summary

Mood disturbance is not only a common abnormality presenting to psychiatrists but is of considerable importance because of the severe consequences that poor recognition or treatment may have in the lives of patients. It is associated with suicide, homicide and reckless behaviour and has potentially significant, undesirable impact on social reputation. *Affect* is a broad term that is used to cover mood, feeling, attitude, preferences and evaluations. In modern usage, it refers to the expression of emotion as judged by the external manifestations that are associated with specific feelings—for example, laughter, crying and fearful appearance. *Mood* is a more prolonged, prevailing state or disposition, whereas *emotion* is often used to refer to spontaneous and transitory experience similar to but not identical to feeling because it need not incorporate the physical accompaniments of the experience. Abnormalities of mood can be classified as follows: (1) morbid states of the basic emotions, including sadness, happiness, fear, anger, surprise and disgust, that can be affected in the intensity, duration, timing, quality of experience, expression and appropriateness to the object or social setting; (2) abnormalities of the physiologic and arousal mechanisms associated with emotions; and (3) abnormalities of the cognitive evaluation of the social world and of the perception of the emotions of others.

I wish to inform you that I have received the cake. Many thanks, but I am not worthy. You sent it on the anniversary of my child's death, for I am not worthy of my birthday; I must weep myself to death; I cannot live and I cannot die, because I have failed so much, I shall bring my husband and children to hell. We are all lost; we won't see each other any more; I shall go to the convict prison and my two girls as well, if they do not make away with themselves because they were born in my body.

A patient of Emil Kraepelin (1905)

Assessing and observing the state of, and changes in, mood are essential in psychiatry but at the same time require skill. Part of the problem has always been the conceptual confusion and lack of cohesive psycho-pathologic theory that has traditionally been associated with disturbance of affect (Berrios, 1985). In a study of patients with unsolved diagnostic problems at the time of discharge from hospital, atypical psychotic depression was found, at follow-up, to be the condition most frequently responsible for doubt (Anstee and Fleminger, 1977). In another study, depressed affect was a major cause of somatic problems without physical pathology (Brenner, 1979). However, the terms used are not standardized nor mutually exclusive. Different languages, in contrast to the names given to physical objects, have an entirely different range of descriptions of mood, so that one is left wondering whether it is just the terms that differ in different cultures or perhaps even the experience of emotion itself. So *Angst* cannot be translated exactly into English with a single equivalent word; neither can *depression* be precisely translated into German. The word *feeling* describes an active experience of somatic sensation, touch, as well as the passive subjective experience of emotion. *Emotion,* according to Whybrow (1997), 'is actually memory and feeling intertwined'. Feelings are also personal convictions, predictive forecasts and social sensibilities. All these nuances of meaning are somewhat different from the associations of the word *mood.*

Traditionally, *feeling* has been used to describe a positive or negative reaction to an experience; it is marked but transitory. *Affect* is a broad term that is used to cover mood, feeling, attitude, preferences and evaluations. In psychiatry, it is customary to limit its use to the expression of emotion as judged by the external manifestations that are associated with specific feelings, for example, laughter, crying or fearful appearance. *Mood* is a more prolonged prevailing state or disposition, whereas *emotion* is often used to refer to spontaneous and transitory experience similar to but

not identical to feeling, as it need not incorporate the physical accompaniments of the experience. In practice, these terms are used more or less interchangeably, a fact that contributes to much confusion.

Mood describes the state of the self in relation to its environment. There is an enormous range of variation of what could reasonably be called *normal* mood. Pathologic mood, that is, mood from which the patient suffers or mood that causes disturbance or suffering to others, also varies a great deal, and the extent to which it is acceptable to others in its expression is different in different social contexts. The clinician has to ask two questions concerning the mood of his patient. First, is the person suffering? Second, is the expression of mood inappropriate in this social setting? Psychopathology of mood is confined to those situations in which there is an affirmative answer to at least one of these questions, and treatment is directed towards improving the mood.

Like other human characteristics, pathology of mood arises in the context of a diathesis. It is the physical constitution that forms the tendency for developing, for example, a prolapsed intervertebral disc; in the mental realm, personality is closely associated with the type, quality and direction of mood. So a person of cyclothymic personality is more prone to morbid states of elation and excessive activity or taciturn dejection and retardation.

Theories of Emotion

The James–Lange theory of emotion was developed independently by William James (1842–1910) and Carl Lange (1834–1900). Simply, it posits that emotions are the result of self-awareness of physical and bodily changes in the presence of a stimulus. William James (1884) wrote:

My theory ... is that the bodily changes follow directly the perception of the exciting fact, and that our feeling of the same changes as they occur is the emotion. Common sense says, we lose our fortune, are sorry and weep; we meet a bear, are frightened and run; we are insulted by a rival, are angry and strike. The hypothesis here to be defended says that this order of sequence is incorrect ... and that the more rational statement is that we feel sorry because we cry, angry because we strike, afraid because we tremble ... Without the bodily states following on the perception, the latter would be purely cognitive in form, pale, colorless, destitute of emotional warmth. We might then see the bear, and judge it best to run, receive the insult and deem it right to strike, but we should not actually feel afraid or angry.

This theory was criticized by Walter Cannon (1871–1945) and Philip Bard (1898–1977). Visceral (physiologic) responses to stimuli are too slow to account for the rapidity of emotions that arise in the presence of appropriate stimuli. In other words, the timeliness of my awareness of the increased heart rate and dry mouth that occur when I am in the presence of a hostile lion is inadequate to explain my fear of the lion. Furthermore, the visceral responses to varying stimuli are similar, yet the emotions may be as disparate as fear, surprise, joy and so on. And injection of adrenaline (epinephrine) is accompanied by visceral changes but not necessarily by emotional change. In addition, animals that have spinal lesions continue to experience emotions. Instead, the Cannon–Bard theory argued that emotion has temporal primacy and that any visceral or behavioural change follows the emotion. In this theory, I see a hostile lion and become fearful. My fearfulness provokes the typical physiologic response of increased heart rate, among others, and the resulting behaviour is that I run off. This theory obviously leaves no room for any cognitive aspect to the origin of emotions.

The other influential theory is Schachter and Singer's (1962) two-factor theory of emotion. The two relevant factors are physiologic arousal and cognition. In this theory, an individual is in a given social context, and they respond to this situation with a physiologic arousal. The meaning attributed to this arousal is determined by their cognitions. If their appraisal is that the context is threatening, then they will feel fear, but if the appraisal is that the situation is funny, then the emotion will be a positive one. This theory has obvious implications for the clinical evaluation of disorders of mood. It specifies that the social context is important, that the cognitions of the individual are relevant and, finally, that careful consideration and description of the accompanying emotion is also important.

Basic Emotions

Ekman and Friesen (1971) have shown that there are six basic emotions that are expressed in the face: anger, disgust, fear, happiness, sadness and surprise. These basic expressions of emotion are universal. Ekman's findings were anticipated by Charles Darwin (1872). It is also the case that despite there being universals in facial expressions of emotions, these expressions are not universal in every regard. In Ekman's fieldwork in Papua New Guinea among the Fore people, there was little distinction between surprise and fear. Furthermore, it is also true that when people experience strong emotions there are display rules that determine who can show which emotion to whom and when. Cultures also differ on which events are likely to produce particular emotions. This is well exemplified by what food one culture regards as a delicacy and what another regards as revolting. The important point is that the general theme is universal; ingesting something repulsive is a cause for disgust (Ekman, 1998).

Communication of Mood

'No man is an Island, entire of itself' (John Donne, 1571–1631), and in no area of life is this more true than that of feelings. Our feelings are very much affected by those around us. They are observable and understandable to other people, and this is not accidental; they are actually signalled as a nonverbal message. The affect itself is not directed towards another person, but the expression of the affect is conveyed both deliberately and unintentionally to others.

One of the most important findings in the past decade has been that of *mirror neurons*. These neurons have been found in primates and birds, and their existence inferred in humans. Mirror neurons fire when an animal performs an action and also when an animal observes the same action performed by another animal. In other words, these neurons mirror the behaviour of another animal. In humans, the relevant neurons are in the premotor cortex and inferior parietal cortex. Rizzolatti and Fadiga (1998) showed that in the macaque monkey there are two distinct groups of neurons in the rostroventral premotor cortex that respond to the observation of grasping objects and grasping actions. The canonical neurons respond specifically to the three-dimensional objects, whereas the mirror neurons respond to the direct observation of the hand actions performed by another animal. Rizzolatti and Craighero (2004) argue that this mirror neuron system underlies imitative learning and is therefore important for the development of human culture and the acquisition of language. More recently, Gallese (2007) proposed that the mirror neuron system is an embodied simulation system wherein we not only see an action, emotion or sensation but form internal representations of these actions, emotions or sensations based on evocations of the same neural systems as when we perform the same actions or experience the same emotions or sensations. Thus by means of this system, the objectified other becomes for us another experiencing self. In other words, empathy and the capacity to understand another person's emotional state have an already identified basis.

Emotions are communicated nonverbally by different parts of the body, for example, by the face (especially the eyes), gesture, posture, tone of voice and general appearance, especially the choice of clothes. While assessing another's affective response, the assessor in part influences it by their own behaviour and disposition. A person who is cheerful on meeting someone else will greet them cheerfully and induce a feeling of cheerfulness, even if transitory, which they then read as the other person being cheerful also. This has important implications in the way that mood is assessed. It would seem that emotion is evaluated empathically. Without having to go through this elaborate argument in words, the observer says to themselves, 'If I felt how I estimate the feelings of that person from their appearance, I would feel very unhappy; they are unhappy'. This is, of course, the empathic method as described earlier, and it takes place spontaneously and without deliberate training. Assessment of others' mood does not need to become verbal to be acted upon. It takes place rapidly and is followed by the appropriate behavioural response from the observer.

Classification of Pathology of Emotions

There is no consensus on how to classify abnormalities of the experience and display of emotions. Cutting (1997) provides a viable framework, which has been adapted for use in this chapter. There are morbid states

BOX 16.1 CLASSIFICATION OF DISORDERS OF EMOTION

ABNORMALITIES OF BASIC EMOTIONS
- Intensity of emotions, including diminution and exacerbation
- Duration, time and quality of experience, including lability of mood, pathologic crying and laughing, parathymia and paramimia
- Expression of emotion, including blunting and flattening of affect
- Appropriateness to object, including phobia

ABNORMALITY OF PHYSIOLOGIC AROUSAL
- Alexithymia

ABNORMALITIES OF EVALUATION OF SOCIAL CONTEXT
- Negative cognitive schemas
- Prosopoaffective agnosia
- Receptive vocal dysprosody

of the basic emotions, including sadness, happiness, fear, anger, surprise and disgust. These basic emotions can be affected in their intensity, duration, timing, quality of experience, expression and appropriateness to the object or social setting. There are abnormalities of the physiologic and arousal mechanisms associated with emotions. Finally, there are abnormalities of the cognitive evaluation of the social world and of the perception of the emotions of others (Box 16.1).

Pathologic Changes in Basic Emotions

CHANGES IN INTENSITY OF EMOTIONS

Most often in psychiatric practice, subjective description of *change* in the experience of emotion is for the worse—a state of dysphoria, meaning the condition of 'being ill at ease'; more rarely, the patient may describe the onset of ecstasy or euphoria. The subjective experience of change of mood can be quantified approximately and represented graphically as in Fig. 16.1, which shows part of a mood chart a previously depressed patient had recorded; he had noticed an association between an acute attack of bronchitis and exacerbation of depressive symptoms.

Diminution of Intensity: Feeling of a Loss of Feeling

This is experienced as a loss of feeling, a deficiency that is all-pervasive, affecting all emotions including sadness, joy, anger, fear and so on. The patient

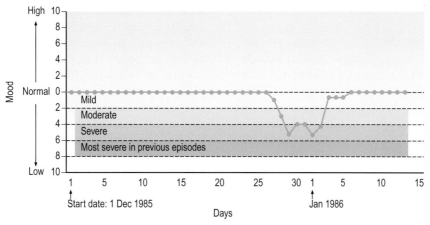

Fig. 16.1 Mood chart kept by a depressed patient who had had acute bronchitis.

resents or does not understand it, suffers very greatly and often feels guilty about the feeling. It is a subjective experience of loss of feelings that were formerly present rather than an objectively observed absence. A depressed young woman said, 'I have no feelings for my children. That is wicked. They are beautiful children'. A person with religious belief may experience this loss of feeling with a religious content: they no longer believe in God. On more detailed eliciting of their subjective experience, they are likely to describe a loss of the feeling of assurance associated with their faith rather than any actual change in the content of their beliefs. This affect occurs particularly in depressive psychosis but also occasionally with personality disorders and schizophrenia. Milder forms are experienced as *depersonalization* or *deaffectualization* (see Chapter 13): the patient complains that their feelings are numbed, diminished, made remote from themself, to which is ascribed the unmelodious word deaffectualization.

Anhedonia

Anhedonia specifically refers to a loss of the capacity to experience joy and pleasure. It is a subset of the diminution of the intensity of emotions. In anhedonia there is a total inability to enjoy anything in life or even get the accustomed satisfaction from everyday events or objects; a 'loss of ability to experience pleasure' (Snaith, 1993). The term was originally introduced by Ribot (1896) and considered to be a prominent symptom of depressive illness by Klein (1974), probably the

best clinical marker predicting response to treatment. This would seem to be a fundamental symptom of depressive illness. A highly intelligent and perceptive man suffering from psychotic depression said, 'I have a sort of uncanny feeling. I know what I am reading is amusing but I am not at all amused by it'. The experience was very well described by J.S. Mill (1806–73):

It was the autumn of 1826. I was in a dull state of nerves, such as everybody is occasionally liable to; unsusceptible to enjoyment or pleasurable excitement; one of these moods when what is pleasure at other times, becomes insipid or indifferent … In this frame of mind it occurred to me to put the question directly to myself, 'suppose that all your objects in life were realized; that all the changes in institutions and opinions which you are looking forward to, could be completely effected at this very instant: would this be a great joy and happiness to you?' And an irrepressible self-consciousness distinctly answered, 'No!' At this my heart sank within me.

Mill (1873)

In Shakespeare's *Hamlet* Hamlet says:

I have of late – but wherefore I know not – lost all my mirth, forgone all custom of exercise; and indeed it goes so heavily with my disposition that this godly frame, the earth seems to me a sterile promontory. This most excellent canopy, the air, look you, this brave o'erhanging firmament, this majestical roof fretted with golden fire – why, it appears no other thing to me than a foul and pestilent congregation of vapours. What piece of work is a man, how noble in reason, how infinite in faculty, in form and moving how express and admirable, in action how like an angel, in apprehension how like a god – the beauty of the world, the paragon of animals! And yet, to me, what is this quintessence of dust? Man delights not me – no, nor woman neither, though by your smiling you seem to say so.

Shakespeare (~1600)

Both extracts indicate the disparity between the absence of the feeling of natural joy that would normally accompany how the world is experienced alongside the preservation of the cognitive appreciation of this lack of emotional response.

Anhedonia as an experience is starting to be deconstructed into its component parts. This deficit in the capacity to experience pleasure is now thought to include impairments in the processes of reward valuation, decision-making, anticipation and motivation. The neural circuits underlying these reward-related mechanisms include the ventral striatum and prefrontal cortical regions (Der-Avakian and Markou, 2012; Gaillard et al., 2013).

Anhedonia is also described as a symptom in schizophrenia, in which it is especially likely to be social—an absence of the ability to feel pleasure in relationships (Cutting, 1985). There is evidence that the hedonic aspects of olfactory experience may be disturbed in schizophrenia. Male patients with schizophrenia failed to attach the appropriate hedonic valence to a pleasant odour, despite correctly perceiving changes in odour intensity in a study where the odour was presented birhinally. In a study in which amyl acetate was presented unirhinally, both males and females with schizophrenia underevaluated the hedonic characteristics at low concentrations and overestimated its hedonic characteristics at concentrations judged to be unpleasant by controls and relatives. These patient-specific findings were not explicable by medication, smoking habit or subjective ratings of odour intensity but rather were associated with increased levels of anhedonia/asociality (Kamath et al., 2013). One of the paradoxes of anhedonia in schizophrenia is that when assessed by 'trait' measures of affect, there are robust and marked deficits in the reported experience of pleasure.

However, when affect is assessed in 'the moment' by laboratory mood-induction procedures, there is no evidence of anhedonia (Cohen et al., 2011; Strauss and Gold, 2012). The reasons for this disjunction are unclear but may include (1) anticipatory hedonic experience deficit, (2) impairment of affective regulation control, (3) encoding-retrieval deficit, (4) representational deficit and (5) social-specific deficits.

It is therefore likely that anhedonia is not a singular, homogenous abnormality in which the inability to experience pleasure equally affects all modalities of experience, but an experience that is composed of different component parts. This conceptualization of anhedonia is given further amplification by a single case report of selective loss of emotional experience in listening to music (Satoh et al., 2011). Pleasure in different kinds of sensory experience may be discrete and open to selective disruption.

Exacerbation of Emotions: Melancholia, Mania and Ecstasy

In affective disorders, the mood is usually the primary focus of the abnormality. The pathology of mood can be manifested as intensification of sadness or joy. In sadness, this may present as feelings of sadness and gloom, despondency, despair or hopelessness. Often, the actual experience is indescribable but recognized as different in character from normal sadness. In other words, the character is qualitatively different from sadness and akin to physical pain:

I was feeling in my mind a sensation close to, but indescribably different from actual pain.

William Styron (1990)

It is a positive and active anguish, a sort of psychical neuralgia wholly unknown to normal life.

William James (1902)

William Styron (1990), in his book about his personal experience of depression, argued that the term *depression* was a weak word for the experience.

'Melancholia' would appear to be a far more apt and evocative word for the blacker forms of the disorder, but it was usurped by a noun with a bland tonality and lacking

any magisterial presence, used indifferently to describe an economic decline or a rut in the ground, a true wimp of a word for such a major illness … Nevertheless, for 75 years the word has slithered innocuously through the language like a slug, leaving little trace of its intrinsic malevolence and preventing, by its insipidity, a general awareness of the horrible intensity of the disease when out of control.

The positive feeling of joy and pleasure can also be intensified. Jamison (1995) described her personal experience of mania:

When you're high it's tremendous. The ideas and feelings are fast and frequent like shooting stars and you follow them until you find better and brighter ones. Shyness goes; the right words and gestures are suddenly there, the power to captivate others a felt certainty. There are interests found in uninteresting people. Sensuality is pervasive and the desire to seduce and be seduced is irresistible … But somewhere this changes … Everything previously moving with the grain is now against – you are irritable, angry, frightened, uncontrollable, and enmeshed in the blackest caves of the mind.

It is clear that the positive, joyful aspect of the elevation of mood can quickly turn into a dysphoric sensation that is uncomfortable and unwelcome, yet that is not a variant of depression. *Euphoria* is a state of excessive unreasonable cheerfulness; it may be manifested as extreme cheerfulness, as described by Jamison in mania, or it may seem inappropriate and bizarre. It is commonly seen in organic states, especially associated with frontal lobe impairment.

Heightened states of happiness such as ecstasy sometimes occur in people with mental illness or abnormality of personality but also occur outside of psychiatry in normal contexts. Ecstatic states can be conceptualized as an altered state of consciousness and can be self-induced in meditation adepts. Jhanas are an example of such a self-induced meditative state characterized by dimming of the awareness of external experience, fading of internal verbalizations, alteration in the sense of personal boundary, intense focus on the object of meditation and increase in joy. This state has been shown to be associated with the activation of cortical processes and of the nucleus accumbens in

the dopamine/opioid reward system (Hagerty et al., 2013).

In neurology, ecstatic states are associated with epilepsy. Fyodor Dostoevsky (1821–81) in his novels, *The Idiot* and *Demons* described ecstatic states based on his own experiences. Gschwind and Picard (2016) define ecstatic seizures as fulfilling the following criteria: (1) the feeling of intense positive emotion termed bliss, (2) enhanced physical well-being and (3) heightened self-awareness or heightened perception of the external world termed clarity. They reported on 52 patients and exemplify these characteristic features drawing from the accounts of these patients. For example, intense serenity and bliss is described as 'the immense joy that fills me is above physical sensations'. 'it is a feeling of total presence, an absolute integration of myself, of unbelievable harmony of my whole body and myself with life, with the world, and with the "All"'; enhanced physical well-being is described as 'something pleasant which fills my inner body, wrapping me, with a rapid crescendo. It is a well-being inside, a sensation of velvet, as I were sheltered from anything negative. I feel light inside, but far from being empty, I feel really present. Something has taken possession of my body, to feel really good'; and heightened self-awareness is described as 'I feel very, very, very present at that time, the consciousness of myself is very increased, rather on a psychic point of view, I am one hundred percent concentrated on myself'. Investigation of these patients suggests that ecstatic experiences arise from a functional network centred on the anterior insular cortex.

Understandably, most psychiatrists writing about the mood state of ecstasy have described its occurrence in patients with psychosis. But ecstatic experience may also be reported in association with minor psychiatric symptoms. The patient may describe a calm, exalted state of happiness amounting to ecstasy, although this tranquil mood state is relatively uncommon and usually short-lived. In schizophrenia, ecstatic mood may be associated with delusions of exaltation, for example, the chronic patient who sat placidly enraptured on a long-stay ward, knowing herself to be the Queen of Heaven and waiting for a messenger to inform her that she was to take over the rule of the world. Ecstatic states, usually with a histrionic flavour, may occur in dissociative disorder and may be associated with religious stigmata (Simpson, 1984). Bizarre, mass hysterical phenomena, often with religious associations, are usually of this type, for example, in the devils of Loudun as described by Aldous Huxley (1952). The social, institutional and group psychological prerequisites for the development of epidemic or mass hysteria (Sirois, 1982) are usually present in these situations, and mismanagement is usually responsible for the development from isolated hysteria in one individual to an epidemic. Ecstasy, solemn elation or excessive exuberant expansiveness may also be seen in epilepsy, as described above, and in other organic states, for example, in general paresis.

Characteristic of ecstasy in psychiatry is that it is self-referent; for example, the flowers of spring 'open for *me*'. There is an alteration of the boundaries of self so that the person may feel 'at one with the universe', or may 'empty myself of all will' so that 'I am nothing but feelings'. The change in ego boundaries does not usually have the aspect of interference with self that accompanies passivity experiences. In ecstasy, the abrogation of self is experienced as being voluntary. Expert knowledge of the abnormal does not preclude ignorance of the normal, and the psychiatrist can never generalize from the sample of people selectively referred to them to the whole of mankind. This discrepancy can become very obvious in the area of *ecstatic* and *religious experience*. There is a need to acknowledge, take into account, have respect for and use in treatment the patient's own subjective experience in this area (Sims, 1994). The psychiatrist sees a most unrepresentative group of those having some form of religious experience, which has been considered to amount to more than 40% of the adult population of the United States, more of whom are males than females, more are stable than unstable and more happy than unhappy.

The anthropology of ecstasy (Lewis, 1971) can be traced through Christian and other cultures and makes contact with recognizable mental illness only at a few points. William James (1902), in *The Variety of Religious Experience*, demonstrated the vast extent of the phenomenology of religion and showed how unwise it would be to equate the surprising with the pathologic. Rodney Stark (1965) in his *A Taxonomy of Religious Experience* included the ecstatic experience as one of the general type of religious experience incorporating awareness of the divine, a sense that the awareness is returned and a deepening of the aforementioned awareness is a sense of personal affective relationship. Stark describes this as 'comparable to the intimacy of friendship, or, perhaps, even courtship. Indeed, a heavily sexual motif runs through the ecstatic writings of Catholic monastics'. For example, '[…] I felt as a wave started at my crown and continued down through my body, out through my feet. I truly felt as if God had passed his hand over me. I felt as if I had been reborn. It was a miracle! I went back to sleep without a care or concern in the World'.

Accounts vary as to the extent of psychopathology among converts to religious groups and sects; it is probably associated with the nature of the group. Thus Ungerleider and Wellisch (1979) found no evidence of severe mental illness in one study, whereas Galanter (1982) described evidence of emotional problems among adherents to Divine Light, the Unification Church, Baba and Subud.

Suggestive indicators for establishing a religious experience as probably associated with psychiatric morbidity are as follows:

- the phenomenology of the experience conforms with psychiatric illness;
- there are other recognizable symptoms of mental disturbance;
- the lifestyle, behaviour and direction of personal goals of the person subsequent to the event are consistent with the natural history of mental disorder rather than with an enriching life experience; and
- such behaviour is consistent with disorders in the person's personality.

With the following signs, the experience is more likely to be intrinsic to the person's belief and less likely to denote psychiatric illness:

- the person shows some degree of reticence to discuss the experience, especially with those they anticipate will be unsympathetic;
- it is described unemotionally with matter-of-fact conviction and appears 'authentic';
- the person understands, allows for and even sympathizes with the incredulity of others;
- the person usually considers that the experience implies some demands on themself; and
- the religious experience conforms with the subject's recognizable religious traditions and peer group.

Finally, for completion, it is worth noting that there is a literature on transcendental sexual experience (Wade, 2001) which includes sex as a route to ecstatic experience. In this study of 86 participants, it was reported that the altered state was independent of orgasm and was considered as a discrete state in its own right and the ecstatic state was experienced as a cosmic force. The experience included transcendence of spatial boundaries, identification with objects and other subjects, among other things.

Intensification of Fear, Anger and Surprise

The intensification of fear and anger is described in Chapter 17. These two basic emotions can occur in pure form but can also complicate the intensification of sadness or joy, so that it is not uncommon for depressed or elated mood to be associated with anxiety or irritability. Morbid surprise is seen in *latah*, a culture-bound disorder described in Malaysia in which there appears to be an exaggerated startle response characterized by a myriad of echo phenomena including echolalia, echopraxia and echomimia. There is also coprolalia, automatic obedience and hypersuggestibility (Bartholomew, 1994). *Hyperekplexia* is a heightened startle reflex that occurs either as a hereditary neurologic condition involving the inhibitory glycine receptor, or as a symptomatic disorder predominantly of epilepsy in which a surprise stimulus provokes a normal startle response that then triggers a focal, usually frontal lobe, seizure (Meinck, 2006). Late-onset cases, without demonstrable pathology, have been reported in which audiogenic, visual or tactile stimuli trigger myoclonic jerks characterized by eye blinking, head flexion, abduction of the upper arms, movement of the trunk and bending of the knees (Hamelin et al., 2004). In addition, the startle reflex can be exaggerated in post-traumatic stress disorder and alcohol withdrawal states (Howard and Ford, 1992).

CHANGES IN TIMING, DURATION AND APPROPRIATENESS TO SITUATION

Timing, Duration and Appropriateness to Situation

The timing and duration of emotions are aspects of the emotional expression that determine whether the emotion is appropriate to its context. In pathologic grief, the timing and duration may be altered such that the grief is delayed or prolonged. Delayed grief is in essence prolongation of the initial numb phase (see discussion later in the chapter). Lability of mood involves both a heightening or an intensification of emotions accompanied by an instability in the persistence of emotions that communicates itself to the observer as an inappropriateness to the social context. It can also appear as a shallowness of emotional expression despite being intense, because it is transitory and can seem not to be deeply felt. It is often a sign of brain damage and is seen after frontal lobe injury or cerebrovascular accident.

Pathologic laughter or crying is usually an unprovoked emotion that does not have an apparent object. In other words, the emotion is not related to any identifiable social situation. Pathologic laughter occurs in epilepsy, in which it is known as *gelastic* epilepsy, but it may also be associated with acquired brain injury. It is commonly associated with pathologic crying, which is also associated with focal brain injury and when it occurs in epilepsy is termed *dacrystic* epilepsy. It is noteworthy that pathologic crying occurs as a discrete condition without pathologic laughter (Poeck and Pilleri, 1963, quoted in Cutting, 1997).

In schizophrenia, Bleuler (1911) described *parathymia* and *paramimia*. In parathymia, patients react to sad news with cheerfulness or even laughter. These patients may become sad or irritated by events to which others will react with indifference or pleasure. Furthermore, the term parathymia is also used for unprovoked or inappropriate bursts of laughter. This particular aspect of parathymia is similar if not identical to pathologic laughter. *Paramimia* refers to the lack of unity between the various modes of expression of emotions:

A female catatonic patient approached one of the female attendants whom she liked and told her in the friendliest manner and in her sweetest tone of voice: 'I really would like to slap your face, people like you are usually called s.o.b.s.'

A woman patient complained bitterly about her 'voices' and body hallucinations; her mouth and her forehead manifested disgust, but her eyes expressed happy eroticism. After a few minutes the mouth also assumed the expression of happiness, while her forehead continued to appear gloomy and wrinkled.

ABNORMALITIES OF EXPRESSION AND APPROPRIATENESS TO OBJECT

Blunting and Flattening of Feeling

The terms *blunting* and *flattening* are used interchangeably to refer to unchanging facial expression, decreased spontaneous movements, poverty of expressive gesture, poor eye contact, affective unresponsivity and lack of vocal inflection (Andreasen, 1979). Thus the terms refer to a composite of features that are related but are not necessarily part of a unified abnormality. *Blunting* implies a lack of emotional sensitivity, such as that displayed by the girl with schizophrenia who, with obvious relish for the sensational effect, took her visitors up to the bedroom to show them her mother who had been dead for 48 hours. *Flattening* is a limitation of the usual range of emotion expressed usually by facial but also bodily gestures. The individual does not express much affect in any direction, although that which is expressed is appropriate in direction. Both blunting and flattening occur in schizophrenia.

Bodily Feelings Associated with Emotion

In the theories of emotion, physiologic changes such as palpitations, dry mouth, sweatiness, and the like have a key determining part in the labelling of emotion. These and other changes can be the sole features of emotional disorder in some individuals. The relationships between mood and somatic symptoms have been discussed in Chapter 14. In a number of cultures and languages, depression is considered to have an anatomic location to such an extent that the mood state and the part of the body become synonymous. Melancholia literally means 'black bile'; similarly, in Urdu the word *jee,* meaning self, describes the hypochondrium anatomically and comes to mean depression, that is, depression is a central assault on the well-being of the self. Changes in bodily feeling are important in a number of conditions. Physical illness frequently precipitates a loss of the accustomed sense of well-being. This is subjectively experienced as a generalized lowering of vitality and may be associated with other psychological abnormalities, for instance hypochondriasis or dissociation. In these settings, the expression of emotional disturbance is likely to emphasize the physical rather than the emotional:

And thence proceeds wind, palpitation of the heart, short breath, plenty of humidity in the stomach, heaviness of heart and heartache, and intolerable stupidity and dullness of spirits. Their excrements or stool hard, black to some, and little. If the heart, brain, liver, spleen, be misaffected, as they usually are, many inconveniences

proceed from them, many diseases accompany … those frequent wakings and terrible dreams, intempestive laughing, weeping, sighing, sobbing, bashfulness, blushing, trembling, sweating, swooning, etc.

Burton (1577–1650), The Anatomy of Melancholia *(1628)*

Vital feelings was a term used by Wernicke (1906) to describe certain somatic symptoms occurring in the affective psychoses. The word *vital* comes from the concept of the *vital self,* which describes the close relationship of the body to awareness of self, the way we experience our bodies and the impression we consider our physical presence makes on others. So, vital feelings are those that make us aware of our vital self. These are the feelings of mood that appear to emanate from the body itself: localized and somatized affect. For example, depressed patients commonly complain of headache. On more informed enquiry, the patient may say, 'it's not exactly a pain, but more an unbearable feeling of pressure like a tight band around the head', 'a feeling of misery, like a black cloud pressing on my head'. The head is the commonest site for vital feelings, but they may also occur in the abdomen—'I have a dull feeling in my bowels, they are slowing down and blocking', in the chest—'it feels like a weight bearing down on my chest, stopping me breathing', in the eyes—'everything looks black, dark and drab; my eyes are heavy, I cannot see properly' or in the legs—'my legs are terribly heavy; I cannot walk I feel so exhausted'. They may occur in other regions of the body, for instance the bladder, the feet, the hair and so on. The features that appear to be constant are the association of the localized body sensation with the prevailing depressed mood; the sensation of weight, tension, heaviness, even depression in the particular organ; and a consequent loss of function—'I cannot think properly … my bowels are blocked'.

Schneider (1920) considered vital feelings to be of paramount diagnostic significance in depressive illness, equivalent to the first-rank symptoms in schizophrenia, the core of cyclothymic depression and autonomic in origin. He considered these feelings to be common in depression. It would seem that Dupré (1913), writing about what he called *coenestopathic states,* was describing the same symptom: 'Coenestopathic states are, indeed, so common as to figure among the most frequent features of the psychoses'. He described *coenaesthesia* as the 'deep but more or less indefinite awareness that we have of our own bodies and the general tone of functional activity'. Coenestopathic states are 'the distressing feelings which emanate from one or other of the coenesthesic areas … a change in the normal quality of physical feeling in certain parts of the body'. They are localized, but there is no local pathogenic lesion. Dupré claimed that coenestopathic states were autonomous and not associated with other psychiatric disorders; but, in describing the affects with which they are associated, he appears to describe affective disorders. The mood of depression may be described as a global loss of vitality in which all functions are affected and all performances depressed.

A change in vital feelings does not occur only in depression. The bizarre feelings that a patient with schizophrenia has about their body is a change in the way they express themself, often further elaborated by delusions. It should be noted that the term *vital* is used rather differently in *vital anxiety states*. These states have been described (López Ibor, 1966) in which the anxiety is thought to be endogenous, developing relatively acutely in people of stable personality.

The depressive content of what phenomenologists would consider to be vital feelings varies very greatly, for example, 'I have turned to stone … I have a feeling of depression in my chest … it is a pain, a knot, a weight … I have a cloud on my head, a feeling of nothingness'. Burns (1971) commented with regard to respiratory vital feelings, 'A striking feature of the breathlessness described by the patients with depression was its fairly sudden onset and cessation, corresponding exactly with the onset and resolution of the depressive illness'.

Trethowan (1979) considered that lowering of vitality is fundamental to the experience of depressive illness. He described this as 'a lowering of vitality which is all-pervasive and leads to a marked loss of ability of the subject to function as he did before he became ill in terms of both mind and body'.

Feelings Attached to the Perception of Objects

Objects may evoke an emotional response in a normal person, for instance, a comfortable feeling of familiarity towards an armchair in which one rests after an energetic walk or apprehensive dislike towards a dentist's chair. This normal affective response may be exaggerated pathologically. Excessive feelings of fear amounting to terror may remain associated with objects. The objects to which affect is attached may not only be physical, inanimate objects but also thoughts, and patterns of thoughts, and people. The occurrence of certain ideas may regularly be associated with specific pathologic emotion, perhaps resulting in phobia (see Chapter 17). Any object of perception may be invested with idiosyncratic affect.

Feelings Directed Towards People

These may be disturbed in a number of ways. Affect may be absent or deadened, increased and excessive or distorted. It may also be ambivalent—both loving and hating, rejecting and overprotecting synchronously. A girl, described in Chapter 14 who was suffering from anorexia nervosa, would take great care to cook enormous meals for her twin sister, to whom she was very close; the sister became grossly obese while the patient vanished almost to a skeleton. In answer to remonstrations about feeding her sister, she said, 'I look horrible, so she should look horrible as well'.

Free-Floating Emotion

This is commonly described in psychiatric disturbance, and in his original description of anxiety neurosis, Freud (1895) considered that the condition was characterized by free-floating anxiety. A powerful affect seems to have no goal and is associated with no object. The patient describes themself as feeling generally anxious, not anxious about anything in particular but just anxious. This free-floating anxiety has somatic and psychological concomitants. It may seem to be localized physically in certain areas of the body. Other free-floating affects occur, such as dread, restlessness, tension, gloom, despondency, euphoria, irritability and so on.

Abnormality of Experience and Physiologic Activity

A speculative hypothesis that clinicians have found helpful is the term *alexithymia,* which was coined by Sifneos (1972) to describe a specific disturbance in psychic functioning characterized by difficulties in the capacity to verbalize affect and elaborate fantasies. This was originally introduced to describe psychosomatic disorders occurring in individuals with difficulty expressing their emotions. The link with absence or diminution of fantasy is a consistent finding (Nemiah and Sifneos, 1970). The communicative style shows markedly reduced or absent symbolic thinking so that inner attitudes, feelings, wishes and drives are not revealed; few dreams and a paucity of fantasies are reported (Taylor, 1984). Thinking is literal, utilitarian and concerned with the minutiae of external events. These individuals have great difficulty in recognizing and describing their own feelings and in discriminating between emotional states and bodily sensations. They show a stiff, robot-like existence, 'almost as if they are following an instruction book'; there may be stiffness of posture and lack of facial expression. They show an impaired capacity for empathy in their interpersonal relationships. Alexithymic characteristics have been found especially among patients with psychosomatic disorders, somatoform disorders, psychogenic pain disorders, substance abuse disorders, post-traumatic stress disorder, masked depression, character neuroses and sexual perversions, but these findings have not been consistently replicated.

The Toronto Alexithymia Scale, which is the most widely used measure of alexithymia, has four factors: difficulty in identifying feelings, externally oriented thinking, difficulty expressing feelings and reduced daydreaming (Kirmayer and Robbins, 1993). The difficulty in identifying feelings and the difficulty in expressing them both appear to be correlated with somatosensory amplification (Nakao et al., 2002). This provides some validation of the idea that alexithymia is the basis for excessive somatization and that this may be caused by undue awareness of discrepant sensations that are then misconstrued as evidence of physical illness.

Somatization in patients with mental disorder can be defined as the selective perception and focus on the somatic manifestations of the disorder with denial or minimization of the affective and cognitive changes (Katon et al., 1982). As a method of expression of emotion, it is frequently reported in transcultural studies, especially in the Indian subcontinent, according to Rack (1982). Murphy and co-workers (1967) studied basic depressive symptomatology in 30 countries and showed how culture changes illness and the way dysphoria is expressed. Bavington (1981), studying depression in a predominantly Pathan culture in Pakistan, found somatization to be expressed in 45% of cases; hypochondriasis was present in 55%, hysterical (dissociative) features in 60%, feelings of guilt in 50%, paranoid ideas in 38%, suicidal thoughts in 75%, diurnal variation in 18%, retardation in 50% and irritability in 80% of depressed patients. Bavington explains these somatic ideas by the presence of vital feelings rather than poverty of language. Mumford (1992) found that patients with psychiatric disorders originating from India and Pakistan typically communicate their distress as somatic symptoms; somatic presentation was common in general hospital settings where psychiatric disorders were often unrecognized and untreated. The use of somatic symptoms and somatic metaphor to communicate emotional distress is found in all languages and cultures. Complaining of emotional dysphoria in terms of somatic symptoms may reflect the limitation of the medical profession in listening to complaints rather than a poverty of language or paucity of verbal expression in the patient.

Abnormalities of Evaluation

The relationship between cognitions and emotions is difficult to disentangle. Initially, it was thought that the emotional state determined the associated cognitions. Thus low mood provoked negative thoughts about the self and the world. However, Beck (Beck 1967; Beck et al., 1979) proposed that a constellation of cognitive errors initiated or maintained depression. These included arbitrary inferences, selective abstractions, overgeneralizations, magnification and minimization. Furthermore, there were cognitive schemas, that is, underlying assumptions about the self, the world and the future, that developed from previous experiences and that habitually influenced how events in the world were appraised and these could induce mood change, either directly or via disruption in self-esteem. This proposal is in line with Schachter and Singer's two-factor theory of emotion, in which cognitions play a central role.

There are also abnormalities of appraisal of the facial or vocal expression of emotions in others.

Prosopoaffective agnosia refers to the selective deficiency in appreciating the emotional expression displayed in the face of others. This abnormality is distinct from prosopagnosia in which only recognition of familiar faces is impaired. It is usually associated with acquired brain disease and has been reported in frontotemporal dementia when it is also associated with impairment of recognition of vocal expression of emotion (Keane et al., 2002); after right thalamic infarct (Vuillemier et al., 1998); and in subjects with right-sided limbic and heteromodal cortical lesions (Weniger and Irle, 2002). It has been reported in autism and Asperger's syndrome, but it is not part of a pervasive impairment of face-processing skills (Hofter et al., 2005). In other words, it occurs in some patients but not in others and dissociates from impairment of face recognition per se.

Prosodic aspects of speech such as pitch, duration and amplitude are part of the nonverbal cues that modify the meaning of the spoken word and indicate the emotional value of an utterance and the intention of the speaker (Mitchell and Ross, 2013). *Expressive emotional prosody* refers to the generation of affect in speech. The mechanisms are unclear but are thought to include bilateral basal ganglia involvement in motor production of speech as a function of affective state and right lateralization of cortical processes in the monitoring and production of acoustic speech parameters (Pichon and Kell, 2013), and the degree to which there is unilateral right-sided or bilateral frontotemporal involvement in *receptive emotional prosody* is uncertain (Witteman et al., 2012). *Receptive emotional dysprosody* refers to the selective deficit in recognizing the emotional tone in speech. This is often associated with *expressive emotional dysprosody,* the impairment of the production of emotional tone in speech. Both abnormalities are found in Parkinson's disease (Caekebeke et al., 1991; Pell, 1996).

The evolutionary relationship between music and language is uncertain, but it is thought that music and language may have a common origin as an emotional protolanguage that remains evident in overlapping functions and shared neural circuitry. In a study of 12 individuals with congenital amusia, a disorder characterized by deficits in acoustic and structural attributes of music, a marked impairment in receptive emotional prosody was demonstrated, suggesting that music and language share mechanisms that trigger emotional responses to acoustic attributes (Thompson et al., 2012).

Abnormality of Mood in Bipolar Disorder

Certainly since the writings of Kraepelin, the apparently opposite mood states of mania and depression have been recognized as occurring in the same illness—frequently at different times and stages of the illness in the same patient, more rarely at the same time in the same patient. Although they are described separately, it is important to realize that these mood states may occur together. Mania and depression are not opposite mood states; they are both pathologic, and the opposite of either would be freedom from morbid emotion. Agitation and overactivity may occur with depression, irritability and a feeling of frustration with mania. A patient, now depressed, having previously been manic, described this: 'The first fine careless rapture has disappeared. I feel more tired and moody'.

Depression of Mood

An additional video for this topic is available ▶ online.

CORE EXPERIENCE: PSYCHOLOGICAL AND PHYSICAL

Depression of mood is common, and depression of such persistence and intensity has to be regarded as illness frequently occurs. There is considerable discussion as to what is the central core of depression. Of course, arguments advocating biochemical, psychodynamic or conditioning factors as initiating causes are not mutually exclusive. Depression affects virtually all physical and psychological functions; for example, using a tachistoscopic method, Powell and Hemsley (1984) were able to show that depression influenced perception.

The word *depression* is a misnomer, as depressive illness may occur without the patient making a complaint of depression as a symptom (*depressio sine depressione*). For this reason, the term *melancholia* may be preferred; although this literally means 'black bile', it has come to be accepted as a medical illness. It was the term used by Lewis (1934) in his classic description of depressive states in a detailed study of 61 cases; this has influenced all subsequent investigation of the condition. Melancholia is the preferred term for Whybrow (1997), who considers that it 'better captures the "veritable tempest in the brain" that marks the experience of inner turmoil and confused thinking as harmony and emotion drain away, often to be replaced by a withered imitation of life'.

The subjective symptoms of depression are very variable. The mood varies from indifference and apathy to profound dejection, despondency and despair. *Anhedonia,* the complete inability to experience pleasure, is a constant feature; it is experienced as joylessness and revealed in facial expression, speech, behaviour, lifestyle and the patient's account of personal experience.

A slowing down of the ability to initiate thought or action is noted by the observer as *retardation.* A patient, describing this after recovery, said, 'it feels as if treacle has been poured into my head through my ears'. Psychic retardation is experienced subjectively as an inability to fulfil normal obligations, as loss of coping. The proneness to self-blame often results in the patient describing themself as lazy and good for nothing. There is a catastrophic lowering of self-esteem as a prominent cognitive component.

Agitation and purposeless restlessness add to the discomfort and to the inability of the depressed person to achieve anything. This anxiety and preoccupation with gloomy thoughts impairs concentration. Diurnal variation of mood is often prominent, with the patient feeling at their worst, and perhaps most suicidal, when they wake early in the morning or, alternatively, somewhat later in the morning. The degree of depression and misery may sometimes successfully be concealed; this is the presentation of *depressio sine depressione* (smiling depression) in a patient who appears not to be depressed in the consulting room but may, much to their doctor's dismay, kill themself. The concealment is probably conscious and may be associated with habitual masking of the expression of emotion or alternatively aimed at avoiding treatment.

Concentration, application and decision-making become difficult, painful and sometimes impossible. The person describes difficulty or impossibility in fantasy and recollection of emotion. This is described as loss of memory and loss of feeling. Often, this loss of mental function makes the patient believe they are 'going mad' or 'losing their mind', a sort of mental hypochondriasis. Physical retardation may become the focus for hypochondriacal beliefs about the body: 'I am constipated … my bowels are totally blocked'. A very depressed middle-aged woman described her bodily feelings thus: 'I have a feeling like having an injection at the dentist's. My face feels numb, but at the same time painful all over'.

Anxiety is a common concomitant with depression and may completely obscure the latter. In agitated depression, agitation and restlessness are extreme and the patient carries a serious risk of suicide. Histrionic behaviour may also obscure the underlying depressive illness. A patient who was actually profoundly depressed kept picking her skin and pulling her hair, saying, 'Look, I can't feel anything when I do this to myself'.

The affect of depression may be localized somatically in vital feelings (described earlier). It may take the form of profound misery or dejection. There is usually a feeling of loss of capacity, helplessness and a feeling that the patient cannot cope. Absence of feelings is often described or it may be described as an inexplicable loss of feelings 'that ought to be there'.

Feelings of guilt and unworthiness are prominent in depressive illness of the endogenous type. This has long been known; for example Plutarch, in the CE 1st century, described a person: 'He looks on himself as a man whom the gods hate and pursue with their anger … "Leave me", says the wretched man, "me the impious, the accursed, hated of the gods, to suffer my punishment".' (Zilboorg and Henry, 1941). On the other hand, Shepherd (1993) considers that guilt feelings did not feature predominantly in depressive states described in pre-Puritan England. The patient may blame themself for having allowed themself to get into this state of mind. They are full of self-reproach and recrimination for all sorts of peccadilloes from the distant past. For all that goes wrong around them they take personal blame; this may be of delusional intensity. Using a scale for the evaluation of feelings of guilt, it was possible to identify two separate components: 'delusional' guilt or shame (experienced in relation to one's actions) and 'affective' guilt (a more general feeling of unworthiness) (Berrios et al., 1992). As well as delusions of guilt and unworthiness, hypochondriacal and nihilistic delusions are relatively common in depression, especially when it occurs in the elderly.

Delusions occur in psychotic depression. It is important to make the distinction between a belief about the state of the world coloured by current mood—'I feel that I must have done something to my brain as I can't think properly', from an actual delusional belief—'I can't think at all, it is impossible, my brain is dead'. The former is a metaphorical statement, the latter a belief held with conviction. In practice, there is often a grey area between frank depressive delusions and emotionally laden views of the world.

Table 16.1 shows the frequency of symptoms, however slight, in depressive illness that were recorded quantitatively using a rating scale in 239 men and 260 women (Hamilton, 1989). It is seen that anxiety is a frequent symptom in depressive illness.

SHAME AND GUILT

Shame and guilt are regarded as self-conscious and moral emotions in that they both involve self-evaluation and play a role in facilitating moral conduct.

They are also emotions that flow from human action, human conduct wherein human beings cause things to happen and whatever results from this conduct can sometimes be regretted or deplored. In essence, these emotions derive from the notion of responsibility, of being an agent who is responsible for the consequences of action and hence can be blamed and/or be disapproved of as an individual.

Williams (1993) wrote: 'The basic experience connected with shame is that of being seen, inappropriately by the wrong people, in the wrong condition. It is straightforwardly connected with nakedness, particularly in sexual connections ... The reaction is to cover oneself or to hide, and people naturally take steps to avoid the situations that call for it'. According to Tangney and Dearing (2002), 'Shame is an extremely painful and ugly feeling that has a negative impact on interpersonal behaviour'. They make the point that shame is associated with the tendency to blame others for negative outcomes and that individuals who are

TABLE 16.1	Frequency of Symptoms in Depressive Illness				
Symptoms	Subjects (%)		Symptoms	Subjects (%)	
Depressed mood	100.0		Depressed mood	100.0	
Loss of interest	99.6		Loss of interest	98.8	
Anxiety, psychic	97.1		Anxiety, psychic	97.8	
Anxiety, somatic	87.4		Somatic, general	94.2	
Insomnia, initial	83.7		Anxiety, somatic	87.3	
Suicide	82.0		Somatic, gastrointestinal	83.5	
Somatic, general	82.0		Suicide	80.4	
Somatic, gastrointestinal	80.3		Insomnia, initial	77.7	
Insomnia, delayed	74.1		Guilt	72.7	
Guilt	71.5		Insomnia, delayed	71.9	
Insomnia, middle	71.5		Weight loss	68.8	
Weight loss	69.0		Agitation	68.1	
Agitation	68.1		Insomnia, middle	66.5	
Libido	59.8		Libido	49.5	
Retardation	52.3		Retardation	43.5	
Hypochondriasis	33.1		Hypochondriasis	25.8	
Loss of insight	28.0		Loss of insight	21.9	
Paranoid symptoms	25.1		Depersonalization	21.1	
Obsessional symptoms	13.3		Obsessional symptoms	20.7	
Depersonalization	10.9		Paranoid symptoms	13.8	
Diurnal variation:	59.4		Diurnal variation:	60.1	
Worse in morning	61.4		Worse in morning	65.5	
Worse in evening	30.7		Worse in evening	25.0	
Worse in afternoon	7.9		Worse in afternoon	9.5	

After Hamilton, M., 1989. Frequency of symptoms in melancholia (depressive illness). Br. J. Psychiatry 154, 201–206, with permission.

shame-prone are also more prone to anger and hostility. Furthermore shame focuses on the self and this is distinct from guilt where the focus is on specific behaviours (Lewis, 1971). Lewis (1971) makes the point that 'the experience of shame is directly about the self, which is the focus of evaluation'. In guilt, the self is not the central object of negative evaluation, but rather the thing done or undone is the focus. In guilt, the self is negatively evaluated in connection with something but is not itself the focus of the experience.

From an anthropologic point of view shame is thought of as arising from public exposure and disapproval of shortcomings or transgression whereas guilt is seen as a private experience deriving from self-generated determination of wrongdoing with the consequent guilt feelings. Nonetheless there is empirical evidence to the contrary—shame can also be experienced in private (Tangney and Dearing, 2002). This is not surprising given the capacity to imagine the absent other in our deliberations. In other words, it cannot be the case that shame can only be experienced when others are physically present because we can imagine the other as present even in their absence. Williams (1993) emphasizes this point 'If everything depended on the fear of discovery, the motivations of shame would not be internalized at all. No one would have a character, in effect, and, moreover, the very idea of there being a shame *culture* [italics in original], a coherent system for the regulation of conduct, would be unintelligible'. Williams goes on to say, 'Even if shame and its motivations always involve in some way or other an idea of the gaze of another, it is important that for many of its operations the imagined gaze of an imagine other will do'.

In Lewis' (1971) account, shame is experienced as a sense of powerlessness and worthlessness in the context of exposure to critical scrutiny, whereas guilt is less painful and less likely to affect self-identity and this is confirmed by Tangney and Dearing's (2002) empirical studies thus making clear that the actual emotional experiences of shame and guilt are distinct. Williams (1993) suggests that the distinction between shame and guilt runs even deeper. He argues that the experience of shame is connected with sight and being seen, whereas 'guilt is rooted in hearing, the sound in oneself of the voice of judgement'. Williams describes the experience of shame as follows:

In my experience of shame, the other sees all of me and all through me, even if the occasion of the shame is on my surface – for instance, in my appearance; and the expression of shame, in general as well as in the particular form of it that is embarrassment, is not just the desire to hide, or to hide my face, but the desire to disappear, not to be there. It is not even the wish as people say, to sink through the floor, but rather the wish that the space occupied by me should be instantaneously empty. With guilt, it is not like this; I am more dominated by the thought that even if I disappeared, it would come with me.

These conceptualizations of shame and guilt are important because they lay the groundwork for furthering our understanding of these emotions in pathologic states. In social anxiety disorder, for example, measures of shame have been shown to be elevated in people with social anxiety whereas guilt was found to be unrelated to social anxiety (Hedman et al., 2013). In a meta-analytic review study, Kim et al. (2011) showed that shame and guilt were equally associated with depression but only when specific types of guilt were considered separately: contextual-maladaptive guilt that involves exaggeration of responsibility for uncontrollable events and generalized guilt involving free-floating guilt divorced from specific contexts were both as likely as shame to be associated depression. From a clinical point of view delusional guilt is often present in severe depression and exaggerated guilt in the context of bereavement. Shame, on the other hand, is prominent in social anxiety.

SUICIDAL THOUGHTS

'I feel as though I want to destroy myself. There is no point in going on.' Suicidal ideas, ruminations and impulses are common. Alvarez (1971) has written a detailed study of suicide from a literary point of view. He is concerned with the background and the reasons for suicide and attempted suicide in many well-known writers, especially poets. He writes about suicide as 'letting go':

I have to admit that I am a failed suicide … Seneca, the final authority on the subject, pointed out disdainfully that the exits are everywhere: each precipice and river, each branch of each tree, every vein in your body will set you free … Yet despite all that, I never quite made it.

The intertwined threads of artistic creativity, manic-depressive illness and suicide have been explored by Goodwin and Jamison (1990).

Both the muse and madness as gifts of the gods have been a recurring theme from earliest times through such 19th-century poets as Browning, Shelley, Coleridge and Byron to the modern American poets such as Sylvia Plath and Anne Sexton, among whom there was found to be a high prevalence of manic-depressive illness and many suicides. In her enlightening study of manic-depressive illness and the artistic temperament, *Touched With Fire,* Jamison (1993) demonstrates differential rates for depressive illness and suicide in poets, artists and other writers and comments on this.

It is no longer satisfactory to simply think of suicidal thoughts or ideas as a unitary phenomenon. Obegi (2019) makes the point that suicidal ideation is itself a composite of thoughts of killing oneself, wishing to be dead, and internal debates about living and dying. Alongside these aspects of suicidal ideation is the degree to which there is suicidal intent, a complex construct that attempts to capture the extent of a person's motivation to die. Next to these issues are ancillary but important features such as psychological pain, feelings of hopelessness, overarousal, readiness and preparedness for suicide, and cognitive rigidity.

House et al. (2020) make the additional point that the term 'ideation' encompasses far more than mere thinking and includes imagining and imagination, a mental state that incorporates images of real or imagined events with a strong visual component. In addition, ideation includes constructing an idea, which involves deliberation, extensive inner dialogue, encompassing the specific details of the potential act and its imagined consequences. Furthermore, they argue that suicidal ideation may be initiated or enhanced by imagining the self-harm or suicide of a third party or suicidal ideation may be reversed or inhibited, for example, by imagining how an attempt may affect the train driver in someone contemplating railway suicide.

The place of psychological pain (psychache/psychalgia) in suicidal ideation and behaviour is starting to be elucidated. A three-dimensional model of psychological pain in suicide describes three components including (1) pain arousal, which is the cognitions about past traumatic experience; (2) painful feelings involving the subjective experience and physiological symptoms and (3) pain avoidance, which is the strong motivation escape from unbearable psychological pain. The suggestion is that suicide results when an individual can no longer endure psychological pain and chooses suicide as the only means of relieving pain. There is some empirical evidence suggesting that individuals who attempt suicide compared with those who have suicidal ideation are more likely to demonstrate a significantly larger cued-P3 amplitude in the punitive condition compared to the reward condition (Song et al., 2020).

There is a role, too, for the degree to which an individual believes that they have or do not have control over their thoughts and in this rumination, the tendency to repetitive and passive fixation on negative emotion and on the potential causes, meaning and consequences of one's distress are linked to suicidal thoughts and behaviours (Rogers et al., 2021). Rumination reflects an impaired ability to disengage from negative emotional and cognitive content rather than merely a tendency to more easily engage with such content and may signal a degree of cognitive rigidity.

Nocturnal cognitive hyperarousal manifest as insomnia has been shown to be associated with suicidal ideation (Kalmbach et al., 2021). This is in line with findings that short sleep duration in farmers is associated with higher suicidal ideation (Oh et al., 2021), that insomnia is associated with suicidal ideation, lifetime suicide attempt in patients with chronic schizophrenia (Miller et al., 2020) and sleep distress, onset insomnia and insufficient sleep is strongly associated with suicidal ideation in university students (Khader et al., 2020).

It is noteworthy that gender seems to mediate the narratives of suicidal thoughts and attempts in military veterans. Females discussed negative self-evaluative processes whereas males discussed a feeling of being overwhelmed by their situation. A female, for example, reported 'I felt like such a failure … No relationship worked. I wasn't productive. I wasn't doing anything that was good. I was just non-existent in an existing world. My self-esteem was so low.' A man reported 'I got to a point, a breaking point. I mean the mind can hold so much and when you deprive your mind of resting, your body of resting and it's always go, go, go then on top of that you experiences in your head recently and emotionally and psychologically … something has to break, there is always a weak link. I feel like at that point I was like "screw this."' The suggestion here is that the content and structure of the inner monologue is determined by gender Denneson et al., 2020).

There are different explanatory hypotheses, such as the integrated motivational-volitional model and the network perspective, aimed at integrating the disparate factors underpinning suicidal ideation and behaviours. These models have in common a recognition that suicidal ideation and behaviours are the end points of complex interactions between different factors (de Beurs et al., 2021). The unanswered questions include how suicidal ideation moves from ideas to action, that is from desire to intent and finally to behaviour. At a simple level, psychological pain and fearlessness about death are associated with desires, plans and preparations for suicide. Specifically, psychological pain and hopelessness are positively associated with the desire to die, but desire is independently associated with fearlessness about death (Marie et al., 2020).

DEPRESSION AND LOSS

Any social situation of transition is associated with some disturbance of emotion (Parkes, 1971). Depression is the affect associated with experience of loss. It is not the intention here to enter into theoretical aspects but to discuss the subjective experience. Parkes (1976) has demonstrated how loss of a person, loss of a limb and even loss of a home are stressful in similar ways, and that there is a mental process going on in which the person is 'making real inside the self events which have already occurred in reality outside'. This process is associated with marked psychic pain and unhappiness. An example of depression associated with the threat of loss of a loved object was a taxi driver who owned his own car, which was the only thing he valued in life. During an episode of profound depression, he polished the taxi to perfection, took it into the garage, connected a pipe to the exhaust of the car, started the engine and killed himself. The dysphoric mood associated with the experience of loss is always exacerbated if there is any sense of guilt or self-blame attached to the circumstances of the loss: 'If

only I had called the doctor in to see Mother earlier; I shall never forgive myself'.

Grief

The immediate experience of loss is shock and numbness. The suddenly bereaved person may say that they cannot believe that it has happened to them. They just feel numb and empty. They may describe depersonalization feelings. There is a tendency to deny that the loss has happened. A woman was referred to a surgeon for a lump in the breast. At operation, the mass was found to be malignant and mastectomy was performed. For several days after the operation, she was unable to accept that the painful area under the dressing signified the loss of her breast rather than a minor excision.

After the initial shock and denial come the pangs of grief. This is an acute feeling of loss, with anxiety prominent, as well as grieving—*anxious searching*. The implications of the experience of loss begin to be realized, and this may cause the person's feelings of anxiety amounting to panic: 'However am I going to cope without him?' The somatic symptoms of anxiety may be present as well as the psychological.

Three distinct patterns of *morbid grief* have been observed (Lieberman, 1978):

1. phobic avoidance of persons, places or things related to the deceased, combined with extreme guilt and anger about the deceased and their death;
2. a total lack of grieving, with anger directed towards others and overidealization of the deceased; and
3. physical illness and recurrent nightmares involving the deceased.

These patterns have relevance for treatment using the behavioural method of *forced* or *guided mourning*.

When the experience of loss has been accepted as a reality, *depression,* the affect appertaining to loss, occurs. The person feels very low and hopeless, perhaps with the lowering of vitality and apathy of depression. They become resigned to their situation but see no way out: 'there is simply no future for me now'. Not surprisingly, this state is often associated with suicidal ideas and impulses, and there is an increased mortality from suicide and other causes in the 6 months subsequent to bereavement (Parkes et al., 1969).

As the state of grieving is resolved, the person gradually overcomes this despairing hopelessness. There is an attitude of mind that results in reorganization and redirection. They gradually make decisions and carry out activities that demonstrate their emotional and intellectual acceptance of the loss and intention to continue their life as congenially as possible, although still remembering the loss. This stage of *resolution* may be postponed for many years, as with Queen Victoria's grieving for Prince Albert.

Parkes (1976) discriminates between the subjective experience of *external loss* and *internal change*. The external loss is shown by pining for the lost object. Anxiety after loss occurs both in bereaved people and in amputees and is associated with anxious searching: a bereaved person used to walk up and down the street wondering if she would see her husband, whom she knew to be dead. In these circumstances, misperception of strangers as being the lost relative may happen. A man whose father had died a long time before thought he heard his father's voice in another room and then realized it was his son. People return to places associated with the lost person or keep articles that belonged to them sacrosanct.

Internal change, with a sense of mutilation, is common to people with different types of loss. Amputees feel themselves to be badly damaged both in their function and in their self-image. Because a man has lost his leg, he will be unable to carry out his previous activities as before and may feel himself to be less of a man. Similarly, the woman with an amputated arm may prefer a cosmetic but useless prosthesis rather than a more functional hook. She may feel the affront to her self-image of a mutilated arm more than the loss of function. Parkes and Napier (1975) stress the social associations of loss in their discussion of prevention and alleviation of the problems resulting from amputation. Widows also describe a feeling of loss within themselves due to their bereavement; there is, of course, often a real loss of status. Those rehoused often described an internal change on moving: 'something of me went when I left the old home'.

Mania

Mania is a word with a long history. Hare (1981) considers that the early descriptions of intellectual deterioration with excitement were made because of the association with organic deterioration from poor general health during the 19th century. As the physical health of the population improved, it was possible to describe separate conditions with different natural histories. However, mania still forms a much higher proportion of affective psychoses occurring puerperally than of affective disorders occurring at other stages of life (Dean and Kendell, 1981).

Mania refers to elation of mood, acceleration of thinking and overactivity. Subjectively, although it may be described as a different state from normal, it is rarely complained of by the patient as a symptom. A young, manic inpatient described his internal state thus: 'I feel hypersuffused with experience … I am developing a close secretarial relationship with Camilla Brown (another young patient) … I feel like a rocket with the blue paper lit, standing in a bottle and just ready to take off'. It has become conventional to refer to all but the most severe cases as suffering from *hypomania*. This is unfortunate because one does not refer to 'hypodepression' and the person using the term *hypomania* often gives the impression that wrong diagnosis is permissible to a greater extent than if the term *mania* had been used.

The early stages of mania may be experienced as enjoyable, even 'wonderful', and an enormous relief from the depression that preceded it. A patient quoted by Whybrow (1997) put it this way: 'In the early stages of mania I feel good – about the world and everybody in it. There's a faster beat; a sense of expectation that my life will be full and exciting'. For this reason, the patient may be reluctant to take medication or to report his condition to his doctor. Later on in manic illness, the patient's experience is usually described as unpleasant and even frightening.

In pure form, it is characterized by excessive cheerfulness, rapid train and association of thought and overactivity. The speed of thinking and the ready ability to form associations results in rapid and apparently sparkling conversation (see Chapter 9). Puns and clang associations abound, for example, in a case quoted by Bingham (1841):

A fine bold lady, well dressed and well known to the officers of a certain house, 'a regular madwoman', as they called her, was brought thither by her friends. She was no sooner announced than every missile and instrument of attack was carefully removed out of her way. She opened the conference by a familiar address to the physician under whose care she had been before and was going to remain, by saying to him, 'Well, Doctor M(orrison), but I beg pardon, I forgot whom I was speaking to – it is Sir A(lexander). Well, Sir A—, since I had the pleasure of seeing you last, I have been benighted, and you have been knighted'.

Kay Redfield Jamison (1995) describes her own experience of mania as follows (previously quoted above but quoted in full here):

When you're high its tremendous. The ideas and feelings are fast and frequent like shooting stars, and you follow them until you find better and brighter ones. Shyness goes, the right words and gestures are suddenly there, the power to captivate others a felt certainty. There are interests found in uninteresting people. Sensuality is pervasive and the desire to seduce and be seduced irresistible. Feelings of ease, intensity, power, well-being, financial omnipotence, and euphoria pervade one's marrow. But, somewhere, this changes. The fast ideas are far too fast, and there are far too many; overwhelming confusion replaces clarity. Memory goes. Humour and absorption on friends' faces are replaced by fear and concern. Everything previously moving with the grain is now against – you are irritable, angry frightened, uncontrollable, and enmeshed totally in the blackest caves of the mind. You never knew these caves were there. It will never end, for madness carves its own reality.

REFERENCES

Alvarez, A., 1971. The Savage God: A Study of Suicide. Weidenfeld & Nicolson, London.

Andreasen, N., 1979. Affective flattening and the criteria for schizophrenia. Am. J. Psychiatry 136, 944–947.

Anstee, B.H., Fleminger, J.J., 1977. Diagnosis 'uncertain': a follow-up study. Br. J. Psychiatry 131, 592–598.

Bartholomew, R.E., 1994. Disease, disorder or deception? Latah as habit in a Malay extended family. J. Nerv. Ment. Dis. 182, 331–338.

Bavington, J., 1981. Depression in Pakistan. Transcultural Psychiatry Society (UK) Workshop, Leeds.

Beck, A.T., 1967. Depression: Clinical, Experimental and Theoretical Aspects. Hoeber, New York.

Beck, A.T., Rush, A.J., Shaw, B.F., Emery, G., 1979. Cognitive Therapy of Depression. Guilford Press, New York.

Berrios, G.E., 1985. The psychopathology of affectivity: conceptual and historical aspects. Psychol. Med. 15, 745–758.

Berrios, G.E., Bulbena, A., Bakshi, N., et al., 1992. Feelings of guilt in major depression: conceptual and psychosomatic aspects. Br. J. Psychiatry 160, 781–787.

Bingham, N., 1841. Religious Delusions. Hatchard, London.

Bleuler, E., 1911. Dementia Praecox: Or the Group of Schizophrenias. International University Press, New York.

Brenner, B., 1979. Depressed affect as a cause of associated somatic problems. Psychol. Med. 9, 737–746.

Burns, B.H., 1971. Breathlessness in depression. Br. J. Psychiatry 119, 39–45.

Burton, R., 1628. The Anatomy of Melancholia. Henry Cripps, Oxford.

Caekebeke, J.F., Jennekens-Schinkel, A., van der Linden, M.E., Buruma, O.J., Roos, R.A., 1991. The interpretation of dysprosody in patients with Parkinson's disease. J. Neurol. Neurosurg. Psychiatry 54, 145–148.

Cohen, A.S., Najolia, G.M., Brown, L.A., Minor, K.S., 2011. The state-trait disjunction of anhedonia in schizophrenia: potential affective, cognitive and social-based mechanisms. Clin. Psychol. Rev. 31, 440–448.

Cutting, J., 1985. The Psychology of Schizophrenia. Churchill Livingstone, Edinburgh.

Cutting, J., 1997. Principles of Psychopathology. Oxford University Press, Oxford.

Darwin, C., 1872. The Expression of the Emotions in Man and Animals. John Murray, London.

de Beurs, D., Bockting, C., Kerkhof, A., Scheepers, F., O'Connor, R., Penninx, B., van de Leemput, I., 2021. A network perspective on suicidal behavior: understanding suicidality as a complex system. Suicide Life Threat Behav. 51 (1), 115–126.

Dean, C., Kendell, R.E., 1981. The symptomatology of puerperal illness. Br. J. Psychiatry 139, 128–133.

Denneson, L.M., Tompkins, K.J., McDonald, K.L., et al., 2020. Gender differences in the development of suicidal behavior among United States military veterans: a national qualitative study. Soc. Sci. Med. 260, 113178.

Der-Avakian, A., Markou, A., 2012. The neurobiology of anhedonia and other reward-related deficits. Trends Neurosci. 35, 68–77.

Dupré, E., 1913. Les cénestopathies, mouvement médical 3–22 (M. Rohde, Trans, 1974). In: Hirsch, S.R., Shepherd, M. (Eds.), Themes and Variations in European Psychiatry. John Wright, Bristol.

Ekman, P., 1998. Afterword. In: Darwin, C. (Ed.), The Expression of the Emotions in Man and Animals. HarperCollins, London.

Ekman, P., Friesen, W., 1971. Constants across cultures in the face and emotion. J. Pers. Soc. Psychol. 17, 124–129.

Freud, S., 1895. On the grounds for detaching a particular syndrome from neurasthenia under the description 'anxiety neurosis. In: Standard Edition of the Complete Psychological Works of Sigmund Freud, vol. III. Translated from the German and under the general editorship of J. Strachey. Hogarth Press, London, pp. 90–115.

Gaillard, R., Gourion, D., Llorca, P.M., 2013. Anhedonia in depression. Encephale 39, 296–305.

Galanter, M., 1982. Charismatic religious sects and psychiatry: an overview. Am. J. Psychiatry 139, 1539–1548.

Gallese, V., 2007. Embodied simulation: from mirror neuron systems to interpersonal relations. Novartis Found. Symp. 278, 3–12.

Goodwin, F.K., Jamison, K.R., 1990. Manic-Depressive Illness. Oxford University Press, New York.

Gschwind, M., Picard, F., 2016. Ecstatic epileptic seizures: a glimpse into the multiple roles of the insula. Front. Behav. Neurosci. 10, 21.

Hagerty, M.R., Isaacs, J., Brasington, L., Shupe, L., Fetz, E.E., Cramer, S.C., 2013. Case study of ecstatic meditation: fMRI and EEG evidence of self-stimulating a reward system. Neural Plast. 2013, 653572.

Hamelin, S., Rohr, P., Kahane, P., Minotti, L., Vercueil, L., 2004. Late onset hyperekplexia. Epileptic Disord. 6, 169–172.

Hamilton, M., 1989. Frequency of symptoms in melancholia (depressive illness). Br. J. Psychiatry 154, 201–206.

Hare, E., 1981. The two manias: a study of the evolution of the modern concept of mania. Br. J. Psychiatry 138, 89–99.

Hedman, E., Ström, P., Stünkel, A., Mörlberg, E., 2013. Shame and guilt in social anxiety disorder: effects of cognitive behaviour therapy and association with social anxiety and depressive symptoms. PLoS One 8, e61713.

Hofter, R.L., Manoach, D.S., Barton, J.J., 2005. Perception of facial expression and facial identity in subjects with social developmental disorders. Neurology 65, 1620–1625.

House, A., Kapur, N., Knipe, D., 2020. Thinking about suicidal thinking. Lancet Psychiatr. 7 (11), 997–1000.

Howard, R., Ford, R., 1992. From the jumping Frenchmen of Maine to posttraumatic stress disorder: the startle response in neuropsychiatry. Psychol. Med. 22, 695–707.

Huxley, A., 1952. The Devils of Loudun. Chatto & Windus, London.

James, W., 1884. What is an emotion? Mind 9, 188–205.

James, W., 1902. The Varieties of Religious Experience: A Study in Human Nature. Longmans, Green, New York.

Jamison, K.R., 1993. Touched with Fire: Manic-Depressive Illness and the Artistic Temperament. Free Press, New York.

Jamison, K.R., 1995. An Unquiet Mind. A Memoir of Moods and Madness. Knopf, New York.

Kalmbach, D.A., Ahmedani, B.B., Gelaye, B., Cheng, P., Drake, C.L., 2021. Nocturnal cognitive hyperaousal, perinatal-focused rumination, and insomnia are associated with suicidal ideation in perinatal women with mild to moderate depression. Sleep Medicine, 81, 439–442.

Kamath, V., Moberg, P.J., Kohler, C.G., Gur, R.E., Turetsky, B.I., 2013. Odor hedonic capacity and anhedonia in schizophrenia and unaffected first-degree relatives of schizophrenia patients. Schizophr. Bull. 39, 59–67.

Katon, W., Kleinman, A., Rosen, G., 1982. Depression and somatization: a review. Part 1. Am. J. Med. 72, 127–135.

Keane, J., Calder, A.J., Hodges, J.R., Young, A.W., 2002. Face and emotion processing in frontal variant frontotemporal dementia. Neuropsychologia 40, 655–665.

Khader, W.S., Tubbs, A.S., Haghighi, A., et al., 2020. Onset insomnia and insufficient sleep duration are associated with suicide ideation in university students and athletes. J. Affect. Disord. 274, 1161–1164.

Kim, S., Thibodeau, R., Jorgensen, R.S., 2011. Shame, guilt, and depressive symptoms: a meta-analytic review. Psychol. Bull. 137, 66–96.

Kirmayer, L.J., Robbins, J.M., 1993. Cognitive and social correlates of Toronto alexithymia scale. Psychosomatics 34, 41–52.

Klein, D.F., 1974. Endogenomorphic depression. Arch. Gen. Psychiatry 31, 447–454.

Kraepelin, E., 1905. Lectures on Clinical Psychiatry, third ed. (T. Johnson, Trans, 1917). W. Wood, New York.

Lewis, A., 1934. Melancholia: a clinical survey of depressive states. J. Ment. Sci. 80, 277–378.

Lewis, H.B., 1971. Shame and Guilt in Neurosis. International University Press, New York.

Lewis, I.M., 1971. Ecstatic Religion: An Anthropological Study of Spirit Possession and Shamanism. Penguin, Harmondsworth.

Lieberman, S., 1978. Nineteen cases of morbid grief. Br. J. Psychiatry 132, 159–163.

López Ibor, J.J., 1966. Neuroses as Mood Disorders. Editorial Gredos, Madrid.

Marie, L., Poindexter, E.K., Fadoir, N.A., Smith, P.N., 2020. Understanding the transition from suicidal desire to planning and preparation: correlates of suicide risk within a psychiatric inpatient sample of ideators and attempters. J. Affect. Disord. 274, 159–166.

Meinck, H.M., 2006. Startle and its disorders. Neurophysiol. Clin. 36, 357–364.

Mill, J.S., 1873. In: Robson, J.M., (Ed.) 1989, Autobiography. Penguin, London.

Miller, B.J., McCall, W.V., Xia, L., et al., 2020. Insomnia, suicidal ideation, and psychopathology in Chinese patients with chronic schizophrenia. Prog. Neuro-Psychopharmacol. Biol. Psychiatry 111, 110202.

Mitchell, R.L., Ross, E.D., 2013. Attitudinal prosody: what we know and the directions for future study. Neurosci. Biobehav. Rev. 37, 471–479.

Mumford, D.B., 1992. Detection of psychiatric disorders among Asian patients presenting with somatic symptoms. Br. J. Hosp. Med. 47, 202–204.

Murphy, H.B.M., Wittkower, E.D., Chance, N.A., 1967. Cross-cultural inquiry into the symptomatology of depression: preliminary report. Int. J. Soc. Psychiatry 13, 6–15.

Nakao, M., Barsky, A.J., Kumano, H., Kuboki, J., 2002. Relationship between somatosensory amplification and alexithymia in a Japanese psychosomatic clinic. Psychosomatics 43, 55–60.

Nemiah, J.C., Sifneos, P.E., 1970. Affect and fantasy in patients with psychosomatic disorders. In: Hill, O.W. (Ed.), Modern Trends in Psychosomatic Medicine, vol. 2. Butterworth, London.

Obegi, J.H., 2019. Rethinking suicidal behaviour disorder. Crisis 40 (3), 209–219.

Oh, J.H., Yoo, J.R., Ko, S.Y., et al., 2021. Relationship between sleep duration and suicidal ideation among farmers: safety for agricultural injuries of farmers cohort study of Jeju, Korea. Saf Health Work 12 (1), 102–107.

Parkes, C.M., 1971. Psycho-social transitions: a field for study. Soc. Sci. Med. 5, 101–115.

Parkes, C.M., 1976. The psychological reaction to loss of a limb: the first year after amputation. In: Howells, J.G. (Ed.), Modern Perception in the Psychiatric Aspects of Surgery. Macmillan, London, pp. 515–533.

Parkes, C.M., Benjamin, B., Fitzgerald, R.G., 1969. Broken heart: a statistical study of increased mortality among widows. Br. Med. J. 1, 740–743.

Parkes, C.M., Napier, M.M., 1975. Psychiatric sequelae of amputation. In: Silverstone, T., Barraclough, B. (Eds.), Contemporary Psychiatry. Headley Brothers, Ashford, pp. 440–446.

Pell, M.D., 1996. On the receptive prosodic loss in Parkinson's disease. Cortex 32, 693–704.

Pichon, S., Kell, C.A., 2013. Affective and sensorimotor components of emotional prosody generation. J. Neurosci. 33, 1640–1650.

Poeck, K., Pilleria, G., 1963. Pathologisches Lachen und Weinen. Art Institut, Orell Füssli.

Powell, M., Hemsley, D.R., 1984. Depression: a breakdown of perceptual defence? Br. J. Psychiatry 145, 358–362.

Rack, P., 1982. Race, Culture and Mental Disorder. Tavistock, London.

Ribot, T., 1896. La Psychologie des Sentiments. Félix Alcan, Paris.

Rizzolatti, G., Craighero, L., 2004. The mirror-neuron system. Annu. Rev. Neurosci. 27, 169–192.

Rizzolatti, G., Fadiga, L., 1998. Grasping objects and grasping action meanings: the dual role of monkey rostroventral premotor cortex (area 5). Novartis Found. Symp. 218, 81–95.

Rogers, M.L., Gorday, J.Y., Joiner, T.E., 2021. Examination of characteristics of ruminative thinking as unique predictors of suicide-related outcomes. J. Psychiatr. Res. 139, 1–7.

Satoh, M., Nakase, T., Nagata, K., Tomimoto, H., 2011. Musical anhedonia: selective loss of emotional experience in listening to music. Neurocase 17, 410–417.

Schachter, S., Singer, J., 1962. Cognitive, social and physiological determinants of emotional state. Psychol. Rev. 69, 379–399.

Schneider, K., 1920. The stratification of emotional life and the structure of the depressive states. Zeitschrift fuer Gesundheitswesen Neurologie und Psychiatrie 59, 281.

Shakespeare, W., 1600. The Oxford Shakespeare Hamlet. Oxford University Press, Oxford.

Shepherd, M., 1993. Historical epidemiology and the functional psychoses. Psychol. Med. 23, 301–304.

Sifneos, P.E., 1972. Short-Term Psychotherapy and Emotional Crisis. Harvard University Press, Cambridge, MA.

Simpson, C.J., 1984. The stigmata: pathology or miracle? Br. Med. J. 289, 1746–1748.

Sims, A., 1994. Psyche' – spirit as well as mind? Br. J. Psychiatry 165, 441–446.

Sirois, F., 1982. Epidemic hysteria. In: Roy, A. (Ed.), Hysteria. John Wiley, Chichester, pp. 101–116.

Snaith, R.P., 1993. Anhedonia: a neglected symptom of psychopathology. Psychol. Med. 23, 957–966.

Song, W., Li, H., Sun, F., Guo, T., Jiang, S., Wang, X., 2020. Pain avoidance and its relation to neural response to punishment characterizes suicide attempters with major depression disorder. Psychiatry Res 294, 113507.

Stark, R., 1965. A taxonomy of religious experience. J. Sci. Stud. Relig. 5 (1), 97–116.

Strauss, G.P., Gold, J.M., 2012. A new perspective on anhedonia in schizophrenia. Am. J. Psychiatry 169, 364–373.

Styron, W., 1990. Darkness Visible. A Memoir of Madness, Cape, London.

Tangney, J.P., Dearing, R.L., 2002. Shame and Guilt. The Guildford Press, New York.

Taylor, G., 1984. Alexithymia: concept, measurement and implications for treatment. Am. J. Psychiatry 141, 725–732.

Thompson, W.F., Marin, M.M., Stewart, L., 2012. Reduced sensitivity to emotional prosody in congenital amusia rekindles the musical protolanguage hypothesis. Proc. Natl. Acad. Sci. U.S.A. 109, 19027–19032.

Trethowan, W.H., 1979. Affective disorders. In: Trethowan, W.H. (Ed.), Psychiatry, fourth ed. Baillière Tindall, London.

Ungerleider, J.T., Wellisch, D.K., 1979. Coercive persuasion (brainwashing), religious cults, and deprogramming. Am. J. Psychiatry 136, 279–282.

Vuillemier, P., Ghika-Schmid, F., Bogousslavsky, J., Assal, G., Regli, F., 1998. Persistent recurrence of hypomania and prosoaffective agnosia in a patient with right thalamic infarct. Neuropsychiatry Neuropsychol. Behav. Neurol. 11, 40–44.

Wade, J., 2001. Mapping of the courses of heavenly bodies: the varieties of transcendental sexual experience. J. Transpers. Psychol. 32 (2), 103–122.

Weniger, G., Irle, E., 2002. Impaired facial affect recognition and emotional change in subjects with transmodal cortical lesions. Cerebr. Cortex 12, 258–268.

Wernicke, C., 1906. Fundamentals of Psychiatry. Thieme, Leipzig.

Whybrow, P.C., 1997. A Mood Apart: Depression, Mania and Other Afflictions of the Self. Basic Books, New York.

Williams, B., 1993. Shame and Necessity. University of California Press, Berkeley and Los Angeles.

Witteman, J., Van Heuven, V.J., Schiller, N.O., 2012. Hearing feelings: a quantitative meta-analysis on the neuroimaging literature of emotional prosody perception. Neuropsychologia 50, 2752–2763.

Zilboorg, G., Henry, G.W., 1941. A History of Medical Psychology. Norton, New York.

Chapter 17

Anxiety, Panic, Irritability, Phobia and Obsession

KEYWORDS

Anxiety
Panic
Phobia
Obsession
Compulsion
Irritability

Summary

Response to *stress* is an integral aspect of human existence, and the alarm reaction sets the context for an understanding of anxiety and anxiety-related disorders. Hence, free-floating anxiety includes experiential features of the alarm reaction but marked out as abnormal by the intensity, the prolonged duration, the trivial nature of the triggering events and finally by the socially disruptive and disabling nature of the experience. Anxiety can be focused on a specified object or situation and this is termed *phobia*; it can occur as paroxysmal and episodic attacks as in panic, or it can be discomforting if unregulated as in obsessive compulsive phenomena:

Montanus speaks of one that durst not walk alone from home for fear that he should swoon or die. A second fears every man he meets will rob him, quarrel with him or kill him. A third dares not venture to walk alone, for fear he should meet the devil, a thief, be sick; fears all old women as witches; and every black dog or cat he sees he suspecteth to be a devil; every person comes near him is malificiated; every creature, all intend to hurt him, seek his ruine; another dares not go over a bridge, come near a pool, rock, steep hill, lye in a chamber where cross beams are for fear he be tempted to hang, drown or precipitate himself. If he be in a silent auditory, as at a sermon, he is afraid he shall speak aloud, at unawares, something undecent, unfit to be said. If he be locked in a close room, he is afraid of being stifled for want of air, and still carries bisket, aquavitae, or some strong waters about him for fear of deliquiums, or being sick; or if he be in a throng, middle of a church, multitude, where he may not well get out, though he sit at ease he is certase affected. He will freely promise, undertake any business beforehand; but when it comes to be performed he dares not adventure, but fears an infinite number of dangers, disasters, etc. … They are afraid of some loss, danger, that they shall surely lose their lives, goods, and all they have; but why they know not.

Robert Burton (1621)

Response to *stress* is an integral aspect of human existence. But what is stress? There are at least three conceptualizations of stress: stress as a stimulus; stress as a response; and stress as an interaction. The notion of stress as a stimulus is modelled on the assumption that it is an external factor that affects an individual, whereas stress as a response locates the stress within the individual. This latter notion was developed by Selye (1907–82), who defined stress as a 'non-specific response of the body to any demand made upon it' (Selye, 1956). The notion of stress as an interaction built on Selye's work and was developed by Lazarus (1922–2002):

A particular relationship between the person and the environment that is appraised by the person as taxing or exceeding his or her resources and endangers his or her well being.

Lazarus and Folkman (1984)

Selye's general adaptation syndrome describes the stress response as comprising three stages: alarm reaction, resistance and exhaustion. The alarm reaction, typically termed the *flight-or-fight response,* involves autonomic arousal mediated by release of catecholamines and is experienced as fear, palpitations or readiness for action, among other things. In the event that the stressor persists, there is decreased release of catecholamines and a switch to release glucocorticoid hormones during the resistance phase. Finally, in contexts of chronic stress, exhaustion is the result with the potential for hypoglycaemia and death.

An understanding of Selye's general adaptation syndrome, particularly the physiologic and experiential aspects of the alarm reaction (flight-or-fight response),

sets anxiety and anxiety-related emotional disturbance in context. The five abnormal phenomena of this chapter are relatively common human experiences and can be construed as emanating from disturbances of the regulation of anxiety. Abnormality in this context is marked out by the severity and intensity of the experience, prolonged duration, occurrence in reaction to what could be considered an inadequate situational stress and the deleterious and disabling effect on social functioning. Each of these phenomena has a normal, even necessary, aspect: it is appropriate to be anxious at the beginning of a speech in public; it is normal for a parent to express irritability when an 8-year-old son breaks a window—it is a necessary learning experience for him; fear is necessary for coping when an individual suddenly discovers oneself to be surrounded by poisonous snakes; meticulous checking and checking again is an important part of learning to be a competent airline pilot; even panic is normal, in a statistical sense, in some situations of extreme mass disaster.

In any modern consideration of anxiety disorders, anxiety, panic and phobia would be included both as states of emotion and as distinct syndromes (Noyes and Hoehn-Saric, 1998). Irritability is a distinct and important mood state that occurs in several conditions, and obsession is both an individual symptom and an essential feature of obsessive compulsive disorder. Superficially, obsession and compulsion can seem unrelated to anxiety, but both can be construed as means of regulating anxiety.

Patients may have insight and present themselves as suffering from 'phobia', 'obsession' or 'anxiety state'. However, the lay meaning of each of these terms is significantly different from their psychiatric use, and it will be more usual for the clinician to diagnose the state from a description of the mood or thought process.

Anxiety

Anxiety is a universal and normal emotion. It is a necessary and adaptive response of the organism to stress. It is clear that levels of arousal relate to the efficiency of an organism's ability to respond appropriately to a task: too little arousal and excessive arousal are both associated with poor performance (this is the Yerkes–Dodson Law) (Yerkes and Dodson, 1908). Lader and

Marks (1971) have discussed the features of anxiety in terms of the emotion being normal or pathologic. In rather concrete terms, a person who discovers that they are sharing a field with a bull feels acutely anxious and runs at top speed for the gate; if, 6 weeks later, when back in the city, they have a panic attack and have to lie down because someone mentions a part of the city called the Bullring, their response is clearly maladaptive and their anxiety pathologic.

More recently, Pine et al. (2021) have described the potential role for two uniquely human cognitive capacities, namely (1) a subjective sense of participating in and re-experiencing remembered events and (2) a limitless capacity to imagine details of future events. It is proposed that the capacity for re-experiencing events allows for lasting memories of an individual's attributes, capacities, past experiences and social relationships. And what the authors term constructive episodic simulation allows for the ability to imagine future events, without temporal limitations and facilitating goal-related behaviour, and promoting goal achievement. The hypothesis is that the evolutionary innovations that made these capacities possible also laid the groundwork for vulnerabilities such as anxiety. Anxiety results from rumination about future harms and failures and a preoccupation with imagined harmful events in the presence of concurrent safety signals. This novel thesis allows for a better understanding of anxiety over and above merely examining the role of cognitive appraisals in the generation of anxiety.

Anxiety may also, arbitrarily, be polarized between *state* and *trait* (Sims and Snaith, 1988). Anxiety state is the quality of being anxious now, at this particular time, probably as a reaction to provoking circumstances. Anxiety trait is the tendency over a long time, perhaps throughout life, to meet all the vicissitudes of life with a habitually excessive degree of anxiety. Anxiety as a description of the experience of normal emotion is not different in quality, only quantitatively, from anxiety state (Hamilton, 1959). Characteristic of the mood of anxiety are feelings of *constriction*. The word *angst* is etymologically associated with the idea of narrowness, stricture, 'straits' and in early usage was located in the praecordium and prominently associated with angina (Sims, 1985). The patient with anxiety state may feel restless, uncertain, vulnerable, trapped, breathless and choked. As well as feeling frightened and worried, hypochondriacal ideas and even feelings of guilt are often prominent. Symptoms of anxiety occur pathologically in *anxiety states* without obvious external cause. The anxiety is not attached to any specific provoking object, and so it is termed *free-floating anxiety*.

There is also a contrast between the experience of anxiety as a subjective emotion and the objective occurrence of physiologic somatic changes normally associated with that affect; some of the commoner symptoms are shown in Box 17.1 (Tyrer, 1982). Tyrer considers irritability to be a symptom *of* anxiety state, but Snaith and Taylor (1985) made the case for irritability being an independent mood state that may be associated with anxiety—or any other mood disorder. Although it is usual to find the psychological and physical aspects of anxiety associated and related in intensity, this may not necessarily be so. The patient may complain of feeling extremely anxious but show minimal somatic expression; in dissociation, marked physical changes have been described when the patient does not complain at all of feeling anxious.

BOX 17.1 SYMPTOMS OF ANXIETY

SOMATIC AND AUTONOMIC
- Palpitations
- Difficulty in breathing
- Dry mouth
- Nausea
- Frequency of micturition
- Dizziness
- Muscular tension
- Sweating
- Abdominal churning
- Tremor
- Cold skin

PSYCHIC (PSYCHOLOGICAL)
- Feelings of dread and threat
- Irritability
- Panic
- Anxious anticipation
- Inner (psychic) terror
- Worrying over trivia
- Difficulty in concentrating
- Initial insomnia
- Inability to relax

From Tyrer, P., 1982. Anxiety. Br. J. Hosp. Med. 27, 109–116, with permission.

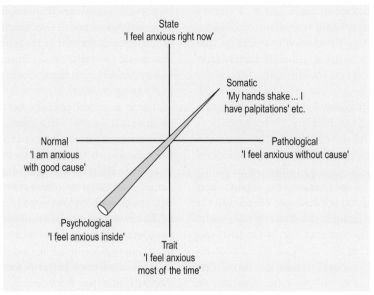

Fig. 17.1 Three-dimensional model of anxiety symptoms.

These three dichotomous aspects of anxiety are represented in Fig. 17.1.

Psychiatric nosology makes a distinction between three principal anxiety syndromes: generalized anxiety disorder, social and specific phobias and panic disorder. Those who suffer from generalized anxiety disorder experience persistent anxiety and worry that is out of proportion to actual events or circumstances (Spiegel and Barlow, 2000). The worry is typically focused on everyday matters, and over time it shifts from item to item; the subject is almost never free from anxiety.

Patients with anxiety disorder describe characteristic ideational components, concentrating on themes of personal danger and especially physical harm (Hibbert, 1984). The 'most important' thought of patients included the following: 'I may panic in front of others', 'I may die of a heart attack while asleep' and 'I am going to have a heart attack'. Fear of physical, psychological or social disaster also occurred during panic attacks. Stressful life experiences in the preceding 12 months, and some physiologic disturbance other than anxiety immediately before the symptoms, were commonly described. These ideas can be construed as *worry*. Worry is now recognized as a cognitive process common during the experience of anxiety. It has been defined as follows:

A chain of thoughts and images, negatively affect-laden and relatively uncontrollable. The worry process represents an attempt to engage in mental problem-solving on an issue whose outcome is uncertain but contains the possibility of one or more negative outcomes. Consequently, worry relates closely to fear process.

Borkovec et al. (1983)

Other psychological functions are affected by acute anxiety. The capacity for reflection is decreased and the field of conscious awareness narrowed; this obviously has survival value for instant physical action but is a disadvantage when planning, reviewing and taking a variety of different factors into consideration are important. The variations of activity with anxiety are seen, for instance, after the experience of disaster: some victims will be numb and inert; others tense, restless and constructively overactive; and others still terrified, almost literally 'petrified', and incapable of sustained activity.

General anxiety is often contrasted with *situational anxiety*, that is, the tendency to become anxious in certain defined situations. This latter is discussed later with phobic states. Under *general anxiety* are included free-floating autonomic anxiety; panic attacks; and the observation during interview that the patient

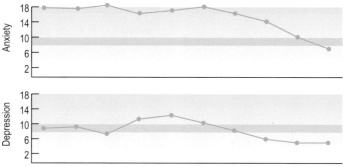

Fig. 17.2 Serial recordings of anxiety and depression in one patient on the Hospital Anxiety and Depression Scale. (From Sims, A.C.P., Snaith, P., 1988. Anxiety in Clinical Practice. John Wiley, Chichester., with permission of John Wiley.)

appears to be anxious, tense, worried or apprehensive. Free-floating anxiety comprises such autonomic components as blushing, 'butterflies in the stomach', choking, difficulty in getting the breath, dizziness, dry mouth, giddiness, palpitations, sweating and trembling, dilated pupils and raised blood pressure; parasympathetic aspects include nausea, vomiting, frequency of micturition and diarrhoea.

The psychological quality of *feeling anxious* or *tense* is more difficult to quantify than its physiologic correlates. Words are idiosyncratic in their meaning, and so there is a tendency to judge the veracity of the patient's statement that they are 'terribly anxious' according to the severity of the autonomic symptoms occurring concurrently. However, it is possible by using serial rating scales to compare the patient's subjective experience at different times; one much-used example of this is the Hospital Anxiety and Depression Scale (Zigmond and Snaith, 1983). Serial recordings of a patient who showed both anxiety and depressive symptoms that responded to treatment at different times are shown in Fig. 17.2. Self-description of anxiety includes worry, brooding, sleeplessness through preoccupation with contents of the thoughts and so on.

PANIC ATTACKS AND DISORDER

Panic attacks occur as discrete episodes of somatic or autonomic anxiety associated with marked psychic anxiety as an extreme sense of fear. The attack ends either with a complete interruption to the patient's current stream of behaviour so that they lie on the floor, rush into the open air, run back into the house or 'collapse' or they terminate their current behaviour voluntarily so that the attack remits more gradually.

In either case, there is something about their mode of activities before the attack that was precipitating panic. The patient makes this association for themself, and they go to elaborate lengths to avoid provoking a panic attack. This may be the antecedent condition for development of a phobic state. The duration of the attack varies from less than a minute to several hours but is normally about 10 to 20 minutes. These attacks may occur many times per day, although usually less frequently. Onset is sudden, with many anxiety symptoms such as palpitations, chest pain or discomfort, choking or smothering feelings, dizziness, feelings of unreality, dyspnoea, paraesthesiae, hot flushes, sweating, faintness, trembling or fear of dying or going mad.

There are distinctions and similarities between panic disorder and generalized anxiety disorder. Forty-one generalized anxiety disorder subjects who had never had panic attacks were compared with 71 subjects with panic disorder (Noyes et al., 1992). The generalized anxiety disorder subjects had an earlier, more gradual onset of symptoms and more often suffered from simple phobias, while the panic disorder subjects tended to report depersonalization and agoraphobia. In general, those with panic disorder had a more severe degree of illness and were more likely to give a history of major depression.

There is growing recognition that there are at least two discrete and distinct experiential subtypes of panic disorder: a respiratory type that is characterized by fear of dying, chest pain and discomfort, shortness of breath, paraesthesias and the sensation of choking and a nonrespiratory type. The respiratory subtype is associated with spontaneous panic experience rather than situationally induced panic. Furthermore, it is

BOX 17.2 SPECIES OF PHOBIA ACCORDING TO RUSH (1798)

- The cat phobia
- The rat phobia
- The insect phobia
- The odour phobia
- The dirt phobia
- The rum phobia
- The water phobia
- The solo phobia
- The power phobia
- The faction phobia
- The want phobia
- The doctor phobia
- The blood phobia
- The thunder phobia
- The home phobia
- The church phobia
- The ghost phobia
- The death phobia

BOX 17.3 SUBDIVISIONS OF PHOBIC NEUROSIS

PHOBIAS OF EXTERNAL STIMULI
- Agoraphobia
- Social phobias
- Animal phobias

PHOBIAS OF INTERNAL STIMULI
- Illness phobias
- Obsessive phobias
- Miscellaneous specific phobias

After Marks, I.M., 1969. Fears and Phobias. Heinemann, London, with permission.

more likely to be provoked in challenge tests by inhalation of 35% carbon dioxide or hyperventilation producing hypocapnic alkalosis (Freire and Nardi, 2012).

PHOBIC STATES

Phobias, or unreasonable fears, have been described for many centuries. For example, Benjamin Rush (1798) defines phobia as 'a fear of an imaginary evil, or an undue fear of a real one' and then produces a list of 18 phobias, partly humorously intended; this is reproduced in Box 17.2. *Agoraphobia* was originally described by Westphal (1871); this condition, literally 'fear of the marketplace', causes very severe disability. Animal phobias have been contrasted by Marks (1970):

If ever we are tempted to think that all phobic states are a unity which reflects the same disorder and aetiology, we can quickly dispel this illusion simply by looking at the startling contrast between animal phobias and agoraphobias. These two conditions differ radically in onset, course, symptomatology, response to treatment and psychological measures.

Solyom et al. (1986) divided the symptomatology of 199 patients into three categories: agoraphobia (80 patients), social phobia (47 patients) and simple phobia (72 patients). Agoraphobia included 'fear of leaving home, of being alone at home or on the street, in crowds, of travelling by car, bus or train'. Social phobia involved anxiety in social situations. Simple phobia described a single but life-disrupting fear, such as of animals, heights, disease, aeroplanes, insects and so on. What is common to all these phobic experiences is that the fear is intense and persistent and that, furthermore, it is provoked by exposure or, the anticipation of exposure, to cues that are clearly discernible and circumscribed objects or situations.

A more comprehensive subdivision of phobic states is contained in Box 17.3 from Marks (1969). Because agoraphobia literally means 'fear of the marketplace', this is frequently appropriate nowadays, as often the most phobic situation for such people is in the supermarket. Agoraphobia is, in fact, a heterogeneous collection of disorders and not an entity; the patient does not only fear a throng of people but has multiple avoidance responses to many stimuli (Snaith, 1991). It includes both those who have a fear of being under public scrutiny, and therefore who avoid public places, and those with illness fears in either a public place where they become noticeable or an exposed place where they will not be able to receive help.

Social phobias are common conditions that have been relatively neglected over recent years (Swinson, 1992). They are particularly likely to occur in association with other disorders of mood or other types of anxiety. There are a variety of different manifestations, but social phobia can be considered to be an extreme variant of shyness. However, avoidance is more typical of the established disorder. It is characterized by excessive fear, self-consciousness and avoidance of social situations due to the possibility of embarrassment or humiliation. Typically the fear focuses on situations where there is the possibility of public performance such as public speaking, eating in public, signing a document under scrutiny or, for men, urinating in a public toilet.

Illness phobia is different from hypochondriacal preoccupation in that, with the former, avoidance occurs. Thus the criteria for phobia, according to Marks (1969), are as follows:

- fear is out of proportion to the demands of the situation,
- it cannot be explained or reasoned away,
- it is not under voluntary control, and
- the fear leads to an *avoidance* of the feared situation.

A 28-year-old married woman said,

My fear problems are worst … I am afraid of catching cancer. I am afraid of catching it from the hospital [radiotherapy hospital] 1 mile away … I bought a scarf from a shop and the assistant frightened me … the look of her, she hardly had any hair and looked very old… I thought I had caught it from her and so I had to wash the house. I cleaned the whole house and it made me poorly. I had to move house because of the hospital and I cannot go back to that shop ever again.

There is also some relationship between phobias, especially agoraphobia, and depression (Schapira et al., 1970). Persistent fear and foreboding, often of a situational nature, may occur with other depressive symptoms. Phobic states, as well as panic disorder, may respond to antidepressant therapy.

Phobias are overpowering and compelling in their nature, dominating the whole of life. Like obsessions, they are repetitive, resisted unsuccessfully, regarded by the subject as senseless and irrational but at the same time as coming from inside of themselves. Some authors therefore describe them as *obsessional fears*. Often compulsive behaviour, such as handwashing, arises out of a phobia, for instance, fear of dirt and contamination. Prominent in the subject's description of their phobia is that they are controlled by it, that the fear is something from inside themself (in no way controlled from outside).

ANXIETY IN OTHER DISORDERS

Obviously, most consideration of anxiety and its different forms and manifestations has been given in the context of the *anxiety disorders*. However, anxiety is a common symptom and is frequently a part of other illnesses, both psychiatric and physical. Among psychiatric conditions, the most frequent comorbidity is with depressive illness; most patients with depression have some anxiety symptoms, most of those with more severe anxiety disorders also have some feelings of depression. Anxiety is a frequent symptom in the prodromal stages of schizophrenia and is also associated with relapse (Tarrier and Turpin, 1992). Anxiety often occurs with organic psychosyndromes, both exacerbating the restlessness of acute organic psychosyndromes or delirium and manifesting as an additional cause of subjective distress in chronic organic states or dementia.

Anxiety is an understandable reaction to physical illness and its consequent distress, pain, physical and social disability and threat to life (Sims and Snaith, 1988). In the following conditions, it may also be a direct expression of the morbid process: hypoglycaemia, hyperthyroidism, phaeochromocytoma, carcinoid syndrome, some cardiac and ictal disorders and states of withdrawal from psychoactive substances. These conditions therefore need to be considered in the differential diagnosis of anxiety, and the component of anxiety in their symptomatology must be dealt with in their treatment.

Irritability

Irritability is defined as a subjective experience that can occur in a variety of physiologic settings, that is, in association with sleep deprivation, hunger or pain and is often conflated with aggression and anger, even though it is conceptually distinct from these constructs (Bell et al., 2021). It is also a feature of disease being found in, for example, mood disorders. Irritability in a patient may be observed by others or experienced subjectively directed towards others (outward) or towards the self (inward). Irritability, outwardly expressed, is considered to be a disorder of mood in its own right and independent of anxiety, depression or other mood state (Snaith and Taylor, 1985): 'Outwardly expressed irritability is an independent mood disorder and not merely one which is symptomatic of states of depression or anxiety'. Outwardly expressed irritability is particularly commonly associated with puerperal mood disorder, whereas inwardly directed irritability was described in those with obsessive compulsive disorder. In the Irritability, Depression and Anxiety Scale, two subscales were developed for irritability (Snaith et al., 1978): outwardly directed irritability and inwardly directed irritability. Snaith and Taylor (1985) have defined irritability for use in the context of psychopathology as:

Irritability is a feeling state characterized by reduced control over temper, which usually results in irascible verbal or behavioural outbursts, although the mood may be present without observed manifestation. It may be experienced as brief episodes, in particular circumstances, or it may be prolonged and generalized. The experience of irritability is always unpleasant for the individual, and overt manifestation lacks the cathartic effect of justified outbursts of anger.

It is a prominent symptom in post-traumatic stress disorder in which it is listed as one of the symptoms of increased arousal. Relatives described an individual survivor of disaster: 'He has completely changed his character. He has become nasty tempered and swears at us all the time.'

The severity of irritability probably has an inverse correlation with age; it occurs in both men and women. It is useful to make a distinction between the subjective mood of irritability and the observation of violent behaviour, although these may overlap. Severe irritability may cause considerable distress to patients, relatives and healthcare professionals; there may be no other psychiatric symptomatology present. The factors that predispose to irritability are not clearly known. 'The state of irritability is primarily a mood which may be translated into behaviour' (Snaith, 1991). It is thought to be related to deficits in reward and threat processing in children and adolescents involving brain regions such as the amygdala and frontal cortices. In adults, it is invariably associated with mood disorders and the amygdala, orbitofrontal cortices and hypothalamus are implicated (Bell et al., 2021).

🜨 Obsessions and Compulsions

▶ **An additional video for this topic is available online.**

There is no necessary association between obsessions or obsessive compulsive disorder and anxiety or any type of anxiety disorder. Isolated obsessions or obsessive compulsive disorder may occur with or without anxiety, with or without depression and with or without personality disorder, anankastic or otherwise. It is a distinct and separate phenomenon.

The patient may be troubled by thoughts that they know to be their own but that they find repetitive and strange; they find they are unable to prevent their repetition. These obsessional thoughts have, according to Lewis (1936), three essential features: a feeling of subjective compulsion, a resistance to it and the preservation of insight. These features distinguish obsession from voluntary repetitive acts and social ceremonies. The word *obsession* is usually reserved for the thought and *compulsion* for the act. The sufferer knows that it is their own thought (or act), that it arises from within themself and that it is subject to their own will whether they continue to think (or perform) it; they can decide not to think it on this particular occasion (but it does and will recur). They are tormented by the fear of what may happen if they disturb the routine. There is no disturbance of consciousness or of the awareness of the possession of their own thought. The person usually functions satisfactorily in other areas of their life uncontaminated by the obsessional thought, but as the obsessions become more severe there is increasing social incapacity and misery that can grossly disrupt their whole lifestyle.

John Bunyan, in his poignant autobiography *Grace Abounding to the Chief of Sinners* (1666), describes gross, obsessional thoughts and ruminations that are connected with, but can be clearly separated from, his underlying religious beliefs. For example:

33. Now you must know, that before this I had taken much delight in ringing, but my Conscience beginning to be tender, I thought that such a practice was but vain, and therefore forced myself to leave it, yet my mind hankered, wherefore I should go to the Steeple house, and look on: though I durst not ring. But I thought this did not become Religion neither, yet I forced my self and would look on still; but quickly after, I began to think, How, if one of the bells should fall: then I chose to stand under a main Beam that lay over thwart the Steeple from side to side thinking there I might stand sure; But then I should think again, Should the Bell fall with a swing, it might first hit the Wall, and then rebounding upon me, might kill me for all this Beam; this made me stand in the Steeple door, and now thought I, I am safe enough for if a Bell should fall, I can slip out behind these thick walls, and so be preserved not with-standing.

34. So after this, I would yet go to see them ring, but would not go further than the Steeple door; but then it came into my head, how if the Steeple it self should fall, and this thought, (it may fall for ought I know) would when I stood and looked on, continually so shake my mind, that I durst not stand at the Steeple door any longer, but was forced to fly, for fear it should fall upon my head.

The *obsessional symptom* and the *religious belief* expressed in this passage are not the same phenomenologically, although they are interconnected. The nature of the obsessional thought is demonstrated in the way that Bunyan felt compelled to think through this elaborate chain of arguments; he resisted his ideas but unsuccessfully. There is no lack of insight into its being his own behaviour. The behaviour was compulsive in that it was the acting out of ambivalent, obsessional notions. There is more than a hint of underlying obsessional personality, for instance, in the numbering of the paragraphs.

A midwife, aged 32, kept thinking after she had finished her spell of duty at hospital that she might have pushed an airway down the throat of a baby that she had delivered. She would telephone the ward repeatedly to check that the infant was well. She frequently made sure that her dog's collar was secure when she was out walking in case he escaped and was killed by traffic. When a little boy and his mother visited her home, she gave him a glass of soda pop. However, she had to drink what she had just poured out for him herself, although she disliked it, to make sure it really was soda pop and not something harmful. The accumulation of more and more symptoms eventually prevented her from working or carrying out any reasonable social life. She knew that these were her own notions, that they were stupid, but she could not stop herself from thinking and performing them.

The compulsive behaviour often provokes further anxiety in the patient, the need both to perform the action and to preserve social acceptability. Although wide areas of life are often implicated in compulsive rituals, it is often striking how the obsessional person omits other areas from their obsessionality. The patient who excoriates their hands by excessive washing and devotes a substantial portion of each day to the pursuit of cleanliness may drive to work in a dirty and ill-serviced car and work in an untidy office! The dilemma of obsessional symptoms remains that they are both reckoned as part of the patient's own behaviour and resisted unsuccessfully, that is, they are under voluntary control but not altogether experienced as voluntary. The patient has an awareness that this particular act or thought is voluntary and can be resisted, with difficulty, but the overall pattern of thinking or behaving is experienced subjectively as inevitable—it is ultimately futile to struggle. The action sometimes 'appears to be against the will of the patient, and often seems to have the quality of disgust or repulsion; this urge to do something yet to be repelled by it, is said to be a singular characteristic of the obsessional state' (Beech, 1974).

Obsession may occur as thoughts, images, impulses, ruminations or fears; compulsions as acts, rituals, behaviours. Schneider's definition (1959) emphasizes that there is no loss of contact with reality: 'An obsession occurs when someone cannot get rid of a content of consciousness, although when it occurs he realizes that it is senseless or at least that it is dominating and persisting without cause'. Thus hallucinations, delusions and mood disturbances cannot be obsessional in form; they are not experienced as senseless, nor is there an attempt to get rid of them. The craving of an alcoholic for their beverage or the abnormal drive of sexual deviation is not compulsive in a strict sense. It is not just that they do not contravene the person's will, although they may dislike themself intensely for having such wishes, in the philias, in particular, the thoughts or urges are welcome and often pleasurable.

Obsessional *ideas* may be simple or complicated. A tune or a few musical notes may become repetitive and be resisted, or a sequence of words, for example, 'the British Socialist Party', may be reiterated irritatingly inside the person's head. The obsessions or compulsions may be more complex and ritualistic. For example, a patient who tried to shut the car door after getting out found this very difficult because they were afraid that the act of shutting would produce unpleasant, obscene, repetitive thoughts. For this reason, they had to go to elaborate lengths to put the car in a certain place, check all the doors before getting out, check them all again after getting out and turn the key while looking in a particular direction.

The *images* of obsessional thinking may be vivid but are always known by the patient to be products of their own mind. These images have been considered by de Silva (1986) to be one of four types.

1. The *obsessional image* depicts repetitively the unwanted intrusive cognition—images of blood flowing, injuries and so on.
2. The *compulsive image* depicts compulsive behaviour by rectifying either an obsessional image—the woman who saw corpses in coffins and had to imagine the same people standing—or an independent compulsive image.
3. The *disaster image* affects compulsive checkers who may not only fear that disaster will occur unless they check but also 'see' the disaster happening in fantasy—the house burning down if the gas taps are not turned off.
4. The *disruptive image* may intrude while compulsive rituals are being carried out and necessitate the ritual being recommenced.

Ruminations are often pseudophilosophical, irritatingly unnecessary, repetitive and achieve no conclusion. A priest has an inner impulse to utter swear words in church, or a mother an impulse to harm her child—both quite frequent complaints of obsessional patients. Reassurance that they will not harm themself or others or act on the impulses can be given to the obsessional, provided it is truly obsessional in form, that they are not concurrently depressed and that there is no coexisting dissocial personality disorder.

The constituent elements of obsessive compulsive experience are said to include the following:

1. a trigger, which is an event or cue that sets off an obsession, a feeling of discomfort or a compulsive urge;
2. an obsession itself;
3. a discomfort that is experienced as a general unease, tension or a sense of guilt;
4. a compulsive urge or drive to carry out a particular behaviour;
5. discomfort reduction;
6. fears of disaster that the patient believes will to come pass but that can be avoided by engaging in compulsive behaviour;
7. inflated sense of responsibility even for events over which the patient has no control;
8. reassurance-seeking behaviour;
9. avoidance of stimuli or situations that may trigger obsessions or compulsions;
10. disruption of social functioning because of the long and complicated compulsions, which are often time consuming and exhausting; and
11. resistance, which was discussed earlier (de Silva, 2003).

Obsessions occur in the context of obsessive compulsive disorder as the major symptom of the condition and are the sole features in about 20% of cases; they also occasionally occur in other circumstances. The depressed patient with obsessional (anankastic) personality may show obsessions and compulsions that clear when their illness is treated. Obsessional states are more common when obsessional personality is present, but this personality type is not a prerequisite. Obsessional symptoms may occur in schizophrenia, when they usually have a bizarre character. Apparent obsessional symptoms may arise de novo in an older person, associated with an organic psychosyndrome. However, the element of resistance characteristic of obsessionality is usually not present. It seems that the person carries out repetitive behaviour to cope with the uncertainties of their life caused by their failing memory and performance. Repetition and stereotyped behaviour in those with learning disability has sometimes been labelled compulsive; however, this is psychopathologically incorrect, as there is no resistance or conflict of urge and repulsion. Similarly, repetitiveness and stickiness of thinking occur with epilepsy, after head injury and with other organic states, but again, this is not truly obsessional in nature.

There is a striking similarity between the clinical presentation of obsessive compulsive disorder in children and adolescents and in adults (Swedo et al., 1989). In 70 consecutive juvenile patients, washing and grooming, repeating, checking and touching rituals were the most frequent compulsions, and obsessions were contamination fears, concerns about disasters happening to the patient or those close to them, symmetry and scrupulousness. Although the condition was frequently familial, the actual presenting symptoms were not shared by relatives, even by monozygotic twins.

There is some evidence that there are categories of obsessive compulsive fears and behaviours that are associated with particular types of threat, or threat domains. These include the aggressive threat domain that concerns fears about one's well-being and that of loved ones; the physical security threat domain that relates to the immediate home environment and includes checking, symmetry and 'just right' symptoms; the environmental cleanliness threat domain that relates to personal hygiene and cleanliness and includes contamination fears and washing and cleaning rituals; and the privation threat domain that relates to essential resources and includes hoarding behaviours (Mathews, 2009). However, this is not the only conceptualization of obsessions. Lee and Kwon (2003) showed autogenous obsessions can be distinguished from reactive obsessions. They describe autogenous obsessions as erupting abruptly into consciousness without identifiable evoking stimuli. This type of obsession is said to be seen as ego-dystonic and aversive and include sexual, aggressive and immoral thoughts or impulses. On the other hand, reactive obsessions are evoked by identifiable stimuli and these stimuli are regarded as realistic and relatively plausible, hence the patient assumes that it makes sense to do something about the thought. These reactive obsessions include thoughts about contamination, possible mistakes or accidents, asymmetry and so on. Lee and Kwon (2003) propose that this conceptualization of obsessions has implications for the subjective experience and for the appraisal and control strategies.

Using a novel semantic linkages approach, Feusner et al. (2021) showed that there are three clusters of themes relating to (1) doubt/checking, (2) contamination/somatic harm/sexual harm and (3) relationship/just right. This study used free-entry data of obsessions from a mobile health treatment platform. Seven thousand unique words representing obsessions from 25,369 individuals from across 108 countries were analysed. The themes partially overlap, as described above, with the previously described themes determined from checklists. The most frequent words were the contamination/somatic/harm words. Obsessions relating to relationships is only starting to be

recognized and include obsessions about partner's flaws, for example, partner's intelligence, social aptitude or morality. Sometimes, it is centred on doubt about whether the relationship is good enough or ideal.

Sexual-oriented obsessions are characterized by unwanted intrusive thoughts, images of ego-dystonic sexual content that may include concerns about child abuse, intimate sexual activity with family, fears related to sexual orientation, inappropriate sexual activity with children or animals and aggressive sexual behaviours (Kuty-Pachecka, 2021). These sexual-oriented obsessions occur in approximately 15% of patients with obsessive compulsive disorder. Often obsessions of this kind are associated with checking or neutralizing behaviours such as contracting specified muscles to check the level of sexual excitement, maintaining sufficient physical distance to ensure that inappropriate physical contact does not take place and undertaking mental actions such as praying. Finally, there is a tendency in sexual-oriented obsessions for there to be hidden methods to neutralize or suppress the obsessions.

Excessive checking is a feature of obsessive compulsive disorder. This usually takes the form of uncertainty about whether a door has been locked, whether a stove has been turned off, even whether, while out driving, an accident resulting in death may have occurred. It is apparent from this account that it is possible to reframe these features of obsessional doubt as problems of recognition memory, thus suggesting that impairment of recognition memory may underlie some of the problems that are present in obsessive compulsive disorder, but the empirical data are not conclusive (Solway et al., 2021).

The role of *disgust* in the psychopathology of anxiety disorders and principally in obsessions and compulsions is gradually being examined and understood. Disgust can be considered an adaptive system that evolved to motivate disease-avoidant behaviours. It is argued that it arose to facilitate the recognition of objects and situations associated with risk of disease and to drive hygienic behaviour. Furthermore, disgust assumed a role in regulating social behaviour by acting to mark prohibited and disapproved behaviours as unacceptable. In this regard, disgust can be conceptualized as a strong and visceral emotion that can arouse powerful affective and behavioural responses. Obsessions and compulsions can be understood in this schema as disorders of disgust systems: patients present with contamination fears, suffer from intrusive thoughts of contamination, engage in excessive sanitation and disinfection of self and the environment (for a fuller exploration and discussion of the place of disgust in psychopathology, see Curtis, 2011). To elaborate, patients with contamination-based obsessive compulsive disorder may perceive themselves as being at greater risk from the effects of contagion, which then promotes harm-reduction behaviours such as cleaning and washing. The absence of illness confirms the rightness of the cleaning and washing behaviours and reinforces the compulsive behaviours. Disgust alongside fear plays an important role in generating and sustaining contamination-based obsessive compulsive disorder. Brady et al. (2021) demonstrated that disgust propensity, disgust sensitivity, perceived infectability and germ aversion are all significantly correlated with contamination-based obsessive compulsive disorder.

REFERENCES

Beech, H.R., 1974. Obsessional States. Methuen, London.

Bell, E., Boyce, P., Porter, R.J., Bryant, R.A., Malhi, G.S., 2021. Irritability in mood disorders: neurobiological underpinnings and implications for pharmacological intervention. CNS Drugs 35, 619–641.

Borkovec, T.D., Robinson, E., Pruzinsky, T., DePree, J.A., 1983. Preliminary exploration of worry: some characteristics and processes. Behav. Res. Ther. 21, 9–16.

Brady, R.E., Badour, C.L., Arega, E.A., Levy, J.J., Adams, T.G., 2021. Evaluating the mediating effects of perceived vulnerability to disease in the relation between disgust and contamination-based OCD. J. Anxiety Disord. 79, 102384.

Bunyan, J., 1666. Grace abounding to the chief of sinners: or, a brief and faithful relation of the exceeding mercy of god. In: Sharrock, R. (Ed.), 1962. Christ, to His Poor Servant John Bunyan. Oxford University Press, Oxford, p. 13.

Burton, R., 1621. The Anatomy of Melancholy, what it Is. With All the Kinds, Causes, Symptomes, Prognostickes, and Several Cures of it by Democritus Junior. Cripps, Oxford.

Curtis, V., 2011. Why disgust matters. Philos. Trans. R. Soc. Lond. B Biol. Sci. 366, 3478–3490.

De Silva, P., 1986. Obsessional-compulsive imagery. Behav. Res. Ther. 24, 333–350.

De Silva, P., 2003. The phenomenology of obsessive-compulsive disorder. In: Menzies, R.G., de Silva, P. (Eds.), Obsessive-Compulsive Disorder. Theory, Research and Treatment. John Wiley, Chichester, pp. 20–36.

Feusner, J.D., Mohideen, R., Smith, S., et al., 2021. Semantic linkages of obsessions: clustering and frequencies of obsessional symptoms from a large international obsessive-compulsive disorder mobile application dataset. J. Med. Internet Res. 23 (6):e25482.

Freire, R.C., Nardi, A.E., 2012. Panic disorder and the respiratory system: clinical subtype and challenge tests. Rev. Bras. Psiquiatr. 34, 32–41.

Hamilton, M., 1959. The assessment of anxiety states by rating. Br. J. Med. Psychol. 32, 50–55.

Hibbert, G.A., 1984. Ideational components of anxiety: their origin and content. Br. J. Psychiatry 144, 613–624.

Kuty-Pachecka, M., 2021. Sexual obsessions in obsessive-compulsive disorder. Definitions, models and cognitive-behavioural therapy. Psychiatr. Pol. 51 (1), 39–52.

Lader, M.H., Marks, I.M., 1971. Clinical Anxiety. Heinemann, London.

Lazarus, R.S., Folkman, S., 1984. Stress, Appraisal, and Coping. Springer, New York.

Lee, H.J., Kwon, S.M., 2003. Two different types of obsessions: autogenous obsessions and reactive obsessions. Behav. Res. Ther. 41, 11–29.

Lewis, A.J., 1936. Problems of obsessional illness. Proc. R. Soc. Med. 29, 325–336.

Marks, I.M., 1969. Fears and Phobias. Heinemann, London.

Marks, I.M., 1970. The classification of phobic disorders. Br. J. Psychiatry 116, 377–386.

Mathews, C.A., 2009. Phenomenology of obsessive-compulsive disorder. In: Antony, M.A., Stein, M.B. (Eds.), Oxford Handbook of Anxiety and Related Disorders. Oxford University Press, Oxford, pp. 56–64.

Noyes, R., Hoehn-Saric, R., 1998. The Anxiety Disorders. Cambridge University Press, Cambridge.

Noyes, R., Woodman, C., Garvey, M.J., et al., 1992. Generalized anxiety disorder versus panic disorder. Distinguishing characteristics and patterns of comorbidity. J. Nerv. Ment. Dis. 180, 369–379.

Pine, D.S., Wise, S.P., Murray, E.A., 2021. Evolution, emotion, and episodic engagement. Am. J. Psychiatry 178 (8), 701–714.

Rush, B., 1798. On the different species of phobia. The weekly Magazine of original Essays, Fugitive Pieces, and Interesting intelligence, Philadelphia. In: Hunter, R., McAlpine, I., 1963. Three Hundred Years of Psychiatry 1535–1860. Oxford University Press, London, pp. 669–670.

Schapira, K., Kerr, T.A., Roth, M., 1970. Phobias and affective illness. Br. J. Psychiatry 117, 25–32.

Schneider, K., 1959. Clinical Psychopathology, fifth ed. Grune and Stratton, New York.

Selye, H., 1956. The Stress of Life. McGraw-Hill, New York.

Sims, A.C.P., 1985. Anxiety in historical perspective. Br. J. Clin. Pract. Suppl. 38, 4–9.

Sims, A.C.P., Snaith, P., 1988. Anxiety in Clinical Practice. John Wiley, Chichester.

Snaith, P., 1991. Clinical Neurosis, second ed. Oxford University Press, Oxford.

Snaith, R.P., Taylor, C.M., 1985. Irritability: definition, assessment and associated factors. Br. J. Psychiatry 147, 127–136.

Snaith, R.P., Constantopoulos, A.A., Jardine, M.Y., McGuffin, P., 1978. A clinical scale for the self assessment of irritability, anxiety and depression. Br. J. Psychiatry 132, 164–171.

Solway, A., Lin, Z., Kaplan, C.M., 2021. Revisiting verbal recognition memory in obsessive-compulsive disorder: a computational approach. J. Psychiatr. Res. 138, 428–435.

Solyom, L., Ledwige, B., Solyom, C., 1986. Delineating social phobia. Br. J. Psychiatry 149, 464–470.

Spiegel, D.A., Barlow, D.H., 2000. Anxiety disorders. In: Gelder, M., Lépez-Ibor, J.J., Andreasen, N.C. (Eds.), New Oxford Textbook of Psychiatry. Oxford University Press, Oxford.

Swedo, S.E., Rapoport, J.L., Leonard, H., Lenane, M., Cheslow, D., 1989. Obsessive-compulsive disorder in children and adolescents. Arch. Gen. Psychiatry. 46, 335–341.

Swinson, R.P., 1992. Phobic disorders. Curr. Opin. Psychiatry. 5, 238–244.

Tarrier, N., Turpin, G., 1992. Psychosocial factors, arousal and schizophrenic relapse. The psychophysiological data. Br. J. Psychiatry 161, 3–11.

Tyrer, P., 1982. Anxiety. Br. J. Hosp. Med. 27, 109–116.

Westphal, C., 1871. Die Agoraphobie: eine neuropathische Erscheinung. Arch. Psychiatr. Nervenkr. 1871 (3), 138–161.

Yerkes, R.M., Dodson, J.D., 1908. The relation of strength of stimulus to rapidity of habit-formation. J. Comp. Neurol. Psychol. 18, 459–482.

Zigmond, A.S., Snaith, R.P., 1983. The hospital anxiety and depression scale. Acta Psychiatr. Scand. 67, 361–370.

Chapter 18

Disorders of Volition and Execution

Chapter Outline

KEYWORDS

Urge
Will
Drive
Movement
Behaviour

Summary

In this chapter, the experience of contentless nondirectional *urge*; natural *instinctual* drive directed towards some target and the *volitional act* with a consciously conceived goal and an awareness of how to achieve it and its consequences are discussed. Abnormalities of urge, instinct, drive and will are some of the most complex in psychopathology. Need is a striving towards a particular object, state or action that is experienced as a desire. Drive is an inclination to satisfy certain primary, that is, innate, needs and as activity, the individual's basic mode of expression. Instinct is an innate pattern of behaviour that leads to drive satisfaction. Will is a goal-directed striving or intention based on cognitively planned motivation. Disturbances of these basic aspects of behaviour occur in both organic and 'functional' psychiatric disorders and are manifest in a variety of ways, including impairments of appetites, impulsivity, aggression, motor disorders and gross behavioural abnormalities.

For I know that in me (that is, in my flesh,) dwelleth
no good thing; for to will is present with me; but how to
perform that which is good I find not.
For the good that I would I do not: but the evil which
I would not, that I do.
Now if I do that I would not, it is no more I that
do it, but sin that dwelleth in me.
I find then a law, that, when I would do good,
evil is present with me …
But I see another law in my members, warring against
the law of my mind, and bringing me into captivity to
the law of sin which is in my members.
      The Epistle of Paul the Apostle to the Romans (1662)

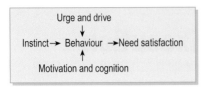

Fig. 18.1 Relationship between instinct, need and behaviour.

This is the most unsatisfactory subject area in clinical psychopathology. The dissatisfaction derives partly from the loss of interest in the subject since the end of the 19th century and the lack of conceptual clarity that has resulted from the impoverished literature but also because of the inherent complexity of the subject. As Berrios (1996) put it, 'The "will" no longer plays a role in psychiatry and psychology. A hundred years ago, however, it was an important descriptive and explanatory concept, naming the human "power, potency or faculty" to initiate action'. Henderson (2005) concurs with this view when he discusses the neglect of volition in the psychiatric literature despite its importance as a concept underlying our understanding of the sense of agency, responsibility and regret. The distinctions between related but distinct concepts such as instinct, urge, impetus, impulse, drive, motivation, will, involuntary and voluntary movements and responsibility have until very recently ceased to be regarded as proper subjects of inquiry. A distinction can correctly but theoretically be drawn between the instinct and thus the desire to carry out an action to satisfy a particular need, the drive and motivation to effect the action and the will to execute the action. All of these are different from the end product, the observable action or behaviour itself (Fig. 18.1).

Urge, Drive and Will and Their Disturbance

Jaspers (1997) distinguishes between the different experiences of primary, contentless nondirectional *urge*; natural *instinctual* drive directed towards some target; and the *volitional act* with a consciously conceived goal and an awareness of how to achieve it and its consequences. Thus for Jaspers, there is a distinction, subjectively, between impulsive acts, awareness of inhibition of will and awareness of loss of will or availability of willpower.

Definitions proposed by Scharfetter (1980) are as follows:
- *Need* (a phenomenological concept): a striving towards a particular object, state or action that is experienced as a desire.
- *Drive:*
  a. as a construct, an inclination to satisfy certain primary, that is, innate, needs;
  b. as activity, the individual's basic mode of expression.
- *Instinct* (a construct): an innate pattern of behaviour that leads to drive satisfaction.
- *Motivation:*
  a. as a phenomenological concept, a more or less clearly experienced mood or affect that is governed by needs and that moves us to actions that satisfy these needs;
  b. as a construct, a hypothetical activating factor.
- *Will* (a phenomenological concept): a goal-directed striving or intention based on cognitively planned motivation.

Scharfetter then describes those primary needs that are innate and not learned as *hunger, thirst, breathing, urination* and *defecation, sleep* and *self-preservation*. Other needs are not essential for survival; their demands can be postponed, and they are more affected by acquired patterns of behaviour, such as sexual need and prosocial need. Secondary needs are acquired and vary with the individual, for example, smoking. Human beings are so complex that although primary needs require rapid satisfaction, they account for only a small proportion of the individual's subjective experience and psychological activity. While I write this, I allow myself to become aware of the primary need for breathing, but I shall not be giving it a thought 10 minutes from now. The acquired primary needs and secondary needs have a greater influence on the individual mental state than innate primary needs.

Drive can be conceived as a state of tension that initiates directed behaviour. In this view, it can either activate or determine selectivity or strength of actions. Hull (1943) introduced the concept of need as a preliminary to introducing the more mechanical concept of drive. For Hull, 'When a condition arises for which action on the part of the organism is a prerequisite to optimum probability of survival of either the individual or the species, a state of need is said to exist' and 'Animals may almost be regarded as aggregations of need. The function of the effector apparatus is to mediate the satiation of these needs. The drive apparatus is synonymous with effector apparatus'. In this scheme, drive has the role of initiating behaviour that satisfies needs.

Instinct may be defined as 'an inherited or innate psychophysical disposition which determines its possessor to perceive and to pay attention to objects of a certain class, to experience an emotional excitement of a particular quality and to act in regard to it in a particular manner or at least to experience an impulse to act' (McDougall, 1908). For Freud, instinct 'appears as a borderline concept, being both the mental representative of the stimuli emanating from within and penetrating to the mind, and at the same time a measure of the demand made upon the energy of the latter in consequence of its connection with the body' (Freud, 1915).

Motivation, as a phenomenological concept, is readily understood by the layman but is ultimately tautologous: 'I do it because I am motivated', 'I am motivated to do it'. However, it is a concept that in psychiatry and psychology we cannot do without. It has both an emotional as well as a cognitive aspect. In other words, it includes the pleasurable rewards that govern and regulate behaviour as well as the reasons proffered for behaviour. There are intrinsic as well as extrinsic motivating factors. Intrinsic factors are those that are internal to the person, and extrinsic factors are those, such as supermarket reward cards, that are external incentives to behave in particular ways. Thus the term motivation refers not only to the goal towards which behaviour is directed but also to emotional states that set it off as well as those that act to reward the behaviour. It also refers to the reasons, justifications or explanations of an action.

Similarly, *will* is a necessary concept but we have great difficulty in comprehending it. Thomas Reid (1710–96), founder of the Scottish School of Common Sense, regarded the will as the power to put into effect our voluntary actions. For Reid (1863), 'all our power is directed by our will, we can form no conception of power, properly so called, that is not under the direction of will. And therefore our exertions, our deliberations, our purposes, our promises, are only in things that depend upon our will. Our advice,

exhortations, and commands, are only in things that depend upon the will of those to whom they are addressed. We impute no guilt to ourselves, nor to others, in things where the will is not concerned'. Other authorities make similar points but emphasize different aspects of will: 'Will has a consciously conceived goal and is accompanied with an awareness of the necessary means and consequences. It implies decision making ability, intention and responsibility' (Jaspers, 1997). Hence, theories of will have implications for notions of moral responsibility, for what being an agent entails and for any description of guilt, shame and punishment. Frith (2013) in his account of volition distinguishes between a first-person and third-person perspective. In the first-person perspective, the experience of volition includes a vivid sense of agency that relies on prior expectations and sensations associated with movement and that is imbued with feelings of responsibility and the possibility of alternative courses of action with the potential for regret given the nature of outcomes. The third-person perspective regards volitional behaviour as internally generated and ultimately unpredictable because it is not determined by immediate environmental contexts.

There are more modern attempts to clarify and delineate the phenomenology of will. Metzinger (2006) makes the point that the experiential content of will is fundamentally difficult to pin down, what he terms *thin* and *evasive* characteristics of the phenomenal content of will. By this, he means the fact that 'will' lacks sensory concreteness unlike, say, vision or taste; that the awareness of the process of 'willing' something is intermittent and not functionally stable; that episodes of 'will' are not temporally segmented and are inherently fuzzy; and finally that the intended goal of 'will' is often less than clear. To amplify these points, Bayne and Levy (2006) wrote:

We typically experience our actions as purposive. We do not simply find ourselves walking towards a door and, on the basis of this, form the belief that we must be intending to open it; instead, we experience ourselves as walking towards the door in order to open it. The sense of goal-directedness can operate at a number of levels. For example, one might experience oneself: walking towards a door in order to open it; opening the door in order to feed the dog; and feeding the dog in order to keep him quiet. The phenomenology of a single action can include the nested purposes for which the action is being performed.

The range of definitions and understandings of the various terms underlines the intrinsic complexity of the subject area and the current absence of a unifying theory or model for making sense of the subject.

Abnormalities of Need, Instinct, Motivation and Will

In terms of the self-description of the subject, any of the following phenomenological abnormalities resulting in observed disturbance of volition may occur. There may be a disturbance of *need,* which may involve hunger, thirst, exploratory behaviour or sleep. An absence of hunger can result in anorexia occurring in chronic physical illness, an increase in hunger causing hyperphagia in Kleine–Levin syndrome and a perversion in pica. Abnormality of thirst can take the form of increased thirst in lithium-induced polydipsia (diabetes insipidus) or of compulsive water drinking in psychosis (Singh et al., 1985), which can result in hyponatraemia. Abnormality of exploratory behaviour can take the form of diminution, which is manifest as lack of curiosity and exploration of the environment. This can be found in schizophrenia and depression. Exploratory behaviour can be increased in mania. Abnormalities of sleep are common and varied. There are different patterns of insomnia, including initial insomnia, which is more often associated with anxiety-based disorders, and early-morning wakening, which is characteristic of depression. Hypersomnia can occur in narcolepsy, Kleine–Levin syndrome and Pickwickian syndrome.

Abnormality of drive can involve diminution, increase or perversion. Diminution of drive towards primary needs occurs in schizophrenia and depression and is probably indistinguishable from abnormalities of need. It is manifest as an absence of the activating tension that initiates behaviour and is observable as apathy. Exacerbation of drive to satisfy sexual need is most prominent in mania but can occur as part of Kleine–Levin syndrome or, indeed, after acquired brain injury or in L-dopa-induced hypersexuality in Parkinson's disease. If drive determines strength and

selectivity of goal of behaviour, then perversion of drive will include such conditions as fetishism.

Abnormality of *motivation* may involve diminution or exacerbation. In schizophrenia and depression, the pleasurable intrinsic motivation that acts as incentive for behaviour may be lost. This is most accurately described as anhedonia, the absence of pleasure in relation to usually pleasurable activities. In mania, it may be increased so that mundane activities become unduly fascinating and rewarding. Disorder of motivation can also be understood as involving the abnormalities of reasoning, justification and explanation, as described in the psychoanalytical literature. This is outside the scope of this book.

Disturbance of *will* can be manifest as loss of volition. As Jeannerod (2006) put it, disorder of volition should only refer to those pathologic conditions in which the ability to make choices, to express preferences, or possibly to experience pleasure and freedom in making these choices or expressing these preferences is affected. This can take the form of impairment of the will to act in schizophrenia and severe depression. It is difficult to distinguish between absence of need, drive, motivation or will. The observable end result is lack of action in the absence of any motor abnormality impairing action. Other abnormalities of will include indecisiveness in depression, ambivalence or ambitendency in schizophrenia. These abnormalities have, at their core, contrasting conceived goals with oscillating decision making that is observable as indecision or alternating and contrasted motor behaviours. Passivity experiences are by definition abnormalities of volition (Box 18.1). Failure of volition as a result of inability to experience pleasure, that is, as a result of anhedonia has been discussed elsewhere (Chapter 16).

ORGANIC CAUSES

Biological drives such as appetite, sleep and thirst are located anatomically in and around the midbrain. Localized disease in this area, of either a structural or biochemical nature, is therefore likely to result in disturbance of drive and hence volition. Hormonal, metabolic and neurophysiologic mechanisms affect volition. Thus the need for food, expressed in hunger and resulting in seeking food, is affected by the state of fullness of the gastrointestinal tract, by the secretion of

BOX 18.1 CLASSIFICATION OF ABNORMALITIES OF NEED, DRIVE, MOTIVATION AND WILL

ABNORMALITIES OF NEED

Appetite
- Absence in anorexia
- Increase, as hyperphagia in Kleine–Levin syndrome
- Perversion in pica

Thirst
- Increase in diabetes insipidus, resulting in polydipsia and in compulsive water drinking, resulting in hyponatraemia

Exploratory Behaviour
- Decrease in schizophrenia and depression
- Increase in mania

Sleep
- Decrease in anxiety and depressive disorders
- Increase in hypersomnia in Kleine–Levin syndrome and Pickwickian syndrome

ABNORMALITIES OF DRIVE
- Decrease in schizophrenia and depression
- Increase in mania
- Perversion in fetishism

ABNORMALITIES OF MOTIVATION
- Diminution, resulting in anhedonia in depression and schizophrenia
- Increase in mania

ABNORMALITIES OF WILL
- Absence or loss, resulting in apathy in schizophrenia and depression
- Oscillating will, resulting in indecisiveness, ambivalence or ambitendency
- Anomalous will in passivity experiences and made actions

insulin from the pancreas and by sensory innervation of the gut wall, as well as by regulation in a putative 'appetite centre'. Physical illnesses have both a specific and a generalized effect on volition.

Excessive appetite (bulimia) may occur with conditions such as tumour affecting the hypothalamus and result in gross obesity, obesity may be associated with hypoventilation and excessive sleeping (hypersomnia) in the Pickwickian syndrome (Burwell et al., 1956), periodic somnolence and intense hunger with voracious overeating occur in the Kleine–Levin syndrome (Critchley, 1962). Excessive thirst and fluid intake (polydipsia) occur with disease of the posterior pituitary or the kidney (nephrogenic diabetes

insipidus, for example, with lithium treatment). Loss of appetite (anorexia) may occur with localized disease of the midbrain, resulting in severe cachexia; however, weight loss is much more common as a general feature of any severe debilitating physical illness.

DISTURBANCE OF VOLITION IN SCHIZOPHRENIA

In schizophrenia, the disturbance of volition is much more at the level of *motivation* or *will* than of *need*. There may be abnormality of appetite with polyphagia and consequent obesity, as occurs in some patients with chronic schizophrenia; however, this is not usual. Patients with schizophrenia who believe that their food is being poisoned may refrain from eating as a consequence; that is, of course, a deliberate act of will. The more conspicuous disturbance, however, is *loss of volition* that results in withdrawal from normal social interaction, for instance, lack of motivation to obtain and continue in employment or diminished sexual drive resulting in decreased fecundity, especially in male patients with schizophrenia.

This symptom was described by Bleuler (1911) as *disturbance of initiative,* according to Lehmann (1967). It is also recognized among the so-called negative symptoms of what Crow (1980) has designated type 2 schizophrenia. The *negative traits*—emotional apathy, slowness of thought and movement, underactivity, lack of drive, poverty of speech and social withdrawal—are a major barrier to effective rehabilitation in chronic schizophrenic patients (Wing, 1978). Although positive symptoms such as delusions, hallucinations and thought disorder are more conspicuous, especially in the earlier stages of a schizophrenic illness, the prognosis is probably affected to a greater extent by the loss of volition.

Andreasen (1982, 1989) has developed an instrument for measuring the negative symptoms of schizophrenia, the Scale for the Assessment of Negative Systems. It is clear that the patient's quality of life and that of their carer are impaired by the consequences of these negative symptoms, especially flatness of affect and loss of volition. What is not so clear is whether they have a subjective awareness of these symptoms or whether they suffer as a result of them. Selten et al. (1993) developed a self-rating scale, the Subjective Experience of Negative Symptoms, to measure the subjective experience of affective flattening, alogia, avolition and apathy, anhedonia and asociality and impaired attention; the scale looks at awareness, causal attribution, disruption and distress.

DISTURBANCE OF VOLITION IN MOOD DISORDERS

Abnormalities of volition in affective illnesses are associated with abnormality of activity, retardation being prominent in depression and overactivity in mania. In depression, motivation is impaired rather than will. A severely depressed managing director continued to worry about their plans for their company, but they found themselves unable to make themselves do anything about it. Loss of motivation occurs alongside loss of other affect. *Anhedonia* (see Chapter 16), or loss of ability to experience enjoyment, is a prominent symptom in depressive illness (Snaith, 1993) that also occurs in schizophrenia. Depressed patients normally describe loss of interest in their previous hobbies and enjoyments in life. This anhedonia can be construed as

part of the loss of motivation to carry out these activities. Such patients also describe lack of appetite and loss of all interest in food; this may result in marked loss of weight.

A 45-year-old male patient, previously highly successful as a salesman, developed severe and persistent depressive symptoms (Sims, 1994). As a result, 2 years before admission he had left his job, his home, his wife and his two children and drifted around the country, being admitted for short periods of time to several psychiatric hospitals. He described his subjective state: 'I feel very anxious, uncomfortable and depressed. It is like having the same person in the same body as me. It is like two different people inside one body. One person is holding back – that's like me. The other person is trying to let go – the other is different, quite strong'. 'Me' was described as 'frightened, depressed, unsure', and the *other person* as 'confident, affable, a great salesman'. 'Self' and his 'other self' are compared in Fig. 18.2. When he was healthy, he was energetic,

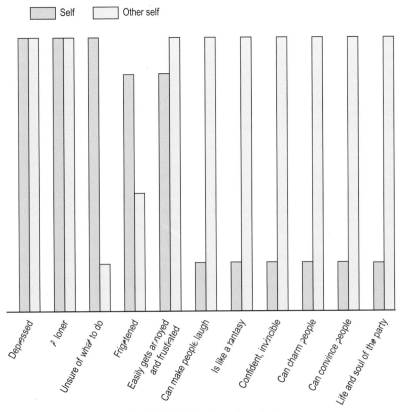

Fig. 18.2 'Myself and my other self.'

an extrovert and able to function well in a pressured situation. When he became depressed, he was miserable, unsure of what to do, frightened and lacking in all energy for any sort of activity. When depressed, he saw 'self' as being his real identity and 'other self' as 'like a fantasy'.

In mania, commonly there is increased activity, a subjective feeling of greater energy, effectiveness and self-confidence; such a person may initiate all sorts of new projects. Manic patients are prone to drink too much alcohol, but they do not usually overeat, perhaps because they are readily distracted and tend to interrupt their meals with other new enterprises. Such people describe it as being easy to make decisions, and their flight of ideas results in starting many tasks that they do not carry through to completion.

An elderly man lived with his wife in a late 19th-century semidetached house in an industrial town. The first intimation of his manic illness was a desperate cry for help from his wife to their family doctor that he was destroying the house. At interview at home, one could see his many uncompleted building projects in the house. He said that he had thought it improper that every time his wife went to the toilet, she should have to go through the backyard, where she could be seen by the neighbours. He had therefore knocked a hole in the wall between the kitchen and toilet to give internal access. Before he could get round to tidying the brickwork and putting in a new door, he had realized that the electric wiring was very old and so he had removed all the cables from the ground floor of the house. He was thinking next of renewing the wiring, but then decided that his wife would like a brand new bathroom. It was at this point that his wife realized that he was ill and consulted their doctor.

Impulsive and Aggressive Acts

The term *impulsivity* is usually reserved for maladaptive behaviour. The behaviour universe thought to reflect impulsivity encompasses actions that appear poorly conceived, prematurely expressed, unduly risky or inappropriate to the situation and that often result in undesirable consequences. When such actions have positive outcomes, they tend not to be seen as signs of impulsivity but as indicators of boldness, quickness, spontaneity, courageousness or unconventionality (Daruna and Barnes, 1993). Eysenck (1993) distinguishes between impulsivity and venturesomeness as follows: 'Our concept of impulsiveness and venturesomeness can best be described by analogy to a driver who steers his car around a blind bend on the wrong side of the road. A driver who scores high on *Imp* never considers the danger he might be exposing himself to and is genuinely surprised when an accident occurs. The driver who scores high on *Vent,* on the other hand, considers the position carefully and decides consciously to take the risk.'

Impulsive acts are 'executed forcefully with no deliberation or reflection, under the influence of a compelling pressure that restricts the subject's freedom of will. Because reflective control or consideration is lacking, the consequences of such acts are not thought out or taken into consideration' (Scharfetter, 1980). It will be seen that this is not an all-or-nothing phenomenon. Voluntary inhibitions will be present to a varying extent from completely preventing the act, modifying it or delaying it to not existing at all when the act takes place unrestrained.

In the past two decades or so, there has been increasing interest in *impulsivity* as a concept as well as in defining a number of impulse control disorders. Impulsivity is seen as a predisposition towards rapid, unplanned reactions to internal or external stimuli and without due regard to the potential negative consequences of these actions for the impulsive individual or for others (Moeller et al., 2001). The essential elements are predisposition, rapid unplanned action and lack of regard for consequences. This suggests that the term is now being used to identify a trait rather than isolated behaviour that is associated with an episode of illness. The current psychological literature, in turn, focuses on behaviourist concepts that are derived from experimental animal models. These schemes identify the features of impulsivity as:
- perseverance of behaviours despite punishment,
- preference for a small but immediate reward over a delayed larger reward, and
- making premature responses or being unable to prevent a response in a response disinhibition attentional paradigm.

Once again, these conceptualizations of impulsivity suggest that impulsivity is a trait.

On the other hand, the older psychiatric literature focused on impulsive behaviour as part of episodes of illness: 'of all the morbid desires, the violent *impulse* [my emphasis] to muscular activity, to bodily movement, is particularly to be noticed, as it is seen, especially in states of mania, as a constant necessity to restless motion hither and thither, beating about, screaming, etc., a state which frequently involves the injury and destruction of what is within reach of the patient, without his having any definite purpose in doing so' and 'the involuntary nature of these acts; the patient often complains that he cannot resist the desire; and further these acts have something instinctive in the manner in which they show themselves; they come on in fits with lucid intervals, they are frequently accompanied by other symptoms of derangement' (Griesinger, 1845). Bleuler (1911) distinguishes between impulsive acts and compulsive acts: 'The action appears to him as something beyond his voluntary control … The patient does something he does not want to do; however he does not offer any resistance.' Thus, in this view, it is resistance to the impulse to act that defines compulsion.

Disorders of impulse control include impairment of control resulting in disinhibition and can be manifest in acquired brain injury, schizophrenia, mania, episodic dyscontrol syndrome and antisocial and emotionally unstable personality disorders. Excessive control of impulses can result in inhibited behaviour and lack of spontaneity present in anxiety-related disorders including avoidant personality disorder.

Aggression is defined as 'a verbal or physical attack on other living creatures or things' (Scharfetter, 1980), and *aggressiveness* as a readiness to be aggressive. In general ethologic terms, this is required by animals for survival and by humans to cope with individual conflicts and problems in their society. However, in a more restricted psychopathologic sense, aggression involves deliberate or reckless damage and destruction and is accompanied by negative emotions such as anger, fear, despair, spite or rage.

The two concepts of aggression that Scharfetter contrasts are an *innate drive* and an *acquired response*. The former theory is followed both by ethologists such as Lorenz (1963) and in classical psychoanalysis in the writings of Freud and of Adler (1929); if aggression is an innate drive, it must find some form of expression.

Learning theory would suppose that aggression is an acquired reaction in response to external stimuli, especially the expression of others' aggressive behaviour, and it is reinforced by the success it achieves.

Examples of impulsive acts follow:

We had a party. On the way home I was seized by an idea out of the blue – swim across the river in your clothes. It was not so much a compulsion to be reckoned with but simply one, colossal, powerful impulse. I did not think for a minute but jumped straight in … only when I felt the water did I realize it was most extraordinary conduct and I climbed out again. The whole incident gave me a lot to think about. For the first time something inexplicable, something quite sporadic and alien, had happened to me.

Jaspers (1997)

A 19-year-old was hospitalized for mutism. She sat motionless for prolonged periods, disinterested in her surroundings, although she appeared alert … She ate and moved slowly but was not stiff. On the second day, suddenly and without warning, she leapt from the chair and grabbed the throat of a passing therapist, severely damaging the therapist's thyroid.

Fink and Taylor (2003)

He complained of headaches, was irritable, and occasionally exploded in a rage with minimal or trivial precipitants. Destruction of property occurred, including holes punched in walls and furniture broken plus poorly coordinated assaults on family members and some neighbours.

Benson and Blumer (1982)

Although impulsivity is often demonstrated by aggression, this is not invariably the case. Gambling, misuse of substances, sexual acts associated with disinhibition and stealing are but some of the behaviours that can occur impulsively.

PSYCHOPATHOLOGY OF IMPULSIVE AND AGGRESSIVE BEHAVIOUR

Criminal acts may arise from delusions of one kind and another, from hallucinations of the various senses, from loss of control, which may act in various different ways; the most difficult point of all to decide upon is the so called impulsive insanity, in which a patient loses self-control, and commits an act, the details of which he remembers, but which he truthfully says he was unable to prevent. Such insane impulses undoubtedly do occur, and I have been consulted by patients who have told me that loss of control of this kind would come upon them like a storm, and that they would seek shelter anywhere to avoid the danger which might arise to themselves or others. It is simple enough when these impulses occur in persons who have suffered from mental unsoundness, but it is much more difficult when the only evidence of insanity is the existence of these impulses; for it may be said that they are but the result of uncontrolled pleasure of power, which is common to all. I should hesitate before accepting impulses, unless I had evidences of insanity in other members of the family, or neuroses such as neuralgia or epilepsy in the patient himself.

Savage (1886)

There is nothing that is likely to result in referral to psychiatric services more quickly than the public exhibition of inexplicable impulsive and aggressive acts. Also, there is nothing more likely to be labelled as madness by the lay public. In practice, such public behaviour is quite commonly associated with mental illness. In a study of mentally disturbed people coming to the attention of the police, there was a tendency for such people to create their disturbance near the city centre rather than at the periphery. Of the situations resulting in the involvement of the police, assault and damage were frequent, but it was the bizarreness of the behaviour that marked the person as being mentally ill; for example, a man who proffered a windscreen wiper as fare for travelling on a bus or a woman who presented herself mute at a hostel. On subsequent admission to the hospital, diagnosis was predominantly of psychotic illness (57%), with schizophrenia accounting for 40% (Sims and Symonds, 1975).

Excessive aggression, and especially unprovoked inappropriate or misdirected aggression, is much more often presented for psychiatric evaluation than a pathologic lack of aggressive behaviour. However, the latter may also be a manifestation of illness. Excessive aggression may be considered both in relation to the underlying psychiatric illness and according to the specific nature of the behaviour.

DIMINISHED AGGRESSION

Decreased aggressiveness may accompany reduced drive; it is seen sometimes in organic, psychotic and psychogenic disturbance. It is frequently associated with apathy in acute organic disorders such as encephalitis or in progressive dementia, although irritability and fractiousness may also occur. Generalized debilitating physical illness is normally accompanied by listlessness and apathy.

In schizophrenia, aggression is usually markedly reduced, with lack of volition and failure to initiate any directed activity; however, unprovoked violence may also occasionally occur. Also in depressive psychosis, reduced aggression is much the most common presentation; however, homicide, quite often associated with suicide, is certainly described among severely depressed individuals with depressive delusions.

A consistently low level of aggressiveness may occur as a personality characteristic, for example, with dependent disorder of personality. It may be seen as part of a neurotic reaction or during adverse life situations, for instance, with the grief of bereavement or the unhappiness of feeling lonely. A certain degree of aggression is necessary for many of the social activities of normal life, and its absence impairs functioning. Pathologic lack of aggression is closely associated with disorder of volition.

Disturbance of Movement and Behaviour

Movement and behavioural disturbances may have crucial diagnostic significance, especially when there is difficulty with verbal explanation. However, as the emphasis of this book is on subjective description of abnormality, these disorders are discussed only briefly. The distinction between movement and behaviour is arbitrary, as will be shown, especially when schizophrenia is considered.

DISTURBANCE OF MOVEMENT AND GESTURE

The term *movement* can be defined as the changing of position in space and is aligned to the term *locomotion,* which implies the act or ability of an organism to transport or move itself from one place to another. There are a number of other associated terms including *action* and *behaviour*. Action is the process of doing something, usually voluntarily, and behaviour consists of an organism's external reactions to its environment. In cognitive psychology it refers to the organism's response given the inputs from the environment through the senses and the requirement to act upon its environment via effector (motor) systems. Behaviour can be influenced by culture, attitudes, emotions, values, ethics, persuasion, coercion and personal constitution.

It is important to distinguish between voluntary and involuntary movement. Voluntary movements have intended goals, that is, they are conscious and deliberate and can be regarded as actions. Involuntary movements, on the other hand, are spontaneous and often automatic. Associated movements such as swinging of the arms during walking is an example of involuntary movements. Eye blinking and some gestures are other examples.

Gestures are little studied but are defined by David McNeill (1992) as 'the movements of the hands and arms that we see when people talk'. According to McNeill, gestures are the spontaneous, involuntary creation of individual speakers and are tightly intertwined with spoken language in time, meaning and function. In this regard, they are an integral part of language as are words, phrases and sentences. There are different types of gestures including iconics, metaphorics, beats, cohesives and deictics. Iconic gestures refer to gestures that have a pictorial aspect representing from the speaker's point of view a dynamic image concurrently with meaning expressed in words. Metaphoric gestures refer to gestures that are similar to iconic gestures except that the pictorial content represents an abstract concept rather than a concrete object or event. Beats refers to gestures that seem like the beating of musical time, moving along the rhythmical pulsation of speech usually in the form of the flick of the hand or finger up and down or back and forth. Cohesive gestures serve to tie together thematically related but temporally separated parts of discourse. And deictic gestures are the familiar pointing that function to indicate objects and events in the concrete world but are also used when there is nothing objectively to point at.

It is important to emphasize how interwoven are speech and gesture. As McNeill (2005) puts it, 'synchronized speech and gesture events comprise virtually unbreakable psycholinguistic units.' The strength of the speech–gesture bond is manifest from the observations that (1) delayed auditory feedback does not interrupt speech–gesture synchrony, (2) gesture inoculates against stuttering and (3) the congenitally blind make gestures to other blind people. Furthermore, McNeill (2005) argues that the integration of gesture with language is an essential part of the machinery that was selected in evolution. In other words, gesture is not a behavioural fossil, an add on to language or an enhancement, but rather it is an indispensable part of language. This is demonstrated by the fact that individuals with amelia (congenital absence of arms) perform gestures with their phantom limbs, and Ian Waterman who had a sudden and total deafferentation of his body from the neck down had preserved gesture morphokinetic accuracy in the presence of topokinetic accuracy. His gestures were co-expressive and synchronized with speech.

Finally, gestures are not signs, salutes or so-called emblems. They are frequent and accompany approximately 90% of utterances, and they seem to occur in similar form across cultures. There is a gesture continuum running from spontaneous gesticulation (what I have been describing above) through to emblems (conventionalized signs such as thumbs up) to pantomime (obligatory absence of speech) and to sign language (McNeill, 2005).

Formal aspects of gestures include (1) timing, synchronization and co-expression with speech; (2) morphokinesis which is the shape of gestures in terms of hand forms and use of space; (3) topokinesis, which is the location of the hands relative to each other, including but not restricted to the approach of one hand by the other; (4) character viewpoint and (5) observer viewpoint.

I have given a relatively detailed description of the formal aspects of gestures above because this subject is little taught or discussed in psychiatry, yet there are reports of abnormalities of gesture and movement in psychiatric disorders with little by the way of introduction of the basics of the subject (see later).

Movement may be increased or speeded up or reduced or slowed down, or it may show various qualitative abnormalities. Some of these disorders of movement are involuntary and are appropriately regarded as neurologic, some are voluntary but carried out unconsciously and some are deliberate actions (of the will). The words used mostly describe the objective characteristics of the action to an outside observer, not the subjective experience of the actor.

These disorders of movement are now considered briefly, starting with abnormalities of increased movement—*agitation* and *hyperactivity,* and decreased movement—*retardation*. The movement disorders of some psychiatric conditions are then described. There are psychiatric sequelae of primary movement disorders including parkinsonism, and often there is disorder of movement associated with conditions that are primarily psychiatric.

Agitation

Agitation implies mental disturbance causing physical restlessness and increased arousal; it is phenomenologically a description of a subjective mood state associated with and resulting in physical expression. The patient may describe their affect as 'feeling agitated', and both they and the external observer see motor restlessness as being logically connected with this. It is demonstrated in many mental states; pathologically, it may occur with affective psychoses, with schizophrenia, with organic psychosyndromes such as senile dementia or with neurotic and personality disorders, especially states of anxiety. Agitation is often a symptom of physical illness, for example, hyperthyroidism or hypoparathyroidism. It is an important component of some states of severe depressive illness. Although retardation is more commonly seen with 'endogenous depression' or melancholia, agitation may occur, either without retardation in alternating phase with retardation, or concurrently with retardation in a *mixed affective state*. *Agitated depression* is an old term for one variant of a severe depressive episode with or without psychotic component. It is alternatively known as *melancholia*. The practical clinical importance of this mood state ensues from the fact that, whereas suicidal impulses may be prevented from expression by retardation, agitation with restlessness may render such behaviour more likely. An early response to treatment after electroconvulsive treatment or effective antidepressant medication may result in the patient becoming less retarded and therefore at greater risk of suicide.

Hyperactivity

This describes the state in which there is increased motor activity, possibly with aggressiveness, over-talkativeness or uncoordinated physical activity. The term is descriptive of behaviour rather than of a subjective psychological state. Restlessness is poorly defined in the psychiatric literature and has diverse and multitudinous causes (Sachdev and Kruk, 1996). Restless hyperactivity or *hyperkinesis* may occur with a variety of different physical assaults on the brain but is especially prominent as a sequela to head injury in children in whom it may be associated with impulsive disobedience and explosive outbursts of anger and irritability (Black et al., 1969); it is also associated with childhood epilepsy when there is brain damage.

Over recent years, the condition of attention deficit/hyperactivity disorder (ADHD), previously described as occurring only in children, has been diagnosed in adults; the childhood disorder does sometimes persist into adult life, but the prevalence of the disorder in adulthood is low compared with that in childhood (Sachdev, 1999). There is a pattern of persistent inattention in all areas of life, overactivity with fidgeting and restlessness and impulsivity with impatience and difficulty in delaying responses. These psychological characteristics result in disturbed behaviour in all areas of life. In adult life, there are persistent difficulties in relationships, usually a poor work record and sometimes also a criminal record. The individual is particularly distractible and prone to be disruptive in a group setting.

Considerable comorbidity in children occurs with conduct disorder, oppositional deficit disorder, mood and anxiety disorders and mental retardation (Biederman et al., 1991). Between 30% and 70% of children who are diagnosed as having ADHD will continue to show symptoms of the condition as adults (Bellak and Black, 1992). In a study of adults with ADHD, both genders had the manifestations of the condition but females who, unlike the situation in childhood, were in the majority had higher rates of depression, anxiety disorders and conduct disorder than normal control subjects (Biederman et al., 1994). This is clearly a condition to which those practising in general adult psychiatry will have to pay more attention.

Retardation

Retardation has two quite different meanings in psychiatry. *Motor retardation*, the sense in which it is used here, implies slowness of the initiation, execution and completion of physical activity; it is frequently associated with retardation of thought, for example, in severe depressive illness. The patient subjectively describes themself as having difficulty with thinking—'my thoughts are slowed up'—and with initiating and carrying out spontaneous activity.

Retardation is so prominent a symptom of the severe endogenous type of depression that in the past it was used to name the condition, *retarded depression*. There is restricted movement, a static posture of dejection and decrease of muscular tone. Gesticulation is reduced, as is the emotional component of facial expression.

Retardation with slowness of motor activity is also seen with other causes of mental slowness, as in various organic psychosyndromes and with physical illnesses. The extreme of retardation—no voluntary movement at all—is known as *akinesis* and occurs with muteness in *stupor.*

Disorder of Movement in Schizophrenia

For the sake of convenience, three types of abnormality may be recognized in schizophrenia: isolated abnormalities of movement and posture, which are now discussed; more complex patterns of disordered behaviour, described later in the chapter; and the presumed effects on movement of the antipsychotic drugs, which are often used in large dosages and for a long time in schizophrenia. Extrapyramidal side effects are described later in this chapter, but brief mention should be made of the *neuroleptic malignant syndrome* with rapid onset of severe generalized muscular hypertonicity with hyperpyrexia and akinetic mutism and autonomic disturbance; death occurs in about 15% of sufferers (Kellam, 1987). Some of the odd motor disorders that occur are described first, and then the disturbances of chronic schizophrenia are mentioned.

Isolated Disorders of Movement and Posture

Catatonia means a state of increased tone in muscles at rest abolished by voluntary activities and thereby distinguished from extrapyramidal rigidity. The syndrome *catatonic schizophrenia* was originally described by Kahlbaum (1873) and is characterized by the presence of the motor disorders described subsequently. In reviewing Kahlbaum's concept, Johnson (1993) considers catatonia, the 'tension insanity', to be a neuropsychiatric syndrome caused by a large variety of organic disease processes manifesting as catalepsy with an abnormal mental state. It is difficult to classify the precise nature of the odd and abnormal posture in catatonic schizophrenia. *Waxy flexibility* (flexibilitas cerea) and *psychological pillow* occur but are both rare conditions. In waxy flexibility, when the limbs of the patient are put into any posture by the interviewer they will be retained in that position for a sustained period (a minute or more). Psychological pillow, when the supine patient's head is maintained a few inches above the bed, may continue for hours. In *stereotypy,* a bizarre uncomfortable-looking posture also may be retained for some hours.

The varied symptoms of catatonia always involve motor activity and posture. There may be hyper- or hypoactivity, mutism, stereotypical posturing and movement, waxy flexibility, stupor and uncontrollable excitement (Fink, 1993). Some variants of catatonia are *lethal (pernicious) catatonia,* with high fever, rigidity and extreme hyperactivity and/or stupor; *neuroleptic malignant syndrome,* with rigidity, fever, autonomic instability and stupor, associated with the use of antipsychotic drugs; *periodic catatonia,* characterized by periods of excitement followed by catatonic stupor; *manic excitement,* with confusion; and *stupor* in the context of delirium. It is now recognized that catatonic movement disturbance is present in disorders other than schizophrenia and has been most recently identified in anti-N-methyl-D-aspartate receptor encephalitis and in self-injurious behaviours in autistic spectrum disorder in childhood (Fink, 2013).

There are two types of abnormal movement in schizophrenia: *idiosyncratic voluntary movements,* or *mannerisms,* and *spontaneous involuntary movements.* Mannerisms are shown in odd, stilted, voluntary movements and patterns of behaviour. The patient may claim to be unaware of these acts or explain them in terms of his delusions.

It is sometimes difficult to distinguish mannerisms from the purposeless movements or postures that are not goal-directed but are carried out in an unvarying way in any individual patient. It is important to attempt to distinguish either of these types of movement from the abnormal movements of *parkinsonian syndromes,* which occur quite frequently in patients with schizophrenia who are treated with typical (first-generation) antipsychotic drugs. *Grimacing* is a common feature in schizophrenia; *Schnauzkrampf* (literally 'snout spasm') is a characteristic facial expression in which the nose and lips are drawn together in a pout.

Abnormality of the *execution of movement* may result from the internal experiences of the schizophrenic patient. At times, they resist stimuli, for example, the interviewer's request to raise their right arm, and show *negativism.* At other times, they demonstrate excessive compliance amounting to *automatic obedience:* not only do they raise their right arm, but they raise the other arm and then stand up with both arms raised in dramatic response to the request. This alternation of cooperation and opposition produces the diffident, unpredictable behaviour of *ambitendency.*

Obstruction is the equivalent in the flow of action to thought blocking in the flow of speech. While carrying out a motor act, the patient stops still in their tracks. After a pause, they continue with the act, or they may proceed to do something else. Usually, they cannot account for their obstruction but may do so in terms of passivity: 'my action was stopped'.

Abnormal movements manifested in the interaction with the interviewer may reveal excessive cooperation or opposition. *Mitgehen, echopraxia, automatic obedience* and *advertence* are symptoms of excessive cooperation. In *Mitgehen* (literally, German, 'to go with'), the interviewer can move the patient's limbs or body by directing them with fingertip pressure, 'as if one was moving an anglepoise lamp' according to Hamilton (1984). When the patient imitates the interviewer's every action, the symptom is called *echopraxia;* this occurs despite the doctor asking them not to. *Automatic obedience* denotes a condition in which the patient carries out every command in a literal, concrete fashion, like an automaton. To demonstrate these symptoms of excessive cooperation, the patient should be asked to resist the interviewer. Mitgehen and echopraxia still occur. This inability to accede to instructions to resist occurs with *forced grasping.* The interviewer presents their hand to be shaken but at the same time asks the patient not to shake it; every time the patient does shake hands, the interviewer has great difficulty in getting their hand away again. In *advertence,* the patient turns towards the examiner when they address them; again, it has a bizarre, exaggerated and inflexible quality.

Opposition occurs as a negative response to all the approaches of the examiner. The patient resists the examiner when the latter attempts to move their limbs. When addressed, the patient turns away—*aversion. Negativism* is not just a refusal by the patient to do what they are asked: it is an active process of resisting all attempts to make contact with them. Opposition may sometimes manifest itself in muteness.

The abnormal movements of schizophrenia are strongly suggestive of neurologic abnormality. In the opinion of Cutting (1985), the movement disorders of schizophrenia including catatonia, perseveration, involuntary movements and disturbed voluntary movements may, in some cases, represent a disorder of conation resulting from hemispheric imbalance. Whether or not Cutting's formulation is correct, there is continuing interest in abnormal movements in schizophrenia that are distinct from those arising from treatment with antipsychotic drugs. Indeed, as we see later, there is a variety of subtle and not so subtle movement disturbances prevalent in schizophrenia that apparently predate treatment.

Disorder of Gesture in Schizophrenia

There appears to be impaired gestural language in schizophrenia. This takes the form of impaired ability to demonstrate a gesture after instruction, the so-called pantomime skill and additionally an impairment in the ability to mimic demonstrated gestures. These problems emphasize impairments in fundamental gestural communicating skills (Walther et al., 2013, 2020). Nonetheless, the skills described in these studies only refer to certain aspects of gesture, namely pantomime skills and the ability to copy demonstrated gestures. It is important to point out that these studies do not refer to the detailed findings and underpinning methodology or concepts described previously, as enunciated by David McNeill. At the most they are investigations of what McNeill terms *emblems* and *pantomime.*

It is noteworthy that Walther and colleagues (2015) specifically refer to gestures that may substitute or aid language comprehension whereas McNeill refers to gestures as integral to language and not add-ons. Walther and colleagues also use the terms *transitive* and *intransitive* gestures. By this they mean that transitive gestures are those that are tool related, simulating specific action in the absence of the object (signalling the use of a comb or a hammer), and intransitive gestures are those overlearned gestures that convey emblematic information such as signalling stop or waving goodbye.

Furthermore, Walther and colleagues argue for a relationship between gestures and praxis. Praxis is the ability to perform skilled and/or learned limb actions, and impairments in this domain are demonstrated by inability to use tools appropriately or inefficiently. These authors claim that praxis also involves the ability to perform meaningful gestures. In their studies they show 18% of patients with schizophrenia had frequent gesture errors, usually minor and including hesitant or sloppy, low-amplitude performance, timing errors as well as inaccurate spatial configurations. Wüthrich and others (2020) show that the impairments in gesture are present in first-degree relatives of patients with schizophrenia although not to the same extent as in the patients. Furthermore, they also demonstrated that, despite improvements in psychopathology, there was deterioration in gesture deficits over time in patients with schizophrenia.

There is evidence that patients with schizophrenia require more time for gesture planning and gesture performance. The patients also presented increased movement per item of gesture and these differences in comparison to the control group were more apparent in the pantomime domain rather than in the imitation domain (Dutschke et al., 2018). In addition, there was evidence that gestural deficits were associated with other abnormalities of motor behaviour such as psychomotor slowing, poor postural control and neurological soft signs.

There is evidence that impairments of gesture performance in patients with schizophrenia are associated with impairments of gestural knowledge and with impairments in nonverbal social perception. The

underlying abnormality linking these deficits appear to be impairments in frontal and motor function (Walther et al., 2015).

Young people at high risk of psychosis are reported to have substantially more mismatch and retrieval gestures than controls (Millman et al., 2014). In this context speech–gesture mismatch refers to gestures that are semantically incongruent with the corresponding lexical content, for example, an individual speaking about 'climbing up a ladder' whilst simultaneously pointing downwards. A retrieval gesture refers to situations when during a pause, an individual is searching for a word or phrase and for example while saying 'The sandwich was almost the very best I ever tasted, it reminded me of that time I was travelling and ate in that café in …[gesture such as grasping air, creating a baton movement]…France!'

In summary, gesture deficit is an emerging area of investigation in psychiatry. The studies to date have failed to fully grasp the detail and complexity of what is already known about gesture in the nonclinical setting.

Motor Disorders in Chronic Schizophrenia
Motor disorder in the mentally ill may be ascribed to the abnormal mental state, to treatment or to independent undiagnosed neurologic disease (Rogers, 1985). Rogers studied motor disorders in 100 extremely chronic psychiatric inpatients, 59 women and 41 men, with a mean length of current admission of 42.8 years. Ninety-two of these patients had had a diagnosis of schizophrenia at some time, and all of them showed some current motor disorder.

Motor disorders are listed under the 10 categories of Table 18.1. These abnormalities are as follows:
- Difficulty with the initiation, efficient execution of or persistence with *purposive motor activity,* resulting in restriction of the motor repertoire available
- *Speech production* with 22 patients usually mute; 25 never initiating spontaneous conversation; 53 showing 'outbursts' of shouting, singing or talking and 51 inarticulate or barely audible at interview
- *Posture* and *tone* with a tendency to flexion associated with varying degrees of rigidity and typically affecting the head or neck

TABLE 18.1 Percentage of Patients with Current Motor Disorder (n = 100)

Motor Disorder	Percentage of Whole Group
Purposive movement	97
Speech production	95
Posture	86
Tone	85
Facial movements or postures	74
Head, trunk or limb movements	67
Activity	64
Stride or gait	48
Eye movements	48
Blinking	38

From Rogers, D., 1985. The motor disorders of severe psychiatric illness: a conflict of paradigms. Br. J. Psychiatry 147, 221–232, with permission.

- *Abnormal movement* or *postures* of *orofacial muscles* with rapid or slow contractions of different muscle groups
- Abnormal movements of the *head, trunk* or *limbs*, which might be brief, jerky and semipurposive in quality
- *Abnormal activity* might occur in outbursts or continuously with behaviour, such as hitting at, stamping, touching or following other people
- *Stride* or *gait* might show shuffling, slowness, not swinging the arms, or turning with head and neck 'in one piece'
- Conjugate deviation of the *eyes*, often up and laterally with deviation of the head in the same direction
- Blinking markedly increased or decreased in rate, sometimes in 'bursts'

Ninety-eight of these 100 patients had had motor disorder recorded before 1955, before there was any treatment with neuroleptic drugs. There was considerable variability between the type of motor disorder recorded before 1955 and observed currently. Disorder of eye movements, tone, gait and blinking were recorded less commonly in the past. Movement disorder in this group of patients was compared between those currently receiving neuroleptic drugs; those not treated for 1 month, 1 year or 5 years; and those never having received medication. With the possible exception of facial movements, which were more frequent in those having received treatment in the past year, there was no difference in the frequency of abnormal movements. In addition to the description of abnormal movements just described, overflow movements have been noted. These are defined as involuntary movements that tend to accompany voluntary movements and are recognized as neurological soft signs and are thought to be characteristic of schizophrenia (D'Agati et al., 2012).

Motor Disorder in Brain Disease

The disturbance of basal ganglia resulting in parkinsonian symptoms has two main causes of relevance to psychiatry: Parkinson's disease and symptoms secondary to exposure to psychotropic drugs. Some of the motor symptoms are similar in these two conditions, but the overall clinical picture differs.

Parkinson's Disease. In Parkinson's disease, as well as motor symptoms, there are often sensory, autonomic and psychiatric abnormalities. Parkinson's original description in 1817 implied an absence of perceptual (as opposed to sensory) abnormality and does not comment on 'psychiatric status', which would then have been an unknown concept.

Primary or secondary sensory abnormalities may occur, and there may be autonomic under- or overactivity. However, the most conspicuous symptoms are in motor function: slowing of emotional and voluntary movement (Walton, 1985); muscular rigidity; akinesia; tremor; and disorders of gait, speech and posture. There is not necessarily any mental change; however, depression is very common (Mindham, 1970), intellectual deterioration may occur and personality disorder is sometimes associated. Psychotic episodes have also been described. A graphic description of the symptoms and subjective experience of parkinsonism is given in Sacks' account *Awakenings* (1973).

Extrapyramidal Side Effects of Antipsychotic Drugs. The extrapyramidal movement disorders produced by antipsychotic drugs are described in detail by Marsden et al. (1986). These include drug-induced parkinsonism with the classic parkinsonian triad of muscle rigidity, tremor and akinesia and such symptoms as abnormalities of gait, speech and posture; excessive salivation; difficulty with swallowing; the characteristic *facies*; and greasy skin. *Akinesia* varies from being mild in degree (dyskinesia) with an immobile, blank, expressionless face; limited movements with loss of such associated motor activity as the arms swinging when walking; and lack of spontaneity to more severe and generalized absence of movement—this may start soon after beginning antipsychotic medication. Cogwheel rigidity and 'pill rolling' of the fingers, tremor of the hands or periorbital tremor may occur but are less common than akinesia. Extrapyramidal side effects of antipsychotic drugs are listed in Box 18.2 (Gervin and Barnes, 2000).

Akathisia, or motor restlessness, occurs frequently. There is a subjective experience of motor unease with a feeling of being unable to sit still and a need to get up and move about and to stretch the legs, tap the feet, or rock the body (Box 18.3). Akathisia may occur at the same time as the akinesia of drug-induced parkinsonism and presents the contrasting state of a subjective urge to move and physical impairment of movement. To distinguish akathisia from other causes of inner restlessness, restlessness of the legs should be found to be especially prominent.

Acute dystonic reactions include a variety of intermittent or sustained muscular spasms and abnormal postures. Dystonia has been defined as 'a syndrome dominated by sustained muscle contractions, frequently causing twisting and repetitive movements, or abnormal postures' (Fahn et al., 1987). There may be protrusion of the tongue, grimacing, oculogyric crises, blepharospasm, torticollis, opisthotonus and other hyperkinetic exaggerated actions of the face, head, trunk or limbs. Owens (1990) has considered the major clinical types of dystonia to be acute dystonias, oculogyric spasms, focal dystonias including torticollis, blepharospasm, writer's cramp and other occupational dystonias, and laryngopharyngeal dystonia, segmental dystonias, generalized dystonia, drug-related (symptomatic) dystonias and psychogenic dystonia.

The frequency of association of so-called tardive dyskinesia, in which repetitive, purposeless movements of the facial muscles, mouth and tongue occur (sometimes with choreoathetotic limb movement and respiratory grunting) with exposure to psychotropic drugs is disputed. There is no doubt that facio-buccolinguomasticatory dyskinesia occurs in many

BOX 18.2 EXTRAPYRAMIDAL SIDE EFFECTS OF ANTIPSYCHOTIC DRUGS

ACUTE MOVEMENT DISORDERS
- Parkinsonism
- Acute akathisia
- Acute dystonia

CHRONIC MOVEMENT DISORDERS
- Tardive dystonia
- Chronic akathisia
- Tardive dyskinesia

From Gervin, M., Barnes, T.R.E., 2000. Assessment of drug-related movement disorders in schizophrenia. Adv. Psychiat. Treat. 6, 332–341, with permission.

BOX 18.3 SUBJECTIVE COMPONENTS OF AKATHISIA

COMMONLY EXPERIENCED
- Sense of inner restlessness
- Mental unease
- Unrest or dysphoria
- Feeling unable to keep still
- An irresistible urge to move the legs
- Mounting inner tension when required to stand still

LESS COMMONLY EXPERIENCED
- Tension and discomfort in the limbs
- Paraesthesiae and unpleasant pulling or drawing sensations in the muscles of the legs

From Gervin, M., Barnes, T.R.E., 2000. Assessment of drug-related movement disorders in schizophrenia. Adv. Psychiat. Treat. 6, 332–341, with permission.

chronic, especially elderly, psychotic patients on neuroleptic medication, but is it causally connected with drugs? The word *tardive* is used because the syndrome was considered to be a late consequence of drug treatment; however, there are cases described in patients who have never received neuroleptic drugs, and the precise relationship remains to be elucidated—it may be simply a late stage of the illness. In practice, the extrapyramidal symptoms secondary to medication are difficult to evaluate and measure by severity—problematic in accounting for aetiologically but important in the satisfactory treatment of the patient. At a 3-year follow-up of psychiatric patients receiving antipsychotic medication, orofacial dyskinesia increased from 39% to 47% of the sample, with a few individuals developing the disorder anew and a few remitting (Barnes et al., 1983). There was an association between dyskinesia and age older than 50 years and the presence of akathisia, but none with the use of antipsychotic drugs; in fact, those on high dosage were unlikely to have the condition. These dyskinesic symptoms also occur in Huntington's chorea and in senile chorea.

Huntington's Chorea

This is a hereditary condition inherited as a Mendelian dominant, which manifests usually in early middle life and is characterized by choreiform movements and dementia. Jerky, rapid, involuntary movements start in the face and upper limbs. Dysarthria and disorders of gait can also occur before intellectual impairment develops. The progressive dementia, with inertia and apathy, may be accompanied by irritability and occasional outbursts of excited behaviour. Occasionally the dementia occurs as the first sign of the illness.

Various psychological abnormalities have been described in the prodromal stage before manifestation of chorea and dementia. These may be anxiety, reactive depression and the features of personality disorder, especially antisocial behaviour. It is not known if this is truly an early symptom of the illness or part of the psychosocial reaction to this appalling and doom-laden condition.

Tics and Gilles de la Tourette Syndrome

Tics are rapid, repetitive, coordinated and stereotyped movements, most of which can be mimicked, and are usually reproduced faithfully by the individual (Macleod, 1987). In Gilles de la Tourette syndrome, multiple tics are accompanied by forced vocalizations that often take the form of obscene words or phrases—*coprolalia* (Lishman, 1997). The condition starts in childhood, before age 16; there are multiple motor tics and unprovoked loud utterances that may amount to shouted obscenities.

The condition is more common in boys than in girls and usually starts between the ages of 5 and 8 years with simple tics. The vocalizations usually begin as unrecognizable sounds but may progress to 'four-letter' swear words. Both tics and utterances are likely to occur with emotional stress. The subject often tries desperately hard not to vocalize the word, and this may be accompanied by considerable anxiety.

An interesting study compared adult sufferers with depressed adults and normal controls on measures of obsessionality, depression and anxiety (Robertson et al., 1993). Gilles de la Tourette syndrome sufferers scored as high as depressives on measures of obsessionality but were intermediate between them and normal subjects for both depression and anxiety.

DISTURBANCE OF BEHAVIOUR

There is no clear demarcation between disturbance of movement and behaviour, and the distinction made here is arbitrary. Thus with parkinsonism and, to an even greater extent, catatonic schizophrenia, an individual abnormal movement may be elaborated into an abnormal pattern of behaviour.

Behavioural Disorders of Schizophrenia

Disorder of movement is characteristic of *catatonia*, in which the patient may become immobilized in one attitude because of increased muscle tone at rest; it is usually seen in schizophrenia but has been described with frontal lobe tumour and some other organic conditions. There are abnormalities of posture and of movement, frequently shown in the actions made in relation to another person—the interviewer. Thus in *waxy flexibility* the posture of the limbs is so described because it is maintained indefinitely after being manipulated into that attitude by the observer. Behaviour, the composite of movements, may also be abnormal, and this is characteristic of *catatonic schizophrenia*, with more than just one isolated abnormality of posture. It has often been commented that the incidence of catatonic schizophrenia has markedly declined. However, Mahendra (1981) has queried the existence of catatonic schizophrenia as a condition with classic Kraepelinian schizophrenic features *and* catatonia in the same patient. He believes many of the patients with catatonia suffered from neurologic disease, perhaps postencephalitis, after epidemic and endemic viral infections. If this were so, the presumed association between schizophrenia and catatonia was accidental.

One could make a vast catalogue of the bizarre and sometimes unpleasant behaviour demonstrated by patients with chronic schizophrenia, but this would never be exhaustive. Certain types of behaviour pattern are described here with examples.

Schizophrenic *stupor* occurs, although rarely. The patient is mute and akinetic, although from the alertness of the eyes and the occasional excursion into abrupt activity or speech, they are clearly conscious. It can be distinguished from depressive or manic stupor by the obvious abnormalities of mood in the stupor of the affective psychoses. A patient with schizophrenia sat mute and motionless with her arms held in stereotyped, twisted posture for hours at a time. This symptom is almost never seen nowadays with adequate treatment of schizophrenic symptoms.

Negativism, as described earlier under motor disorders, may influence the behaviour of the patient substantially. A schizophrenic patient was interviewed in prison. He was brought to the door of the doctor's examination room. When the doctor invited him to enter, he took two steps backwards. To get him to enter, the doctor had to ask him to go away. When the doctor put his hand out to shake hands, the patient put his hand behind his back and reversed behind the desk. He would not sit down until he was politely asked to remain standing.

Excitement may occur associated with catatonia but can also be seen without this state; sometimes a patient is mute and motionless for a time and then unpredictably becomes overactive and aimlessly destructive. A chronic schizophrenic patient, normally calm, would suddenly and unaccountably rush headlong across the ward and charge head first into the wall. On occasion this behaviour was directed at a window, and he had cut himself severely on the glass in the past.

Impulsive behaviour may not always be manifested as excitement; it may be carried out in contradistinction to the patient's habitual behaviour. A normally respectable and tranquil elderly female patient would suddenly and unpredictably make sexual assaults on unsuspecting male visitors to the hospital.

Hoarding is a common feature in chronic schizophrenics and is not confined to those in institutions. A patient used to put insects and pieces of rubbish found around the hospital, such as cigarette ends and small pieces of string, into a small tin. She did not appear to use her assortment but was constantly collecting more items.

Water intoxication due to grossly excessive water drinking has been described in schizophrenia, although it may occur, but much less commonly, in almost any psychiatric disorder (Ferrier, 1985). The symptom is potentially dangerous (Singh et al., 1985) and can even result in death from hyponatraemia often associated with convulsions. The water drinking may be explained by the patient in terms of delusions, or there may be a failure of the normal thirst–fluid intake homeostatic mechanism or both.

There may be *mannerisms* and idiosyncrasies of behaviour as well as of single movements. One totally mute male chronic patient used to retire to the top of a remote staircase above a ward where he ingeniously and delicately cut keys that would open any door in the hospital. He would exchange these for cigarettes with other patients, despite remaining utterly silent.

Gross self-neglect has been described, especially among elderly reclusives who have sometimes been well educated, intelligent and wealthy. This syndrome has, rather unfortunately, been called the *Diogenes syndrome* after the Greek philosopher who rejected social norms and worldly luxuries (Clark et al., 1975). An early case was described by Daniel Hack Tuke (1874) of a rich old man, 'mad Lucas', who died in a filthy state half-naked and alone in his decaying mansion. He remained as a hermit for 25 years, continually terrified that his younger brother would seize his house and kill him. He and similar recluses usually suffer from a paranoid schizophrenic illness, although the term *Diogenes syndrome* itself is purely descriptive (Aquilina, 1992).

Multitudinous other forms of abnormal behaviour are manifested in schizophrenia. Flagrant stealing occurs sometimes with a manneristic flavour, such as the hospital inpatient who 'stole' bedsprings, much to the discomfort of the occupants. Unprovoked aggression and 'nastiness' sometimes occur. Patients may exhibit childish naughtiness or grotesque dirtiness, and self-immolation and suicide have occasionally occurred. This may take place in obedience to auditory hallucinations or as part of a delusion. One patient regularly heard a voice that instructed him to jump out of the window; he was prevented on many occasions but finally took the reinforced window frames with him in leaping to his death.

Behavioural Signs of Emotional Disturbance

Psychiatrists have learned that they must *listen* to their patients; it is also important to *observe* them and form useful, testable hypotheses from these observations. Internal medicine has, traditionally, made great diagnostic use of physical signs, and psychiatry also would do well to use behavioural signs as possible indicators, not positive proof, of psychological disturbance. Trethowan (1977) has noted, in addition to the evidence for catatonia and parkinsonism, the following *behavioural*, as opposed to neurologic, signs, which may be of value diagnostically in psychiatry:

- *The handshake* may be limp and lifeless, as in the asthenic adolescent or sufferer from simple schizophrenia or vice-like as in mania. The hand of the schizophrenic patient with negativism may be withdrawn when the interviewer offers theirs, or the manic or personality disordered patient may insist on shaking hands, contrary to the doctor's intention.

- *Other forms of hand behaviour* that may be significant include bitten or picked nails, clenched hands with blanched knuckles and restless fidgeting with the fingers; all of these may indicate acute or chronic anxiety. Heavily cigarette-stained fingers obviously reflect the large number of cigarettes smoked and the extent to which each cigarette is consumed; this may demonstrate a degree of tension. Tremor may reveal alcoholism with alcohol withdrawal. In 'Trethowan's wedding ring sign', a woman during history taking unconsciously reveals her marital difficulties by constantly sliding her wedding ring on and off her finger.

- *The feet* may be used for restless pacing in agitated depression. Akathisia, as described earlier, with an inability to keep the feet still may indicate excessive medication with phenothiazine drugs.

- *Depressive facies* and *posture* sometimes lead to diagnosis before the patient speaks. The patient may be slumped in the chair with a fixed expression of unmitigated grief on their face and prominent 'crow's foot' between the eyebrows. Trethowan (1977) has commented on the greatly reduced blink rate with severely retarded depressives.

- *Clothing* in mania may be distinctive and suggestive of both the diagnosis and the hypereroticism that sometimes accompanies it. Hair, makeup and dress may be unequivocal demonstrations of manic mood: 'Thus Stella, normally a fairly modest girl, appeared one day in my consulting room wearing an all-black outfit consisting of net stockings, a mini-skirt which extended barely to vulva level, and a top with so deep a cleavage as almost to expose her umbilicus. As if this were not enough, she had stuffed her red, white and blue jubilee panties into the top of her open handbag, for all to see' (Trethowan, 1977).

- *Stroking the cheek* may be an indicator of emotional distress, as described by Gillett (1986): 'During the initial history taking and assessment, there was one over-ridingly important emotive issue, as evident from observation of her body language signs. When she spoke of her son dying at the age of three, her body stiffened, the muscle tension in her face increased, as if trying to stifle expression, lacrimation increased (though only just perceptibly), and her voice rose in pitch and wavered. She then lightly stroked her right cheek with the tip of her fore-finger, as if wiping away an imaginary tear—a common sign which usually indicates a desire to cry at the same time as a wish not to show it'.

This list is far from exhaustive. The point is that clinicians should use their eyes and their previous clinical experience to form hypotheses in observation that they can subsequently test in the history or examination of mental state.

REFERENCES

Adler, A., 1929. Problems of Neuroses. Kegan Paul, Trench, Trubner, London.

Andreasen, N.C., 1982. Negative symptoms in schizophrenia. Definition and reliability. Arch. Gen. Psychiatry 39, 784–788.

Andreasen, N.C., 1989. Scale for the Assessment of Negative Systems (SANS). Br. J. Psychiatry 155 (Suppl. 7), 53–58.

Aquilina, C., 1992. Diogenes syndrome. Psychiatr. Bull. 16, 573.

Barnes, T.R.E., Kidger, T., Gore, S.M., 1983. Tardive dyskinesia: a three year follow-up study. Psychol. Med. 13, 71–81.

Bayne, T., Levy, N., 2006. The feeling of doing: deconstructing the phenomenology of agency. In: Sebanz, N., Prinz, W. (Eds.), Disorders of Volition. MIT Press, Cambridge, MA, pp. 49–68.

Bellak, L., Black, R.B., 1992. Attention-deficit hyperactivity disorder in adults. Clin. Ther. 14, 138–147.

Benson, D.F., Blumer, D., 1982. Psychiatric Aspect of Neurologic Disease, vol. 2. Grune and Stratton, New York.

Berrios, G.E., 1996. The History of Mental Symptoms. Cambridge University Press, Cambridge.

Biederman, J., Faraone, S.V., Spencer, T., Wilens, T., Mick, E., Lapey, K.A., 1994. Gender differences in a sample of adults with attention deficit hyperactivity disorder. Psychiatry Res. 53, 13–29.

Biederman, J., Newcorn, J., Sprich, S., 1991. Comorbidity of attention deficit hyperactivity disorder with conduct, depressive, anxiety, and other disorders. Am. J. Psychiatry 148, 564–577.

Black, P., Jeffries, J.J., Blumer, D., Wellner, A., Walker, A.E., 1969. The post-traumatic syndrome in children. In: Walker, A.E., Caveness, W.F., Critchley, M. (Eds.), The Late Effects of Head Injury. Thomas, Springfield.

Bleuler, E., 1911. Dementia Praecox or the Group of Schizophrenias (J. Zinkin, Trans, 1950). International Universities Press, New York.

Burwell, C.S., Robin, E.D., Whaley, R.D., Bickelmann, A.G., 1956. Extreme obesity associated with alveolar hypoventilation – a Pickwickian syndrome. Am. J. Med. 21, 811–818.

Clark, A.N.G., Manikar, G.D., Gray, I., 1975. Diogenes syndrome: a clinical study of gross neglect in old age. Lancet 1, 366–373.

Critchley, M., 1962. Periodic hypersomnia and megaphagia in adolescent males. Brain 85, 627–656.

Crow, T.J., 1980. Molecular pathology of schizophrenia: more than one disease process? Br. Med. J. 280, 66–68.

Cutting, J., 1985. The Psychology of Schizophrenia. Churchill Livingstone, Edinburgh.

D'Agati, E., Casarelli, L., Pitzianti, M., Pasini, A., 2012. Neuroleptic treatments and overflow movements in schizophrenia: are they independent? Psychiatry Res. 200, 970–976.

Daruna, J.H., Barnes, P.A., 1993. A neurodevelopmental view of impulsivity. In: McCown, W.G., Johnson, J.L., Shure, M.B. (Eds.), The Impulsive Client: Theory, Research and Treatment. American Psychological Association, Washington, DC.

Dutschke, L.L., Stegmayer, K., Ramseyer, F., Bohlhalter, S., Vanbellingen, T., Strik, W., Walther, S., 2018. Gesture impairments in schizophrenia are linked to increased movement and prolonged motor planning and execution. Schizophr Res 200, 42–49.

Epistle of Paul the Apostle to the Romans, 1662. Chapter 7, 18–23, Authorized Version.

Eysenck, S.G.B., 1993. The 17: development of a measure of impulsivity and its relationship to the superfactors of personality. In: McCown, W.G., Johnson, J.L., Shure, M.B. (Eds.), The Impulsive Client: Theory, Research and Treatment. American Psychological Association, Washington, DC.

Fahn, S., Marsden, C.D., Calne, B., 1987. Classification and investigation of dystonia. In: Marsden, C.D., Fahn, R.S. (Eds.), Movement Disorders 2. Butterworth, London.

Ferrier, I.N., 1985. Water intoxication. Br. Med. J. 291, 1594–1596.

Fink, M., 1993. Catatonia: a treatable disorder, occasionally recognized. Direct. Psychiatry 13, 1–8.

Fink, M., 2013. Rediscovering catatonia: the biography of a treatable syndrome. Acta Psychiatr. Scand. Suppl. 441, 1–47.

Fink, M., Taylor, M.A., 2003. Catatonia: A Clinician's Guide to Diagnosis and Treatment. Cambridge University Press, Cambridge.

Freud, S., 1915. Instincts and their vicissitudes. Translated by J Riviere and General Editor J Strachey. In: Collected Papers, vol. 4. Hogarth Press, London.

Frith, C., 2013. The psychology of volition. Exp. Brain Res. 229, 289–299.

Gervin, M., Barnes, T.R.E., 2000. Assessment of drug-related movement disorders in schizophrenia. Adv. Psychiat. Treat. 6, 332–341.

Gillett, R., 1986. Short term intensive psychotherapy – a case history. Br. J. Psychiatry 148, 98–100.

Griesinger, W., 1845. Mental Pathology and Therapeutics (C.L. Robertson, J. Rutherford, Trans, 1882). William Wood and Co, New York.

Hamilton, M., 1984. Fish's Schizophrenia, third ed. John Wright, Bristol.

Henderson, S., 2005. The neglect of volition. Br. J. Psychiatry 186, 273–276.

Hull, C.L., 1943. Principles of Behaviour. Appleton-Century-Crofts, New York.

Jaspers, K., 1997. General Psychopathology (J. Hoenig, M.W. Hamilton, Trans). The Johns Hopkins University Press, Baltimore.

Jeannerod, M., 2006. From volition to agency: the mechanism of action recognition and its failures. In: Sebanz, N., Prinz, W. (Eds.), Disorders of Volition. MIT Press, Cambridge, MA, pp. 175–192.

Johnson, J., 1993. Catatonia: the tension insanity. Br. J. Psychiatry 162, 733–738.

Kahlbaum, K.L., 1873. Die Katatonie, oder das Spannungs Irresein. In: Catatonia (Y. Levi, T Pridan, Trans, 1973). Johns Hopkins University Press, Baltimore.

Kellam, A.M.P., 1987. The neuroleptic malignant syndrome, so called: a survey of the world literature. Br. J. Psychiatry 150, 752–759.

Lehmann, H.E., 1967. Schizophrenia. In: Freedman, A.M., Kaplan, H.I. (Eds.), Comprehensive Textbook of Psychiatry. Williams and Wilkins, Baltimore.

Lishman, W.A., 1997. Organic Psychiatry, third ed. Blackwell Scientific, Oxford.

Lorenz, K., 1963. On Aggression (M. Latzke, Trans, 1966). Methuen, London.

Macleod, J., 1987. Davidson's Principles and Practice of Medicine, thirteenth ed. Churchill Livingstone, Edinburgh.

Mahendra, B., 1981. Where have all the catatonics gone? Psychol. Med. 11, 669–671.

Marsden, C.D., Mindham, R.H.S., MacKay, A.V.P., 1986. Extrapyramidal movement disorders produced by antipsychotic drugs. In: Bradley, P.B., Hirsch, S.R. (Eds.), The Psychopharmacology and Treatment of Schizophrenia. Oxford University Press, Oxford.

McDougall, W., 1908. An Introduction to Social Psychology. Methuen, London.

McNeill, D., 1992. Hand and Mind. The University of Chicago Press, Chicago.

McNeill, D., 2005. Gesture and Thought. The University of Chicago Press, Chicago.

Metzinger, T., 2006. Conscious volition and mental representation: toward a more fine-grained analysis. In: Sebanz, N., Prinz, W. (Eds.), Disorders of Volition. MIT Press, Cambridge, MA, pp. 19–48.

Millman, Z.B., Goss, J., Schiffman, J., Mejias, J., Gupta, T., Mittal, V.A., 2014. Mismatch and lexical retrieval gestures are associated with visual information processing, verbal production, and symptomatology in youth at high risk for psychosis. Schizophr. Res. 158 (1–3), 64–68.

Mindham, R.H.S., 1970. Psychiatric symptoms in parkinsonism. J. Neurol. Neurosurg. Psychiatry 33, 188–191.

Moeller, F.G., Barratt, E.S., Dougherty, D.M., Schmitz, J.M., Swann, A.C., 2001. Psychiatric aspects of impulsivity. Am. J. Psychiatry 158, 1783 1817 93.

Owens, D.G.C., 1990. Dystonia – a potential psychiatric pitfall. Br. J. Psychiatry 156, 620–634.

Reid, T., 1863. In: Hamilton, W. (Ed.), The Works of Thomas Reid. Maclachlan and Stewart, Edinburgh.

Robertson, M.M., Channon, S., Baker, J., Flynn, D., 1993. The psychopathology of Gilles de la Tourette's syndrome: a controlled study. Br. J. Psychiatry 162, 114–117.

Rogers, D., 1985. The motor disorders of severe psychiatric illness: a conflict of paradigms. Br. J. Psychiatry 147, 221–232.

Sachdev, P., 1999. Attention deficit hyperactivity disorder in adults [editorial]. Psychol. Med. 29, 507–514.

Sachdev, P., Kruk, J., 1996. Restlessness: the anatomy of a neuropsychiatric symptom. Aust. N. Z. J. Psychiatry 30, 38–53.

Sacks, O.W., 1973. Awakenings. Duckworth, London.

Savage, G., 1886. Insanity and Allied Neuroses: Practice and Clinical. Cassell, London.

Scharfetter, C., 1980. General Psychopathology: An Introduction. Cambridge University Press, Cambridge.

Selten, J.P.C.J., Sijben, N.E.S., van den Bosch, R.J., Omloo-Visser, J., Warmerdam, H., 1993. The subjective experience of negative symptoms: a self-rating scale. Compr. Psychiatry 34, 192–197.

Sims, A., 1994. Myself and my other self: the 'double phenomenon' in neurotic disorders. In: Sensky, T., Katona, C., Montgomery, S. (Eds.), Psychiatry in Europe: Directions and Developments. Gaskell, London.

Sims, A.C.P., Symonds, R.L., 1975. Psychiatric referrals from the police. Br. J. Psychiatry 127, 171–178.

Singh, S., Padi, M.H., Bullard, H., Freeman, H., 1985. Water intoxication in psychiatric patients. Br. J. Psychiatry 146, 127–131.

Snaith, R.P., 1993. Anhedonia: a neglected symptom of psychopathology. Psychol. Med. 23, 957–966.

Trethowan, W.H., 1977. Psychiatry's physical signs. World Med. 16, 19–21.

Tuke, D.H., 1874. The hermit of red Coats' green. J. Ment. Sci. 20, 361–372.

Walther, S., Mittal, V.A., Stegmayer, K., Bohlhalter, S., 2020. Gesture deficits and apraxia in schizophrenia. Cortex 133, 65–75.

Walther, S., Stegmayer, K., Sulzbacher, J., et al., 2015. Nonverbal social communication and gesture control in schizophrenia. Schizophr. Bull. 41 (2), 338–345.

Walther, S., Vandellingen, T., Müri, R., Strik, W., Bohlhalter, S., 2013. Impaired pantomime in schizophrenia: association with frontal lobe. Cortex 49, 520–527.

Walton, J., 1985. Brain's Diseases of the Nervous System, ninth ed. Oxford University Press, Oxford.

Wing, J.K., 1978. Reasoning about Madness. Oxford University Press, Oxford.

Wüthrich, F., Pavlidou, A., Stegmayer, K., et al., 2020. Nonverbal communication remains untouched: no beneficial effect of symptomatic improvement on poor gesture performance in schizophrenia. Schizophr. Res. 223, 258–264.

Chapter 19

Disorder of Aesthetic Perception and Praxis

Chapter Outline

KEYWORDS

Aesthetics
Beauty
Obsessive compulsive disorder
Tourette syndrome
Body dysmorphic disorder
Schizophrenia
Mood disorder

Summary

Abnormalities of aesthetic perception and aesthetic praxis are yet to be fully recognized and described. This chapter introduces concepts and develops the frameworks to further our understanding of aesthetics and reviews some of the evidence for an evolutionary and scientific basis of aesthetic perception and praxis. The newly emerging findings of the relationship between psychiatric disorders and fundamental aspects of aesthetic perception, including abnormalities of symmetry, form and face perception, are discussed. The understanding of how mood disorders impinge on the perception of landscapes is examined. Finally, the rudimentary understanding of the impact of disease on the production of visual art, particularly of how frontotemporal dementia and primary progressive aphasia influence the production of visual art, is described.

As little as art is to be defined by any other element, it is simply identical with form. Every other element can be negated in the concept of form, even aesthetic unity, the idea of form that first made the wholeness and autonomy of the artwork possible.
    Theodor Adorno (1903–69), Aesthetic Theory (1997)

The beauty of art presents itself to sense, to feeling, to perception, to imagination; its sphere is not that of thought, and the apprehension of its activity and its productions demand another organ than that of the scientific intelligence…And lastly, the source of artistic creations is the free activity of fancy, which in her imagination is more free than nature's self.

Georg Wilhelm Friedrich Hegel (1770–1831), Aesthetics: Lectures on Fine **Art (1975)**

Aesthetics is concerned with the nature of beauty, the underlying principles that determine why we come to find some things beautiful and others unattractive or indeed, ugly. The subject is not restricted to what influences our taste in matters of visual perception but also how music, poetry, theatre and the physical environment affect us and how we respond emotionally to engagement with these experiences. It is true that visual perception, specifically the visual arts, have been extensively investigated and will be the focus of this chapter. It is not generally appreciated how fundamental matters of taste and aesthetically pleasing perceptions are to human individual and social life. Furthermore, the ways in which abnormalities of aesthetic perception and practice are expressed in psychiatric disorders are rarely discussed or investigated. In this chapter, I will introduce relevant conceptual and empirical findings about aesthetic perception and practice with a view to classifying and exemplifying abnormalities of aesthetic perception and practice in psychopathology.

The term *aesthetics* itself derives from the Greek *aistehetikos* meaning aesthetic, sensitive, sentient, pertaining to sense perception. This very clearly puts aesthetics in the domain of perception. Nonetheless, studies of aesthetics also focus on how artists imagine, create and perform art. This means that aesthetics is also concerned with *praxis*, the practice of art. It goes without saying that artists are as concerned with the making of art as with what impact the artistic artefact will have on the aesthetic judgement of the person who is engaging with the piece of art.

Alexander Gottlieb Baumgarten (1714–62), a German philosopher, is usually credited with the first definition of the term aesthetics as the 'science of sensible knowledge', and his preoccupation was to determine the cognitive conditions for the appreciation of beauty, thereby laying the foundations for the modern examination of the fundamental principles and values

underpinning our appreciation of beauty. It is worth noting though that discussions regarding the nature of beauty in the Western tradition go back at least to Plato (428/427–348/347 BCE). Aristotle (384–322 BCE) in *Poetics* applies the term *mimesis* to define what it is that characterizes art and makes the point that it is rhythm, language or harmony that either singly or jointly constitute mimesis. And, for Aristotle, it is mimesis that distinguishes man from other living creatures. Furthermore, the quality of a work of art is determined by the structural union of its parts such that if any one part is displaced or removed, the whole will be disjointed or disturbed. The problem with Aristotle's approach is that there is no agreed feature that exemplifies what harmony, for example, is or how to decide what structural union is. This problem is true for other writers including Horace (65-8 BCE) and Longinus who do no more than give instructions on how to produce great art, instructions that are, in the end, merely general principles that are of little utility in practical life.

Immanuel Kant (1724–1804), in *Critique of Judgment* (1790/2000), wrote about the key distinguishing features of the judgement of beauty. These were:

- A disinterested approach to beautiful objects; and he meant by this that we take pleasure in something because we find it beautiful rather than judging it beautiful because we find it pleasurable.
- Beautiful objects seem universal and necessary by which is meant that beauty behaves as if it were a universal and necessary property of an object, like its weight or chemical composition, but that these properties are features of the human mind as there is nothing in the object itself that makes it beautiful.
- Beautiful objects seem to be purposive but without purpose and that they ought to affect us as if they had a purpose.

Kant identifies form as what is fundamental to aesthetic judgements, and form refers to shape, arrangement and rhythm but excludes content such as colour, tone, etc. This is the beginning of the attempts to define some fundamental characteristics that may be said to underpin our judgement of beauty.

Kant's approach laid the groundwork for modern conceptualizations of aesthetics and the nature of beauty. There is a growing consensus that there is understandable and discoverable basis to our responses to beautiful objects, and this is the goal of scientific and evolutionary studies of aesthetics. Gustav Theodor Fechner (1801–87) showed that the shape and dimension of objects determine whether and how far we find them pleasing. For example, he demonstrated that the golden ratio (0.62), which is the ratio of a rectangle's width to length, was the most appealing to the eye. He wrote:

When an object of our contemplation undergoes random variation in size and shape, then all things being equal, the mean values seem to be preferred from the aesthetic point of view or appears with the character of predominant pleasantness as the normal value in comparison with the others, which, according to their degree of variation from the mean, can appear less pleasing or, if certain limits are exceeded, even displeasing. (Kirk, 2014).

This approach suggests that there are features that are intrinsic to visual objects that influence our aesthetic responses, and that these features lie somewhere between the simple and the increasingly complex. Following this approach, Daniel Berlyne proposed a theory about the way in which artworks arouse emotions by novelty, complexity, surprisingness, uncertainty and incongruity (Berlyne, 1971). This bottom-up approach culminates in Zeki's (1998) proposal that:

(T)he general function of art [is] a search for the constant, lasting, essential, and enduring features of objects, surfaces, faces, situations, and so on, which allows us not only to acquire knowledge about the particular object, or face, or condition represented on the canvas but to generalize, based on that, about many other objects and thus acquire knowledge about a wide category of objects or faces.

A full critical examination of Zeki's proposal is outside the scope of this book (see Bergeron and Lopes, 2012). There is the sense in which features of objects in the external world are judged to be pleasing, that is, to be beautiful because of their interaction with aspects of neural and cognitive processing within the visual cortex, and, as such, art evokes the sense of wonder, even of sublimity by these intrinsic features.

If it is accepted that the foregoing is true, then Coss (2003) makes the point that there is a role for natural selection on visual-pattern recognition and

associated physiological arousal underpinning aesthetic perception. For this to work efficiently, there must be (1) specificity of initial pattern recognition, (2) recognition of visual-pattern significance in the appropriate organism–environment context, (3) emotional significance that emerges in this context and (4) successful expression of appropriate action in dealing with this visual pattern. Furthermore, a taxonomy of aesthetic adaptations has been proposed (see Thornhill, 2003, for detailed discussion):

- Aesthetic valuation of landscape features
- Aesthetic valuation of nonhuman animals
- Aesthetic valuation of acoustic behaviour of nonhuman animals
- Aesthetic judgements arising from daily or seasonal environmental cues that signal a need to change behaviour
- Aesthetic valuation of human bodily form
- Aesthetic valuation of social status cues
- Aesthetic valuation of social scenarios
- Aesthetic valuation of skill
- Aesthetic judgement of food
- Aesthetic judgement of ideas

This taxonomy and proposed domains of interest allow us to begin to consider what the nature of the psychopathology of aesthetic perception may look like.

Further consideration of, for example, the nature of aesthetic valuation of habitat affordances involves features of the habitat that are markers of the physical environment that afford survival as refuge sites or prospect sites. In this scheme, prospect refers to the ability to survey the landscape and refuge to the ability to hide when in danger. The presence of environmental structures that allow prospect views would have increased the likelihood of spotting resources such as water and food and of recognizing approaching threats such as predators, etc. (Ruso et al., 2003). Landscape features that tend to be perceived and assessed as beautiful include the perception of types of trees such as acacias with broad moderately layered canopies as the most attractive trees and of scenes with water that sparkles and ripples while reflecting sunlight or moonlight being regarded as beautiful. These features of water are thought to be relevant to the perception of glossy and sparkling surfaces as attractive (Coss, 2003).

Sexual selection of aesthetic preferences for male beards, male voice, facial attractiveness, female hips and breasts have all been investigated. It is accepted that symmetrical faces are rated as more attractive than asymmetrical ones, and neotenic female faces are also rated as sexually attractive. The role of a low female waist-to-hip ratio in mate choice is still uncertain—this is indicative of a small waist and large hips, possibly signalling the existence of significant energy reserves (Skamel, 2003). Neonate features such as large eyes and a small nose convey an exaggerated appearance of youthfulness, freshness, naïveté and openness suggesting fitness as a beneficiary of resources. Hence the preference for neotenic female faces. In addition to bodily traits that are integral to the body, there are also controllable modifications of appearance such as clothing, use of cosmetics, orthodontics, hair styling and colouring, scarification, tattooing, body piercing, use of jewellery, clothing, head and feet shaping during infancy, cosmetic surgery and fattening or dieting that can alter judgements of physical attractiveness (Cunningham and Shamblen, 2003).

Ramachandran's universal laws of aesthetics are an attempt to identify underlying principles that determine what the features are that determine why particular visual objects are aesthetically pleasing (Ramachandran and Seckel, 2014). These laws underpin the appreciation of visual objects but profoundly influence how artists construct their works. In other words, an understanding of these implicit rules is at play in art practice. These laws include (1) *grouping* in which there are groupings of items in clusters of, for instance, a blue sky is reflected in the blue robes of the people in a painting; (2) *symmetry*; (3) peak *shift effect* in which the more an object resembles the underlying form the more pleasing it is. This is exemplified in female figures that are more feminine than real females by the exaggeration of breasts, hips and the typically feminine triple flexion poise; (4) *isolation*, which is the simplification of an object to mere part of it as a representation and (5) *perceptual problem-solving*, which is associated with the rewarding discovery of a hidden object as in a puzzle.

Abnormal Aesthetic Perceptions

FORM PERCEPTION
Symmetry

The centrality of valuation of symmetry in the appreciation of beauty is well established. The underlying rationale for its importance is yet to be fully understood. There is the possibility that symmetry of the face and body is a sign of physical fitness, including the absence of disease and of infections, and a sign of normal early development. Secondly, there is also the possibility that symmetry signals a distinction between inanimate and animate objects.

Radomsky and Rachman (2004) argue that in obsessive compulsive disorder there is a compulsion to order and arrange one's surrounding so as to avoid disorderly surroundings and to ensure that objects are arranged in 'exactly the right way'. This feature of obsessive compulsive disorder is thought to indicate a heightened preference for symmetry. Patients often say that they need to ensure that their belongings are in exactly the right place before they can proceed with their day. In their study designed to develop a psychometric scale, the Symmetry, Ordering and Arranging Questionnaire, Radomsky and Rachman (2004) identified a number of items including:

- It is important that my belongings are placed in a symmetrical and evenly distributed way.
- The wall hangings (pictures, posters, etc.) in my home must be exactly even or straight.
- I feel compelled to arrange objects so that they are balanced and evenly spaced.

A 45-year-old female patient could not leave her house for work in the morning until she had ensured that the curtains were exactly perpendicular and the edges were symmetrical and parallel to each other. This preoccupation and compulsion meant that she was often late for work.

Summerfeldt and colleagues (2015) showed that individuals who scored highly on items for a sense of incompleteness, better known as *not-just-right experience* (including dissatisfaction with whether one's perceptions, actions or intentions have been adequately achieved) have higher levels of self-perceived symmetry-related concerns and behaviours and displayed greater aesthetic sensitivity demonstrated by heightened preferences for symmetry in images. These 'not-just-right' experiences have also been reported in Tourette syndrome (Neal and Cavanna, 2013). In Tourette syndrome this is exemplified by compulsions involving counting, symmetry and 'just right' thoughts or actions (Cavanna and Rickards, 2013). For example, a 25-year-old female patient presented with the compulsion to intentionally move her other limb in response to an involuntary tic in the first. This was intended to 'balance' the movements, illustrating the need for symmetry.

Body dysmorphic disorder is defined, in part, by recourse to the concept of beauty and ugliness as it turns on the preoccupation with an imagined defect in appearance that leads to significant distress, implicitly because the defect is perceived as ugly, that is, not beautiful. Hence, it is not surprising, perhaps, that it is in body dysmorphic disorder that a heightened sensitivity to symmetry is most obvious. It is often reported that patients with body dysmorphic disorder have a preoccupation with 'uneven' or 'asymmetrical' eyebrows, eyes, hair or other body areas (Hart and Phillips, 2013). So, for example, some patients complain of asymmetrical beard growth, chin being too prominent and asymmetrical, cheekbones being asymmetrical, one tooth larger than another, etc. (Phillips, 2005). And it is not merely that there is a preoccupation with symmetry but that there is also aesthetic sensitivity, a combination of an ability to differentiate between aesthetic proportions, heightened emotional response to beautiful or ugly images, and aesthetic valuation comprising standards, images and identity. Veale and Lambrou (2002) hypothesized that patients with body dysmorphic disorder are more likely to have greater aesthetical perceptual skills compared to other people and that this results in a greater emotional response in reaction to their negative evaluation of themselves in comparison with others. Lambrou et al. (2011) showed that patients with body dysmorphic disorder were like a group of individuals who had trained in art and design in having clear notion of the criteria of beauty defined by symmetry, that they showed a greater awareness of their aesthetic facial proportions and this facility extended to other people's faces and to buildings too. In addition, patients with body dysmorphic disorder and the art and design group, in this study, displayed a higher attractiveness standard

probably due to their increased understanding of aesthetic proportions. It is noteworthy that Hübner et al. (2015) did not find that patients with body dysmorphic disorder have enhanced general aesthetic perceptual sensitivity.

Furthermore, Veale and colleagues (2002) reported that patients with body dysmorphic disorder compared to other psychiatric patients were five times more likely to have aesthetic interest and/or skills. This relationship between body dysmorphic disorder and heightened preference for symmetry and thereby to the notion of 'aestheticality' is drawn from Harris' notion of 'aestheticality' as a trait that is linked to higher emotional response to beauty or ugliness (Harris, 1982) and that has relevance in the context of plastic/cosmetic surgery.

In summary, obsessive compulsive disorder, Tourette syndrome and body dysmorphic disorder are three conditions in which a heightened aesthetic sensitivity seems to, at the least, play a part. For the present, there are no reported phenomena that are based on a diminution of aesthetic sensitivity.

Shape of Objects

Zeki's proposal regarding the fundamental role of the visual perceptual system to our perception and aesthetic evaluation points to the fact that nonhuman objects in the world are likely to be evaluated as beautiful based on their intrinsic features. Much of the neurology of visual object perception deals with sensory awareness of objects, perception of objects, their recognition including naming and ability to use to the objects, in for example, visual agnosia. Boutoleau-Bretonnière et al. (2016) studied 15 individuals with probable behavioural variant frontotemporal dementia and compared them with 15 healthy adults with a view to investigate the emotional judgement of artwork by patients with behavioural variant frontotemporal dementia. The artwork targets were 32 abstract paintings. Patients with behavioural variant frontotemporal dementia reported absent emotional response to the artworks, and the paintings were more likely to be judged ugly and unpleasant by the patients. The authors conclude that patients with behavioural variant frontotemporal dementia have a preserved ability to make aesthetic judgments but an inability to experience emotional response to artworks. There was a link between finding the paintings as unpleasant and finding them ugly.

Faces

The previous discussion with respect to symmetry concerns in obsessive compulsive disorder, Tourette syndrome and body dysmorphic disorder focused on judgements of beauty as determined by symmetry. It is notable though that faces are not only evaluated with reference to symmetry to determine their beauty but also to other features such as their closeness to an averaged face. Thus in experimental studies, participants preferred a composite averaged face to the faces of actual individuals. This suggests that distinguishing features such as large noses, etc. would be negatively evaluated. In addition to this, it is also true that neotenic features such as large eyes and small chins are preferred in females and, finally, that the absence of skin blemishes is highly valued.

Dentofacial aesthetics focusses on frontal aspects of the face including the aesthetics of teeth, the smile, and the harmony of the face as well the lateral aspect of the face as designated by the face in profile. The features of relevance in lateral aspect include the length of the nose, the prominence of the soft tissues of the chin, the ratio of the nose to the lips and the inclination of the maxillary incisors. Romsics et al. (2021) report that dental students showed a preference for female faces with less prominent/slightly retruded chin and an anteriorly shifted maxillary arch. As for the nose, the preference was not in isolation for the length of the nose, but it was the harmony of the nose and chin that overrode the importance of the individual dimensions. Lambrou et al. (2011) demonstrated that in body dysmorphic disorder, there was greater concern about the skin, whole face, eyes, nose and hair on head compared with control groups comprised of people with and without aesthetic training. In addition, there were concerns too about calves, thighs, hips, bottom, waist/abdomen, breast/chest, back, shoulders, arms and hands but these individual areas were only of significance when they were grouped into upper body, lower body and shape of whole body (see later for further discussion about evaluation of human bodily form). The subjective descriptions included misshapen nose, hair never right, eyes too small, lines around the mouth, crooked teeth, sunken cheeks, dark circles under the eyes, lips too thin, etc. (Phillips, 2005).

The important role of the skin in determining the aesthetic value of the self is exemplified by the statements made by dermatology patients in a study of body dysmorphic disorder presenting to dermatology. Statements included 'Acne bothers me a lot; in general, I feel ugly'; These spots make me ugly and I have low self-esteem; I don't want to go out'; 'Before there was no spot, and now there is this horrible one on my face'; 'The lesions appear on the face, they are ugly and everyone stares'; 'Wrinkles and blemishes really bother me, I can't look in the mirror'; 'I have many wrinkles, my skin is ugly'; 'I used to be beautiful, but now I'm old and I feel ridiculous'; 'I don't like the wrinkles around my eyes, especially when I smile' (Morita et al., 2021). These statements illustrate the importance of what Ramachandran and Seckel (2014) refer to as the 'smoothness and suppleness of youthful oestrogen-charged skin' and departures from this aesthetic ideal is highly negatively valued.

Finally, neotenia can itself be a sought-after ideal form. A young man sought surgery from maxilla-facial surgeons, requesting to have his upper jaw reduced in size, because he believed that his upper jaw was too prominent. He also requested that his low jaw be made less chiselled and more rounded. In addition, he wanted his laryngeal prominence reduced in size. The underlying desire was for androgyny, because it was more aesthetically pleasing, but this desire did not arise either in the context of gender dysphoria or homosexual preference.

But perhaps even more surprising is subjective descriptions of abnormal aesthetic perception of the face and sometimes, too, of the body. This is illustrated by statements such as the following: *There's a clash between what I see and what I think. I think my worries are ridiculous. But I see it!' (italics in the original); 'I sometimes think I don't see my face correctly, that I'm like my mother after she had a stroke'* (Phillips, 2005).

AESTHETIC ADAPTATIONS

Valuation of Landscape Features

The valuation of landscape features such as open ground that is sparsely populated by trees with a wide canopy resembling the ancestral human origins in the East African savannah and with visible sources of water are positively valued and regarded as beautiful. As described previously, this is understood according to the Prospect and Refuge theory, as probably due to the survival value of these landscape features. It is well recognized that this sense of beauty can be attenuated or indeed abolished in severe depression where the patients often remark that looking at nature no longer provokes the usual sense of warmth, charm or beauty as it previously did. In their narrative review of the term anhedonia, De Fruyt et al. (2020) quote from classical descriptions of depression in textbooks by Bevan Lewis, Kraepelin, Henderson and Gillespie and Aubrey Lewis' classical description of melancholia to show that the visual representation of the physical environment is attenuated, lacking in vigour, and gives no ready delight to the patient.

This abnormality is best exemplified by Aubrey Lewis (1934):

[I]n a clinic such as that at Heidelberg, where most of the patients are peasants from the Palatinate, or Baden, one is amazed at the frequency with which depressive patients mention this failure to enjoy the sight of their fields, the sky and trees and the flowers as one of the most distressing of their symptoms, a deprivation most keenly felt (my italics for emphasis).

Aubrey Lewis includes this anomaly within his description of feelings of unreality and depersonalization. De Fruyt and colleagues (2020) include it within the ambit of anhedonia.

What is important is that the underpinning abnormality that is relevant here is directly linked to the usual normative predisposition to evaluate particular types of physical natural environments as beautiful and evocative of pleasure.

Valuation of Human Bodily Form

Much of the work on the aesthetics of bodily form examines the role of evolution in determining what is perceived as physically attractive. I have discussed the features of faces that are recognized as influencing our perception of beauty. I now turn to the body. Cunningham and Shamblen (2003) make the point that in females, visible breasts and hips that convey reproductive health and strength and that suggest fitness to fulfil sex responsibilities are recognized as important. In males, thick eyebrows, a large chin and shoulders are important and senescence features such as male pattern baldness, grey hair convey social maturity, reduced competitiveness and fitness as a mentor. The absence of senescence features increases romantic attractiveness.

Anorexia nervosa is perhaps a condition that has been most discussed with regard to the aesthetic valuation of bodily form. For example, Julian Robinson wrote, *'Today, in this … quest for beauty and an admired social identity, men and women of the Western world … diet to the point of anorexia, have parts of their intestines surgically removed, so as to reduce the waistline and lower their caloric intake, or have their buttocks, breasts, and thighs or nose reshaped'* (Robinson, 1998). It is important to recognize the role of culture in determining the relationship between female body weight and curvaceousness (see Cunningham and Shamblen, 2003, for a full discussion). Cultural preferences for slenderness are associated with reliable and effectively distributed food supply, with education and professional success, and may also indicate sex ratios that suggest a poor marriage market for females. Cunningham and Shamblen (2003) conclude that *'as long as the job market is good, focusing on controllable aspects of one's life, such as grooming oneself to be slender for one's career, seems more adaptive than dressing for romantic partners who may not materialise'*. In this schema, some women emphasize their self-control and de-emphasize their sexuality to the point of anorexia.

It is in the misapprehension of body size and overestimation of body weight and body form that abnormality of aesthetic perception is most obvious in anorexia nervosa. Slade and Russell (1973) showed that patients with anorexia nervosa overestimated the width of their bodies in comparison with normal female controls and that this attribute did not extend to the perception of physical objects. Furthermore, this attribute was less pronounced in judging the size of a female model, and there was no difficulty in estimating the height of a model or their own height. The overestimation was true for all bodily regions including face, chest, waist and hips. It is now established that this tendency is not restricted to people with anorexia nervosa (Cash and Deagle, 1997; Slade, 1988). What is more remarkable is the degree that this overestimation flies in the face of the physical reality of a malnourished and grossly underweight person.

One of Hilde Bruch's (2001) patients, Bert, was 180 pounds when he decided to go on a diet.

[W]hen his weight was down to one hundred twenty-six pounds and everybody admired him, said he looked great, something happened; he suddenly could not see how he looked. Until then he had watched his size dwindle and noticed that he looked slimmer from week to week. Now he actually feared that he would get fat again, and he actually saw himself larger, though the figure on the scale indicated that he had lost more weight. He drastically cut down on his previous diet, stopped watching the scale, and was frantically preoccupied with becoming fat again. He claims that he saw himself swelling up.

There is a further aspect to the picture of anorexia nervosa, namely that the dieting results in a prepubertal bodily form, and this approximates the idealized form suggested by neoteny, even if it is a markedly exaggerated pursuit. Writing about one of her patients, Hilde Bruch (2001) reported:

She was also troubled about seeing her body change. From childhood on, she felt it was not 'nice' to look like a woman, that her tissues would bulge, that the female body was not beautiful. Her mother was in her forties when Joyce was born, and she had no memory of how her older sisters had looked as teenagers or how she had felt about them. In order to avoid the sagging flesh later on, she decided as an adolescent to avoid the curves and roundness of her own development. She wanted to have a body as good as it could possibly be, which meant to her to be thin. She brought her weight down to seventy pounds, taking inordinate pride in being so slim, with no curves, and in having achieved this herself.

In males, broader shoulders and chests are rated as more sexually attractive than average male physiques. Nonetheless, 'pumped-up' body builder physique is not highly sexually attractive to most females. Furthermore, rates of body building increase in times of economic stress when males feel under threat and the hyper masculine body idea may be an attempt to shore up masculine anxiety (Cunningham and Shamblen, 2003). This fundamental understanding of the aesthetics of masculine bodily form is probably relevant in muscle dysmorphia, a condition in which disturbed body image is associated with disordered eating and excessive exercising (see Chapter 14).

ABNORMAL AESTHETIC PRAXIS

The art of the mentally ill has been written about, published and studied since Philippe Pinel (1745–1826) wrote about two patients who drew and painted, in his *Medical Treatise on Mental Disorder or Mania* in 1801 (Beveridge, 2001). Other contributors to this subject include John Haslam (1764–1844), WAF Browne (1805–85) and Cesare Lombroso (1835–1909). The question that the art of the mentally ill raises, as Beveridge, puts is 'Is there anything distinctive about the work of the mentally ill?'

Various authors have taken differing positions on this question. Paul Meunier (1873–1957), writing under the pseudonym Marcel Reja, thought that the art of the mentally ill was primitive in character, whereas Walter Morgenthaler (1882–1965) thought that art by the mentally ill might assist our understanding of the roots of creativity and Hans Prinzhorn (1886–1933) argued that the artistic work of the mentally ill should not be examined for diagnostic clues, but rather it should be recognized as works by individuals.

Increased Artistic Production

Silvano Arieti (1914–81) in his book *Interpretation of Schizophrenia* noted that patients with schizophrenia paint more frequently than expected given the general level of inactivity observed in schizophrenia. He accounted for this impression by the fact that the monotony and consequent boredom of asylum life triggers artistic output even in people with modest talent. Another possible explanation that he put forward was artistic production was a means of restoring or compensating for the psychological loss and emptiness attendant on schizophrenia (Arieti, 1974).

Miller and colleagues in a series of papers (Miller et al., 1996, 1998; Miller and Miller, 2014) have shown that some individuals who suffer from left-sided frontotemporal dementia, with predominant temporal involvement, develop new onset of visual art productivity. These patients appear to have left anterior temporal lobe dysfunction. Miller et al. (2000) reported on 12 patients with frontotemporal dementia who had new or preserved musical or visual ability. These patients manifested musical or visual talents but never verbal talents. The authors report that the artistic works lacked a symbolic or abstract component and that painters copied or remembered realistic landscapes, animals or people or perfected visual designs. They concluded that their findings suggested recall of previously learned information or images. The authors also report that the artists approached their works with a high degree of focus, fixated on their compositions, obsessively working and reworking their creations almost to the detriment of other aspects of their lives. Often the preoccupying nature of the artistic creation was associated with other behaviours such as coin collecting, spitting, tooth picking and copying the Bible. Miller and Miller (2014) hypothesized that preserved right-sided and posterior functions and spared dorsolateral and medial cortices were needed to be able to appreciate, integrate and create a composition.

Seeley et al. (2008) report on a single case study of an individual, Anne Adams, who suffered from primary progressive aphasia. In the decade before her language deficits became overt, she developed an intense drive to produce visual art. She is reported as creating expressive transmodal art, such as rendering music in paint. As her aphasia progressed her art moved in the direction of photorealism. There was evidence of increased grey matter volume and hyperperfusion in right posterior neocortical areas despite severe degeneration of left inferior frontal-insular, temporal and striatal regions. Her increased artistic ability is thought to demonstrate released inhibition or paradoxical facilitation.

In summary, the role of neuropathology and/or psychopathology in facilitating aesthetic praxis is yet to be fully unravelled.

Content of Visual Art Production

Cesare Lombroso in his study of 108 patients concluded that there were recognizable features in the art of the mentally ill, namely eccentricity, symbolism, minuteness of detail, obscenity, uniformity and absurdity (Beveridge, 2001). Emil Kraepelin (1856–1926) wrote in *Dementia Praecox and Paraphrenia* that:

In the drawings of patients also there invariably appears on the one hand incoherence, on the other hand

persistence [italics in the original] of impulse to movement. Fig 10 reproduces one of the senseless, childish drawings which a patient produced in large numbers; there are wonderful combinations of strokes and flourishes with hints of stereotypy ... there were endless variations of the same recurring fundamental form.

Kraepelin (1919)

Arieti's contribution was not dissimilar to Kraepelin's. He argued that regression which is part of the natural process of schizophrenia rekindles fantasies and motivational impulses, finding actualization on paper or canvas. He claims that the works are rigid, schematic, stereotypical, confused, irregular and freedom-seeking. He concludes 'schizophrenic art is the result of a struggle between motivational impulses and the specific ... cognitive media available to the patient. The sudden availability of primary process forms and the disinhibition of wishes and aspirations become substitutes for the technique, skill, and commitment that many patients never had before they became ill' (Arieti, 1974).

It is plain from the foregoing that psychiatrists who comment on the art of the mentally ill have little or no training in art criticism or in art history, and their comments are suspect given the absence of expertise in art criticism. This is not to say that art critics' views are unproblematic. Beveridge examines this and, using Jean Dubuffet (1901–85) as an example, wrote:

There is in the writings of Dubuffet a curious paradox in which, on the one hand, the mentally ill are accorded special abilities, and, on the other, the existence of such a thing as mental illness is denied. Further, there is another paradox in which psychiatrists are derided for reducing people to diagnostic categories, while the writings hail patients as schizophrenic and as the undisputed masters of the genre.

Beveridge (2001)

Finally, as already hinted at in the preceding section, sometimes there is an attempt to use the quality of the artwork as a proxy for the severity or as evidence of clinical deterioration (see the case of Anne Adams). The danger of this approach is exemplified in the examination of Louis Wain, the Edwardian cat-painter who spent his last years in London mental hospitals and whose artwork was used as evidence for clinical diagnosis and mental disintegration when, in fact, Wain was simply experimenting with design; the most bizarre images were not necessarily produced while he was most ill (Beveridge, 2001).

In summary, we are not yet at the stage when the content of the artwork of people with mental illness can be used as evidence of psychopathology, nor is it possible, at present, to conclusively draw attention to forms that are systematically abnormal and that point to underlying but covert disrupted mechanisms.

REFERENCES

Adorno, T., 1997. Aesthetic Theory (R. Hullot-Kentor, Trans.). Bloomsbury, London.

Arieti, S., 1974. Interpretation of Schizophrenia. Basic Books, New York.

Berlyne, D.E., 1971. Aesthetics and Psychobiology. Appleton-Century-Crofts, New York.

Bergeron, V., Lopes, D.M., 2012. Aesthetic theory and aesthetic science: prospects for integration. In: Aesthetic Science: connecting minds, brains, and experience. Shimamura A.P., Palmer, S.E.,(Eds). Oxford University Press, Oxford.

Beveridge, A., 2001. A disquieting feeling of strangeness? The art of the mentally ill. J. R. Soc. Med. 94 (11), 595–599. https://doi.org/10.1177/014107680109401115.

Boutoleau-Bretonnière, C., Bretonnière, C., Evrard, C., 2016. Ugly aesthetic perception associated with emotional changes in experience of art by behavioural variant of frontotemporal dementia patients. Neuropsychologia 89, 96–104.

Bruch, H., 2001. The Golden Cage: The Enigma of Anorexia Nervosa. Harvard University Press, Cambridge.

Cash, T.F., Deagle III, E.A., 1997. The nature and extent of body–image disturbances in anorexia nervosa and bulimia nervosa: a meta–analysis. Int. J. Eat. Disord. 22 (2), 107–126.

Cavanna, A.E., Rickards, H., 2013. The psychopathological spectrum of Gilles de la Tourette syndrome. Neurosci. Biobehav. Rev. 37 (6), 1008–1015.

Coss, R.G., 2003. The role of evolved perceptual biases in art and design. In: Voland, E., Grammer, K. (Eds.), Evolutionary Aesthetics. Springer, Berlin, pp. 69–130.

Cunningham, M.R., Shamblen, S.R., 2003. Beyond nature versus culture: a multiple fitness analysis of variations in grooming. In: Voland, E., Grammer, K. (Eds.), Evolutionary Aesthetics. Springer, Berlin, pp. 201–237.

De Fruyt, J., Sabbe, B., Demyttenaere, K., 2020. Anhedonia in depressive disorder: a narrative review. Psychopathology 53, 274–281.

Harris, D.L., 1982. Cosmetic surgery—where does it begin. Br. J. Plast. Surg. 35 (3), 281–286.

Hart, A.S., Phillips, K.A., 2013. Symmetry concerns as a symptom of body dysmorphic disorder. Journal of Obsessive-Compulsive and Related Disorders 2 (3), 292–298.

Hegel, G.W.F., 1975. (T.M. Knox, Trans.). Aesthetics: Lectures on Fine Art, vol. 2. Oxford University Press, Oxford.

Hübner, C., Wiesendahl, W., Kleinstäuber, M., Stangier, U., 2016. Facial discrimination in body dysmorphic, obsessive-compulsive and social anxiety disorders. Psychiatr. Res. 236, 105–111.

Kant, I., 1790/2000. Critique of Judgment (P. Guyer & E. Matthews, Trans.). Cambridge University Press, Cambridge.

Kirk, U., 2014. The modularity of aesthetic processing and perception in the human brain. In: Shimamura, A.P., Palmer, S.E. (Eds.), Aesthetic Science: Connecting Minds, Brains, and Experience. Oxford University Press, Oxford, pp. 318–336.

Kraepelin, E., 1919. Dementia Praecox and Paraphrenia (R.M. Barclay, Trans.). Medical Book Company, Chicago.

Lambrou, C., Veale, D., Wilson, G., 2011. The role of aesthetic sensitivity in body dysmorphic disorder. J. Abnorm. Psychol. 120 (2), 443.

Lewis, A.J., 1934. Melancholia: a clinical survey of depressive states. J. Ment. Sci. 80 (329), 277–378.

Miller, Z.A., Miller, B.L., 2014. A cognitive and behavioural neurological approach to aesthetics. In: Shimamura, A.P., Palmer, S.E. (Eds.), Aesthetic Science: Connecting Minds, Brains, and Experience. Oxford University Press, Oxford, pp. 356–374.

Miller, B.L., Ponton, M., Benson, D.F., Cummings, J.L., Mena, I., 1996. Enhanced artistic creativity with temporal lobe degeneration. Lancet (London, England) 348 (9043), 1744–1745.

Miller, B.L., Boone, K., Cummings, J.L., Read, S.L., Mishkin, F., 2000. Functional correlates of musical and visual ability in frontotemporal dementia. Br. J. Psychiatr. 176 (5), 458–463.

Miller, B.L., Cummings, J., Mishkin, F., et al., 1998. Emergence of artistic talent in frontotemporal dementia. Neurology 51 (4), 978–982.

Morita, M.M., Merlotto, M.R., Dantas, C.L., Olivetti, F.H., Miot, H.A., 2021. Prevalence and factors associated with body dysmorphic disorder in women under dermatological care at a Brazilian public institution. An. Bras. Dermatol. 96 (1), 40–46.

Neal, M., Cavanna, A.E., 2013. Not just right experiences" in patients with Tourette syndrome: complex motor tics or compulsions? Psychiatr. Res. 210, 559–563.

Phillips, K.A., 2005. The Broken Mirror. Oxford University Press, Oxford.

Radomsky, A.S., Rachman, S., 2004. Symmetry, ordering and arranging compulsive behaviour. Behav. Res. Ther. 42 (8), 893–913.

Ramachandran, V.S., Seckel, E., 2014. Neurology of visual aesthetics. In: Shimamura, A.P., Palmer, S.E. (Eds.), Aesthetic Science: Connecting Minds, Brains, and Experience. Oxford University Press, Oxford, pp. 375–389.

Robinson, J., 1998. The Quest for Human Beauty: An Illustrated History. WW Norton, New York, NY.

Romsics, L., Segatto, A., Boa, K., et al., 2021. Patterns of facial profile preference in a large sample of dental students: a cross-sectional study. Int. J. Environ. Res. Public Health 18 (16), 8554.

Ruso, B., Renninger, L., Atzwanger, K., 2014. Human habitat preferences. In: Voland, E., Grammer, K. (Eds.), Evolutionary Aesthetics. Springer, Berlin, pp. 279–294.

Seeley, W.W., Matthews, B.R., Crawford, R.K., Gorno-Tempini, M.L., Foti, D., Mackenzie, I.R., Miller, B.L., 2008. Unravelling Bolero: progressive aphasia, transmodal creativity and the right posterior neocorte. Brain, 131(Pt 1) 39–49.

Skamel, U., 2003. Beauty and sex appeal: sexual selection of aesthetic preferences. In: Voland, E., Grammer, K. (Eds.), Evolutionary Aesthetics. Springer, Berlin, pp. 174–200.

Slade, P.D., 1988. Body image in anorexia nervosa. Br. J. Psychiatr. 153 (52), 20–22.

Slade, P.D., Russell, G.F.M., 1973. Awareness of body dimensions in anorexia nervosa: cross-sectional and longitudinal studies. Psychol. Med. 3 (2), 188–199.

Summerfeldt, L.J., Gilbert, S.J., Reynolds, M., 2015. Incompleteness, aesthetic sensitivity, and the obsessive-compulsive need for symmetry. J. Behav. Ther. Exp. Psychiatry. 49, 141–149.

Thornhill, R., 2003. Darwinian aesthetics informs traditional aesthetics. In: Voland, E., Grammer, K. (Eds.), Evolutionary Aesthetics. Springer, Berlin, pp. 9–35.

Veale, D., Ennis, M., Lambrou, C., 2002. Possible association of body dysmorphic disorder with an occupation or education in art and design. Am. J. Psychiatr. 159 (10), 1788–1790.

Veale, D.M., Lambrou, C., 2002. The importance of aesthetics in body dysmorphic disorder. CNS Spectr. 7 (6), 429–431.

Veale, D., Ennis, M., Lambrou, C., 2002. Possible association of body dysmorphic disorder with an occupation or education in art and design. Am. J. Psychiatr. 159 (10), 1788–1790.

Zeki, S., 1998. Art and the brain. Daedalus 127 (2), 71–103.

VARIATIONS OF HUMAN NATURE

Chapter 20

The Expression of Disordered Personality

Chapter Outline

KEYWORDS

Personality
Personality disorder
Paranoid personality disorder
Schizoid personality disorder
Dissocial personality disorder
Emotionally unstable personality disorder
Histrionic personality disorder
Anankastic personality disorder
Anxious (avoidant) personality disorder
Dependent personality disorder

Summary

Personality is the unique way that an individual expresses themselves. It includes their characteristic gait, their mode of experiencing the world and reacting to it. Their typical affective responses, their conduct and moral attitude, what values guide them and what they do, what they create and how they act. Abnormalities of personality on the other hand are enduring patterns of experience and behaviour affecting cognition, affect, interpersonal functioning and impulse control that are inflexible, pervasive and lead to clinically significant impairment. It is important to emphasize that the types of abnormal personality currently described are at most tentative and inconclusive attempts to render in words complex aspects of human functioning. The categories have clinical utility but are problematic for many reasons including lack of reliability, validity and instability over time.

But the impressions and actions of human beings are not solely the result of their present circumstances, but the joint result of those circumstances and of the characters of the individuals: and the agencies which determine human character are so numerous, (nothing which has happened to the person throughout life being without its portion of influence), that in the aggregate they are never in any two cases exactly similar. Hence, even if our science of human nature were theoretically perfect, that is, if we could calculate any character as we can calculate the orbit of any planet, from given data; still, as the data are never all given, nor even precisely alike in different cases, we could neither make positive predictions, nor lay down universal propositions.

                              John Stuart Mill (1811)

In the preceding quote from a *System of Logic,* Mill states succinctly the difficulty of forming a theory of personality that is useful in clinical practice in *predicting* behaviour. Nonetheless, theories of personality abound. Jaspers' (1997) definition of personality is as good a place to start as any other definition:

We see the personality in the particular way an individual expresses himself, in the way he moves, how he experiences and reacts to situations, how he loves, grows jealous, how he conducts his life in general, what needs he has, what are his longings and aims, what are his ideals and how he shapes them, what values guide him and what he does, what he creates and how he acts. In short, personality is the term we give to the individually differing and characteristic totality of meaningful connections in any one psychic life.

There is an implicit but erroneous notion that a description of personality somehow captures all that there is to say about a person. Reflection makes obvious that it is impossible to describe the totality of any human being in a single, simple term. Furthermore, as Jaspers remarked, 'The personality as understood is not what an individual actually is but an empirical and inconclusive phenomenon' that is limited in its scope precisely because human beings are free to act in the world and 'at any moment freedom can have birth and give everything a different meaning'. Descriptions of personality, in other words, are tentative and fragile. The individual's life and choices are not fixed and predetermined by any description that we may have. Every individual has an infinite reality and potential. Our feeble attempts at description are mainly to make communication between practitioners efficient.

Attempts at classifying personality fall into two main categories: nomothetic and idiographic. The nomothetic approach assumes that human beings only vary to the degree in which they share certain traits or personality dimensions. On the other hand, the idiographic approach assumes that human beings are unique individuals and the theories here point to the characteristics that make individuals unique and distinctive. Sadly, there is a gulf between psychological personality theories such as that by figures such as Gordon Allport (1897–1967), Hans Eysenck (1916–97) and Raymond Cattell (1905–98) and the approach that is favoured by psychiatrists that deals predominantly with abnormalities of personality.

The term *personality disorder* is an abstraction built on several tenuous theories. It is an untidy concept, but it carries clinical usefulness. The way in which the term has been developed and its relationship with *neurosis* is dealt with elsewhere (Sims, 1983). The intention here is only to discuss the effects that different types of personality have on actions and behaviour. The clinician builds on a profile for personality disorder. This leads to a characteristic pattern of behaviour that allows us, to some extent, to predict their future actions and to describe what makes this individual different. The clinical designation of personality is purely descriptive and carries no theoretical implications, otherwise there is a logical flaw in describing personality type in terms of consistent behaviour and at the same time claiming the *type* accounts for definite patterns of behaviour. Acute and detailed observation of the characteristics of personality and its evaluation is a useful psychiatric skill that has, regrettably, been much neglected for many years.

These characteristics of behaviour, including the capacity for and nature of relationships with other people, are brought together to describe *traits* or *personality types*; obviously, to be clinically relevant these traits must have implications for the functioning of the individual. The distinction between *trait*, the predisposition associated with personality, and *state*, the current mental condition, is very important. These classifications of personality disorder, based on such lists of traits, were categorized by Schneider (1923) and more recently in *International Classification of Diseases* (10th revision [ICD-10]; World Health Organization, 1992) and in *Diagnostic and Statistical Manual of Mental Disorders* (5th edition [DSM-5]; American Psychiatric Association [APA], 2013). Certain characteristics have clinical significance, such as the degree to which the person is aware of the feelings and is sensitive to the judgements of other people. Abnormal personality is found when a personality trait considered to be clinically significant is present to either too small or too great an extent to conform statistically with the mass of mankind. The concepts of personality and personality disorder were discussed by Tantam (1988), and more recently personality disorder has been reviewed by Tyrer and Stein (1993). There are considerable problems with the descriptions of types of personality disorders. The most significant are the lack of specificity in the definitions of personality disorders, the excessive comorbidity among personality disorders, the questionable validity of the identified categories and the instability of these diagnostic terms over time (Skodol, 2012). Furthermore, it is recognized that part of the problem with the current classification system is the unsatisfactory nature of personality typologies and the need for an integration of dimensional thinking into how personality and personality disorder are conceptualized. This development in thinking about personality disorders is also drawing attention to the need to base discussions about personality disorder on what is understood about normal personality traits. This has led to an evaluation of the Five-Factor model of personality as a potential foundation for a theory of abnormal personality (Widiger et al., 2012). The Five-Factor model of personality includes neuroticism, extraversion, openness, agreeableness and conscientiousness as the relevant factors. The hope is that an integration of normal and abnormal personality within a common hierarchical structure would allow for a more precise and individualized description of personality structure for each individual (Widiger et al., 2012) but this hope is not widely shared (Paris, 2013).

A different approach to the classification of personality disorders that is starting to gain traction is that proposed by Crawford et al. (2011). They emphasize the point that categorical methods that utilize personality disorder typologies do not take account of the wide variations in terms of personality disturbance and associated disturbance. They emphasize how prevalent personality disorders are within the adult population, estimating it to be approximately 10%, and that it influences response to treatment of mental disorder as well as the long-term outcome of disorders (Tyrer and Evans, 2000). Their proposal is to do away

with the current personality disorder typologies and to classify all personality disorders along a single dimension ranging from normal personality on one end to severe personality disorder at the other (Tyrer et al., 2015). The intention seems to be to replace typologies by five dimensions of severity along five nomothetic trait domains including asocial, emotionally unstable, obsessional (anankastic), anxious/dependent and dissocial groups and additionally to provide a simple algorithm for clinical use (Tyrer et al., 2011). There is little doubt that there are serious problems with personality typologies but whether a dimensional approach as proposed will solve the problems is yet to be determined.

Abnormality of personality at present is probably best described in terms of trait. What then is *personality disorder*? Here Schneider's definition is a good starting point: 'Personality disorder is present when that abnormality of personality causes either the patient himself or other people to suffer' (Schneider, 1958). Alternatively, from *DSM-5* (APA, 2013): 'An enduring pattern of inner experience and behaviour that deviates markedly from the expectations of the individual's culture'. This pattern is manifested in two or more of the following areas: cognition, affectivity, interpersonal functioning or impulse control. The enduring pattern is inflexible and pervasive across a broad range of personal and social situations. The enduring pattern leads to clinically significant distress or impairment in social, occupational or other important areas of functioning. The pattern is stable and of long duration, and its onset can be traced back at least to adolescence or early childhood.

- A highly conscientious and meticulous post office sorter was promoted to foreman sorter after many years' reliable service. The appropriate response might have been to be pleased at the increased pay and to spend the first week's increment before receiving it. However, this man was fearful about the promotion. He worried that he might not be able to cope with the job, that he might not be able to persuade the men in his charge to sort letters to his own high standards, that he would not be able to mix socially with his superiors and equals, that he would make a fool of himself and that other people would laugh at him. He became miserable, anxious and lacking confidence, and he had to stop work. Because of his abnormal, obsessional (anankastic) personality, he responded to the stress of promotion by becoming acutely distressed and developing depressive symptoms.

- A bland and plausible confidence trickster extracted without compunction the means of subsistence from an elderly widow. Their psychopathic blunting of appreciation for the way others would experience their behaviour and their consequent feelings resulted in them causing suffering to others.

Personality abnormality is a part of the individual's constitution. Whether it manifests as personality disorder depends to a considerable extent on social circumstances. A highly abnormal personality that in one situation may be considered criminal psychopathy and be possessed by a convicted prisoner, in another situation will be the driving force in a highly successful and relatively creative political revolutionary. Personality in an individual cannot be divorced from its social and cultural setting. Indeed, some have argued that the personality disorder constructs that we currently utilize are derived from and calibrated against Western middle-class cultural norms (Mulder, 2012).

Having ascertained whether personality disorder is present, its type should be categorized using an accepted system. However, a caution is needed here. It is often extremely difficult to fit people into arbitrary categories of personality, and the whole topic of classification is still highly unsatisfactory. It may be much better to use a few descriptive sentences for the personality, and probably it is best to combine description with categorization. The systems used in *ICD-10* and *DSM-5* can be recommended; the typological classification of personality disorder introduced by Tyrer and Alexander (1979) was also satisfactory but has not been widely used. Table 20.1 is a composite of these classifications. They all start from the same bases: the definition of personality, the evaluation of abnormality and the observation of certain influential and regularly occurring traits. Tyrer and Alexander's five discrete categories of abnormal personality followed from a cluster analysis of personality data and is therefore a simplification of *ICD-9* (World Health Organization, 1977), which itself was based originally on Schneider. *DSM-IV* and *DSM-5* have certain different terms that have proved important in American psychiatry, although they are not necessarily found helpful elsewhere. These include *narcissistic* personality disorder, which is discussed later in this chapter; *avoidant,* which is similar to *anxious* personality disorder in *ICD-10;* and *schizotypal* personality disorder, which *ICD-10* classifies with *schizophrenia, schizotypical* and *delusional disorders.*

TABLE 20.1 **Comparison of Personality Types**		
Tyrer and Alexander(1979)[a]	**ICD-10**[b]	**DSM-IV**[c]
	F60.0 Paranoid	Paranoid
Schizoid	F60.1 Schizoid	Schizoid
Sociopathic		Schizotypal
	F60.2 Dissocial	Antisocial
	F60.3 Emotionally unstable	
	.30 Impulsive	
	.31 Borderline	Borderline
	F60.4 Histrionic	Histrionic
Anankastic	F60.5 Anankastic	Obsessive compulsive
Dysthymic	F60.6 Anxious	Avoidant
Passive dependent	F60.7 Dependent	Dependent
	F60.8 'Other'	Narcissistic

[a]Tyrer and Alexander (1979).
[b]World Health Organization (1992).
[c]American Psychiatric Association (1994).

The following descriptions are based on the categorization found in *ICD-10*. It is important to realize that these categories are not mutually exclusive: mixed personality types are more frequent than a single personality type in pure form. Readers in the United Kingdom or in countries influenced by British psychiatry should be aware of an ongoing source of confusion perpetuated by recent discussion of the legal and administrative aspects concerning 'dangerous people with severe personality disorder' (Mullen, 1999; Haddock et al., 2001). In descriptive psychopathology, this debate is almost entirely concerned with dissocial personality disorder, but those taking part in the discussion tend to ignore other personality types, thus causing confusion for the assessment and classification of those with other personality disorders such as anankastic or anxious avoidant personality disorder. This can result in inappropriate treatment or lack of treatment being administered by mental health professionals and unjustifiable stigmatization being experienced by the sufferers.

Paranoid Personality Disorder

The essential feature of this type of personality disorder is self-reference, the proper psychiatric sense of the word *paranoid;* such people misinterpret the words and actions of others as having special significance for, and being directed against, themselves. Theoretically, self-referent ideas could imply that others are always noticing them in an admiring and benevolent way; in practice, such people would not consult a psychiatrist and those presenting in psychiatry have ideas of persecution. They mistrust other people and are very sensitive and suspicious, believing that others are against them and that what they say about them is derogatory. There are active and passive types of paranoid personality disorder; both types feel that others are 'getting at them' but their response differs.

The active paranoid personality manifests suspiciousness and is hostile and untrusting. Such a person is quarrelsome, litigious, quick to take offence, intensely suspicious and sometimes violent; they will go to enormous lengths to defend their rights or to address real or imagined injustices. They are extremely vigilant and tenacious in taking precautions against any perceived threat. This is the sort of person who will march fearlessly across a field of young corn because they see there is a public right of way on the map and the farmer has no right to violate this. They repudiate blame and may be regarded by others as devious, scheming and secretive. Such a person is intensely jealous of what they regard as their own belongings, which may be people as well as objects, and they spend a lot of time planning to 'get their own back'. They may be self-important and fanatical. Morbid jealousy may be shown, and such a person may be involved in acts of violence because of imagined injustice. Such a personality may find creative expression in social and political life but is likely to be very destructive within the family. A patient commented on this ruefully, 'I have scarcely talked to my wife for the last 10 years', because of his succession of court cases against those with whom he came into contact.

A person with passive paranoid personality faces the world from a position of submission and humiliation. They assume that whatever happens to them will be damaging. Like the active type, they are suspicious, sensitive and self-referent and misconstrue circumstances and other people. They believe that other people will dislike them and that they will ultimately let them down. However, they accept 'the slings and arrows of outrageous fortune' passively, bowing to the inevitable; they are vulnerable and frequently feel humiliated and unable to initiate any assertive activity. Other people tend to take advantage of them, thus fulfilling their pessimistic expectations.

A frequent manifestation of psychopathology within the context of paranoid personality is the presence of an overvalued idea (see Chapter 8). This, alternatively described as a fixed idea (*idée fixe*), is a belief that might seem reasonable both to the patient and to other people. However, it comes to completely dominate the person's thinking and life, and, instead of testing its validity, they tend to consider that every circumstance of life substantiates it; it becomes the basis for action that is sometimes aggressive or self-destructive. It is quite distinct phenomenologically from both *delusion* and *obsessional ideas.*

Schizoid Personality Disorder

This personality disorder is characterized by a lack of need for, and defect in, the capacity to form social relationships. Such people show withdrawal from social involvement, emotional coolness and detachment and indifference to the praise, criticism and feelings of other people.

These individuals are 'loners' with a disinclination to mix, and they appear somewhat aloof. They lack tender feelings, have little interest in sexual experience and are not interested in the company of others. They are not depressed in mood, nor are they shy or sensitive towards other people, but they are solitary and prefer not to be involved in social occupations. Their interests and hobbies usually tend to increase their isolation from other people, as they are more interested in things, objects and machines.

Close relatives may complain of the subject's emotional detachment, an inability to inspire strong feelings in others, a lack of any real sense of pleasure, oddness and eccentricity and callous indifference to others' suffering. In a follow-up of former schizoid subjects, they were found to use psychological constructs less than a control group, and this pointed to the schizoid individuals' lack of empathy (Chick et al., 1979).

Those with schizoid personality and poor social adjustment have been considered more likely to develop schizophrenia. In a large study based on the previous personality assessment of 50,054 male recruits to the Swedish army, aspects of personality were found to be risk factors for the subsequent development of schizophrenia (Malmberg et al., 1998).

Dissocial Personality Disorder

The essential, phenomenological abnormality of dissocial (asocial, antisocial or psychopathic) personality disorder is primarily one of empathy. There is a defect in the capacity to appreciate other people's feelings, especially in comprehending how other people feel about the consequences of this person's own actions. This personality type, or abnormality, includes those people considered to suffer from psychopathic personality within the meaning of the Mental Health Act, 1983 (Bluglass, 1983). A normal person is prevented most of the time, by shame or by their capacity for empathy, from carrying out unpleasant actions towards other people. They do not want to be disliked and feel keenly how it would be passively to be the recipient

of such behaviour. It is this inability to feel for themself the discomfort that others experience as a result of their antisocial activities that appears to be absent in the psychopath. Despite such comprehensive descriptions as that of Cleckley (1941), in *The Mask of Sanity*, and others, there are still considerable doubts as to whether this personality type forms a distinct category, and if it does, whether it should be considered within or outside psychiatry. This is succinctly expressed by Wooton (1959): psychopaths are 'extremely selfish persons and no one knows what makes them so'.

The confusion of terminology is explained partly by the varied nature of presentation; partly by the conflicting desires of professionals not to stigmatize and also not to cast blame on those who cannot control their actions; and partly by the requirements of classification for different professional groups and settings—lawyers, criminologists, psychiatrists, psychologists and so on. A comprehensive account of diagnostic issues, developmental history and methods of treatment is to be found in Dolan and Coid (1993).

The concept of *moral derangement* was introduced by Benjamin Rush (1812), and of *moral insanity* by Prichard (1835), who considered this to occur among criminals who showed loss of feeling, of control, and of ethical sense, equivalent to mental disease but at a different level. It is important to stress that not all psychopaths are criminal, nor are all criminals psychopathic. Henderson (1939) described *creative, inadequate* and *aggressive psychopathy*, citing Lawrence of Arabia as an example of a creative psychopath. Dissocial personality disorder, with conspicuous lack of conscience and human sympathy, is found more often in males than in females.

This personality disorder should not be diagnosed unless the subject is older than 18 years. However, in childhood or adolescence, many of the following may have been demonstrated by the person subsequently diagnosed as dissocial: truancy, expulsion or suspension from school for misbehaviour, delinquency, running away from home, persistent lying, repeated casual sexual intercourse, repeated drunkenness, substance abuse, theft, vandalism, school performance below expectation, repeated violation of rules at home and school and fighting. Of course, such behaviour may occur in normal children, especially with social deprivation, but it is their persistence and the presence of so many of these signs of disturbed behaviour that may predict subsequent psychopathy. There is also debate concerning the manifestation of attention deficit disorder in childhood and subsequent antisocial behaviour in young adult life (Hinshaw, 1994).

Such a person may be meaninglessly cruel, callous, aggressive and emotionally cold, rejecting social norms and showing irresponsibility in their relationships. They are often unable to maintain consistency at work, with frequent unemployment, changes of occupation, absenteeism and poor relationships. Similarly, there are unsatisfactory relationships with sexual partners, with a history of several separations or divorces, promiscuity with heterosexual or homosexual preferences, desertion and repeated marital arguments. Poor parenting results in conspicuous physical and psychological problems among their children, and the individual's aggressiveness may result in child abuse with nonaccidental injury. As they age, they are less likely to be in conflict with the law and less likely to be violent, but their affectionless inability to see the consequences of their actions and the way other people suffer because of them remains destructive within the family and in other institutions. There is a failure to accept society's norms as regards social behaviour, drugs and alcohol and personal property. A lengthy criminal record is frequently seen because they fail to learn from their experiences (Craft, 1966). Such a person may feel miserable and even suicidal when discovered in an unacceptable act, but this does not amount to the normal sense of feeling guilt. There is a failure to identify with the victim.

The definition of psychopathy proposed by Whiteley (1975) is as follows. The psychopath is an individual:

1. who persistently behaves in a way that is not in accord with the accepted social norms of the culture or times in which they live;
2. who appears to be unaware that their behaviour is seriously at fault; and
3. whose abnormality cannot be readily explained as resulting from the 'madness' we commonly recognize nor from 'badness' alone.

Failure to plan ahead and failure to honour obligations, for example, matrimonial or financial commitments, are repeated. There is a disregard for truth and also for safety, both for the individual themself and for others.

Emotionally Unstable Personality Disorder

IMPULSIVE TYPE

This personality disorder is not often encountered. The essential feature is liability to intemperate and uncontrolled outbursts of mood, most frequently violent anger but occasionally inconsolable grief, extreme anxiety or uproarious hilarity. It is usually aggressiveness that brings individuals with this disorder to the attention of the psychiatrist; with very slight provocation, they may have become irritable and on occasions violent. They are treated with extreme circumspection by other people, and their ill humour therefore becomes reinforced as it enables them to get their own way. They may exploit other people's fears of them to achieve their objectives, for example, the arbitrarily violent husband whose wife is completely dominated by him through fear. Such personalities are disruptive and unpopular.

Those with this personality structure behave normally for most of the time and only occasionally explode in impulsive irritability, which is more common in younger people and may appear in either sex (Snaith and Taylor, 1985). In the system of classification advocated by Tyrer and Alexander, this personality type is not retained as distinct but combined with paranoid and asocial personality to form a category of *sociopathic personality disorder.*

BORDERLINE TYPE

This very confused diagnostic term has been used variously to describe a group of apparently neurotically disturbed patients who became psychotic while undergoing psychoanalysis; an enduring, unstable and vulnerable personality structure; and a group of patients who 'almost' had schizophrenia (Anonymous, 1986). It is considered that at least five of the following should be present for the diagnosis to be made (*DSM-5*; APA, 2013):

- frantic efforts to avoid real or imagined abandonment;
- a pattern of unstable and intense interpersonal relationships;
- identity disturbance in areas such as self-image, gender identity or long-term goals;
- impulsivity or unpredictability in areas that are potentially self-damaging;

- recurrent suicidal behaviour, gestures or threats or self-mutilating behaviour;
- affective instability due to a marked reactivity of mood;
- chronic feelings of emptiness;
- inappropriate intense anger or difficulty in controlling anger; and
- transient, stress-related paranoid ideation or severe dissociative symptoms.

Although psychodynamically inclined psychiatrists have used this category extensively, there appears to be no phenomenological thread linking the very different criteria that are required for its diagnosis. Carrasco and Lecic-Tosevski (2000) have described it as the most controversial of all personality disorders and 'best understood as a heterogeneous syndrome manifested by ego-syntonic affective instability and impulsivity (behavioural dyscontrol) and propensity to cognitive-perceptual distortions in the context of chronically unstable interpersonal relationships'. Both genetic factors and early childhood adversity are implicated in its aetiology with implications for the neural circuits that regulate affect, behaviour and cognition (Hooley et al., 2012).

Histrionic Personality Disorder

The word *histrionic* is derived from 'playing on the stage'; it is a better term than *hysterical* for this disorder, which is characterized by theatrical behaviour, craving for attention and excitement, excessive reaction to minor events and outbursts of mood, especially temper tantrums. In summarizing the descriptions of 22 authors, De Alarcon (1973) found the greatest agreement for hysterical personality disorder in the following features: histrionic behaviour, egocentricity, emotional lability, excitability, dependency, suggestibility and seductiveness.

Characteristic of the disturbance of histrionic personality is the nature of relationships with limited ability to experience profound affect and communicate such feelings. There is a shallowness and lability of emotion, and this is seen by others as lacking in genuineness, even though they are superficially charming—'the life and soul of the party'. They form excellent and rapid acquaintanceships with new people, but they have great difficulty sustaining a close long-term, mutually rewarding, exclusive relationship.

Mood is fluctuating and inconsistent, and they display towards other people a craving for attention, affection and appreciation. They are seen as egocentric, self-indulgent and inconsiderate of others. There is often extreme but superficial involvement with many different people in a short space of time, and such a person is seen as being manipulative, vain and demanding; the manipulativeness is often ineffectual and self-destructive. They are often superficially found very attractive and achieve their short-term goals while being unable to sustain long-term relationships; for instance, marriage frequently ends in divorce. They may be dependent and helpless, constantly seeking reassurance and the approval of others. Gestures of self-harm, dissociative conversion symptoms and abuse of alcohol and other drugs are common. Depressive symptoms are also frequently encountered, especially when a breakdown of relationships occurs. In a hospital study of those with histrionic personality disorder, Thompson (1980) found 83% of subjects to be female; there was a clear association with depression, drug overdoses, self-mutilation, abuse of alcohol and a history of criminality and sometimes violence. Tyrer and Alexander do not regard this as a distinct personality disorder but combine it with dependent personality disorder in a category of *passive dependence*.

Anankastic Personality Disorder

Anankastic personality traits in moderate amount are valuable in society and for the success of the individual; they are frequently observed in professionals such as lawyers or doctors. However, when these are developed to an abnormal extent and interfere with the person's functioning, personality disorder is present and is characterized by perfectionism, rigidity, sensitivity, indecisiveness, a lack of capacity to express strongly felt emotion and excessive conscientiousness. The anankast's pervading sense of insecurity is associated with extreme self-doubt and feelings of sensitivity concerning how other people view them.

Perfectionism and excessive attention to detail interfere with the overall grasp of subjects or situations. There is gross preoccupation with rules, efficiency, trivial details, procedures and protocol. One patient was making lists of the lists she had previously set herself. She could not throw away a list until everything on it had been completed and, as some of the items on the lists were things that she wished to remind herself to do regularly, she was accumulating such an ever-increasing number of lists as to be unmanageable. Efficiency and perfection are aimed at, but the excessively detailed manner in which the attempt to achieve them is made undermines the possibility of success. Often, extreme orderliness in one area of life results in chaos in another, for example, the medical practitioner who kept the top of his desk in immaculate tidiness but tipped all his case notes and other papers into the back of his car.

Rigidity in patterns of behaviour is characteristic. The individual values accuracy and thoroughness highly and respects other obsessional people for these qualities. They tend to keep fixed times and live to a regular programme, altered only with the greatest misgivings. These constraints are extended to other people in that they insist that they submit to their way of doing things. There is often a lack of awareness of the feelings in others evoked by their behaviour. This anankastic control of other people is typified by Mrs Ogmore-Pritchard in Dylan Thomas' *Under Milk Wood* (1954), who imposes on her dead husband the dictum 'I must put my pyjamas in the drawer marked pyjamas … I must take my cold bath which is good for me'.

The anankast is extremely sensitive to the criticism, real or suspected, of other people; the slightest censure is 'taken very much to heart'. This awareness of other people's opinion makes them a conformist, not prepared to step out of line, always wishing 'to keep up with the Joneses'. They are rigid, formal and self-controlled, not only in their public business but also at home and with their more intimate relationships. Insecurity about their abilities and their relationships makes the anankast indecisive. They doubt their own capacity and only too easily find themself agreeing in secret with those who criticize him. They vacillate and have great difficulty in making choices, constantly looking at situations from different points of view, 'weighing up the pros and cons'. They often find themself in a position of ambivalence and may overcompensate for this indecisiveness by making arbitrary decisions that then become immutable on

insufficient evidence, or they may compensate for their legalistic rigidity by flaunting the law ostentatiously. Even in this, their basic perfectionism is still manifest. The anankast finds the initiation or completion of any activity difficult, but hard work is highly prized, and they are therefore prepared to carry on the middle part of the task indefinitely.

There is a need for formality, and their feelings of sensitivity about how other people view them results in restricted ability to express tender emotion. They are unduly conventional, serious and formal. Stinginess may be shown both with money and with the expression of feelings. Such a person actually experiences strong affect but is quite unable to express this appropriately towards other people.

The different facets of the anankastic personality disorder are, of course, interlocked. As traits of personality, they are seen frequently, not least among members of the medical profession. However, developed as a personality disorder, this way of life may be incapacitating, especially the indecisiveness and inability to express strong emotion. Depression, obsessive compulsive disorder, eating disorder and hypochondriasis are not uncommonly associated with this abnormality of personality (Samuels and Costa, 2012).

Anxious (Avoidant) Personality Disorder

This is a disorder of *trait,* whereas anxiety disorder is a disorder of *state* (see Chapter 17). There is often free-floating anxiety that is exacerbated by any overt predisposing cause. Such people often find the public side of life, for example, at work, very much more stressful than the private side, within the family. *Trait* anxiety is present when the development of the individual's personality results in some level of abnormal anxiety being a persistent background part of their constitution (Sims and Snaith, 1988); this could alternatively be described as anxious temperament or anxiety-prone personality. Such people describe themselves as 'born worriers'.

This personality disorder is characterized by persistent and pervasive feelings of terror and apprehension; a belief that one is socially inept, unattractive or inferior; excessive preoccupation with criticism and rejection by others; hesitancy in new social relationships; restriction of lifestyle because of the need for security; and avoidance of those social situations that might provoke disapproval (*ICD-10*; World Health Organization, 1992).

Dependent Personality Disorder

The dependent personality is characterized by feelings of inadequacy concerning self and dependence on other people. There is gross lack of self-confidence, initiative and drive. Such a person is unable to react to the changing demands of life and allows other people, sometimes one other person, to assume responsibility for major areas of life. They may function reasonably well and appear inconspicuous when carried along through life by a dominant close relationship. However, when external stress occurs they lack confidence, are unable to cope and crave long-term support and encouragement from relatives, a close friend, their family doctor, their social worker, their minister, their employer or their surrounding social organizations. They may, for example, flourish in the armed forces but be unable to adjust to civilian life.

Such people tend to go through life with one dominant dependent relationship; for a man, this may be initially his mother and subsequently his wife, who takes over his mother's role. Crises resulting in psychiatric referral may occur when a parent dies or becomes incapable, his marriage breaks down, he loses his job, after detection in crime or after physical illness. It is usually only after such situations that a person with this type of personality disorder comes to the attention of the caring professions. Dependence amounts to passive compliance with the aims and demands of the more dominant partner. There is a lack of vigour in maintaining aims and goals and in attempting to achieve these. They may describe themselves as depressed, but it is more a feeling of inertia and an inability to cope with their problems than the symptoms of affective disorder. Originally, this personality disorder was conceptualized as arising out of problematic early parent–child relationships but pathologic dependency is now seen as stemming from a perception of the 'self' as weak accompanied by the belief that other people are comparatively competent and confident. As a result of this the individual becomes preoccupied with obtaining and maintaining relationships with potential caregivers (Bornstein, 2012).

Persistent Mood Disorders

In the *ICD-9* (World Health Organization, 1977), these conditions were classified as disorder of personality. However, in the *ICD-10*, they have been listed as a sub-category of affective disorders because they are genetically related to mood disorders and sometimes respond to the same methods of treatment. They are retained in this chapter because they conform with the psychopathology of personality disorders. Akiskal (1993) has made a convincing case for depressive personality to be returned to the generic category of personality disorders rather than being classified with *axis 1 mood (affective) disorders*. There is a persistent lifelong abnormality of mood, not amounting to illness, as opposed to those reactive or endogenous disturbances of affect that are of shorter duration and are regarded as illness. The most frequent types of affective personality disorder show excessive lability of mood or persistent depressive stance towards life. Other abnormalities of personality may occur, such as persistent hypomania, but these rarely present to the psychiatrist.

Those with *cyclothymia* show marked fluctuations of mood. For instance, for a day or a week they may be optimistic, energetic, creative and garrulous, then for a period they may become gloomy, morose, taciturn and unable to turn themselves to any useful activity. These cycles may be linked to other biological rhythms such as the menstrual cycle; they may, however, appear out of the blue, apparently unprovoked. A premorbid cyclothymic personality is thought to predispose to manic-depressive psychosis. Certainly, Goodwin and Jamison (1990), in a study of manic-depressive illness and creativity, found that among poets especially there was an excess of cyclothymic personality, depressive illness and suicide.

Dysthymia is manifested by all-pervasive and permanent gloom and apprehension. It leads to the diagnostic quandary: 'is this depressive state or depressive trait?' Such people are usually gentle and sensitive; they take themselves and their activities seriously; they are often safety-conscious and hypochondriacal in disposition. An acquaintance with this personality structure coined aphorisms that revealed his mental state, such as 'there is no situation in life so bad as to be incapable of further deterioration' or 'every silver lining has its cloud'.

Other Personality Disorders

DSM-5 (APA, 2013) includes two other personality disorders. They are briefly described here for completeness.

NARCISSISTIC PERSONALITY DISORDER

This is categorized by a grandiose sense of self-importance or uniqueness; preoccupation with fantasies of unlimited success, power, brilliance, beauty or ideal love; an exhibitionistic need for constant attention and admiration; indifference, anger or humiliation in response to criticism or indifference from others and characteristic disturbances in interpersonal relationships, such as feelings of entitlement to special favours, taking advantage of other people, relationships with others that alternate between the extremes of over-idealization and devaluation and lack of empathy.

AVOIDANT PERSONALITY DISORDER

This personality disorder is, in fact, close to the anxious personality disorder of *ICD-10*; it is characterized by excessive sensitivity to rejection, humiliation or shame. There is unwillingness to enter into a relationship unless the person receives strong guarantees of uncritical acceptance. There is social withdrawal despite a need for affection and acceptance, and the person has very low self-esteem, devaluing their own achievements, and is very aware of their personal shortcomings. Such people are exquisitely sensitive to the way they believe others will react to them.

In *DSM-5*, the helpful notion of three *clusters* of personality types is based on descriptive similarities. Cluster A includes *paranoid, schizoid* and *schizotypal personality disorders*. In cluster B are *antisocial, borderline, histrionic* and *narcissistic personality disorders*. Cluster C contains *avoidant, dependent* and *obsessive compulsive personality disorders*. In practice, of course, patients may show features from different clusters, and the validity of this subclassification is still being questioned.

Why is a text on psychopathology concerned with personality classification and disorder? The accurate observation and delineation of personality characteristics is valuable in clinical practice for diagnosis, prognosis and the rational planning of treatment. The skills of a trained psychopathologist are ideally suited to the observation of consistent personality traits and forming an opinion unprejudiced by preconceived theoretical considerations.

REFERENCES

Anonymous, 1986. Management of borderline personality disorders [leading article]. Lancet 2, 846–847.

Akiskal, H.S., 1993. Proposal for a depressive personality (temperament). In: Tyrer, P., Stein, G. (Eds.), Personality Disorder Reviewed. Gaskell, London.

American Psychiatric Association, 1994. Diagnostic and Statistical Manual of Mental Disorders, fourth ed. American Psychiatric Association, Washington, DC.

American Psychiatric Association, 2013. Diagnostic and Statistical Manual of Mental Disorders, fifth ed. American Psychiatric Association, Washington, DC.

Bluglass, R.S., 1983. A Guide to the Mental Health Act, 1983. Churchill Livingstone, Edinburgh.

Bornstein, R.F., 2012. Dependent personality disorder. In: Widiger, T.A. (Ed.), The Oxford Handbook of Personality Disorders. Oxford University Press, Oxford.

Carrasco, J.L., Lecic-Tosevski, D., 2000. Specific types of personality disorder. In: Gelder, M., López-Ibor, J.J., Andreasen, N.C. (Eds.), New Oxford Textbook of Psychiatry. Oxford University Press, Oxford.

Chick, J., Waterhouse, L., Wolff, S., 1979. Psychological construing in schizoid children grown up. Br. J. Psychiatry 135, 425–430.

Cleckley, H.M., 1941. The Mask of Sanity. Kingston, London.

Craft, M., 1966. Psychopathic Disorders. Pergamon Press, Oxford.

Crawford, M.J., Koldobsky, N., Mulder, R., Tyrer, P., 2011. Classifying personality disorder according to severity. J. Personal. Disord. 25, 321–330.

De Alarcon, R.D., 1973. Hysteria and hysterical personality disorder. Psychiatr. Q. 47, 258–275.

Dolan, B., Coid, J., 1993. Psychopathic and Antisocial Personality Disorders: Treatment and Research Issues. Gaskell, London.

Goodwin, F.K., Jamison, K.R., 1990. Manic-Depressive Illness. Oxford University Press, New York.

Haddock, A., Snowden, P., Dolan, M., Parker, J., Rees, H., 2001. Managing dangerous people with severe personality disorder: a survey of forensic psychiatrists' opinions. BJPsych Bull. 25, 293–296.

Henderson, D.K., 1939. Psychopathic States. Norton, New York.

Hinshaw, S.P., 1994. Attention Deficits and Hyperactivity in Children. Sage, Thousand Oaks, CA.

Hooley, J.M., Cole, S.H., Gironde, S., 2012. Borderline personality disorder. In: Widiger, T.A. (Ed.), The Oxford Handbook of Personality Disorders. Oxford University Press, Oxford.

Jaspers, K., 1997. General Psychopathology (J. Hoenig, M.W. Hamilton, Trans). The Johns Hopkins University Press, Baltimore.

Malmberg, A., Lewis, G., David, A., Allebeck, P., 1998. Premorbid adjustment and personality in people with schizophrenia. Br. J. Psychiatry 172, 308–313.

Mill, J.S., 1811. third ed. A System of Logic, vol. II. John W. Parker, London.

Mulder, R.T., 2012. Cultural aspects of personality disorder. In: Widiger, T.A. (Ed.), The Oxford Handbook of Personality Disorders. Oxford University Press, Oxford.

Mullen, P.E., 1999. Dangerous people with severe personality disorder. Br. Med. J. 319, 1146–1147.

Paris, J., 2013. The Intelligent Clinician's Guide to the DSM-5. Oxford University Press, Oxford.

Prichard, J.C., 1835. A Treatise on Insanity and Other Disorders Affecting the Mind. Sherwood, Gilbert and Piper, London.

Rush, B., 1812. Medical Inquiries and Observations upon the Diseases of the Mind. Kimber and Richardson, Philadelphia.

Samuels, J., Costa, P.T., 2012. Obsessive-compulsive personality disorder. In: Widiger, T.A. (Ed.), The Oxford Handbook of Personality Disorders. Oxford University Press, Oxford.

Schneider, K., 1923. Psychopathic Personalities. 1958. Cassell, London.

Schneider, K., 1958. Clinical Psychopathology, fifth ed. Grune and Stratton, New York, p. 1959.

Skodol, A.E., 2012. Diagnosis and DSM-5: work in progress. In: Widiger, T.A. (Ed.), The Oxford Handbook of Personality Disorders. Oxford University Press, Oxford.

Sims, A.C.P., 1983. Neurosis in Society. Macmillan, Basingstoke.

Sims, A., Snaith, R., 1988. Anxiety in Clinical Practice. John Wiley, Chichester.

Snaith, R.P., Taylor, C.M., 1985. Irritability: definition, assessment and associated factors. Br. J. Psychiatry 147, 127–136.

Tantam, D., 1988. Personality disorders. In: Granville-Grossman, K. (Ed.), Recent Advances in Clinical Psychiatry, vol. 6. Churchill Livingstone, Edinburgh.

Thomas, D., 1954. Under Milk Wood. Dent, London.

Thompson, D.J., 1980. A Comprehensive Study of Hysterical Personality Disorder. MSc thesis, University of Manchester.

Tyrer, P., Alexander, J., 1979. Classification of personality disorder. Br. J. Psychiatry 135, 163–167.

Tyrer, P., Crawford, M., Mulder, R., et al., 2011. The rationale for the reclassification of personality disorder in the 11th revision of the International Classification of Diseases. Personal. Ment. Health 5, 246–259.

Tyrer, P., Evans, K., 2000. Personality disorders. Principles of Medical Biology 14, 451–461.

Tyrer, P., Reed, G.M., Crawford, M.J., 2015. Classification, assessment, prevalence, and effect of personality disorder. Lancet 385, 717–726.

Tyrer, P., Stein, G., 1993. Personality Disorder Reviewed. Gaskell, London.

Whiteley, J.S., 1975. The psychopath and his treatment. In: Silverstone, T., Barraclough, B. (Eds.), Contemporary Psychiatry. Headley Brothers, Ashford.

Widiger, T.A., Samuel, D.B., Mullins-Sweatt, S., Gore, W.L., Crego, C., 2012. An integration of normal and abnormal personality structure: the five-factor model. In: Widiger, T.A. (Ed.), The Oxford Handbook of Personality Disorders. Oxford University Press, Oxford.

Wooton, B.F., 1959. Social Science and Social Pathology. Allen and Unwin, London.

World Health Organization, 1977. International Statistical Classification of Diseases, Injuries and Causes of Death, Ninth Revision. World Health Organization, Geneva.

World Health Organization, 1992. The ICD-10 Classification of Mental and Behavioural Disorders: Clinical Description and Diagnostic Guidelines. World Health Organization, Geneva.

DIAGNOSIS

Chapter 21

Psychopathology and Diagnosis

Chapter Outline

KEYWORDS

Diagnosis
Health

Summary

Diagnosis allows the naming, defining and identification of a singular malady so that it can become an object for consideration, comparison, explanation and control. It is therefore self-evident that the diagnostic process is fundamental to the practice of psychiatry. The importance and relevance of psychopathology is that it is the constellation of abnormal phenomena that are elicited by the clinical interview, reinforced by the phenomenological approach, that constitute psychiatric syndromes. In other words, psychopathology is the foundation upon which clinical psychiatry is built.

'There's glory for you!' 'I don't know what you mean by "glory",' Alice said. 'I meant, there's a nice knock-down argument for you!' 'But "glory" doesn't mean "a nice knock-down argument",' Alice objected. 'When I use a word,' Humpty Dumpty said in a rather scornful tone, 'it means just what I choose it to mean, – neither more nor less.'

Lewis Carroll, Through the Looking Glass (1872)

Diagnosis is much more than a word plucked out of the air and pinned on to a hapless 'patient'. It conveys meaning about the antecedents of the present state, about other conditions that are similar and, most important of all, about what is likely to happen in the future and, therefore, what should be done about it. Diagnosis is a means of communication between doctors; it should encompass a full formulation (see Chapter 2) rather than just a single word used in an idiosyncratic manner.

The importance of making a diagnosis and the range of diagnoses are as great in psychiatry as in the rest of medicine; the conceptual differences between different diagnostic categories are actually greater, as *mental disorders* include situational, social, emotional and psychological disturbance as well as physical illness. Understandably, most of the medical illnesses that have been described are based on signs or symptoms; this is true also for psychiatry. There is therefore a very close association between the observation and classification of 'symptoms in the mind' (Burton, 1621) and psychiatric diagnosis.

The importance with which diagnosis is regarded in psychiatry has developed alongside the introduction of effective remedies for many conditions. There has been a substantial change in the attitude of psychiatrists since Stengel wrote in 1959 that there was 'almost general dissatisfaction with the state of psychiatric classification, national and international'. Much of the progress made has arisen directly from the more careful application of descriptive psychopathology, for instance, Kendell (1975). Schwartz and Wiggins (1987) have shown that to make a diagnosis an experienced clinician uses a mechanism of *typification:* 'This more fundamental capacity to recognize various mental disorders arises, not through mastering conceptual definitions, but rather through directly encountering individual patients who manifest these disorders. Through such direct encounters we learn the typical forms of the various mental disorders. We learn what is distinctive to each condition and how to distinguish these conditions from one another'. This process of 'typification' seeks to recognize what is emblematic of different conditions, what is unusual but yet representative, and what is untypical and so highly unusual as to be uncharacteristic. Thus the detailed examination of psychopathologic functions that forms the substance of this text is a prerequisite to this, the first step for clinical diagnosis in psychiatry.

Abnormal phenomena, then, are the foundation of the diagnostic process. Diagnosis allows the naming, defining and identification of a singular malady so that it can become an object for consideration, comparison, explanation and control (Sadler, 2004).

In general medicine, diagnosis is based on the complete clinical process: detailed history taking, examination of the patient and carrying out appropriate special investigations. This is true also for psychiatry. However, because of the limitations of its subject, this book does not deal with physical examination nor with physical (radiologic, laboratory) or psychological (psychometric) investigations.

Concepts of Health and Psychopathology

The late Peter Sedgwick (1981) made the important point that 'disease is a human invention … there are no illnesses or diseases in nature', hence the quotation at the beginning of this chapter. He rightly pointed out that human beings describe potato blight as a disease solely because they want to grow potatoes: 'if man wished to cultivate parasites (rather than potatoes) there would be no "blight" but simply the necessary foddering of the parasite crop'. Sedgwick claimed that it was the human social meaning attached to the fracture of a septuagenarian femur that constituted illness or disease.

Out of his anthropocentric self-interest, man has chosen to consider as 'illness' or 'diseases' those natural circumstances which precipitate the death (or the failure to function according to certain rules) of a limited number of biological species; man himself, his pets and other cherished livestock, and the plant varieties he cultivates for gain or pleasure.

Such arguments point us to the fact that medicine is not 'objective, scientific' applied biology but is necessarily value-laden. This is true of the disruption of the internal state that 'patients' bring as 'complaints' to the doctor and true also of those complaints that the doctor regards as 'symptoms'. For Sedgwick (1982), all diseases start as illness states recognized as such because of the negative value attached to the symptoms or complaints.

All illness, whether conceived in localized bodily terms or within a larger view of human functioning, expresses both a social value judgement (contrasting a person's condition with certain understood and accepted norms) and an attempt at explanation (with a view to controlling the disvalued condition).

Another view of the effect of social values on the presentation of illness is the notion of the *sick role* as developed by Talcott Parsons (1902–79) (1951a). Whatever the underlying causes of conditions, the role that the subject themself, the patient, chooses to play and the role that is forced on them by those around them because of their illness are highly significant in the way their symptoms manifest. Parsons (1951b) argued that health is included in the functional needs of the individual member of society so that, from the point of view of the functioning of the social system, too low a general level of health or too high an incidence of illness is dysfunctional. Disease in this formulation incapacitates the effective performance of social roles, and there is therefore social interest in the alleviation of disease. To put this in another way, disease is not purely or merely a natural phenomenon but a state of disturbance of the total human being, including the state of the organism as a biological system and of their personal and social adjustments, including their ability to fulfil social roles.

This approach introduces the notion that behavioural deviance itself can be the source of disease. Yet how is such deviance to be recognized and defined? Social deviance can be recognized by self-definition. The individual may come to hold the belief that they have a problem or there may be a societal reaction that indicates that an individual's behaviour constitutes a problem. Societal reaction of this type might occur when a community comes to recognize a person's inability or reluctance to respond in a particular expected way. According to David Mechanic (1968),

'the view taken of the deviant depends in large part on the frame of reference of the observer and the extent to which the deviant appears to be able or willing to control his responses. The evaluator views the act within the context of what he believes the actor's motivation to be. If the action appears reasonable in terms of the assumed motivation of the actor, there is a very good chance that deviant behaviour will be defined in terms of the goodness–badness dimension. If the behaviour appears to be peculiar and at odds with expectations of how a reasonable person might be motivated, such behaviour is more likely to be characterized in terms of the sickness dimension'.

The problem with this is self-evident. Disease definition in this formulation seems significantly prone to error and subjective judgement and is liable to be used as a tool of social control.

With regard to self-definition of illness, people differ in the way they perceive, evaluate and act on or fail to act on the symptoms they experience. Mechanic (1986) has called this *illness behaviour.* This is influenced by the salience of the complaint, the degree to which it disturbs social roles, the folk understanding of the seriousness and consequences of the complaint or implied disease, and the competing claims on the person's time and resources.

Somatic or psychological symptoms do, of course, frequently occur without any evidence of organic disease. When attempting to describe and classify such symptoms, it is helpful to establish a phenomenological basis; conditions are recognized because of the particular characteristics of the patient's complaints, not because of some presumed theoretical notion of cause. The bizarre lengths that result from the application of a preformed theory of disease aetiology to symptoms, rather than developing from *symptoms* to *theory*, is admirably illustrated in Engelhardt's (1981) essay *'The disease of masturbation'.* In the 19th century, masturbation was widely believed to produce many signs and symptoms including dyspepsia, constriction of the urethra, epilepsy, blindness, vertigo, loss of hearing, headache, impotence, loss of memory, insanity, cardiac arrhythmia, rickets, leucorrhoea in women, conjunctivitis and generalized weakness, and it was held to be a dangerous disease entity.

Lewis (1953) pointed out that mental illness could be characterized in terms of psychopathology: 'disturbance of part functions as well as general efficiency'. The term *Part functions* refers to the different aspects of psychological experience and behaviour described in previous chapters: memory, perception, forming beliefs and so on. Thus Lewis saw a disturbance in perception, for example hallucination, as a reason for establishing a *case* of mental illness—on psychopathologic grounds. This approach antedated Christopher Boorse's contribution to our understanding of the nature of mental disorders. His distinction between disease and illness is deservedly influential. He argued that an organism is *healthy* to the degree that it is not diseased. And, he defined a *disease* as a type of internal state of an organism that interferes with some function that contributes to survival and reproduction. In addition, that the disease state is not simply in the nature of the species; that is, it is either atypical of the species or, if typical, mainly due to environmental causes. Diseases become illnesses only when they satisfy certain further, and normative, conditions. A disease is an illness only if it is serious enough to be incapacitating and therefore is regarded as undesirable, a title for special treatment and a valid excuse for normally criticizable behaviour. For Boorse, mental functions such as perceptual processing, intelligence and memory clearly serve to provide information about the world that can guide effective action. Drives serve to motivate it. Anxiety and pain function as signals of danger, language as a device for cultural co-operation and cognitive enrichment, and so on. He concludes: 'it seems certain that a few of the recognized mental disorders are genuine diseases, whether mental or physical. Even without any knowledge of the relevant functional systems, one can sometimes infer internal malfunction immediately from biologically incompetent behaviour'. Finally, Boorse thought that diseases are what doctors treat and illnesses are what people suffer from (Boorse, 1976).

Use of Symptoms to Form Diagnostic Categories

The relationship between signs and symptoms in psychiatry was discussed in Chapter 1. Traditionally, symptoms have been divided into those causing suffering and pain (distress) and those causing loss of function (disability). When the only disharmony is between the individual and their society, the disturbance is not regarded as mental illness. For the great majority of mental disorders, diagnostic classification is made according to the profile of symptoms presented. Exceptions to this are as follows:

- when the aetiology is known, for example, dementia in human immunodeficiency virus disease;
- when the genetic basis and structural pathology are known, for example, Huntington disease; and
- when cause is hypothesized to result from a process without conclusive evidence, for example, dissociative fugue.

Descriptive psychopathology is almost atheoretical in nature and thus allows the development of a generally descriptive diagnostic terminology.

Symptoms are collected into constellations that commonly occur together to form the *syndromes* of mental illness. It is usual to make a distinction between *illness,* with a definite onset after normal health, and the *lifelong* characteristics of learning disability or personality disorder.

Another fundamental distinction often made by psychiatrists and based ultimately on psychopathology

is that between *psychoses* and *neuroses*. Psychoses 'are major mental illness. They are exceedingly hard to define although they are usually said to be characterized by severe symptoms, such as delusions and hallucinations, and by lack of insight' (Gelder et al., 1983); there is loss of contact with reality. It is probable that the everyday use of the concept of psychosis by clinicians is based on the notion of 'unitary psychosis'; the development of this concept has been discussed by Berrios and Beer (1994). Neurosis 'is a psychological reaction to acute or continuous perceived stress, expressed in emotion or behaviour ultimately inappropriate in dealing with that stress'; phenomenological characteristics held in common by neurotic patients include disturbances of self-image, of the experience of relationships and, often, bodily symptoms without organic cause (Sims, 1983). Although the term neurosis has fallen out of favour, the concepts that the term refers to are still important as organizing principles: an understandable reaction to stress; the emotional disturbance is a variant of normal response, possibly only exaggerated in degree and intensity; a condition in which insight is retained; and finally the extent of disruption to personality and self-identity is minimal.

Psychiatric diagnosis is often hierarchical, organic syndromes taking precedence over functional psychoses, these over neuroses and neuroses over situational or adjustment reactions. A patient with schizophrenia and super-added anxiety will usually receive only the diagnosis of schizophrenia. This can be a considerable disadvantage in practice for planning treatment programmes as, for instance, the prognosis of chronic schizophrenia may be determined more by the presence of neurotic symptoms than by the response of schizophrenic symptoms to treatment (Cheadle et al., 1978). Foulds (1976) used this hierarchical approach to establish a system of classification of *personal illness,* with *delusions of disintegration* at the apex, taking priority over intervening levels down to *dysthymic states* as the lowest level.

An example of *categorical* classification is shown in Box 21.1. Various noncategorical methods of classification have also been used. In the *dimensional* approach as advocated by Eysenck (1970), the variations of presentation of mental illness are accounted for on just three dimensions: psychoticism, neuroticism and

BOX 21.1 CLASSIFICATION OF MENTAL DISORDERS

PSYCHOSES

- Organic disorders:
  - Acute organic syndrome
  - Chronic organic syndrome (dementia)
  - Dysamnestic syndrome
- Schizophrenia:
  - Schizoaffective disorders
  - Paranoid states
- Affective disorders:
  - Mania
  - Depressive disorder

NEUROSES AND RELATED DISORDERS

- Neuroses:
  - Depressive neurosis
  - Anxiety neurosis
  - Phobic neurosis
  - Obsessional neurosis
  - Hysteria
  - Depersonalization syndrome
  - Nonspecific and mixed
- Personality disorders
- Adjustment disorder
- Other disorders:
  - Sexual dysfunction and sexual deviations
  - Alcohol and drug dependence
  - Miscellaneous syndromes
  - Psychological factors associated with medical conditions
- Mental retardation
- Disorders specific to childhood

After Gelder, M., Gath, D., Mayou, R., 1983. Oxford Textbook of Psychiatry. Oxford University Press, Oxford, with permission of Oxford University Press.

extroversion/introversion. *Multiaxial* classification codes different sets of information separately.

THE PRESENT STATE EXAMINATION

An example of psychiatric phenomenology applied in nosologic research is the development of the Present State Examination (PSE; Wing et al., 1974): 'The Present State Examination (PSE) schedule is a guide to structuring a clinical interview, with the object of assessing the present mental state of adult patients suffering from one of the neuroses or functional psychoses.' It aims to enquire about the patient's condition and subjective state and to record this information as symptoms. When there is conflict between clinical and statistical judgements, clinical judgement is allowed to prevail. Symptoms are aggregated into a list of

syndromes. The classification of symptoms is carried out on a programme known as 'Catego', which reduces the 500 PSE items to a maximum of six descriptive categories and thence into one descriptive group for the individual patient.

An aim of the PSE has been to determine whether there are clinically recognizable symptoms on which all psychiatrists can agree and label in the same way. Wing et al. (1974) pose two questions:

First, whether certain psychological and behavioural phenomena which have generally been thought by psychiatrists to be symptoms of mental illnesses can be reliably recognized and described, irrespective of the language and culture of the doctor or patient; secondly, whether rules of classification can be specified with such precision that an individual with a given pattern of symptoms will also be allocated to the same clinical grouping.

Thus the PSE starts from a psychopathologic standpoint. The interviewer is trained to note the presence or absence of listed symptoms in the glossary. Groups of symptoms are collected together into syndromes by use of computerized Catego class. The end product of the PSE is diagnosis as a research tool based on phenomenology and available for study by other workers in other cultures. An example of the relationship between syndromes and symptoms in the PSE is shown in Fig. 21.1.

This example of an excerpt from the PSE involves the terms used for the symptoms of schizophrenia. The *nuclear syndrome* of Wing et al. (1974) is composed of Schneider's (1958) first-rank symptoms. The symptoms they listed as comprising this syndrome in the ninth edition of the PSE are *thought intrusion, thought insertion, thought broadcast, thought commentary, thought withdrawal, voices about the patient, delusions of control, delusions of alien penetration* and *primary delusions.* They make the useful point that *thought insertion* is likely to be rated with a false positive if the examiner does not have the symptom in mind but some general approximation to it. *Voices about the patient* implies nonaffective verbal hallucinations heard by the subject talking about him in the third person. *Delusions of control* refers, of course, to passivity experiences. *Delusions of alien forces penetrating or controlling* the mind

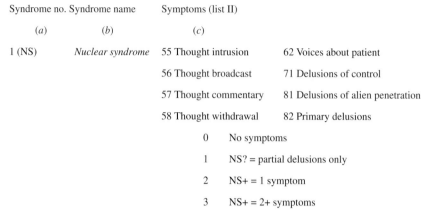

Syndrome no. (a)	Syndrome name (b)	Symptoms (list II) (c)	
1 (NS)	*Nuclear syndrome*	55 Thought intrusion	62 Voices about patient
		56 Thought broadcast	71 Delusions of control
		57 Thought commentary	81 Delusions of alien penetration
		58 Thought withdrawal	82 Primary delusions
		0	No symptoms
		1	NS? = partial delusions only
		2	NS+ = 1 symptom
		3	NS+ = 2+ symptoms

Fig. 21.1 Excerpt from the Present State Examination. (From Wing, J.K., Cooper, J.E., Sartorius, N., 1974. The Measurement and Classification of Psychiatric Symptoms: an Instruction Manual for the PSE and Category Program. Cambridge University Press, Cambridge, with permission.**)**

or body is a special form of symptom already listed as belonging to the nuclear syndrome. By *primary delusions*, Wing et al. imply *delusional perception* and give the example of a patient undergoing liver biopsy who came to believe, as the needle was inserted, that they had been chosen by God.

The 10th edition of the PSE was further developed into the Schedules for Clinical Assessment in Neuropsychiatry (SCAN; Wing et al., 1990), which then mapped into the diagnostic categories in *International Classification of Diseases* (World Health Organization, 1992) and *Diagnostic and Statistical Manual of Mental Disorders*, 3rd revised edition (American Psychiatric Association, 1987). The emphasis placed here on the PSE is intended because it is such a direct application of descriptive psychopathology to psychiatric diagnosis (Table 21.1).

Postscript

Fundamental to psychiatry is the need to understand what the patient is experiencing. Eisenberg (1986) has succinctly summarized the aspirations of the biological school of psychiatry: 'For every twisted thought there is a twisted molecule.' Ironically, if this association were to be achieved it would make the need for expert phenomenological skills more, rather than less, important, as it is likely to remain, from the patient's point of view, more comfortable to have their thoughts than their molecules explored. At the opposite pole of psychiatry, psychodynamics, there is also great value in descriptive psychopathology, unembellished by interpretation, as a starting point for further understanding.

USES OF PSYCHOPATHOLOGY

It has been said of William of Ockham, who so courageously navigated the murky and dangerous waters of medieval philosophy and science, that he was 'an empiricist refusing to stretch knowledge beyond the bounds of ascertainable experience' (Leff, 1958). This is the position of descriptive psychopathology: aiming not to draw conclusions beyond the subjective experience of the patient and its judicious exploration by the interviewer. Every psychiatrist uses phenomenology to some extent, but it is a much more valuable tool if used rigorously.

The four practical applications of descriptive psychopathology, then, are as follows.

- *Communication.* It enables clinicians to speak and write to each other about the problems of their patients in a mutually comprehensible way. This is clearly of value both in clinical practice and for research.
- *Diagnosis.* Psychiatric diagnosis is based to a considerable extent on psychopathology, and this is wholly appropriate, especially until there is more evidence for aetiology and underlying pathology for the different conditions.
- *Therapy.* The method of empathy, that is using phenomenology to explore the patient's subjective experience, is a rational way of establishing a therapeutic relationship. It enables the therapist

TABLE 21.1 First-Rank Symptoms of Schizophrenia[a] and Symptoms from the Present State Examination[b]

First-Rank Symptom	Equivalent Symptom from Present State Examination
Delusional	
Delusional percept	Primary delusion
Auditory Hallucinations	
Audible thoughts	Thought echo or commentary
Voices arguing or discussing	Voices about the patient
Voices commenting on the patient's action	Voices about the patient
Thought Disorder: Passivity of Thought	
Thought withdrawal	Thought block or withdrawal
Thought insertion	Thought insertion
Thought broadcasting (diffusion of thought)	Thought broadcast or thought sharing
Passivity Experiences: Delusion of Control	
Passivity of affect ('made' feelings)	Delusions of control
Passivity of impulse ('made' drives)	Delusions of control
Passivity of volition ('made' volitional acts)	Delusions of control
Somatic passivity (influence playing on the body)	Delusions of alien penetration

[a]Schneider, K. 1958. Clinical Psychopathology, fifth ed. (M.W. Hamilton, Trans, 1959). Grune and Stratton, New York.
[b]Wing, J.K., Cooper, J.E., Sartorius, N., 1974. The Measurement and Classification of Psychiatric Symptoms: an Instruction Manual for the PSE and Category Program. Cambridge University Press, Cambridge.

acknowledgement of the value of psychopathology by lawyers and doctors.

The patient's symptoms, their sufferings, are a logical starting point for the doctor's sympathy, curiosity and therapeutic endeavour. To start elsewhere turns medicine on its head and, ultimately, one arrives in a topsy-turvy world like Samuel Butler's *Erewhon* (1872), where 'illness of any sort is considered … to be highly criminal and immoral; and that I was liable, for catching cold, to be had up before the Magistrates and imprisoned for a considerable period' and 'if a man forges a cheque, or sets his home on fire or robs with violence from a person, or does any such things that are criminal in our own country, he is either taken to a hospital and is carefully tended at the public expense, or if he was in good circumstances, he lets it be known to all his friends that he is suffering from a severe fit of immorality … and they come and visit him with great solicitude'. You may think this is too far-fetched; however, the less pleasant aspects of this certainly appear to have been the situation for some of the dissidents in psychiatric custody in the previous USSR (Bloch and Reddaway, 1977).

The ultimate aim of psychiatry is not, of course, knowledge, but to help people to function and feel better; phenomenology is a valuable therapeutic tool. Ideally, it gives the patient, in their doctor, a person who understands what they are feeling but does not try to explain causes in terms of theory, which the patient may find unconvincing. The patient often has a great sense of relief when the doctor, however falteringly, describes back to them the symptoms, or the internal experience, that they, the patient, have found so difficult to describe.

NEED FOR RESEARCH

Psychopathology was introduced into psychiatry before the current emphasis on quantification, population surveys and experimental method. It is now imperative both for the further development of descriptive psychopathology and, more importantly, for continued progress in psychiatric research that more rigorous research methods be applied. Phenomenology has a place in psychiatric research that has not yet been fully exploited. It forms a logical bridge between research findings emanating from clinical and applied psychology and the increasing

to understand the subjective experience of their patient and will give the patient confidence in further entrusting the secrets of his internal environment to the therapist.

- *The law.* Descriptive psychopathology is the only reasonable way of determining what is mental illness and what are the differences between mental illnesses from a forensic point of view. Mutual enlightenment in the area between the law and psychiatry, where there is at present so much misunderstanding, will result from a clearer knowledge of disordered neuroanatomy—physiology and chemistry—that is resulting from more sophisticated methods of neuroimaging and assay. This is the direction that research in descriptive psychopathology should go.

Investigation of the experience of the individual has to be linked to an understanding of their biology, and it is also important to assess how normal phenomena are distributed within the population. The scientific bases of psychiatry include, as well as biological and behavioural sciences, epidemiology and phenomenology. Recognition of homogeneity includes both the symptoms within an individual patient and the features of an affected population. The PSE has been discussed earlier as a method of quantifying psychopathologic information.

To introduce experimental methods into research in descriptive psychopathology will sometimes involve single case studies in which variables that have been evaluated phenomenologically are altered. For example, Green and Preston (1981) amplified the quiet whispering of a chronic schizophrenic patient during the time they were auditorily hallucinated. They whispered at the same time as they heard voices, and the content of their vocalization corresponded to what the voices were reported to have said, thus demonstrating the disturbance of boundaries of self found in schizophrenia. This type of investigation has been extended further, and there are several examples in this book (see Chapters 7 and 11). There has been a danger in that some other psychological studies, not quoted here, have used phenomenology imprecisely and hence vitiated the significance of their findings.

An interesting development in research based on descriptive psychopathology is the application of particular psychological techniques to specific phenomenological entities. Examples of this are the use of cognitive behaviour therapy in the treatment of persistent auditory hallucinations (Bentall et al., 1994) and more general application of psychological interventions in schizophrenia (Haddock and Lewis, 1996).

It is important that progress in the treatment of patients and in research that advances in biological aspects of psychiatry are assisted by accurate psychiatric diagnosis based on phenomenology that is both reliable (i.e., capable of reproduction by the same interviewer at a different time or by different interviewers) and quantifiable. Never were the skills of the clinical phenomenologist more necessary or more likely to yield beneficial results both in understanding and in therapy. The introduction of improved neuropsychiatric methods of investigation increases the need for reliable findings from descriptive psychopathology rather than rendering it obsolete. Jaspers (1997) commented, 'phenomenology, though one of the foundation stones of psychopathology, is still very crude'. This is still true, but it is now high time that descriptive psychopathology became more sophisticated.

Phenomenology takes the doctor's art and discipline of observation inside their patient's mind. David Hume (1804) described the absence of physical examination in medicine in his essay *Of Polygamy and Divorces*. He tells of the physician brought into the Grand Signior's seraglio in Constantinople.

He was not a little surprised in looking along a gallery to see a great number of naked arms standing out from the sides of the room. He could not imagine what this could mean; until he was told that those arms belonged to bodies which he must cure without knowing any more about them than what he could learn from the arms. He was not allowed to ask a question of the patient, or even of her attendants, lest he might find it necessary to enquire concerning circumstances which the delicacy of the seraglio allows not to be revealed. Hence physicians in the east pretend to know all diseases from the pulse, as our quacks in Europe undertake to cure a person merely from seeing his water.

Psychiatry must now come out of the seraglio and use all available information in the service of its patients, including phenomenology, for diagnosis, for understanding and for treatment.

REFERENCES

Bentall, R.P., Haddock, G., Slade, P.D., 1994. Cognitive behaviour therapy for persistent auditory hallucinations: from theory to therapy. Behav. Psychother. 25, 51–56.

Berrios, G.E., Beer, D., 1994. The notion of unitary psychosis: a conceptual history. Hist. Psychiat. V 13–36.

Bloch, S., Reddaway, P., 1977. Russia's Political Hospital. Gollancz, London.

Boorse, C., 1976. What a theory of mental health should be. J. Theory Soc. Behav. 6, 61–84.

Burton, R., 1621. The Anatomy of Melancholy, what it Is. With All the Kinds, Causes, Symptoms, Prognostickes, and Severall Cures of it by Democritus Junior. Cripps, Oxford.

Butler, S., 1872. Erewhon. Cape, London.

Carroll, L., 1872. Through the Looking Glass, and what Alice Found There. Macmillan, London.

Cheadle, A.J., Freeman, H.L., Korer, J., 1978. Chronic schizophrenic patients in the community. Br. J. Psychiatry 132, 221–227.

Eisenberg, L., 1986. Mindlessness and brainlessness in psychiatry. Br. J. Psychiatry 148, 497–508.

Engelhardt, H.T., 1981. The disease of masturbation: values and the concept of disease. In: Caplan, A.L., Engelhardt, D.T., McCartney, J.J. (Eds.), Concepts of Health and Disease. Addison-Wesley, Reading.

Eysenck, H.J., 1970. A dimensional system of psychodiagnosis. In: Mahrer, A.R. (Ed.), New Approaches to Personality Classification. Columbia University Press, New York, pp. 169–207.

Foulds, G.A., 1976. The Hierarchical Nature of Personal Illness. Academic Press, London.

Gelder, M., Gath, D., Mayou, R., 1983. Oxford Textbook of Psychiatry. Oxford University Press, Oxford.

Green, P., Preston, M., 1981. Reinforcement of vocal correlates of auditory hallucinations using auditory feedback: a case study. Br. J. Psychiatry 139, 204–208.

Haddock, G., Lewis, S.W., 1996. New psychological treatments in schizophrenia. Adv. Psychiatr. Treat. 2, 110–116.

Hume, D., 1804. Essays and Treaties on Several Subjects, vol. 1. Bell and Bradfute, Edinburgh.

Jaspers, K., 1997. General Psychopathology (J. Hoenig, M.W. Hamilton, Trans). The Johns Hopkins University Press, Baltimore.

Kendell, R.E., 1975. The Role of Diagnosis in Psychiatry. Blackwell, Oxford.

Leff, G., 1958. Medieval Thoughts. Penguin, Harmondsworth.

Lewis, A.J., 1953. Health as a social concept. Br. J. Sociol. 4, 109–124.

Mechanic, D., 1968. Medical Sociology. The Free Press, New York.

Mechanic, D., 1986. The concept of illness behaviour: culture, situation and personal predisposition. Psychol. Med. 16, 1–7.

Parsons, T., 1951a. Illness and the role of the physician: a sociological perspective. Am. J. Orthopsychiatry 21, 452–460.

Parsons, T., 1951b. The Social System. The Free Press, New York.

Sadler, J.Z., 2004. Values and Psychiatric Diagnosis. Oxford University Press, Oxford.

Schneider, K., 1958. Clinical Psychopathology. In: (M.W. Hamilton, Trans, 1959), fifth ed. Grune and Stratton, New York.

Schwartz, M.A., Wiggins, O.P., 1987. Typifications: the first step for clinical diagnosis in psychiatry. J. Nerv. Ment. Dis. 175, 65–77.

Sedgwick, P., 1981. Illness – mental and otherwise. In: Caplan, A.L., Engelhardt, H.T., McCartney, J.J. (Eds.), Concepts of Health and Disease: Interdisciplinary Perspectives. Addison-Wesley, Reading, pp. 119–130.

Sedgwick, P., 1982. Psycho Politics. Harper and Row, New York.

Sims, A.C.P., 1983. Neurosis in Society. Macmillan, London.

Stengel, E., 1959. Classification of mental disorders. Bull. World Health Organ. 21, 601–603.

Wing, J.K., Babor, T., Brugha, T., et al., 1990. SCAN: schedules for clinical Assessment in Neuropsychiatry. Arch. Gen. Psychiatry 47, 589–593.

Wing, J.K., Cooper, J.E., Sartorius, N., 1974. The Measurement and Classification of Psychiatric Symptoms: An Instruction Manual for the PSE and Category Program. Cambridge University Press, Cambridge.

World Health Organization, 1992. The ICD-10 Classification of Mental and Behavioural Disorders: Clinical Description and Diagnostic Guidelines. World Health Organization, Geneva.

Self-Assessment 1

Instructions

Each set of numbered items is followed by five lettered options. Select the ONE lettered option that is BEST in each case.

Chapter 1

Descriptive psychopathology is:
  a) The study of ego defence mechanisms that underlies behaviour change
  b) Concerned with the selection, delimitation, differentiation and description of abnormal psychological phenomena
  c) Directly the outcome of analysing the content of dreams
  d) A method of describing the interaction between doctors and patients
  e) An introspective system of understanding and describing abnormal cognitions

Empathy in descriptive psychopathology is:
  a) Achieved by precise, insightful, persistent and knowledgeable exploration of the patient's experience
  b) A communication technique aimed at putting the patient at ease
  c) Metacommunication
  d) The basis of sympathy for the patient's situation
  e) An aspect of transference

The term *understanding* in psychopathology:
  a) Derives from Freud's structural theory of the psyche
  b) Describes the causal mechanisms underlying abnormal experiences
  c) Has no limit in the capacity to describe and comprehend experience
  d) Derives from Dilthey's conception of the distinction between the sciences and humanities
  e) Has no place in contemporary psychiatry

Chapter 2

Specific communication skill techniques include the following EXCEPT:
  a) Summary statements
  b) Attentive listening
  c) Normalizing statements
  d) Looped questions
  e) Open questions

Aspects of observation of appearance and behaviour include the following EXCEPT:
  a) Posture
  b) Gesture
  c) Talk
  d) Facial expression
  e) Self-hygiene

Assessment of insight involves the following domains EXCEPT:
  a) Fluency of talk
  b) Recognition of subjective psychological change
  c) Attribution of the change to pathology
  d) Recognition of need for treatment
  e) Compliance with treatment

Chapter 3

Automatism is characterized by the following EXCEPT:
  a) Involuntary behaviour
  b) Behaviour that is inappropriate to the circumstances
  c) Complex and coordinated behaviour
  d) Unimpaired judgement
  e) Apparently purposeful and directed behaviour

Mania à potu is a syndrome characterized by the following EXCEPT:
  a) Insomnia
  b) Total or partial amnesia for the aberrant behaviour
  c) Alcohol consumption
  d) Senseless violence
  e) Prolonged sleep

Delirium is a condition characterized by the following EXCEPT:
- a) Insidious onset
- b) Global impairment of cognitive functions
- c) Reduced level of consciousness
- d) Impaired attention
- e) Disordered sleep–wake cycle

Chapter 4

Dreams:
- a) Occur in non–rapid eye movement (REM) sleep
- b) Are associated with paralysis
- c) Involve an accentuation of self-awareness
- d) Involve consolidation of spatial and temporal connections
- e) Are synonymous with night terror

Kleine–Levin syndrome is characterized by:
- a) Severe hypersomnia
- b) Sleep paralysis
- c) Short REM latency
- d) Hypnogogic hallucinations
- e) Cataplexy

Attention:
- a) Is the focusing of consciousness on any aspect of experience
- b) Is synonymous with concentration
- c) Involves disinhibition of memory
- d) Is distinct from vigilance
- e) Relies solely on active processes

Chapter 5

The following are TRUE of confabulation EXCEPT:
- a) It is a false memory
- b) It is associated with organic amnesia
- c) It can involve embellishment of actual memories
- d) It is typically 'fantastic' in nature
- e) Suggestibility is a prominent feature

Short-term memory:
- a) Is an unlimited capacity system
- b) Comprises a central action system
- c) Involves a 'phonological loop' that holds memory traces for up to 5 minutes
- d) Involves a visuospatial scratch pad that allows for manipulation of visual information
- e) Cannot be distinguished from attention

Long-term memory functions include the following EXCEPT:
- a) Registration
- b) Retention
- c) Repression
- d) Retrieval
- e) Recall

Chapter 6

Formal characteristics of time include all of the following EXCEPT:
- a) Duration
- b) Sequence
- c) Synchrony
- d) Rhythm
- e) Bidirectionality

Déjà vu experience is an example of abnormality of:
- a) Rhythm
- b) Sense of uniqueness of time
- c) Time duration
- d) Temporal order
- e) Direction of time

Features of seasonal affective disorder include the following EXCEPT:
- a) Hypersomnia
- b) Insomnia
- c) Craving for carbohydrates
- d) Overeating
- e) Lethargy

Chapter 7

Abnormalities of the elementary aspects of visual perception include the following EXCEPT:
- a) Palinopsia
- b) Macropsia
- c) Hemacropsia
- d) Palinacousis
- e) Achromatopsia

In synaesthesia the following are TRUE EXCEPT:
- a) The perception of a sensory object is presented in another sensory modality
- b) The perception occurs in peri-personal space
- c) Music to colour transformations occur
- d) Elaboration of form constants is a feature
- e) Emotional distress is a common accompaniment

Formal characteristics of images include the following EXCEPT:
a) Images are not clearly delineated
b) Images have a character of objectivity
c) Images appear in inner subjective space
d) Images are actively created
e) Images dissipate rapidly and have to be re-created

Chapter 8

The following are examples of primary delusions EXCEPT:
a) Autochthonous delusions
b) Delusional percept
c) Persecutory delusions
d) Delusional atmosphere
e) Delusional memory

Secondary delusions are:
a) Secondary to other abnormal experiences
b) Understandable in the light of the patient's social context
c) Not held with conviction
d) Amenable to counterargument
e) Transient

Delusions are examples of:
a) Perseveration
b) Impairment of consciousness
c) False perception
d) False beliefs
e) Autoscopy

Chapter 9

Schneider's first-rank symptoms include the following EXCEPT:
a) Somatic hallucinations
b) Audible thoughts
c) Passivity experiences
d) Thought withdrawal
e) Thought insertion

Delusions of control of thought include EXCEPT:
a) Thought broadcasting
b) Thought echo
c) Thought insertion
d) Thought withdrawal
e) Thought blocking

The term *circumstantiality* refers to:
a) Flight of ideas
b) Loosening of association
c) Concrete thinking
d) Over-inclusive thinking
e) Impedance of flow of thinking by unnecessary detail

Chapter 10

Recognized abnormalities of language in schizophrenia include the following EXCEPT:
a) Lack of use of cohesive ties
b) Alogia
c) Neologism
d) Clang associations
e) Telegony

The Cloze technique is a measure of:
a) Predictability of speech
b) The proportion of the number of different words to the total number of words
c) Cohesive ties
d) Rules of proposition
e) Fluency of language

Primary sensory dysphasia is:
a) The inability to produce names or sounds at will
b) A gross disturbance of words and syntax resulting in unintelligible speech
c) A disorder of indistinct speech
d) The loss of comprehension of the meaning of words
e) The inability to read with understanding

Chapter 11

Insight in schizophrenia has been shown to be positively correlated with the following EXCEPT:
a) The likelihood of developing depression
b) The likelihood of hospitalizations
c) Compliance with treatment
d) Long-term outcome
e) Working memory

Valid measures of insight must take into consideration the following EXCEPT:
a) The multidimensional aspect of insight
b) The relationship of insight to affect
c) The influence of cultural factors

d) The variation of insight across different symptom domains
e) The added value of behavioural observations

Insight involves all of the following EXCEPT:
a) Awareness of change
b) Recognition of illness in others
c) Attribution of change to illness
d) Recognition of the need for treatment
e) Cooperation with treatment

Chapter 12

Autoscopy can involve all of the following EXCEPT:
a) Feeling of presence
b) Failure to perceive self in a mirror
c) Visual hallucination of internal organs within bodily space
d) Visual hallucination of exact copy of the self in mirror image
e) Projection of the observing self in extrapersonal space

Ego vitality is:
a) Awareness of being an agent
b) Awareness of unity and coherence of self
c) Awareness of being
d) Awareness of continuity of self over time
e) Awareness of boundaries to the self

Nihilistic delusion is an example of:
a) Disorder of ego boundary
b) Disorder of continuity of self over time
c) Disorder of activity
d) Disorder of vitality
e) Disorder of unity of self

Chapter 13

Definitive features of depersonalization include the following EXCEPT:
a) The experience is pleasant
b) There is a feeling of strangeness
c) It is a subjective experience
d) Insight is preserved
e) It can affect bodily sensation

Depersonalization has shown to consist of a number of components including the following EXCEPT:
a) Perceptual alteration

b) Unreality of surroundings
c) Temporal integration
d) Unreality of self
e) Emotional numbing

Depersonalization is known to be associated with the following EXCEPT:
a) Lysergic acid diethylamide (LSD)
b) Cannabis
c) Mescaline
d) Sensory deprivation
e) Narcolepsy

Chapter 14

Individual determinants of hypochondriasis include the following EXCEPT:
a) Feelings of disgust
b) Preoccupation with bodily function
c) Serious illness or injury in childhood
d) Fear of infection
e) Fascination with the Internet

Mass psychogenic illness:
a) Occurs most commonly in young males
b) Often starts in a child of low status in the peer group
c) Affects most severely the most adjusted people
d) Symptoms spread by line-of-sight transmission
e) Is unaffected by media response

The concepts of *conversion* and *dissociation* suggest:
a) That physical symptoms can only have an organic basis
b) That causation is unconscious
c) That symptoms carry no obvious advantage for the patient
d) That symptoms are unlikely to be psychologically meaningful
e) That the patient is acting a part

Chapter 15

Pain asymbolia:
a) Presents with absent pain response
b) Is associated with increased thermal sensitivity
c) Is associated with hyperhidrosis
d) Presents with self-stimulation
e) Is usually an acquired disorder that occurs after vascular lesions

Pain associated with psychopathology is:
  a) Better localized
  b) Clearly delineated along recognized neuroanatomic distribution
  c) Easy for the patient to describe
  d) Constant and unremitting
  e) Tends to be provoked by definite agents

Central pain (thalamic syndrome):
  a) Presents with a cutting sensation
  b) Is activated by cutaneous stimulation
  c) Presents as hypoalgesia
  d) Is unaffected by temperature change
  e) Does not present with allodynia

Chapter 16

Alexithymia refers to:
  a) Inability to experience pleasure
  b) Reacting to sad news with laughter
  c) Absence of unity between different modes of experience of emotions
  d) Inability to verbalize affect and elaborate fantasy
  e) Selective deficiency in correctly appraising vocal expression of emotion

Ekman's basic emotions include all of the following EXCEPT:
  a) Anger
  b) Disgust
  c) Fear
  d) Jealousy
  e) Sadness

Mood is defined as:
  a) A positive or negative reaction to an experience
  b) A prolonged prevailing inner state or predisposition
  c) A spontaneous and transitory experience in response to an experience
  d) The external behavioural manifestation of inner state
  e) An evaluative attitude towards an object

Chapter 17

The respiratory subtype of panic disorder is characterized by all of the following EXCEPT:
  a) Fear of dying
  b) Chest pain and discomfort
  c) Shortness of breath
  d) Provocation by inhalation of 35% carbon dioxide
  e) Induced by specific situations

Selye's general adaptation syndrome includes one of the following stages:
  a) Shock and numbness
  b) Sadness
  c) Guilt and hostility
  d) Flight-or-fight response
  e) Resolution

The constituent elements of obsessive compulsive phenomenon include all of the following EXCEPT:
  a) Inflated sense of responsibility, even for events over which the patient has no control
  b) Avoidance of cues likely to trigger obsession
  c) Fear of disaster that the patient believes will come to pass
  d) Resistance
  e) Increased discomfort following compulsive act

Chapter 18

Abnormal movement in catatonia include all of the following EXCEPT:
  a) Waxy flexibility
  b) Psychological pillow
  c) Stereotypy
  d) Cataplexy
  e) Mitgehen

Motivation can be defined as:
  a) Innate disposition that determines what objects to attend to in the world
  b) A state that initiates directed action
  c) A striving towards an object that is experienced as a desire
  d) A reward system that governs and regulates behaviour
  e) The power to put into effect voluntary action

Impulsivity involves all of the following EXCEPT:
  a) Predisposition towards rapid, unplanned action
  b) Lack of regard for consequences
  c) Preference for delayed larger reward over small but immediate reward
  d) Perseverance of behaviour despite punishment
  e) Inability to prevent response in response disinhibition attentional paradigm

Chapter 19

Abnormalities of form perception include which of the following:
- a) Heightened preference for symmetry
- b) Marked reduction in preference for symmetry
- c) Reduced emotional response to beauty
- d) Reduced preference for neotenic facial features
- e) Reduced aesthetic valuation of distinguishing facial features

Aesthetic valuation of landscape features is affected in:
- a) Anxiety
- b) Behavioural variant frontotemporal dementia
- c) Depression
- d) Obsessive compulsive disorder
- e) Tourette syndrome

Development of new onset visual art production is associated with:
- a) Midline brain lesions
- b) Left anterior temporal lobe lesions
- c) Left posterior temporal lobe lesions
- d) Occipital lobe lesions
- e) Dorsolateral frontal lobe lesions

Chapter 20

Paranoid personality disorder can be defined as a disorder in which:
- a) An individual mistrusts others and is unduly suspicious
- b) There is a lack of need for and defect in capacity to form relationships
- c) A defect in empathy is evident
- d) Uncontrollable outbursts of intemperate and uncontrolled mood occurs
- e) Theatrical behaviour and craving for attention occurs

In dependent personality disorder, all of the following features occur EXCEPT:
- a) Lack of self-confidence
- b) Perfectionistic disposition
- c) Craving for support and encouragement of others
- d) Difficulty in coping with changing demands of life
- e) Presence of a dominant close relationship

The following conditions have been shown to be frequently associated with anankastic personality disorder EXCEPT:
- a) Eating disorder
- b) Hypochondriasis
- c) Alcohol dependence syndrome
- d) Obsessive compulsive disorder
- e) Recurrent depressive disorder

Chapter 21

Illness behaviour is influenced by all of the following EXCEPT:
- a) Salience of the complaint
- b) Extent of disturbance of social roles
- c) Cultural understanding of the seriousness of the complaint
- d) Competing claims on the sufferer's resources
- e) The underlying biology of the condition

All the following individuals have made contributions to our understanding of health and disease EXCEPT:
- a) Christopher Boorse
- b) Aaron Beck
- c) Peter Sedgwick
- d) Talcott Parsons
- e) David Mechanic

Practical applications of psychopathology include all of the following EXCEPT:
- a) Communication between clinicians
- b) Cognitive neuroscience research
- c) Diagnosis
- d) Nosology
- e) Therapy

Self-Assessment 2

Instructions

Each set of matching questions consists of a list of 10 lettered options (A–J) followed by four numbered items. For each numbered item, select the appropriate lettered option. Each lettered option may be selected only once.

Chapters 3 and 4

A. Confusion
B. Coma
C. Delirium
D. Disorientation
E. Hypersomnia
F. Insomnia
G. Oneiroid state
H. Parasomnia
I. Stupor
J. Twilight state

1. A 75-year-old female patient is found wandering the streets. On examination, she does not know the date, day, time, season, where she is or her own address.
2. An 18-year-old male patient presents with a history of several irresistible periods of drowsiness during the day. At night he reports periods when he is fully awake but unable to move his limbs.
3. The partner of a 25-year-old male patient accompanies him to the outpatient appointment. She reports that he talks in his sleep, wanders aimlessly in the bedroom for a few minutes at night and has no recollection of these incidents.
4. A 47-year-old female patient with a history of recurrent depression is admitted in a mute state. She is immobile but fully conscious and alert. She is able to make eye contact but does not respond to any attempt at verbal communication.

Chapter 5

A. Anterograde amnesia
B. Confabulation
C. Cryptoamnesia
D. Dissociative fugue
E. False memory
F. Ganser state
G. Perseveration
H. Pseudologia fantastica
I. Recovered memory
J. Retrograde amnesia

1. A 20-year-old male patient was involved in a road traffic accident. He sustained a head injury. He was only able to recall events that happened approximately 5 minutes before the collision.
2. A 20-year-old male patient presented in prison while on remand. When examined, he responded to questions about the date and the capital of France with approximate answers and disorientation for time and place.
3. A 45-year-old male patient was involved in an accident at work where he sustained a serious head injury and lost consciousness. On regaining his consciousness, he could only recall events that happened approximately 36 hours after the incident.
4. A 57-year-old male patient with an established history of impairment of short-term memory in the context of alcohol abuse responded to questions about how he had spent the previous day with objectively false accounts that included embellishments and intrusions from previous occasions.

Chapter 7

A. Imagery
B. Palinopsia
C. Macropsia

D. Micropsia
E. Paraprosopia
F. Alloaesthesia
G. Pelopsia
H. Dyschromatopsia
I. Teleopsia
J. Metamorphopsia
1. A 45-year-old man presents with a complaint that he first saw a black cat at the corner where his drive joined the main street. After this, for the next 72 hours or so, he kept seeing the same cat at various times and situations. What is the term for this experience?
2. A 19-year-old man with a recent diagnosis of schizophrenia complained that the faces of people looking at him would suddenly look different, as if they were pulling faces at him. Sometimes, the faces would appear sinister, lopsided and strange. What is the term for this experience?
3. A 25-year-old female patient with a history of complex focal seizures complained of scenes and objects becoming smaller before a seizure. What is this experience termed?
4. A 25-year-old male patient complained that objects look far away. He found this surprising and distressing. What is this experience termed?

Chapter 8

A. Delusional percept
B. Delusional intuition
C. Delusional memory
D. Delusional atmosphere
E. Secondary delusion
F. Overvalued idea
G. Delusion of love
H. Delusional misidentification
I. Delusion of persecution
J. Delusional jealousy
1. A 20-year-old male patient was admitted into hospital after an attack on his father. He reported that his father had been replaced by a robot who looked almost exactly like him but was definitely not him. He feared that this 'robot' had malignant intentions and that his life was in danger. What is this belief called?

2. A 40-year-old female patient complained that her local priest was sending her secret messages, declaring his feelings for her. She complained that, although he was the father of her child, he was yet to visit them.
3. A 21-year-old female patient suddenly became convinced that she was the rightful heir to the throne of Norway. She was not Norwegian by birth or ancestry. When asked the reason for this belief, she said that she had suddenly come to this realization. She denied any other unusual experience.
4. A 54-year-old male patient with a longstanding history of schizophrenia reported persistent and stressful auditory verbal hallucinations of derogatory and threatening content. The voices would often tell him that he deserved to be killed and that new immigrants into his local area from Romania were going to murder him. He then held a firm belief that he was at risk from immigrants, particularly Romanians. This belief was held with conviction and was impervious to counterargument.

Chapter 9

A. Fantasy thinking
B. Imaginative thinking
C. Conceptual thinking
D. Circumstantial thinking
E. Thought block
F. Concrete thinking
G. Over-inclusive thinking
H. Thought insertion
I. Thought withdrawal
J. Audible thought
1. A 21-year-old male university student described spending a lot of time thinking about the future and about the possibility of becoming a famous musician, becoming rich and being able to live in a mansion in Florida.
2. A 25-year-old female patient, newly admitted into hospital, complained that her thoughts were being interfered with. She was particularly distressed by the experience of having thoughts manipulated and taken from her.

3. In a test, a 19-year-old patient with a diagnosis of schizophrenia responded to a question as follows: 'Which of the following are essential parts of a room: walls, chairs, floor, window?' 'Chairs'.

4. A 57-year-old female patient said, 'I was starting to feel high, so I tied dumb-bell weights round my ankle'.

Chapter 10

A. Aphonia
B. Logoclonia
C. Echolalia
D. Paragrammatism
E. Nominal dysphasia
F. Asyndesis
G. Metonym
H. Jargon aphasia
I. Receptive dysphasia
J. Neologism

1. A 65-year-old, right-handed male patient who was recovering from a left-sided stroke was unable to follow the verbal command, 'Take the paper with your left hand, fold it in two and put it on the floor'.

2. A 25-year-old patient said, 'Phlogons have invaded my lungs turning first sideways and now medways'.

3. A 64-year-old male patient with a long-standing history of schizophrenia replied to the question, 'What have you got in your cup?' 'A fluid that while being colourless turns dark on brewing'.

4. A 72-year-old male patient with a diagnosis of Parkinson's disease said, 'I'm star …, star …, starting to think of mo …, mo …, mo …, moving house'.

Chapter 14

A. Misoplegia
B. Dysmorphophobia
C. Palinaptia
D. Alloaesthesia
E. Exosomesthesia
F. Microsomatognosia

G. Macrosomatognosia
H. Muscle dysmorphia
I. Paraschemazia
J. Aschemazia

1. A 23-year-old male patient presented with the belief that his muscles were too small, a preoccupation with physical build, excessive exercising and disturbed eating.

2. A 56-year-old female patient complained of hating her left hand. Although it looked normal, she said that she hated it and had always wished that it were different in size, shape and feel.

3. A 27-year-old male patient presented with a long-standing belief that his face was ugly, in particular, his nose, which he thought was far too large and crooked. Objectively, his nose was not excessively large or crooked.

4. A 40-year-old female patient presented with the complaint that she could continue to feel her toothbrush in her hands for up to 15 minutes after she used it.

Chapter 16

A. Anhedonia
B. Echolalia
C. Hyperekplexia
D. Coenaesthesia
E. Prosopoaffective agnosia
F. Receptive emotional dysprosody
G. Cyclothymia
H. Ecstasy
I. Echomimia
J. Alexithymia

1. An 8-year-old male patient presented with a history of heightened startle reflex characterized by eye blinking, head flexion, abduction of the upper arms, movement of the trunk and bending of the knees in response to a loud noise.

2. A 40-year-old female patient with a history of recurrent depression and current depression gave a history of inability to experience pleasure in her usual hobbies and interests, as well as a general inability to experience any feeling.

3. A 36-year-old male patient presented to the local dental hospital with an aching pain in both sides of the lower jaw radiating to the temporomandibular joints and to the neck. In response to the question, 'How are you feeling in your spirits?', he seemed puzzled and asked for the question to be repeated. He then said, 'My body is heavy and I am aching all over'.

4. A 75-year-old male patient with a diagnosis of Parkinson's disease spoke in a monotonous voice. In addition he seemed not to recognize the emotional meaning of variations in tone of voice.

Chapter 17

A. Anxiety
B. Anankastic personality
C. Compulsion
D. Disgust
E. Irritability
F. Panic
G. Phobia
H. Obsession
I. Rumination
J. Social phobia

1. A 32-year-old female patient presented with discrete episodes of intense and extreme fear.

2. A 23-year-old female patient presented with excessive fear, self-consciousness and avoidance of social situations due to the possibility of embarrassment or humiliation.

3. A 27-year-old male accountancy trainee presented with a history of repetitive and intrusive thoughts about cleanliness and hygiene, which were associated with increasing tension and worry and which he recognized as his own thoughts. He tried to resist these thoughts but found that they became even more urgent and intrusive.

4. A 32-year-old female patient who had recently given birth presented with a 6-week history of temper outbursts, feelings of hostility towards her husband, an unpleasant feeling of distress and impatience with her children.

Chapter 18

A. Akathisia
B. Anhedonia
C. Catatonia
D. Drive
E. Impulsivity
F. Instinct
G. Kleine–Levin syndrome
H. Motivation
I. Urge
J. Will

1. A 21-year-old male recently diagnosed with schizophrenia and treated with risperidone complains of motor restlessness, inner agitation and an inability to sit still.

2. A 17-year-old male patient is brought to the attention of his general practitioner because he newly recognized a problem with gambling, drinking excessively and misusing cannabis. In addition, he is reported as prone to losing his temper and liable to say things he later regrets.

3. A 21-year-old male patient presented with a history of episodes of excessive sleeping (up to 15 hours a day), excessive eating, increased sexual libido, low mood and transient persecutory beliefs.

4. A 28-year-old female patient presented for the first time with markedly slowed movements, sometimes resulting in immobility, strange postures and muteness. On examination, she allows her upper limbs to be put in uncomfortable postures that she holds for long periods of time.

Self-Assessment 1: Answers

Chapter 1

Descriptive psychopathology is:
- b) Concerned with the selection, delimitation, differentiation and description of abnormal psychological phenomena

Descriptive psychopathology is distinct from psychodynamic psychopathology and hence does not deal with ego defence mechanisms nor analysis of dreams. It is not dependent on an understanding of abnormal cognitions, which is a characteristic of cognitive behavioural theories. Finally, it is not about the nature of the interactions between the doctor and patient.

Empathy in descriptive psychopathology is:
- a) Achieved by precise, insightful, persistent and knowledgeable exploration of the patient's experience

Empathy is a procedural method in descriptive psychopathology. It is a term that focuses on the way a clinician comes to a full understanding of the patient's abnormal subjective experience. It is distinct from sympathy and does not rely on transference.

The term *understanding* in psychopathology:
- d) Derives from Dilthey's conception of the distinction between the sciences and humanities

Understanding is a technical term that is drawn from Dilthey's appreciation of the difference between the sciences and the humanities. In science, Dilthey argues, 'we come to give explanations of the nature of the relationships between observations, whereas in the humanities we come to a psychological understanding of how different states unfold.'

Chapter 2

Specific communication skill techniques include the following EXCEPT:
- d) Looped questions

Communication skills are foundational to clinical inquiries. Summary statements allow the clinician to communicate to the patient what they have learnt from the clinical interview. The clinical interview is dependent on attentive listening, which is signalled to the patient by eye contact, demonstrable interest in the patient's account, body posture, encouraging noises and comments and responses that indicate accurate comprehension. Normalizing statements are statements that suggest that unusual beliefs, thoughts or actions are not only peculiar to the patient but also common enough even if not universal. Open questions are questions that allow for answers that open up a subject rather than close them down and are better at the beginning of clinical interviews. There are no such questions as 'looped questions'.

Aspects of observation of appearance and behaviour include the following EXCEPT:
- c) Talk

Talk is an aspect of the mental state examination that deals with speech and the content of speech. All the other items refer to observable aspects of appearance and behaviour.

Assessment of insight involves the following domains EXCEPT:
- a) Fluency of talk

Insight is a term that has specific meaning in relation to the mental state examination and is determined by recognition of change that is understood by the patient as due to abnormality, that requires treatment and, finally, involves acceptance of treatment.

Chapter 3

Automatism is characterized by the following EXCEPT:

d) Unimpaired judgement

Automatism is a term that refers to states that are usually found in epilepsy and are defined as occurring in the context of clouding of consciousness, which occurs during or immediately after a seizure. The individual retains control of posture and muscle tone and performs simple and complex movements and actions without being aware of what is happening. Occasionally, the automatism is terminated with a grand mal convulsion.

Mania à potu is a syndrome characterized by the following EXCEPT:

a) Insomnia

Mania à potu, or pathological intoxication, is a syndrome that presents as an outburst of uncontrollable rage and excitement leading to destructive actions against persons or property. It is regarded as behaviour that is out of character for the individual, the duration is short and there is subsequent amnesia for the event.

Delirium is a condition characterized by the following EXCEPT:

a) Insidious onset

Delirium is an abrupt change in conscious awareness and attention accompanied by changes in cognition, perception, psychomotor behaviour, sleep–wake cycle and emotion. It has a rapid onset, diurnal variation and recovery within 4 weeks.

Chapter 4

Dreams:

b) Are associated with paralysis

Paradoxical sleep or rapid eye movement (REM) sleep is associated with bursts of jerky, rapid eye movements that is referred to as REM sleep. When people are awakened during these periods, they recall detailed mental life and characterize the experience as dreaming. REM sleep is accompanied by abolition of muscle tone and loss of stretch reflexes, hence a sensation of paralysis. Dreams are distinct from night terrors.

Kleine–Levin syndrome is characterized by:

a) Severe hypersomnia

Kleine–Levin syndrome is a rare syndrome of periodic somnolence often lasting for days or weeks at a time and associated with intense hunger. Symptoms include irritability, excitement and restlessness. Somnolence is the most conspicuous symptom.

Attention:

a) Is the focusing of consciousness on any aspect of experience

Attention is an aspect of cognition. It refers to the ability to attend to specific sensory input. It has a limited capacity, and there are three distinct attentional abilities, namely, disengagement, shifting and engagement. *Disengagement* is the ability to move attention from a specific stimulus, *shifting* is the ability to move attention from one target stimulus to another and *engagement* refers to the ability to lock attention to a new sensory stimulus.

Chapter 5

The following are TRUE for confabulation EXCEPT:

d) It is typically 'fantastic' in nature

Characteristic features of confabulation include falsely retrieved memory often containing false details; the patient is unaware that they are confabulating and unaware of the existence of memory deficits; the patient may act on the confabulation, and this phenomenon is more apparent in autobiographical memory. There are two types: spontaneous and provoked. In the spontaneous type, the content may be fantastic, but this is not typically the case.

Short-term memory:

d) Involves a visuospatial scratch pad that allows for manipulation of visual information

Short-term memory refers to that aspect of memory function that allows for some information to be passed on from sensory memory before being transferred to long-term memory. It is a limited capacity system that can handle six to seven bits of information. Items can be stored for up to 30 seconds.

Long-term memory functions include the following EXCEPT:

c) Repression

Short-term memory refers to that aspect of memory function that allows for some information to be passed on from sensory memory before being transferred to long-term memory. It is a limited capacity system that can handle six to seven bits of information. Items can be stored for up to 30 seconds.

Chapter 6

Formal characteristics of time include the following EXCEPT:

e) Bidirectionality

Formal characteristics of time include duration, sequence, synchronicity and rhythm. There is implicit in our notion of experienced time an arrow of time that moves from the past through the present to the future. Hence there is no bidirectionality.

Déjà vu experience is an example of abnormality of:

b) Sense of uniqueness of time

Déjà vu is an alteration in the experience of the uniqueness of time. This experience is such that novel events seem to be familiar as if they have already been previously experienced.

Features of seasonal affective disorder include the following EXCEPT:

b) Insomnia

Seasonal affective disorder is characterized by repeated episodes of depression occurring at the same time of the year, usually in late winter or spring. Features include anxiety, irritability, hypersomnia, increased appetite and weight gain. There are also reports of lethargy and craving for carbohydrates.

Chapter 7

Abnormalities of the elementary aspects of visual perception include the following EXCEPT:

d) Palinacousis

Palinacousis is an abnormality of elementary auditory perception in which there is persistence of a sound beyond the actual period of the auditory sensation.

The following are TRUE of synaesthesia EXCEPT:

e) Emotional distress is a common accompaniment

Synaesthesia is a conscious experience that is involuntary. There are several variants including musical notes to colour synaesthesia. The perceptions are said to occur in peri-personal space. Some of the perceptions are thought of as elaborations of form constants.

Formal characteristics of images include the following EXCEPT:

b) Images have a character of objectivity

Images are characterized by several formal characteristics including occurring in inner subjective space, lacking the character of objectivity, being effortfully created, dissipating rapidly and not having the clarity and vividness of normal perceptions.

Chapter 8

The following are examples of primary delusions EXCEPT:

c) Persecutory delusions

Primary delusions are regarded as occurring without any antecedent and, as such, being ultimate. The current convention is to include autochthonous delusion, delusional percept, delusional atmosphere and delusional memory as examples of primary delusions. The importance of primary delusions is that they are thought to be pathognomonic of schizophrenia in the absence of organic brain disease.

Secondary delusions are:

a) Secondary to other abnormal experiences

Secondary delusions are best conceptualized as being secondary to other abnormal experiences such as mood disturbance. They are held with conviction and are resistant to counterargument as all delusions are. They are not transient and are distinguished from overvalued ideas as not being understandable in the light of the patient's social context, personality or personal history.

Delusions are examples of:
d) False beliefs
Delusions are defined as being false beliefs that are held with extraordinary conviction, are resistant to counterargument and are not comprehensible given the patient's social, cultural, and educational background.

Chapter 9

Schneider's first-rank symptoms include the following EXCEPT:
a) Somatic hallucinations
Schneider's first-rank symptoms include audible thoughts, passivity experiences (made experiences), thought withdrawal and thought insertion. Somatic hallucinations are not part of Schneider's first-rank symptoms.
Delusions of control of thought include:
b) Thought echo
Delusions of control include abnormal experiences in which the patient experiences a breakdown in their ego boundaries and in which the accompanying experience of having their agency controlled by external forces results in the experience of being a passive recipient of undue influence. It includes such experiences as thought insertion, thought withdrawal, and some examples of thought broadcasting and thought blocking.
The term *circumstantiality* refers to:
e) Impedance of flow of thinking by unnecessary detail
Circumstantiality is the inclusion of unnecessary detail in response to inquiries. It is as if the patient is unable to separate the figure from the ground or see the wood for the trees. It can sometimes be conflated with over-inclusive thinking that refers to the inability to maintain conceptual boundaries and is demonstrable on testing. Flight of ideas occur in manic episode and loosening of association in schizophrenia. *Concrete thinking* is a term that refers to a loss of the abstract attitude that was thought to be demonstrable by the interpretation of proverbs.

Chapter 10

Recognized abnormalities of language in schizophrenia include the following EXCEPT:
e) Telegony
Several authors have shown abnormalities of language use in schizophrenia. These abnormalities include the lack of cohesive ties, alogia (an example of poverty of content of speech), neologisms and clang associations. Telegony is a now discredited theory of heredity.
The Cloze technique is a measure of:
a) Predictability of speech
The Cloze technique is an experimental statistical method for determining redundancy in speech. It shows how predictable speech is when some words are omitted from speech. In schizophrenia, the omitted words are unpredictable and difficult to guess.
Primary sensory dysphasia is:
d) The loss of comprehension of the meaning of words
Primary sensory aphasia is an abnormality of comprehension of language and not a disorder of the production of language.

Chapter 11

Insight in schizophrenia has been shown to be positively correlated with the following EXCEPT:
a) The likelihood of hospitalizations
Insight is associated with working memory, compliance with treatment, likelihood of developing depression and long-term outcome. Superficially it may be thought of as being associated with hospitalizations through its effects on compliance with treatment, but this has yet to be shown.
Valid measures of insight must take into consideration the following EXCEPT:
b) The relationship of insight to affect
Insight is a complex and multidimensional concept. It has cultural aspects to it, and levels of insight vary across illness domains and are informed by observations of behaviour outside of clinical interview. There is a relationship between insight and positive affect,

but this does not have a direct bearing on the measurement of insight.

Insight involves all of the following EXCEPT:

b) Recognition of illness in others

The definition of insight does not include the recognition of illness in others.

Chapter 12

Autoscopy can involve all of the following EXCEPT:

c) Visual hallucination of internal organs within bodily space

Autoscopy refers to a complex set of experiences involving duplication of the self. This includes feeling of presence, negative heautoscopy (inability to perceive the self in a mirror), internal autoscopy (perceiving internal organs outside), autoscopic hallucination and heautoscopy proper. What is clear is that in internal autoscopy the perception is outside of bodily space.

Ego vitality is:

c) Awareness of being

Ego vitality is one of the formal characteristics of the self. It refers to the experience of being alive that is prior to the sense derived from feedback from our viscera. Other features of the self include agency, unity and coherence; continuity over time and awareness of boundaries of the self.

Nihilistic delusion is an example of:

d) Disorder of vitality

Nihilistic delusion is a disorder of the sense of vitality, of being alive. It occurs despite there being no abnormality of the sensory inputs from the body, the continuing presence of action and full conscious awareness of being alive.

Chapter 13

Definitive features of depersonalization include the following EXCEPT:

a) The experience is pleasant

Depersonalization is an experience of strangeness and of unreality. It is described in 'as if'

terms. The experience is extremely unpleasant and distressing.

Depersonalization has shown to consist of a number of components including the following EXCEPT:

c) Temporal integration

Components of depersonalization include emotional numbing, changes in bodily experience, changes in visual experience, changes in auditory experience, changes in tactile experience, etc. There are distortions in the experience of time, but there is no disturbance of temporal integration.

Depersonalization is known to be associated with the following EXCEPT:

e) Narcolepsy

Depersonalization has been reported in the context of use of drugs such as LSD, cannabis and mescaline and in sensory deprivation. It has not been reported in narcolepsy.

Chapter 14

Individual determinants of hypochondriasis include the following EXCEPT:

e) Fascination with the Internet

Hypochondriasis is the subjective and undue awareness of physical symptoms that are then interpreted as evidence of serious illness. Determinants include history of physical illness in childhood, preoccupation with bodily functions, fear of infection and the use of the Internet to research symptoms and possible diagnoses. However, fascination with the Internet per se is not a determinant of hypochondriasis.

Mass psychogenic illness:

d) Symptoms spread by line-of-sight transmission

Mass psychogenic illness commonly occurs in young females, starting in a girl of high status in her peer group who is unhappy and affecting those most psychologically vulnerable. Symptoms often spread by line-of-sight transmission and are influenced by social concerns and media response.

The concepts of *conversion* and *dissociation* suggest:

    b) That causation is unconscious

    Conversion and dissociation are understandable in the context of theories of unconscious motivation. The notion of the unconscious is necessary in understanding the mechanism and processes underlying the observed abnormalities. There is no evidence of deliberate or intentional action to dissemble. Symptoms are psychologically determined, causation is unconscious and the symptoms carry some sort of advantage for the patient (the so-called *primary* or *secondary gain*).

Chapter 15

Pain asymbolia:

    a) Presents with absent pain response

    Pain asymbolia is a condition in which situations that ought to cause pain do not. It can occur as a congenital or acquired disorder. It is usually associated with autonomic neuropathies, including anhidrosis. Other features include lack of thermal sensitivity, self-stimulation, intellectual disability, recurrent fever secondary to anhidrosis and failure to thrive.

Pain associated with psychopathology is:

    d) Constant and unremitting

    Psychogenic pain is said to be more diffuse and less well localized. The pain is more persistent and constant and less likely to be provoked by readily identifiable agents. It is also usually associated with underlying disturbance of mood, and the quality of the pain is less well described.

Central pain (thalamic syndrome):

    b) Is activated by cutaneous stimulation

    Central thalamic pain is experienced as a spontaneous burning sensation that can be activated by cutaneous stimulation or temperature changes. It can also present with tactile or cold allodynia. It is intractable and occurs in the setting of cerebrovascular accident, multiple sclerosis and spinal cord injury.

Chapter 16

Alexithymia refers to:

    d) Inability to verbalize affect and elaborate fantasy

    Alexithymia is a term coined by Sifneos. It refers to a specific disturbance characterized by difficulties in the capacity to verbalize affect and to elaborate fantasies. Anhedonia is the inability to experience pleasure. *Incongruous affect* is the term for responding to a given situation with inappropriate emotional response. *Receptive emotional dysprosody* is the term that refers to the selective deficit in recognizing emotional tone in speech.

Ekman's basic emotions include all the following EXCEPT:

    d) Jealousy

    Ekman and colleagues showed that there are six basic emotions that are expressed in facial displays. These include anger, disgust, fear, happiness, sadness and surprise. Jealousy is a composite emotion and is not one of the basic emotions.

Mood is defined as:

    b) A prolonged prevailing inner state or predisposition

    Mood is a prolonged prevailing state or disposition. It is usually distinguished from emotion that is construed as a transitory and spontaneous experience. *Affect* is a broad term that covers mood, emotion, feeling attitude, preferences and evaluations. In contemporary psychiatry it refers to the observable expressions of emotion.

Chapter 17

The respiratory subtype of panic disorder is characterized by all of the following EXCEPT:

    e) Induced by specific situations

    The respiratory type of panic disorder is associated with spontaneous panic experience rather than situationally induced panic. It is more likely to be induced by inhalation of 35% of carbon dioxide. It is characterized by fear of dying, chest pain, shortness of breath, etc.

Selye's general adaptation syndrome includes one of the following stages:

    d) Flight-or-fight response

    Selye's general adaptation syndrome conceived of stress as a nonspecific response of the body to any demand put on it. It describes three stages, namely, alarm reaction, resistance and, finally, exhaustion in the context of chronic stress. The alarm reaction is experienced as fear, palpitations and readiness for action and is best known as the flight-or-fight response.

The constituent elements of obsessive compulsive phenomenon include all of the following EXCEPT:

    e) Increased discomfort following compulsive act

    Obsessive compulsive phenomenon is characterized by repetitive and intrusive thoughts or actions that arise from within the individual and are recognized as being subject to their will. There is a sense of subjective compulsion, resistance to the feeling of compulsion and preservation of insight. Usually, the compulsive act ameliorates tension and anxiety.

Chapter 18

Abnormal movement in catatonia includes all of the following EXCEPT:

    d) Cataplexy

    In catatonia there is increased muscular tone at rest. This is abolished by voluntary action and distinguishes catatonia from extrapyramidal rigidity. Well-recognized features are waxy flexibility, psychological pillow, stereotypy and mitgehen. Cataplexy is a feature of narcolepsy.

Motivation can be defined as:

    d) A reward system that governs and regulates behaviour

    Motivation is a concept that attempts to explain what it is that activates action and behaviour as in 'What is the motivation for travelling to Paris?' As a phenomenological concept, it is experienced as a mood or affect that is governed by needs and that moves to actions that satisfy needs. It is distinguishable from the terms *need, drive, instinct* and *will*.

Impulsivity involves all of the following EXCEPT:

    c) Preference for delayed larger reward over small but immediate reward

    Impulsivity is usually used to refer to maladaptive behaviour. Impulsive acts are poorly conceived, prematurely expressed, unduly risky and liable to produce undesirable consequences. They are associated with rapid, unplanned reactions to stimuli and without due regard to potential negative consequences. In experimental paradigms, impulsive actions have been shown to persist despite punishment, to be more likely to occur with preference for small but immediate rewards and to occur as premature responses in disinhibition attentional paradigms.

Chapter 19

Abnormalities of form perception include which of the following:

    a) Heightened preference for symmetry

    Abnormalities of form perception include disturbances in the perception of symmetry, emotional responses to artworks and preference for neotenic features of faces, especially of female faces. Heightened preference for symmetry is one of the most investigated subjects, and there is evidence of increased preference in obsessive compulsive disorder, Tourette syndrome and dysmorphic body disorder.

Aesthetic valuation of landscape features is affected in:

    c) Depression

    Aesthetic valuation of landscapes is a fundamental aspect of the way that we respond to the physical environment. Prospect and Refuge theory demonstrates the evolutionary basis of this aspect of psychology. There is demonstrable abnormality in depression. There are no reports of abnormality in anxiety, behavioural variant frontotemporal dementia, obsessive compulsive disorder or Tourette syndrome.

Development of new onset visual art production is associated with:

    b) Left anterior temporal lobe lesions

    Abnormalities of aesthetic praxis are only starting to be recognized. There is some evidence that there might very well be increased artistic production schizophrenia. The most robust findings are in association with frontotemporal dementia in which the evidence links lesions in the left anterior temporal lobes with this phenomenon.

Chapter 20

Paranoid personality disorder can be defined as a disorder in which:

    a) An individual mistrusts others and is unduly suspicious

    Paranoid personality disorder is characterized by mistrust of other people, suspiciousness and a tendency to be quarrelsome and litigious. There is high vigilance against any perceived threat, and there may be undue sensitivity to slights. Inability to establish relationships is not a key feature. There is no impairment of empathy, and uncontrollable outbursts of anger is not a feature.

In dependent personality disorder all of the following features occur EXCEPT:

    b) Perfectionistic disposition

    Dependent personality disorder is characterized by feelings of inadequacy associated with undue dependency on others. There is a lack of self-confidence and a tendency to avoid taking responsibility. Coping with the demands of a stressful life is compromised, and there seems to be a need to form a relationship with a dominant person. Perfectionism is not a feature of dependent personality disorder.

The following conditions have been shown to be frequently associated with anankastic personality disorder EXCEPT:

    c) Alcohol dependence syndrome

    Anankastic personality disorder is associated with perfectionism, rigidity, indecisiveness and excessive conscientiousness. It is also associated with depression, obsessive compulsive disorder, eating disorder and hypochondriasis.

Chapter 21

Illness behaviour is influenced by all of the following EXCEPT:

    e) The underlying biology of the condition

    Illness behaviour is influenced by the salience of the complaint, the degree the complaint disturbs social roles, folk understanding of the seriousness and potential consequences of the complaint and the competing claims on the person's time and resources. The underlying biology of the complaint does not have significant influence on illness behaviour.

All of the following individuals have made contributions to our understanding of health and disease EXCEPT:

    b) Aaron Beck (well known to psychiatrists as creator of cognitive behavioural therapy and not an authority on concept of illness and disease)

    Boorse, Sedgwick, Parsons and Mechanic have all contributed to our understanding of the nature of health and disease. Beck is best known for his work on cognitive behavioural therapy.

Practical applications of psychopathology include all of the following EXCEPT:

    d) Nosology

    Psychopathology has direct influence on communication between clinicians in providing a language to classify and categorize abnormal phenomena. This role of psychopathology is foundational to cognitive neuroscience, especially about the understanding of phenomena such as delusions, hallucinations and thinking disorders. Diagnostic categories rely on accurate assessments of abnormal phenomena, and of course treatment naturally flows out of diagnosis. However, nosology deals with the classification of diseases including causes, effects, symptoms and natural history. In this regard, nosology is distinct from psychopathology.

Self-Assessment 2: Answers

Chapters 3 and 4

1. A 75-year-old female patient is found wandering the streets. On examination she does not know the date, day, time, season, where she is or her own address.

   D. Disorientation

   Disorientation is manifest as disturbance of orientation to time, place and person. This is assessed by determining whether the patient is aware of the day, date, time of day, season, current place and who it is that is conducting the interview. Disorientation is important in determining whether a chronic organic brain disease such as dementia or an acute organic brain disease such as delirium is present.

2. An 18-year-old male patient presents with a history of several irresistible periods of drowsiness during the day. At night he reports periods when he is fully awake but unable to move his limbs.

   E. Hypersomnia

   Hypersomnia, also described as excessive somnolence, is present in several disorders such as Kleine–Levin syndrome, narcolepsy and seasonal affective disorder.

3. The partner of a 25-year-old male patient accompanies him to the outpatient appointment. She reports that he talks in his sleep, wanders aimlessly in the bedroom for a few minutes at night and has no recollection of these incidents.

   H. Parasomnia

   Parasomnias are disorders of arousal and sleep-stage transition that consist of abnormal sleep-related movements, behaviours, emotions, perceptions, dreaming and autonomic nervous system functioning that accompany sleep.

4. A 47-year-old female patient with a history of recurrent depression is admitted in a mute state. She is immobile but fully conscious and alert. She is able to make eye contact but does not respond to any attempt at verbal communication.

   I. Stupor

   Stupor is a symptom complex, and the central feature is a reduction in, or absence of, relational functions including action and sleep. It is distinct from coma. It is characterized by mutism and akinesis.

Chapter 5

1. A 20-year-old male patient was involved in a road traffic accident. He sustained head injury. He was only able to recall events that happened approximately 5 minutes before the collision.

   J. Retrograde amnesia

   Retrograde amnesia is the loss of memory for events preceding the onset of brain injury. It is demonstrable as an impairment of retrieval but is thought to reflect impairment of retention/ storage.

2. A 20-year-old male patient presented in prison while on remand. When examined, he responded to questions about the date and the capital of France with approximate answers and disorientation for time and place.

   F. Ganser state

   Ganser state was first described in 1898, and the typical features include approximate answers (vorbeigehen), clouding of consciousness with disorientation, recent history of head injury or physical illness, hallucinations and amnesia. Sometimes there are hysterical features including somatic conversion symptoms.

3. A 45-year-old male patient was involved in an accident at work where he sustained a serious head injury and lost consciousness. On re-

gaining his consciousness, he could only recall events that happened approximately 36 hours after the incident.

A. Anterograde amnesia

Anterograde amnesia is a deficit in memory for events following the onset of a clinical disorder such as a head injury. It is demonstrable in impairment of retrieval but represents problems with registration/encoding.

4. A 57-year-old male patient with an established history of impairment of short-term memory in the context of alcohol abuse responded to questions about how he had spent the previous day with objectively false accounts that included embellishments and intrusions from previous occasions.

B. Confabulation

Confabulation is characterized by falsely retrieved memory often containing false details. Confabulation is not intentionally produced. There are two types, namely, spontaneous and provoked. It is seen as part of Korsakov's syndrome.

Chapter 7

1. A 45-year-old man presents with a complaint that he first saw a black cat at the corner where his drive joined the main street. After this, for the next 72 hours or so, he kept seeing the same cat at various times and situations. What is the term for this experience?

B. Palinopsia

Palinopsia is persistence of a visual stimulus beyond the actual presentation of the visual object.

2. A 19-year-old man with a recent diagnosis of schizophrenia complained that the faces of people looking at him would suddenly look different, as if they were pulling faces at him. Sometimes the faces would appear sinister, lopsided and strange. What is the term for this experience?

E. Paraprosopia

Paraprosopia is a disorder of visual perception in which distortion of perceived faces takes place.

3. A 25-year-old female patient with a history of complex focal seizures complained of scenes and objects becoming smaller before a seizure. What is this experience termed?

D. Micropsia

Micropsia is a condition in which visual hallucinations of small objects are reported.

4. A 25-year-old male patient complained that objects looked far away. He found this surprising and distressing. What is this experience termed?

G. Pelopsia

Pelopsia is a condition in which visual perception of objects is reported as further away than is expected.

Chapter 8

1. A 20-year-old male patient was admitted into hospital after an attack on his father. He reported that his father had been replaced by a robot who looked almost exactly like him but was definitely not him. He feared that this 'robot' had malignant intentions and that his life was in danger. What is this belief called?

H. Delusional misidentification

Delusional misidentification is the general term for a group of conditions including Capgras syndrome, Frègoli syndrome, syndrome of subjective doubles and syndrome of inter-metamorphosis. These conditions are united by the concept of doubles. The example is one of Capgras syndrome: the patient believes that a familiar person has been replaced by an impostor.

2. A 40-year-old female patient complained that her local priest was sending her secret messages, declaring his feelings for her. She complained that, although he was the father of her child, he was yet to visit them.

G. Delusion of love

Delusion of love/Clérambault syndrome/Erotomania are terms for the delusional belief of being loved by a person, usually someone unattainable. It is associated with stalking behaviours and sometimes with hostility and violent behaviour.

3. A 21-year-old female patient suddenly became convinced that she was the rightful heir to the throne of Norway. She was not Norwegian by birth or ancestry. When asked the reason for this belief, she said that she had suddenly come to this realization. She denied any other unusual experience.

B. Delusional intuition

Delusional intuition is another term for autochthonous delusion. It is an example of primary delusion. It describes a delusion that arises suddenly, de novo, and that is grasped in one stage as opposed to the two-staged delusional percept. It is probably best understood as the emergence of new meaning or belief.

4. A 54-year-old male patient with a long-standing history of schizophrenia reported persistent and stressful auditory verbal hallucinations of derogatory and threatening content. The voices would often tell him that he deserved to be killed and that new immigrants into his local area from Romania were going to murder him. He then held a firm belief that he was at risk from immigrants, particularly Romanians. This belief was held with conviction and was impervious to counter-argument.

E. Secondary delusion

Secondary delusion is best understood as arising in the context of other abnormal phenomena such as hallucinations or abnormality of mood.

Chapter 9

1. A 21-year-old male university student described spending a lot of time thinking about the future, about the possibility of becoming a famous musician, becoming rich and able to live in a mansion in Florida.

A. Fantasy thinking

Fantasy thinking is an example of normal thinking involving the creation of new images or ideas that are not dependent on external events.

2. A 25-year-old female patient, newly admitted into hospital, complained that her thoughts were being interfered with. She was particularly distressed by the experience of having thoughts manipulated and taken from her.

I. Thought withdrawal

Thought withdrawal is a disorder of the control of thinking. It can also be construed as an example of passivity experiences. It involves the belief or experience of having thoughts withdrawn from the patient's mind. It relies on the underlying assumption that thoughts are akin to physical objects that can be removed and that the boundaries of the self are permeable, thus making it possible for others to manipulate contents of the mind.

3. In a test, a 19-year-old patient with a diagnosis of schizophrenia responded to a question as follows: 'Which of the following are essential parts of a room: walls, chairs, floor, window?' 'Chairs'.

G. Over-inclusive thinking

Over-inclusive thinking is a term developed by Cameron to describe a phenomenon that was shown on testing patients with schizophrenia in which conceptual boundaries seemed to be impaired.

4. A 57-year-old female patient said, 'I was starting to feel high, so I tied dumb-bell weights round my ankle'.

F. Concrete thinking

This phenomenon was thought to reflect the loss of the abstract attitude in patients with schizophrenia. It was said to be demonstrable in the response of patients to interpretation of proverbs.

Chapter 10

1. A 65-year-old, right-handed male patient who was recovering from a left-sided stroke was unable to follow the verbal command, 'Take the paper with your left hand, fold it in two and put it on the floor'.

I. Receptive dysphasia

This is an impairment in comprehension of spoken speech demonstrable in the loss of the meaning of words.

2. A 25-year-old patient said, 'Phlogons have invaded my lungs, turning first sideways and now medways'.

J. Neologism

Neologism is the term for the invention of new words or the unusual use of words to signify something novel. It is reported in schizophrenia.

3. A 64-year-old male patient with a long-standing history of schizophrenia replied to the question, 'What have you got in your cup?' 'A fluid that whilst being colourless turns dark on brewing'.

G. Metonym

Metonymy refers to the use of the name of one thing to represent something related to it such as referring to businesspeople as a bunch of suits. In psychiatry it is often used to describe responses to inquiries that demonstrate an understanding of the question but that are descriptions of the expected answer.

4. A 72-year-old male patient with a diagnosis of Parkinson's disease said, 'I'm star …, star …, starting to think of mo …, mo …, mo …, moving house'.

B. Logoclonia

Logoclonia is a term referring to the spastic repetition of syllables that occurs in parkinsonism.

Chapter 14

1. A 23-year-old male patient presented with the belief that his muscles were too small and a preoccupation with physical build, excessive exercising and disturbed eating.

H. Muscle dysmorphia

Muscle dysmorphia is a term to describe the belief that one's muscles are poorly developed with the consequent excessive exercising, disturbed eating and sometimes abuse of steroids.

2. A 56-year-old female patient complained of hating her left hand. Although it looked normal, she said that she hated it and had always wished that it were different in size, shape and feel.

A. Misoplegia

Misoplegia is a term to describe hatred of a body part that is not founded on an objective change in the size, shape or physical feel of the body part.

3. A 27-year-old male patient presented with a long-standing belief that his face was ugly, in particular his nose that he thought was far too large and crooked. Objectively, his nose was not excessively large or crooked.

B. Dysmorphophobia

Dysmorphophobia/dysmorphic body disorder are terms for the abnormal belief of personal ugliness. The belief can relate to the face or to the nose or teeth or chin. Other body parts including breasts and buttocks can also be the object of dislike.

4. A 40-year-old female patient presented with the complaint that she could continue to feel her toothbrush in her hands for up to 15 minutes after she used it.

C. Palinaptia

Palinaptia is the experience of persistence of tactile sensation beyond the duration of the actual stimulus.

Chapter 16

1. An 8-year-old male patient presented with a history of heightened startle reflex characterized by eye blinking, head flexion, abduction of the upper arms, movement of the trunk and bending of the knees in response to a loud noise.

C. Hyperekplexia

Hyperekplexia is heightened startle reflex characterized by eye blinking, head flexion, abduction of the upper arms, movement of the trunk and bending of the knees in response to a loud noise. It occurs as a feature of hereditary neurological condition involving glycine receptors or in epilepsy in which the startle reflex provokes a seizure.

2. A 40-year-old female patient with a history of recurrent depression and current depression gave a history of inability to experience pleasure in her usual hobbies and interests, as well as a general inability to experience any feeling.

A. Anhedonia

Anhedonia is a term that refers to the inability to experience pleasure. It can extend to the inability to experience any feeling. It is typically present in severe depression.

3. A 36-year-old male patient presented to the local dental hospital with an aching pain in both sides of the lower jaw radiating to the temporomandibular joints and to the neck. In response to the question, 'How are you feeling in your spirits?', he seemed puzzled and asked for the question to be repeated. He then said, 'My body is heavy and I am aching all over'.

J. Alexithymia

Alexithymia is a term that refers to a specific difficulty in the capacity to verbalize affect and to elaborate fantasies.

4. A 75-year-old male patient with a diagnosis of Parkinson's disease spoke with a monotonous voice. In addition, he seemed not to recognize the emotional meaning of variations in tone of voice.

F. Receptive emotional dysprosody

Receptive emotional dysprosody refers to the selective deficit in recognizing emotional tone in speech.

Chapter 17

1. A 32-year-old female patient presented with discrete episodes of intense and extreme fear.

F. Panic

Panic attacks occur as discrete episodes of somatic or autonomic anxiety associated with marked psychic anxiety as an extreme sense of fear.

2. A 23-year-old female patient presented with excessive fear, self-consciousness and avoidance of social situations due to the possibility of embarrassment or humiliation.

J. Social phobia

Social phobia can be conceived as an extreme form of shyness. It is manifest as excessive fear, self-consciousness and avoidance of social situations and fear of embarrassment or humiliation.

3. A 27-year-old male accountancy trainee presented with a history of repetitive and intrusive thoughts about cleanliness and hygiene, which were associated with increasing tension and worry and which he recognized as his own

thoughts. He tried to resist these thoughts but found that they became even more urgent and intrusive.

H. Obsession

Obsessions are repetitive and recurrent thoughts, ruminations or images that are recognized by the patient as deriving from their own mind. The obsessions are usually resisted but usually with increasing tension and anxiety.

4. A 32-year-old female patient, who had recently given birth presented with a 6-week history of temper outbursts, feelings of hostility towards her husband, an unpleasant feeling of distress and impatience with her children.

E. Irritability

Irritability is considered as a mood in its own right. It is characterized by reduced control over temper. This results in verbal or behavioural outbursts. It may be brief or chronic in duration. It is usually unpleasant for the patient and can be disruptive to relationships.

Chapter 18

1. A 21-year-old male recently diagnosed with schizophrenia and treated with risperidone complains of motor restlessness, inner agitation and an inability to sit still.

A. Akathisia

Akathisia is manifest as a subjective experience of motor unease with the accompanying feeling of being unable to sit still. There is a feeling of wanting to stretch the legs, stand up, tap the feet or rock the body. There is a distressing inner feeling of restless.

2. A 17-year-old male patient is brought to the attention of his general practitioner because he newly recognized a problem with gambling, drinking excessively and misusing cannabis. In addition, he is reported as prone to losing his temper and liable to say things he later regrets.

E. Impulsivity

Impulsivity is a maladaptive behaviour involving poorly conceived actions that are prematurely expressed, unduly risky and without due regard to consequences.

3. A 21-year-old male patient presented with a history of episodes of excessive sleeping (up 15 hours a day), excessive eating, increased sexual libido, low mood and transient persecutory beliefs.
G. Kleine–Levin syndrome

Kleine–Levin syndrome is characterized by episodes of hypersomnolence. In addition, there is excessive eating, irritability, cognitive impairment, apathy, derealization and hypersexual behaviour. Other psychiatric symptoms such as depression, anxiety, delusions and hallucinations may occur.

4. A 28-year-old female patient presented for the first time with markedly slowed movements, sometimes resulting in immobility, strange postures and muteness. On examination, she allows her upper limbs to be put in uncomfortable postures that she holds for long periods of time.
C. Catatonia

Catatonia is a state of increased muscle tone at rest that is abolished by voluntary action. It includes features such as waxy flexibility, psychological pillow, mitgehen, negativism, automatic obedience and mutism.

Index

Page numbers followed by 'f' indicate figures, 't' indicate tables, and 'b' indicate boxes.